National Physical Therapy
Examination and
Board Review

Annie Burke-Doe, PT, MPT, PhD

Professor
West Coast University
Los Angeles, California

Mark Dutton, PT

New York   Chicago   San Francisco   Athens   London   Madrid   Mexico City
Milan   New Delhi   Singapore   Sydney   Toronto

National Physical Therapy Examination and Board Review

1 2 3 4 5 6 7 8 9   LWI   23 22 21 20 19 18

ISBN 978-1-260-01062-6
MHID 1-260-01062-7

Notice

Medicine is an ever-changing science. As new research and clinical experience broaden our knowledge, changes in treatment and drug therapy are required. The authors and the publisher of this work have checked with sources believed to be reliable in their efforts to provide information that is complete and generally in accord with the standards accepted at the time of publication. However, in view of the possibility of human error or changes in medical sciences, neither the authors nor the publisher nor any other party who has been involved in the preparation or publication of this work warrants that the information contained herein is in every respect accurate or complete, and they disclaim all responsibility for any errors or omissions or for the results obtained from use of the information contained in this work. Readers are encouraged to confirm the information contained herein with other sources. For example and in particular, readers are advised to check the product information sheet included in the package of each drug they plan to administer to be certain that the information contained in this work is accurate and that changes have not been made in the recommended dose or in the contraindications for administration. This recommendation is of particular importance in connection with new or infrequently used drugs.

This book was set in Adobe Garamond Pro by Cenveo® Publisher Services.
The editors were Michael Weitz and Kim J. Davis.
The production supervisor was Richard Ruzycka.
Project management was provided by Radhika Jolly of Cenveo Publisher Services.

Library of Congress Cataloging-in-Publication Data

Names: Burke-Doe, Annie, author. | Dutton, Mark, author.
Title: National physical therapy examination and board review / Annie
    Burke-Doe, PT, MPT, PhD, Professor, West Coast University, Los Angeles,
    California, Mark Dutton, PT.
Description: New York : McGraw-Hill Education, [2019] | Includes
    bibliographical references and index.
Identifiers: LCCN 2018037778 (print) | LCCN 2018038694 (ebook) | ISBN
    9781260010633 (ebook) | ISBN 1260010635 (ebook) | ISBN 9781260010626
    (paperback) | ISBN 1260010627 (paperback)
Subjects: LCSH: Physical therapy—Examinations, questions, etc. | Physical
    therapy—Study guides. | BISAC: MEDICAL / Physical Medicine &
    Rehabilitation.
Classification: LCC RM701.6 (ebook) | LCC RM701.6 .B87 2019 (print) | DDC
    615.8/2076—dc23
LC record available at https://lccn.loc.gov/2018037778

Contents

Authors

Norman C. Belleza, PT, DPT
Assistant Professor
University of St. Augustine
San Marcos, California [Chapter 1]

Annie Burke-Doe, PT, MPT, PhD
Professor
West Coast University
Los Angeles, California [Chapters 4-7, 10]

Chris Childers, PT, MS
Board Certified Geriatric Clinical Specialist
Assistant Professor
University of St. Augustine
San Marcos, California [Chapters 8, 9]

Heather Scott David, PT, EdD, MPT, NCS
Assistant Professor
University of St. Augustine
San Marcos, California [Chapter 3]

Mark Dutton, PT [Chapter 2]

Christopher J. Ivey, PT, MPT, OCS, SCS, ATC, MS
Assistant Professor
University of St. Augustine for Health Sciences
San Marcos, California [Chapter 2]

Kristen Johnson, PT, EdD, MS
Board Certified Specialist in Neurologic Physical Therapy
Associate Professor
University of St. Augustine for Health Sciences
San Marcos, California [Chapter 3]

Joanne Laslovich, PT, MA, DPT
Associate Professor
University of St. Augustine for Health Sciences
San Marcos, California [Chapter 1]

Rolando Lazaro, PT, PhD, DPT, GCS
Associate Professor
Department of Physical Therapy
California State University
Sacramento, California [Chapters 4-7]

Ellen Lowe, PT, PhD, MHS
Fellow of the American Physical Therapy Association
Educational Leadership Institute
Director of Clinical Education/Associate Professor
Franklin Pierce University
Goodyear, Arizona [Chapter 8]

Jim Mathews, PT, DPT, MBA, GCS
Assistant Professor
Assistant Program Director
University of St. Augustine for Health Sciences
San Marcos, California [Chapter 9]

Kayla Smith, PT, DSc, OCS, COMT
Associate Professor
University of St. Augustine for Health Sciences
San Marcos, California [Chapter 2]

Preface

This manual is your guide to prepare you for the National Physical Therapy Examination (NPTE) and earning your licensure. This guide includes insights from professional physical therapists (PT) on each component of the exam, encompassing a review of NPTE contents to best prepare you for successful exam results. The exam covers a broad range of topics, from special populations to the body's main organ systems and how they interact to non-system components, outlining professional responsibilities and ethics.

This NPTE guide was written to parallel the exam and offers concise information on broad topics to help you study effectively; however, this is not the only resource you should utilize when preparing for the exam. Many resources are available to ensure you are revisiting the foundation of information you have reviewed as a part of your PT program, including your old materials from your program and other recognized online sources. This study guide will help you understand the test and its contents by providing an overview of each subject covered, along with many practice question opportunities with multiple choice questions about the subjects on which you will be tested.

THE EXAM

The Federation of State Boards of Physical Therapy (FSBPT) describes the PT exam as a measure of the knowledge and abilities of entry-level physical therapists. It consists of 250 items to be answered in 5 hours. The questions within each section of test content are drawn from an examination item bank after ensuring they are high-quality and psychometrically sound. The PT content outline can be found on the website of the Federation of State Boards of Physical Therapy at: http://www.fsbpt.org/FreeResources/NPTEDevelopment/NPTEContent.aspx.

Introduction: Test Administration and What to Expect

Schedule your test here: https://www.prometric.com/en-us/clients/fsbpt/Pages/landing.aspx.

The test is administered by a proctor in several testing locations. The proctor will ensure all protocols are enforced. It is a good idea to call the testing location and ask any specific questions about the facility and what to bring and what not to bring.

Usually personal items are not allowed. This includes, but is not limited to, purses, bags, loose clothing, electronics, and food and beverages.

Make sure to arrive at your Prometric examination a minimum of 30 minutes before your scheduled exam time. As a general guide, you will need two forms of identification—this should be verified by your examination location. According to the FSBPT website, one form of ID must be government issued, such as a passport, driver license, or state ID card; a secondary form of ID must be preprinted with your name and contain your signature. A credit card with your signature will satisfy this secondary requirement; a Social Security card does *not* satisfy this requirement. Both forms of ID must match exactly to the first and last name on your "Authorization to Test" letter issued by FSBPT. If you are denied admittance to the examination due to any problem with your identification, you will forfeit your Prometric fee and will be required to register for another fixed-date administration.

The PT exam is 5 hours long and is broken down into five blocks of 50 questions. These are structured as "mini exams" and follow the basic content outline as the blueprint for the larger examination. During the test there are two types of breaks: scheduled and unscheduled. The PT exam will have one scheduled 15-minute break after two blocks of 50 questions have been completed. You are also able to have three unscheduled breaks. An unscheduled break can be taken between 50-question blocks during the time that the "unscheduled break" screen is visible. The timer will continue during unscheduled breaks; however, the scheduled break is not counted toward your 5-hour examination time.

Not all items are scored. Pretest questions are included on each examination to see if these questions meet standards to be included in future exams. These pretest questions will not be graded, and will be dispersed randomly within the exam. For additional information, see https://www.fsbpt.org/FreeResources/NPTECandidateHandbook/TakingtheExamination.aspx#requirements%20originalAttribute=.

NPTE EXAM PREPARATION STRATEGIES

How much time should I spend preparing?
Preparation time can vary from student to student, so it is important to accurately assess how much time it will take you to study all of the topics that will be covered in the NPTE exam. As you look over the topics, identify the areas for which you will need the most review time and the areas in which you need the least time, to help prioritize your studying. To start, look at your current schedule. How much time you can devote to studying? What are your current responsibilities, and how much time does that eliminate from your study time? What amount of time can you commit to each day or in total each week to study? Ensure you are giving yourself enough time to master each topic. Sticking to a schedule will help you pace yourself efficiently and allot for time to revisit topics that need additional review.

Use proper note-taking and critical reading strategies
As you well know by now, using proper note-taking and critical reading strategies that have worked for you in the past will make your time more effective and allow you to optimize the time you are spending. Review the sections of this guide to ensure you understand the high-yield terms. Think about how questions could be formed based on the topics. Think about how you would explain certain concepts to another person. These are effective strategies to enhance your learning.

Test-taking strategies for multiple choice questions
Use of the multiple choice test-taking strategies to help eliminate one or more of the possible answers can help improve your overall exam performance. After reading the question completely and determining what is being asked, rule out the wrong answer or answers. Use your existing knowledge rule out any option that is clearly wrong. Sometimes working backward by looking over the answers first and then looking at the question can also be helpful. Pay attention to absolute words like *always, all, only, must*, or *never*, because these can determine what is being asked and help an option stand out. Finally, recognize responses that are opposites. One of the two is commonly the answer.

Seek other sources
If more help or insight is needed into a particular topic, you can explore other resources to master it. From your old notes, former instructors, and online sources, the resources are limitless. Some students form study groups to better prepare for the exam, especially if you recently ended your program.

Practice timed tests

The NPTE is timed and taking timed practice test will assist you in your preparation. This will allow you to see how quickly you progress through questions and will let you know if it is necessary to shorten your time per question to ensure you do not run out of time to allow for you to review after you have answered your question to confirm you have selected the best answer.

Take the breaks

As noted earlier, there are scheduled breaks. Use this time during the test to rest your mind, get water, or move your legs. Breaking up the sitting time over the 5-hour exam will benefit you.

Don't forget to breathe

It is important to keep your composure and remain focused. The brain performs best when it is well oxygenated and when you are not experiencing nerves or anxiety. Preparation before the exam will also help calm your nerves, but on the day of the exam make sure to breathe deeply in between questions or any time you start to feel anxious.

Cardiac, Vascular, and Pulmonary Systems

Norman Belleza and Joanne Laslovich

■ CLINICAL APPLICATION OF FOUNDATIONAL SCIENCES

OVERVIEW

In understanding the human body movement system, the principles of moving blood, nutrients, ions, oxygen (O_2), carbon dioxide (CO_2), metabolic byproducts, and waste, producing electrical gradients, and generating differences in pressure are fundamental in the functioning of the cardiac, vascular, and pulmonary systems. In terms of physiology, it is the action at the cellular level of these organ systems that allows for the transport, movement, and functioning of the systems in everyday life, activity, and exercise. In addition, the introduction and use of pharmacological agents has an influence on the movement of these systems when needed in instances of pathology and/or disease.

ANATOMY AND PHYSIOLOGY OF THE CARDIAC AND VASCULAR SYSTEMS

Chambers of the Heart

There are four distinct chambers of the heart (Figure 1–1). The chambers' work can be divided into two pairs that essentially serve as two pumps to the lungs (pulmonary circulation) and to the rest of the body (systemic circulation). The action of the heart and myocardium moves and circulates blood throughout the body.

High-Yield Terms to Learn

Action potential	The basis for nerve impulses when cell membrane reaches threshold potential.
Angina pectoris	Chest pain that is related to ischemia of the myocardium.
Apnea	Cessation of breathing after an expiration, interrupted by eventual inspiration or becomes fatal.
Atherosclerosis	Disease of the arteries characterized by plaque deposits of fatty materials on the inner walls of the vessel.
Automatic rhythmicity	Property of cardiac nodal tissue to self-excite, which leads to automatic action potentials and heart contraction.
Bradypnea	Slow rate, shallow or normal depth, regular rhythm (as in drug overdose).
Chronotrophy	Changes or influences that increase or decrease heart rate.
Cor pulmonale	Right-side heart failure as a result of pulmonary hypertension causing acute and chronic pulmonary disease.
Crackles/rales	Adventitious breath sounds that can be heard over areas of the lung where there are accumulated fluids or collapsed alveoli.
	There is partial reopening of the alveoli during inspiration.
Cyanosis	Bluish coloration of skin, tissues, or membranes.
Dead space	When air does not reach into the alveoli or airways within the lungs.

High-Yield Terms to Learn (*continued*)

Dyspnea	Shortness of breath.
Effective refractory period	Timeframe when tissue cannot generate additional incoming action potentials.
Eupnea	Normal rate, depth, and rhythm of breathing.
Frank–Starling law	Observation that increased stretching and preloading of the heart causes an increase in heart contractility.
Hemoptysis	Presence of blood produced from coughing.
Hyperpnea	Increased breathing due to increased depth, but usually not increased rate.
Ionotrophy	Changes or influences that increase or decrease heart contractility.
Orthopnea	Shortness of breath caused by lying in flat position.
Oxygen diffusing capacity	Measure of the rate at which oxygen can diffuse from the pulmonary alveoli into the blood.
Pulmonary ventilation	The process of drawing air into and out of the lungs.
Perfusion	Amount of blood flow to a given region.
Respiration	The process of gas exchange with the atmosphere and cells of the body.
Shunt	When blood does not flow to a region.
Sinus rhythm	Any rhythm of the heart established by impulses from the SA node.
Stridor	A high-pitched sound caused by obstruction of the larynx or trachea heard during inspiration and expiration.
Tachypnea	Increased breathing rate, usually shallow with regular rhythm (as in restrictive lung pathologies).
Wheezing	A music-pitch-like continuous sound heard due to narrowing in the airway.

- **Right atrium (RA):** Receives blood from the systemic circulation via the superior and inferior vena cave. Also receives blood from the coronary sinus (coronary circulation).
- **Right ventricle (RV):** Delivers blood received from the RA in the lungs and the pulmonary system via the pulmonary artery.
- **Left atrium (LA):** Receives oxygenated blood from the lungs and the pulmonary system via four pulmonary veins.
- **Left ventricle (LV):** Delivers the blood received from the LA to the rest of the body (systemic circulation) via the aorta.

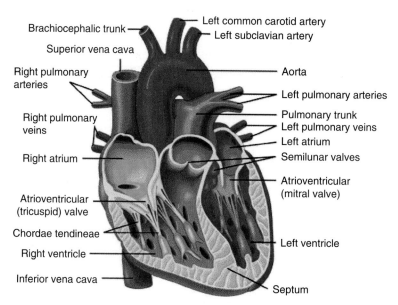

FIGURE 1-1 Internal view of the heart. (From https://i.pinimg.com/originals/ac/a0/d1/aca0d11a36c6f07206d703c5d2eadf7a.gif.)

- Atrioventricular (AV) valves: Prevent backflow of blood from the ventricle back into the atria. The AV valves are reinforced by structures called chordae tendineae and papillary muscles.
  - Tricuspid valve is found on the right side of the heart between the RA and RV.
  - Bicuspid valve (mitral valve) is found on the left side of the heart between the LA and LV.
- Semilunar (SL) valves: Prevent backflow toward the ventricles.
  - Pulmonary valve: Prevents backflow into the RV from the pulmonary artery.
  - Aortic valve: Prevents backflow into the LV from the aorta.

Movement of Ions, Electrical Activity, and Conduction of the Heart

Cardiac tissues of the heart maintain ionic gradients that favor the influx and efflux of different ions that regulate heart contraction and conduction. Through the action of active and passive ion pumps, the heart regulates these activities. The movement of ions in and out of the cardiac tissue such as cardiac muscle tissue (myocytes) and nodal (nervous) tissue produces heart contractility and conductivity. Calcium, potassium (K^+), and sodium (Na^+) have varying roles in heart activity. At resting potential K^+ tends to efflux, while in contrast the gradient favors a Na^+ and Ca^+ influx as shown in Figure 1–2.

Cardiac Nodal Tissue Action Potential

Automatic rhythmicity refers to the property of cardiac nodal tissue to self-excite, which leads to automatic **action potentials** and heart contraction. There are a total of five phases (Phase 0–Phase 4) to recognize in the events of cardiac nodal conduction and muscle contraction. Figure 1–3 is a representation of nodal tissue **action potentials**.

Phase 4   **Resting Potential:** Figure 1–3 demonstrates that there is a constant depolarization toward the threshold. Several factors contribute to this increased net positivity inside the cell. There is a decline in the efflux of K^+, due to decreased K^+ permeability. This retention of K^+ causes a climb in the intracellular positivity. In addition, there is an increase in Na^+ permeability. This causes an influx of Na^+, which further increases the net positivity within the cell. Further, the contributions of

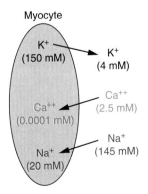

FIGURE 1–2 Cardiac cell ion concentration gradients.

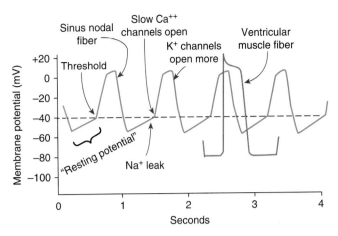

FIGURE 1–3 Rhythmical discharge of sinus nodal fiber. (From Hall JE. *Guyton and Hall Textbook of Medical Physiology.* 12th ed. Philadelphia, PA: Saunders Elsevier; 2011, Figure 3.)

K^+ and Na^+ cause the biased opening of voltage-gated Ca^+ channels which herald the next phase.

Phase 0   **Upstroke:** In Figure 1–3, there is an increased positive movement from threshold at approximately –40mV. The opening of voltage-gated Ca^+ channels brings on this depolarization. The influx of Ca^+ causes depolarization beyond threshold toward the top of the action potential.

Phase 1   **Spike:** This phase is absent in cardiac nodal tissue but is present in cardiac muscle tissue action potentials.

Phase 2   **Plateau:** In Figure 1–3, at the top of depolarization is a relative "flattening" of the wave pattern, which is a prolonged plateau phase. This is caused by the continuing influx of Ca^+ that is countered by the opening of K^+ channels that cause K^+ efflux.

Phase 3   **Repolarization:** In Figure 1–3, the decline and drop toward resting potential is from the continued efflux of K^+. At the end of repolarization, action from Na^+/K^+ pumps and Ca^+ pumps return the cell to resting potential.

Cardiac Muscle Tissue Action Potential

The characteristics of depolarization and repolarization in cardiac muscle tissues differs from those of nodal tissue. There are a total of 5 phases, described below, in ventricular muscle action potential.

Phase 4   **Resting Potential:** Figure 1–4 demonstrates that there is a lower resting potential in cardiac muscle tissue compared to cardiac nodal tissue. Several factors contribute to this increase in negativity inside the cell. There is an increase in K^+ permeability, which results in an efflux of K^+. This loss of positive charge causes the intracellular membrane to become more negative. There is a slight increase in permeability to Na^+ and Ca^+, which causes in an influx of these ions. This aids in preventing the resting potential from becoming increasingly more negative or hyperpolarized due to the loss of K^+.

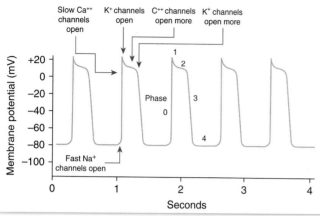

FIGURE 1–4 Ventricular muscle action potential. (From Hall JE. *Guyton and Hall Textbook of Medical Physiology*. 12th ed. Philadelphia, PA: Saunders Elsevier; 2011, Figure 4.)

Phase 0 **Upstroke:** Since we are now looking at cardiac muscle tissue, there is no inherent property for automatic rhythmicity. Therefore, the arrival of a stimulus or action potential from nodal tissue is required for cardiac muscle to undergo an action potential. Unlike nodal tissue, it is the opening of fast voltage–gated Na⁺ channels that causes the upstroke in action potential.

Phase 1 **Spike:** In Figure 1–4, there is a characteristic spike that represents this phase. At the peak of depolarization in Phase 0, there is a brief opening of K⁺ channels, and then the channels mostly close. This brief window causes K⁺ to efflux and there is a drop in positive charge within the tissue.

Phase 2 **Plateau:** At the end of Phase 1, there is relative "flattening" of the wave pattern, which is a prolonged plateau phase. This is caused by increasing permeability of Ca^+, and this influx of Ca^+ is countered by the opening of K⁺ channels, which cause K⁺ efflux. The plateau phase is an important feature in cardiac muscle physiology that increases the time for the **effective refractory period**, also known as the absolute refractory period. If there were an arrival of another **action potential** during the refractory period, this would not cause another heart contraction. This prevents summation and tetany of cardiac muscle, which would have consequential effects on heart function if it were to occur.

Phase 3 **Repolarization:** In Figure 1–3, the decline and drop toward resting potential is from the continued efflux of K⁺. At the end of repolarization, actions from Na⁺/K⁺ pumps and Ca^+ pumps return the cell to resting potential.

Conduction System

The conduction system of the heart is illustrated in Figure 1–5.

Sinoatrial Node

The sinoatrial (SA) node is an area of specialized tissue located on the right atrium near the opening of the superior vena cava. Also known as the pacemaker of the heart, the SA node automatically creates **action potentials** 70 to 80 times per minute in the normal adult.

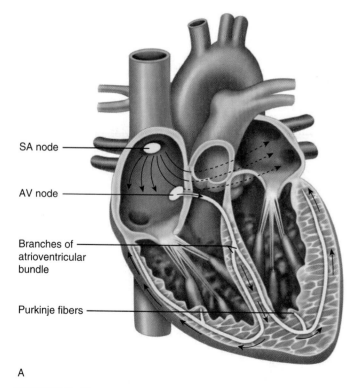

SA node

AV node

Branches of atrioventricular bundle

Purkinje fibers

A

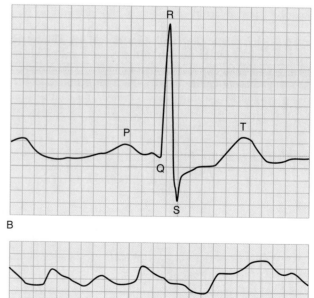

B

C

FIGURE 1–5 Conduction system of the heart. (From http://facweb.bhc.edu/academics/science/robertsk/biol101/heart_files/image010.jpg.)

Atrioventricular Node

Conduction continues along internodal pathways from the SA node to another area of specialized tissue called the AV node. There is a 0.1-second delay that occurs that allows the atria to contract first to empty all blood into the ventricles before the ventricles contract.

AV Bundle

The distal portion of the AV node passes into the area known as the AV bundle, also known as the bundle of His. This is located at the interventricular septum. Gap junctions do not connect the atria and ventricles. The only conduction between the atria and ventricles is via the AV bundle.

Right and Left Bundle Branches

The AV bundle divides into the right and left bundle branches and follows along the length of the interventricular septum and toward the apex of the heart.

Purkinje Fibers

The right and left bundle branches continue into enlarged Purkinje fibers that extend from the apex and around the ventricles and lateral heart walls. The conduction system causes heart contraction from the apex, and then up in a superior direction to direct blood toward the aorta and the pulmonary trunk.

Electrocardiogram (ECG or EKG)

- P-Wave represents atrial depolarization
- QRS wave or complex represents ventricular depolarization (atrial repolarization is masked by the QRS wave)
- T-Wave represents ventricular repolarization
- PR interval represents the time for conduction to travel from atria to the Purkinje fibers
- QT interval represents the time of ventricular activity from depolarization to repolarization

Figure 1–6 shows the waveforms in a normal ECG.

Coronary Artery Circulation

The coronary arteries deliver blood to the heart muscle for oxygenation of the tissues. Figure 1–7 shows the right and left coronary arteries and their branches.

Regulatory Influences on the Heart

A. Sympathetic Innervation

The cardiac acceleratory center (CAC) is a specialized area located in the medulla oblongata. When the body requires increased blood flow such as in exercise or a fight-or-flight response, there are several areas that the CAC can affect. With influences over the SA and AV node, the CAC can increase heart rate; this is known as a positive **chronotrophic** effect. In addition, influences over the

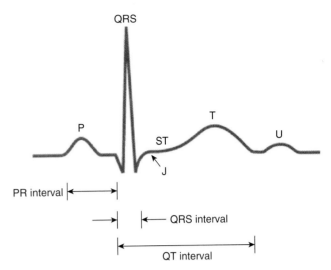

FIGURE 1–6 Electrocardiogram normal waveform. (From http://accessmedicine.mhmedical.com/data/books/harr/harr_c228f002.gif.)

cardiac muscle can increase the strength of heart contraction; this is termed a positive **ionotrophic** effect.

B. Parasympathetic Innervation

The cardiac inhibitory center (CIC) also is located in the medulla oblongata and has influences on the heart via the vagus nerve (cranial nerve X). The primary influence of the CIC is directed only toward the SA and AV node and regulates heart rate. Unlike the CAC, the CIC does not have direct links to cardiac muscle to have an effect on contractile strength. With increased parasympathetic input, the heart rate decreases, which produces a negative chronotrophic effect.

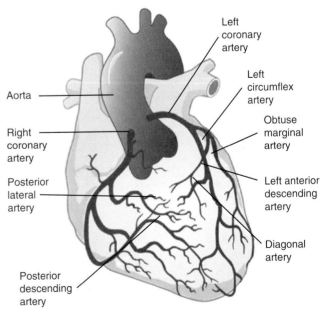

FIGURE 1–7 Coronary artery circulation. (From http://accessanesthesiology.mhmedical.com/data/books/2152/longnecker3_ch47_f002.png.)

C. Sensory Input

Sensory input for regulation of the cardiovascular system is received through a number of sensory receptors. Central and peripheral chemoreceptors as well as baroreceptors help to monitor the changing needs of blood volume, needs for O_2, and pressure.

Peripheral chemoreceptors are located in the aorta and carotid artery. These receptors detect changes in blood pH, hydrogen (H^+), O_2, and CO_2. When CO_2 increases and/or O_2 decreases, pH decreases (pH acidosis), and this causes an increased response for increased cardiac output. Conversely, when CO_2 decreases and/or O_2 increases, pH increases (pH alkalosis), and this calls for a decrease in cardiac output.

Central chemoreceptors are located in the medulla and are sensitive to changes in H^+ ion concentration. Only dissolved gases can diffuse past the blood-brain barrier. In the presence of increased CO_2 levels in the peripheral blood, CO_2 then can cause an increase in H^+ ion concentrations in the brain. Central chemoreceptors would detect these changes in H^+ concentrations.

Baroreceptors are located in the carotid artery and aorta. Changes in blood pressure and blood volume cause a response to counter these changes. The body's response has several mechanisms that counter these changes in a number of ways, which may include either increasing or decreasing cardiac output, heart contractility, heart rate, vasoconstriction, and vasodilation.

The Cardiac Cycle

The cardiac cycle is a group of cardiac events that occur from the beginning of one heartbeat to the beginning of the next beat. Two phases of the cycle, diastole (the relaxation period of the heart), and systole (the contraction period) are illustrated in Wiggers diagram in Figure 1–8.

Cardiac Hemodynamics

A. Cardiac Output

The amount of measured blood that is ejected from a single ventricular contraction is referred to as stroke volume (SV). In a normal male adult, this is approximately 70 mL. Cardiac output is a product of SV and heart rate. Hence, a person with a heart rate of 60 beats per minute (bpm) and SV of 70 mL per stroke would have 4200 mL/min, or 4.2 L per minute. By increasing either the SV (or increasing heart contractility) or the heart rate, cardiac output correspondingly increases. In addition, it is important to note that SV is a product between end-diastolic volume (EDV) and end-systolic volume (ESV). This amount is normally 120 mL. Whereas EDV is the amount of blood that enters the ventricle at the end of diastole, ESV is the amount of blood that remains in the ventricle after a full contraction. This range is normally approximately 70 mL. Therefore, SV is approximately 70 mL. Many varying factors can play a role in cardiac output dynamics that can increase or decrease the amount of EDV or ESV, which in turn affects SV.

B. Preload

Preload is the amount of blood volume that enters into the ventricle at the end of ventricular diastole. The degree to which the

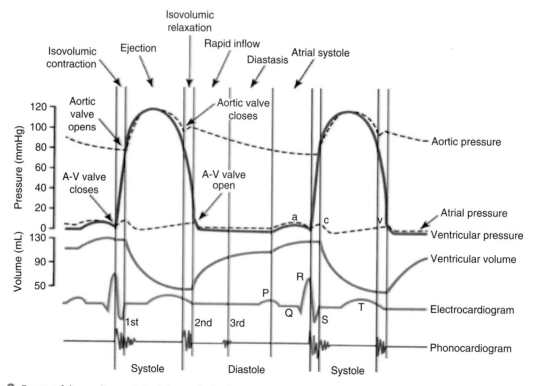

FIGURE 1–8 Events of the cardiac cycle for left ventricular function—also known as Wiggers diagram. (From Guyton AC, Hall JE. *Textbook of Medical Physiology.* 11th ed. Philadelphia, PA: Saunders; 2006.)

heart muscle can stretch just before a contraction influences pre-load. To a certain extent within physiological limits, an increase in preload will have a net increase in SV. This phenomenon is known as the **Frank–Starling law** of the heart, where it was observed that increased stretching and preloading of the heart causes an increase in heart contractility. The primary factor that can drive preload is the amount of venous return received by the ventricles.

C. Heart Contractility

Contractility is described by the contractile force exerted at a given muscle length. The ventricle at rest is shorter than the optimal length for a contraction. Stretching of the ventricle by increasing preload will positively create a stronger contraction and SV as pre-viously described. Other extrinsic and intrinsic factors can influ-ence contractility. In a sympathetic response, there is increased contractility. Other influences such as certain hormones, ions, and pharmaceutical agents can also regulate contractility.

D. Afterload

Where preload is a measure of the amount or volume of blood, afterload is a distinctly different measure by looking at the amount of pressure exerted from the pulmonary and arterial system back toward the aortic and pulmonary SL valves. Therefore, afterload represents the amount of force that must be overcome to open these valves in order to eject blood. Normally this pressure is 80 mmHg in the aortic valve and 10 mm in the pulmonary trunk.

Vascular System

Blood is moved through the body along two major circuits delivering nutrients, oxygenated enriched blood, and carrying deoxygenated blood back to the heart via systemic circulation. Pulmonary circulation involves carrying deoxygenated blood from the heart to the lungs and carrying blood back to the heart via pul-monary veins. There are five major classes of blood vessels of the cardiovascular system: arteries, arterioles, capillaries, venules, and veins. Figure 1–9 illustrates the cardiovascular circulatory system.

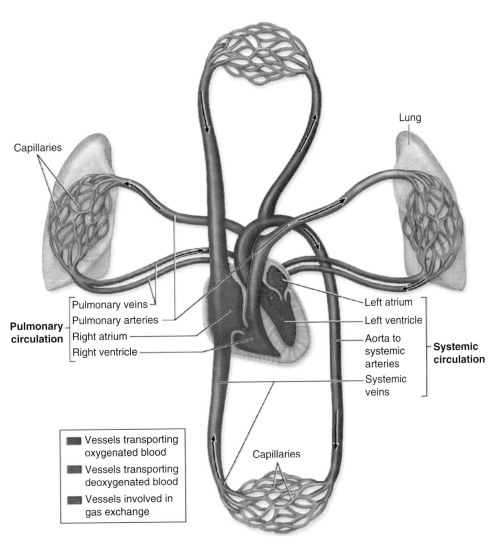

FIGURE 1–9 Cardiovascular circulatory system. (From https://accessmedicine.mhmedical.com/data/books/mesc13/mesc13_c011f001.png.)

Arteries

Arteries consist of the aorta and the main peripheral branching arteries. These vessels carry O_2 from high pressure areas to low pressure areas, carrying vital O_2 to the tissues throughout the body. There are varying amounts of elasticity and extensibility in arteries. The pulmonary artery carries deoxygenated blood from the RV to the lungs for oxygenation.

Arterioles

Arterioles are the smallest of the arteries, measuring between 0.3 mm and 10 μm in diameter. Their most important feature is the presence of vascular smooth muscles that can change the diameter and regulate blood flow. This is an important regulator of blood pressure and flow by changing the vessel diameter to direct and reroute blood flow using the properties of vasodilation and vasoconstriction where needed.

Capillaries

Capillaries are the smallest of vessels that allow for exchange of gases, fluids, ions, and nutrients to and from the blood to the tissues and cells throughout the body. The vessels are usually 1 mm to 10 μm in thickness.

Venules

Capillaries join to form venules that range from 8 to 100 μm in diameter. Venules carry unoxygenated blood back to the heart. Venules and veins have a large capacity to hold blood and serve as the primary blood reservoir; 64% of the systemic circulation is found in these vessels.

Veins

Blood pressure in veins is very low when compared to the arterial system. Therefore, an important feature of one-way valves helps to prevent backflow and pooling of blood en route to the right atrium of the heart. There are both superficial and deep veins, with the deep veins corresponding with an artery in the same area and often sharing the same name (ie, femoral, axillary, tibial, etc.). Venous circulation and blood return is aided by skeletal muscle contractions, gravity, and the movement from respiratory function.

ANATOMY AND PHYSIOLOGY OF THE PULMONARY SYSTEM

The pulmonary system functions to move O_2 and CO_2 in the process of respiration. **Respiration** is defined as the process of gas exchange with the atmosphere and cells of the body. In order for respiration to take place, the involvement of both the cardiac system and the pulmonary system moves and exchanges gases from the atmosphere and to the tissues. A number of exchanges occur in the processes of external and internal respiration.

External Respiration

This process involves the drawing of air in and out of the lungs. This is also called **pulmonary ventilation**. Air is drawn into the lungs during inspiration and removed from the lungs during expiration. Gas exchange occurs in the lungs with the movement of O_2 into and removal of CO_2 out of the blood. The cardiac system carries oxygenated blood to the body and CO_2 is transported from the body tissues to the lungs.

Internal Respiration

The delivery of O_2 and CO_2 between body tissue cells and the blood is called internal respiration. When the cellular processes of O_2 and CO_2 are used, this is called cellular respiration.

General Anatomy and Structure

The right lung is larger and has three lobes (superior, middle, and inferior) separated by a horizontal and oblique fissure. The left lung is smaller due to accommodation of the heart within the cardiac notch. The oblique fissure separates the two left lobes (superior and inferior). The inferior aspect of the lungs is bordered by the diaphragm. This large dome-shaped muscle is the major muscle involved in inspiration. Figure 1–10 represents the surface anatomy of the lungs.

Atmospheric air is inspired and expired in the upper airways of the nose or mouth. Air is warmed and filtered by the mucosal layers in the nasal cavity. The nose and mouth come together in the pharynx. The larynx leads to the trachea. The epiglottis serves as a flap to direct only air toward the lungs. Vocal cords in the larynx are involved in the formation of speech.

The trachea divides into primary left and right bronchi that enter each lung. Multiple divisions of the bronchi down to microscopic bronchioles that are one cell thick form the bronchial tree. At the level of respiratory bronchioles, alveolar sacs and alveoli comprise the respiratory unit where respiration occurs.

Pleura of the Lungs

The innermost layer that directly lines the lungs is called the visceral pleura. The outermost layer that interfaces with the inner surface of the rib cage, diaphragm, and mediastinum is called the parietal pleura. The potential space between these layers is intrapleural space, and a serous pleural fluid aids in the movement of these layers across each other during respiration.

Breathing Mechanics

Inspiration

Ventilation is the process of moving air into and out of the lungs. The diaphragm plays the principal role in inspiration. The dome shape of the diaphragm contracts, flattens, and moves downward when it is innervated by the phrenic nerve. Contributing to inspiration are the external intercostals that pull the rib cage upward and outward. This creates increased volume in the thoracic cavity and pressure inversely decreases. This internal negative pressure draws air into the lungs.

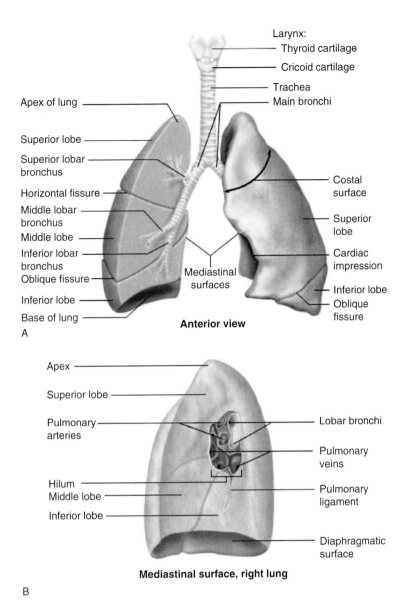

FIGURE 1-10 Lungs–surface anatomy. (From http://slideplayer.com/slide/7523978/24/images/29/Lungs+-+Surface+Anatomy.jpg.)

When more air is required due to increased workload, accessory muscles contribute to deeper breathing and increased breathing rate. The scalenes and sternocleidomastoid serve as accessory muscles, as do the levator costarum and serratus muscle. If the upper extremities are fixed distally, the trapezius, pectoralis major and minor, and serratus can aid as accessory muscles to inspiration.

Expiration

In normal resting expiration, it is important to note that there is no active muscle involvement. Passive forces allow the lungs to deflate and expire air. There is a normal elastic recoil in the lung tissue due to the presence of elastic fibers that are stretched on inspiration. Surface tension along the alveoli also contributes to the tendency of the lungs and alveoli to deflate.

When there is increased demand on respiration and air needs to be quickly expelled, the internal intercostals, abdominal muscles, and quadratus lumborum can aid as accessory muscles to expiration.

Lung Volumes and Capacities

SKILL KEEPER: LUNG VOLUMES

When a patient starts to exercise, breathing rate and depth increase. What are the changes that occur to the different lung volumes with increased activity in healthy individuals?

Figure 1–11 shows the maximum lung volumes and capacities. The normal ranges for lung volumes and capacities measured in

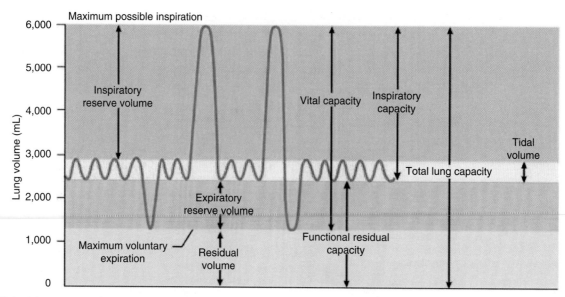

FIGURE 1–11 Lung volumes and capacities. (From http://images.slideplayer.com/25/7594504/slides/slide_51.jpg.)

liters of oxygen of a healthy individual are presented in the chart below.

Lung Volumes	Normal Ranges
Tidal volume (TV)	0.4–1.0 L
Inspiratory reserve volume (IRV)	2.5–3.5 L
Expiratory reserve volume (ERV)	1.0–1.5 L
Residual volume (RV)	0.8–1.4 L

Lung Capacities	Normal Ranges
Inspiratory capacity (IC) • TV + IRV	2.9–4.5 L
Functional residual capacity (FRC) • ERV + RV	1.8–2.9 L
Vital capacity (VC) • TV + IRV + ERV	3.0–5.0 L
Total lung capacity (TLC) • TV + IRV + ERV + RV	4.7–6.4 L

Gas Exchange

At sea level, the pressure that surrounds us is 760 mmHg. This is sometimes expressed as 1 atmospheric unit. Atmospheric air has a composition of 78% nitrogen, 21% O_2, and 0.4% CO_2 in addition to other trace amounts of gases. The represented amount of pressure of each gas is termed the partial pressure of that gas. For instance, O_2 is 21% of atmospheric pressure. Atmospheric pressure is 760 mmHg, and O_2 represents 21% of the composition. Therefore, O_2 is 160 mmHg of atmospheric pressure. The pH of blood indicates the presence or absence of H^+ ions in the body.

The normal range for blood pH is 7.36 to 7.44. The normal range for CO_2 in the blood is 36 to 44 mmHg. Bicarbonate (HCO_3^-) is normally 23 to 30 meq/mL. An increase in HCO_3^- increases pH, and a decrease in HCO_3^- decreases body pH.

Ventilation and Perfusion

Ventilation (Ve) occurs when air enters into the alveoli. **Perfusion** (Q) represents the amount of blood flow to an area. Optimal respiration occurs when there is adequate ventilation and perfusion.

Some air does not reach down to the alveoli or to the terminal ends of the bronchial tree where respiration takes place. This is referred to as anatomical **dead space**. Some air does reach the alveoli, but there may be poor perfusion to this area. This is referred to as alveolar dead space or physiologic dead space.

Anatomical **shunt** refers to blood vessels that do not interact with the terminal respiratory units of the bronchial tree, where there is no gas exchange. Physiologic shunt occurs when there is good perfusion at the alveoli but the alveoli does not have ventilation.

The relationship between ventilation and perfusion can be expressed as a ratio of V/Q. Position of the body and various disease states can affect this ratio. In the upright position, the top of the lungs, or apex, receives greater amounts of ventilation. The bottom of the lungs has decreased ventilation. Conversely, perfusion, which is gravity dependent, is greater at the base of the lungs and less at the top (apex) of the lungs. Changing positions (ie, supine and side-lying) changes these zones and ratios of V/Q.

Oxygen and Carbon Dioxide Transport

Oxygen is not as soluble in water as CO_2. Therefore approximately less than 2% of O_2 is dissolved in the blood plasma. Hemoglobin is a specialized protein that contains iron that helps to bind and carry O_2. Ninety-eight percent of the O_2 is carried by hemoglobin. The combination of O_2 and hemoglobin is called oxyhemoglobin.

CO_2 is transported in the body through several different mechanisms. The following chemical equation describes CO_2 transport:

$$H_2O + CO_2 \leftrightarrow H_2CO_3 \text{ (carbonic acid)} \leftrightarrow H^+ \text{ (hydrogen ion)} + HCO_3^- \text{ (bicarbonate)}$$

CO_2 has a higher solubility than O_2, and therefore it can dissolve directly into the plasma. Some of the CO_2 is converted to H^+ and HCO_3^- which are directly dissolved in the plasma. CO_2 is also able to bind to hemoglobin, and 23% of CO_2 is transported as carbaminohemoglobin. The majority of CO_2 is transported as HCO_3^- that is produced from the red blood cells through a process using the enzyme carbonic anhydrase. Seventy percent of CO_2 transport occurs from this process.

Control of Breathing

Specialized groups of neurons gather in neuronal pools in the pons and the medulla to regulate breathing as shown in Figure 1–12. These centers are categorized as the dorsal respiratory group (DRG) and the ventral respiratory group (VRG), both located in the medulla. The pneumotaxic center and the apneustic center are located in the pons.

> ### SKILL KEEPER: NEUROLOGICAL CONTROL OF BREATHING
>
> *A patient has sustained injuries from a motor vehicular accident and as a result is in a coma with a traumatic brain injury. If the patient was experiencing erratic and random breathing rate and depth, what type of injury might this be indicative of?*

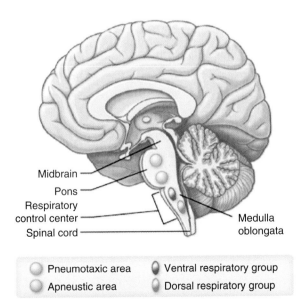

Midbrain
Pons
Respiratory control center
Spinal cord
Medulla oblongata

- ○ Pneumotaxic area
- ○ Apneustic area
- ● Ventral respiratory group
- ○ Dorsal respiratory group

FIGURE 1–12 Respiratory control center in the medulla oblongata and pons. (From https://fadavispt.mhmedical.com/data/books/2182/exercphys_ch6_f008-1.png.)

Dorsal Respiratory Group

The DRG is involved in inspiration by causing excitation of the diaphragm via the phrenic nerve and the external intercostals via the external intercostal nerve. These are the primary muscles in normal inspiration.

Ventral Respiratory Group

The VRG is involved in motor control of expiration and inspiration when there is increased demand for respiration, such as in exercise. Recall that expiration in normal rested conditions is a passive process and no muscle activity is needed in the lungs for recoil and expelling of air under normal breathing conditions.

Pneumotaxic Center

The pneumotaxic center controls the rate and depth of breathing by inhibiting the activity of the DRG. The pneumotaxic center essentially serves as an on/off switch for the DRG. In addition, the pneumotaxic center inhibits activity of the apneustic center.

Apneustic Center

The apneustic center prolongs the activity of the DRG by increasing the depth and slowing the rate of inspiration.

Sensory Input

Various receptor types monitor the environment of the body to regulate breathing dynamics. Baroreceptors monitor pressure changes and chemoreceptors are sensitive to changes in pH, H^+, HCO_3^-, O_2, and CO_2 levels. Input from irritant receptors and stretch receptors also regulate ventilation and respiration. Various reflexes and responses from the input of these receptors are relayed to the brain for adjustments in breathing.

ANATOMY AND PHYSIOLOGY OF THE LYMPHATIC SYSTEM

General Anatomy and Structure

The lymphatic system, similar to the cardiac and vascular systems, is involved in the movement of fluids throughout the body. In the capillary dynamics of the cardiovascular system, not all the fluid that is filtered out of the capillaries is reabsorbed by the venules. Remaining fluid in the tissues is picked up by the lymphatic system, and once collected in the lymph vessels is called lymph. Lymph re-enters cardiovascular circulation either via the right lymphatic duct that drains the upper right quadrant of the body, or thoracic duct which drains the remaining areas of the body as shown in Figure 1–13.[1]

The lymphatic system is comprised of a network of lymphatic vessels, capillaries, nodes, and larger vessels. The lymphatic system performs several essential roles. First, it transports excess fluid that is collected in the interstitial spaces of body tissues that was not reabsorbed, which can be up to 3 liters per day. Without this system, there would be increased swelling

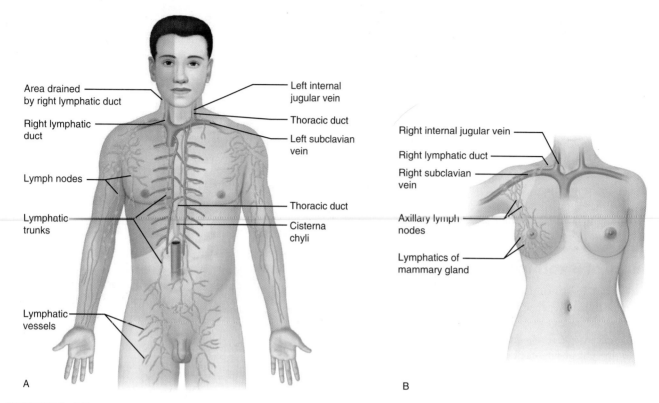

FIGURE 1–13 Lymphatic system drainage via the right lymphatic and thoracic ducts. (From https://image.slidesharecdn.com/chapter16-lymphaticsystemandimmunity-110728070145-phpapp01/95/chapter-16-lymphatic-system-and-immunity-9-728.jpg?cb=1311836704.)

in the extremities, heart, and lungs. A second function is that lymph transports undigested fats that cannot be transported by the blood. A third function is the lymphatic system serves as the structural basis for the immune response. A number of cells mediate the immune response. Lymphocytes and phagocytic cells serve as the body's defense against foreign invaders and disease. The body can also initiate inflammation as an additional measure of the immune response. The immune response is not extensively reviewed in this section. The primary focus is on the system's role on the movement of fluids as it relates to cardiac and vascular function.[1]

Lymphatic System Organization and Movement

The lymphatic system is comprised of a network of lymphatic capillaries that form microscopic tubes called lymphatic pathways. These vessels operate under very low pressure with a series of one-way valves to prevent backflow. Contractions of smooth muscle and skeletal muscle, as well as changes in thoracic pressure from the pulmonary system, help to keep lymph fluid moving. Buildup of fluid in the tissue is called edema. In instances of lymph node removal, such as breast cancer, removal of axillary lymph nodes can cause upper extremity lymphedema.[1]

Proteins do not enter easily into cardiovascular vessels but readily transport into the lymphatic system. Lacteals are found in the small intestines lining the digestive tract and absorb digested fats and carry them into the venous system. Lymph collects in the larger lymphatic vessels and is carried to specialized organs called lymph nodes. The lymph node and its components are shown in Figure 1–14.[1]

There are hundreds of lymph nodes throughout the body that house a large number of lymphocytes and macrophages to mediate the immune response to fight invading microorganisms. Movement of the lymph through the vessel system and delivery to lymph nodes allows the body to maintain surveillance on the quality of the blood and the overall state of health throughout the body.[1]

PHARMACOLOGY AS RELATED TO THE CARDIOVASCULAR/PULMONARY SYSTEM[2]

SKILL KEEPER: PHARMACOLOGICAL MANAGEMENT OF HYPERTENSION (HTN)

What are the mechanisms of diuretic medications that are used to manage HTN? When diuretics are not effective in managing chronic HTN, what other medications might be prescribed and what are their effects?

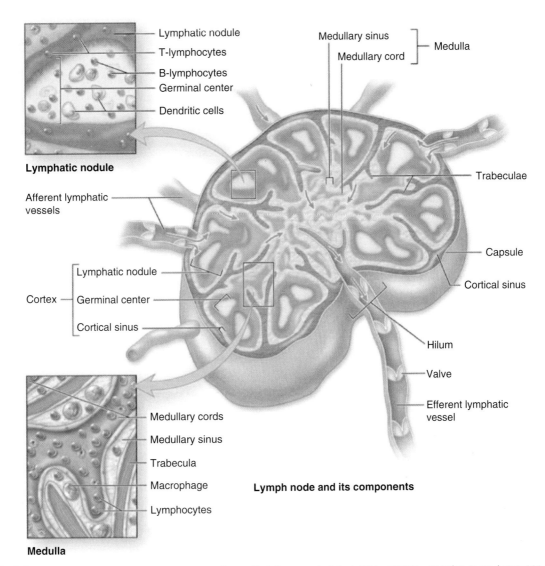

Lymphatic nodule
- Lymphatic nodule
- T-lymphocytes
- B-lymphocytes
- Germinal center
- Dendritic cells

Medullary sinus
Medullary cord
Medulla

Trabeculae

Capsule

Cortical sinus

Hilum

Valve

Efferent lymphatic vessel

Afferent lymphatic vessels

Cortex
- Lymphatic nodule
- Germinal center
- Cortical sinus

Medulla
- Medullary cords
- Medullary sinus
- Trabecula
- Macrophage
- Lymphocytes

Lymph node and its components

FIGURE 1–14 Lymph node and its components. (From https://i.pinimg.com/originals/63/ea/55/63ea5543f05e0e59cb190e801e556408.jpg.)

A. Primary or Essential Hypertension

Various drugs, classified by the mechanism of action, are employed to address hypertension (HTN). The action of the pharmaceutical intervention can have an effect on (a) blood volume, (b) vascular smooth muscle tone, (c) angiotensin, and (d) sympathetic nervous system effects.

Diuretics—Loss of fluid from the blood has a decreased net effect on blood volume and lowers blood pressure.

- Thiazide group
  - Hydrochlorothiazide for mild to moderate HTN
- Loop diuretics
  - Furosemide (Lasix)
  - Bumetanide (Bumex)

Sympathetic nervous system control—Pharmacological drugs can regulate the amount of sympathetic flow to the cardiovascular system. This influence can control several aspects including heart rate, contractile force of the cardiac muscle, cardiac output, venous tone, and total peripheral resistance.

- Central nervous system sympathetic regulation of cardiac output and vascular resistance
  - Examples: Clonidine, methyldopa
  - Side effects: Salt retention
- Beta blockers
  - Examples: Propranolol, atenolol, metoprolol, carvedilol, and newer drug nebivolol
  - Affect cardiac output

Vasodilators—Vasodilation is achieved by affecting the amount of tone in the smooth muscles of the vascular system. Factors that cause vasodilation include blocking of Ca^+ channels, increase in the presence of nitric oxide (NO), opening of K^+ channels (which leads to increased hyperpolarization within the cell), or activation of dopamine receptors.

- Calcium channel blockers
  - Examples: Nifedipine, verapamil, diltiazem
  - Compensatory salt retention of the body is decreased with the use of these drugs, and therefore they are often used for treatment of chronic HTN
- Infused IV drugs used in emergency cases
  - Nitroprusside, diazoxide, and fenoldopam
  - Cause membrane hyperpolarization or dopamine receptor activation

Angiotensin and renin inhibitors

- Angiotensin-converting enzyme (ACE) inhibitors: Decrease amount of angiotensin II and decrease vasoconstriction and production of aldosterone (a hormone from the kidneys that promotes salt and water retention)
  - Examples: Lisinopril, captopril, benazepril (Lotensin)
  - Side effects: Chronic cough, hyperkalemia, and possible renal damage
  - Contraindications: During pregnancy due to damage to renal system of developing fetus
- Angiotensin II blockers
  - Valsartan, irbesartan, and candesartan

B. Angina Pectoris
Nitrates

- Nitrates are the most important therapeutic drug in the treatment of insufficient O_2 delivery to the coronary arteries.
- Duration: Can range from 10 to 20 minutes to 8 to 10 hours.
- Delivery route: Sublingual or transdermal.
- Action
  - Release of NO within smooth muscle. Relaxation of the muscle in the vascular system causes vasodilation.
  - Most importantly, the effect is more on the venous system than on the arterial vessels. Increasing venous diameter causes more blood to stay within the venous system. This in turn reduces the amount of blood returning to the right atrium. This causes a decrease in preload and the heart has to work less, resulting in an ultimate decrease in O_2 need for the heart.
  - Relaxation of the arterial vessels decreases total peripheral resistance and there is a decrease in afterload. In response, the heart has to work less to deliver blood from the ventricles. Decrease in heart work also decreases the O_2 demands of the heart.
  - To a lesser degree, nitrates can also cause dilation of the coronary vessels and can reverse the spastic restrictions to the coronary arteries delivering blood and O_2 to the heart.

Calcium channel blockers—These drugs were discussed earlier in the treatment of HTN due to the ability to cause vasodilation. These drugs also are effective in the treatment of **angina pectoris**.

- Examples: Nifedipine, diltiazem, verapamil.
- Specifically, these drugs block L-type Ca^+ channels. Calcium is important in the interaction of actin and myosin in muscle contraction. The decreased presence of intracellular Ca^+ causes decreased interaction of these filaments and thus promotes decreased muscle contraction in smooth muscle. The net effect is vasodilation.
- A newer drug, ranolazine, has an effect on Ca^+, but is not a Ca^+ channel blocker like the drugs described above. This medication acts on decreasing intracellular Na^+ which also causes the cell to remove intracellular Ca^+ and therefore decreases heart contractility.

Beta blockers

- This class of drugs was discussed in the treatment of HTN as well.
- Examples: Propranolol, atenolol.
- Block sympathetic nervous system flow and decrease heart rate and contraction, and cardiac output. Decreased heart work also decreases the pressure exerted by the heart.
- In the same manner, beta blockers provide antianginal benefits by decreasing the O_2 demands of the heart. Though not effective in acute angina, these medications are used in prophylactic treatment in conjunction with nitrates. This may help to mitigate angina during exercise.

C. Heart Failure

This is the progressive decline in heart function due to disease, with a resultant decrease in cardiac output. The various pathways of intervention include the use of diuretics to remove salt and water, reducing afterload with ACE inhibitors, decreasing sympathetic input through beta blockers, and decreasing preload and afterload by promoting vasodilation.

Digoxin

- Digoxin is also known as digitalis and is used commonly throughout the United States.
- Action
  - Decreases activity of the Na^+/K^+ ATPase, which effects the Na^+ pump of the cell.
  - Decreases the removal of Na^+ and increases its intracellular presence.
  - Increases intracellular Ca^+ and is stored in the sarcoplasmic reticulum.
  - Increases strength of heart contraction.
  - Increases heart rate (**chronotrophy**) and increases the rate of fire in the electrical properties of the heart. Though there is increased **inotrophy**, digoxin has not demonstrated decreases in mortality rate.
- Prescribing the use of other medications such as diuretics, ACE inhibitors, and vasodilators has been shown to be more efficacious with less risk of undesired side effects and toxicity. Some toxic symptoms include heart arrhythmias, nausea, vomiting, and diarrhea. Cardiac depression may also occur, leading to cardiac arrest.

Diuretics

- Different classification of drugs are used for various heart pathologies.
- Diuretics are considered first in cases of systolic and diastolic heart failure.

- Furosemide is used immediately for severe edema or pulmonary congestion.
- Thiazide is used for milder cases of heart failure.

Angiotensin antagonists

- Used for HTN but also for heart failure
- Examples: Losartan, captopril
- Reduce aldosterone, vasoconstriction, and amount of heart work via lower blood volume and afterload resistance

Beta blockers

- Seem counterproductive to decrease heart contraction in heart failure; however, long-term studies show these drugs slow the progression of chronic heart failure
- Can be used in cardiomyopathy
- Not used for treatment of acute heart failure

Vasodilators

- Used in acute severe failure with congestion
- Increasing preload through increased venous return and decreasing afterload resistance results in increased efficiency of the heart
- Especially effective when heart failure is a result of chronic increased afterload, such as hypertension and a recent myocardial infarct
- Examples: Hydralazine, isosorbide dinitrate
- Shown effective in treating heart failure in African Americans

D. Antiarrhythmic Drugs

Arrhythmias are caused by an abnormality in automaticity or conduction. Pharmacological agents are classified or grouped by the ion channels that are influenced by the mechanism of action of the drug. These include (a) Na^+ channel blockers, (b) beta-adrenoreceptor blockers, (c) K^+ channel blockers, and (d) Ca^+ channel blockers.

Sodium channel blockers

- Sodium channel blockers can shorten **action potentials** (APs) or lengthen APs in heart conduction
- Examples
  - Amiodarone slows speed of conduction and prolongs APs. This drug is classified as both a Na^+ channel blocker and a K^+ channel blocker.
  - Lidocaine is introduced by IV or via intramuscular injection.

Beta blockers

- Used to treat arrhythmias after myocardial infarction (MI)
- Decrease movement of Ca^+ and Na^+ and reduce abnormal pacemakers
- Have been shown to be effective in reducing chronic heart failure
- Examples: Propanolol, esmolol

Potassium channel blockers

- The blocking of K^+ channels prolongs AP, increases the time for repolarization, and increases the **effective refractory period**.

This prevents the heart from responding to additional APs such as ventricular tachycardia.
- Example: Amiodarone.
- Side effects: Depositing microcrystals in the cornea and skin, affects to the thyroid, paresthesia, and tremors.

Calcium channel blockers

- Effective at managing AV nodal tachycardia
- Examples: Verapamil, diltiazem
- Side effects: Decreased cardiac contractility, prolonged AV conduction, and decreased blood pressure
- Should not be used in cases of ventricular tachycardia

E. Asthma and Chronic Obstructive Pulmonary Disease (COPD)

Acute bronchoconstriction can be treated with various classifications of drugs. Bronchodilators such as β_2 agonists, muscarinic antagonists, and theophylline are used effectively to manage these pathologies. In cases of chronic asthma, long-term management with corticosteroids is employed.

Beta-adrenoreceptor agonists

- Delivery route: Inhalation via pressurized canister or nebulizer treatment
- Side effects: Skeletal tremor, tachycardia, and cardiac arrhythmias
- Short-acting
  - Examples: Albuterol, terbutaline, metaproterenol
  - Duration: No more than 4 hours
- Long-acting
  - Examples: Salmeterol, formoterol, indacaterol, vilanterol
  - Duration: Up to 12 hours
  - Recommended for prophylactic intervention

Methylxanthines

- Naturally occurring forms: Caffeine from coffee, theophylline from tea, and theobromine from cocoa
- Theophylline prescribed medically for asthma and COPD
- The result produced by theophylline is bronchodilation and increased contractile force of the diaphragm
- Examples: Aminophylline, roflumilast, pentoxifylline
- Side effects: GI irritation and tremors. More severe effects in overdosage can include insomnia, nausea, arrhythmias of the heart, and seizure activity.

Muscarinic antagonists

- Block muscarinic receptors, inhibit bronchoconstriction; mediated by the vagus nerve (parasympathetic nervous system).
- First-response drugs in acute bronchoconstriction are beta-agonist drugs such as albuterol. However, in COPD, the use of muscarinic antagonists may be preferred and may be more effective with fewer side effects.
- Delivery route: Aerosol.
- Examples: Ipratropium, tiotropium, aclidinium.

Corticosteroids

- Commonly considered first-line pharmaceutical interventions to treat moderate to severe asthma.
- Decrease inflammation and allergic response.
- Minimize bronchoconstriction.
- Used for children who do not respond to the use of beta agonists. Considered appropriate to mitigate deleterious chronic inflammation and damage from longstanding asthma.
- Delivery route: Aerosol.
- Examples: Beclomethasone, budesonide, dexamethasone, flunisolide, fluticasone, mometasone.
- Less harmful then prednisone and hydrocortisone:
  - Prednisone and hydrocortisone are used in severe cases and when other interventions are unsuccessful.
  - These drugs act by reducing arachidonic acid synthesis and inhibiting COX-2 expression.
  - Side effects: Frequent use can cause adrenal suppression and changes in the pharynx natural bacteria, leading to candidiasis. These effects can be countered by alternating the dosage of the medication to higher doses every other day.

Leukotriene antagonists

- Receptor blockers that inhibit leukotrienes that are involved in late inflammatory response.
- Prevent bronchoconstriction during exercise and antigen reaction.
- Examples: Montelukast, zafirlukast.
- These drugs are not as effective in managing severe asthma; therefore corticosteroids are more commonly used.

EFFECTS OF ACTIVITY AND EXERCISE ON THE CARDIOVASCULAR/ PULMONARY SYSTEM

A. Exercise Effects on Respiration

Oxygen use and pulmonary ventilation during exercise—
The resting O_2 consumption for a young male at rest is approximately 250 mL/min. This can be increased on average to the numbers in the following chart:

	mL/min
Untrained average male	3600
Athletically trained average male	4000
Male marathon runner	5000

From Hall JE: *Guyton and Hall Textbook of Medical Physiology*. 12th ed. Philadelphia, PA: Saunders Elsevier; 2011, 1036.

The chart demonstrates that O_2 consumption can be increased significantly by nearly 20-fold when comparing an average male to a well-conditioned athlete.[3]

VO₂ max and effects of exercise training—
In a study of gains in VO_2 max by Fox in 1979, the effects of progressive athletic training on VO_2 max was measured at 7 and 13 weeks. It was surprising that results demonstrated only an increase of approximately 10% of VO_2 max overall. Also, there was little variance in frequency of training when comparing 2 times to 5 times a week. Marathon runners are able to improve O_2 consumption by up to 45% more than the untrained athlete. This may be linked by genetic determination as well as body type and relative ratio of body mass to lung capacity. Individuals with distinct advantages may self-select for marathon and longer-distance sports. However, it is likely that years of training may account for large increases in VO_2 for marathon runners versus short-term training, as demonstrated in the study.[3]

Oxygen-diffusing capacity of athletes—
The measure of the O_2-diffusing capacity is the amount of O_2 that crosses through the respiratory membrane and enters into the blood each minute. The following chart demonstrates diffusing capacities in various individuals:

	mL/min
Non-athlete at rest	23
Non-athlete during maximal exercise	48
Speed skaters during maximal exercise	64
Swimmers during maximal exercise	71
Oarsman during maximal exercise	80

From Hall JE: *Guyton and Hall Textbook of Medical Physiology*. 12th ed. Philadelphia, PA: Saunders Elsevier; 2011, 1037.

There are several significant findings. The first is the greater than twofold increase from a non-athlete at rest to during maximal exercise. Physiologically, this occurs because at rest, many pulmonary alveoli are poorly perfused or not perfused at all. During exercise, there is a large increase in blood flow. In maximal exercise, all pulmonary capillaries are perfused. This increases surface area exposing blood to O_2. Second, there is a threefold or greater increase in O_2-diffusing capacity in well-trained athletes. Is this because persons with higher O_2-diffusing capacities choose these sports, or is it because endurance training improves this ability? The mechanisms of how this occurs is unknown; however, it is most likely linked to effects of long-term endurance training activities that increase a person's O_2-diffusing capacity.[3]

Exercise effects on blood gases—
During exercise, there is an increased demand for O_2 by muscles throughout the body. It might be thought that this increase in demand would cause a decrease in O_2 levels and increase in CO_2 in the blood. However, this is not normally what occurs. In fact, O_2 and CO_2 levels remain near normal. This demonstrates the body's increased respiratory capacity to adjust in a large range to maintain adequate aeration. Significant changes in blood gases are not necessary to prompt a change in respiration. Instead, stimulation of the

respiratory centers at the brain stem can regulate these changes. Movement of the joints and muscles can cause sufficient sensory input to the respiratory centers, and in turn the brain can match the exact needs to maintain blood gas levels at or near normal.[3]

B. Exercise Effects on the Cardiovascular System

Effects of training and exercise on the heart and cardiac output—The tables below compare cardiac output, heart rate, and SV among various individuals and circumstances. From rest to exercise, cardiac output in an untrained individual can be increased more than four times resting. An average marathoner can increase this almost six times greater, while well-seasoned athletes can increase this to nearly seven to eight times more, ranging from 35 to 40 L/min.[3]

	L/min
Cardiac output in young man at rest	5.5
Maximal cardiac output during exercise in young untrained man	23
Maximal cardiac output during exercise in average male marathoner	30

From Hall JE: *Guyton and Hall Textbook of Medical Physiology.* 12th ed. Philadelphia, PA: Saunders Elsevier; 2011, 1038.

	Stroke Volume (mL)	Heart Rate (beats/minute)
Resting		
Non-athlete	75	75
Marathoner	105	50
Maximum		
Non-athlete	110	195
Marathoner	162	185

From Hall JE: *Guyton and Hall Textbook of Medical Physiology.* 12th ed. Philadelphia, PA: Saunders Elsevier; 2011, 1039.

According to the data, marathoners have about a 40% greater maximum cardiac output over untrained persons. During exercise, there is hypertrophy of the skeletal muscle and a 40% increase in heart chamber size and mass. The enlarged heart affords decreased heart rate (HR) for marathon athletes because the SV is greater when compared to the non-athlete.[3]

During exercise, SV increases from 105 to 162 mL while heart rate increases from 50 to 185 bpm. These changes represent an increase of 50% and 270%, respectively. This demonstrates that heart rate by and large accounts for the greater contribution in increasing cardiac output during strenuous exercise. SV reaches a ceiling effect at approximately 50% of the maximum of heart rate. Therefore, any remaining increase in cardiac output is attributed to increased heart rate. Figure 1–15 shows the approximate stroke

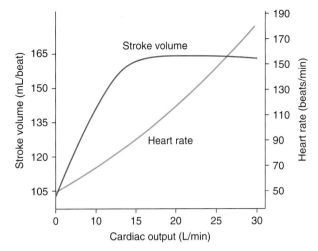

FIGURE 1–15 Approximate stroke volume output and heart rate at different levels of cardiac output in a marathon athlete.

volume and heart rate at different levels of cardiac output in a marathon athlete.[3]

Relationship of cardiac performance and VO₂ max—The respiratory system has a much greater capacity and reserve than does the cardiovascular system. In maximal exercise, the cardiovascular system is at nearly 90% of capacity. In contrast, the respiratory system is about 65% of maximum ventilation. Because of this, the cardiovascular system is the primary limiter of VO_2 max. The 40% gains in cardiac output in marathon runners serves as the single most important physiological benefit of the training regimen of marathon runners.[3]

■ EXAMINATION

OVERVIEW

The physical therapist uses the results of tests and measures to determine whether an individual has an adequate ventilatory pump and O_2 uptake/CO_2 elimination system to meet O_2 demands at rest, during movement, and during the performance of purposeful activity as well as whether the cardiovascular pump, circulation, O_2 delivery, and lymphatic drainage system are adequate to meet the body's demands at rest and with activity. Measures will also determine the appropriateness of an individual's responses to increased O_2 demand, the state of musculoskeletal balance and skeletal alignment, and the individual's environment. Responses are monitored at rest, during activity, and after activity, and may indicate the presence or severity of an impairment, activity limitation, participation restriction, or disability.

VITAL SIGN ASSESSMENT

Heart Rate or Pulse

- Locations: Heart rate is most accurately measured at the cardiac apex, where the point of maximal impulse (PMI) can

TABLE 1–1 **Normal ranges for physiological variables for unwell children.**

Age	Approximate Weight (kg)	Systolic Blood Pressure (mmHg)	Heart Rate (beats/minute)	Respiratory Rate (breaths/minute)
Term	3.5	60–105	110–170	25–60
3 months	6	65–115	105–165	25–55
6 months	8	65–115	105–165	25–55
1 year	10	70–120	85–150	20–40
2 years	13	70–120	85–150	20–40
4 years	15	70–120	85–150	20–40
6 years	20	80–130	70–135	16–34
8 years	25	80–130	70–135	16–34
10 years	30	80–130	70–135	16–34
12 years	40	95–140	60–120	14–26
14 years	50	95–140	60–120	14–26
17+ years	70	95–140	60–120	14–26

The Royal Children's Hospital, Melbourne, Australia, Clinical Practice Guideline: Normal Ranges for Physiological Variables; cited July 16, 2018. Available from: https://www.rch.org.au/clinicalguide/.

be palpated. Table 1–1 presents the normal pulse ranges for children. Pulses can be palpated using two to three fingers (not the thumb) at various locations: carotid, axillary, brachial, radial, femoral, popliteal, posterior tibial, and dorsalis pedis pulse, and can be graded on a 4-point scale as seen in Table 1–2.

- Tachycardia is defined as greater than 100 bpm and can be a normal response to exercise, or abnormal in disease processes. Bradycardia is defined as less than 60 bpm. Elite athletes may have lower resting heart rates.

Respiration

- Observe rate, depth, and rhythm of breathing.
- Normal respiratory rate in adults is 12 to 20 bpm. Late childhood is 15 to 25 bpm. Early childhood is 20 to 40 bpm. Newborns are 30 to 60 bpm.

TABLE 1–2 **Pulse 4-point scale.**

Grade	Description
0	Absent
1+	Palpable, but thready and weak; easily obliterated
2+	Normal, easily identified; not easily obliterated
3+	Increased pulse; moderate pressure for obliteration
4+	Full, bounding; cannot obliterate

From https://i.pinimg.com/236x/e9/ef/36/e9ef360e7e46d2ea3ab2220b5672b496--google-search-nursing.jpg.

- Various breathing patterns: **Eupnea** (normal), **bradypnea**, **tachypnea**, **hyperpnea**, Cheyne–Stokes, air trapping, apneustic, pursed-lip, Kussmaul, Biot, and ataxic.

Pulse Oximetry (SpO$_2$)

- A specialized sensor typically placed on ear lobe or finger measures arterial O$_2$ saturation.
- Normal ranges are 95% to 100%.
- Activity should stop if SpO$_2$ drops below 90% in acutely ill patients. Patients with chronic lung disease should stop if below 85%.
- Consult with physician for possible need for supplemental O$_2$ for patients with low SpO$_2$ levels during activity or mobility tasks.

Blood Pressure

- Hypotension results when blood pressure (BP) is lower than the expected normal. BP is not adequate to maintain proper perfusion/oxygenation. Can be caused by bed rest, drugs, shock, heart arrhythmias, myocardial infarction.
- Orthostatic hypotension is considered a drop in systolic BP of more than 20 mm Hg or a diastolic drop of more than 10 mm Hg when patient moves from supine to standing position. Healthy and unhealthy blood pressure ranges are presented in Table 1–3.

Temperature

- Note temperature changes in the body—increased warmth, or areas that are cool to touch.

TABLE 1–3 Healthy and unhealthy blood pressure ranges.

Blood Pressure Category	Systolic mmHg (upper #)		Diastolic mmHg (lower #)
Normal	Less than 120	and	Less than 80
Elevated	120–129	and	Less than 80
High blood pressure (hypertension) stage 1	130–139	or	80–89
High blood pressure (hypertension) stage 2	140 or higher	or	90 or higher
Hypertensive crisis (consult your doctor immediately)	Higher than 180	and/or	Higher than 120

Reprinted with permission https://www.heart.org/-/media/files/health-topics/high-blood-pressure/hbp-rainbow-chart-english-pdf-ucm_499220.pdf ©2018 American Heart Association, Inc.

- Changes in skin coloration or loss of hair may also accompany temperature differences in skin or in extremities.

Pain

Angina

- Differentiate between noncardiac- or cardiac-origin pain.
- Assess patient's complaint of angina such as:
  - Description (throbbing, aching, strong, sharp, dull)
  - Frequency
  - Onset
  - Triggering events
  - Time of day
  - What alleviates symptoms (activity, cessation of activity, medication)
  - Take special note of any referred pain symptoms that could be cardiac in nature

Patient can rate angina using a standardized scale as shown in Table 1–4. Patient can also rate exertion by using the Borg scale or modified Borg scale to rate exertion during activity (Table 1–5).

TABLE 1–4 Angina rating scale.

1. Mild, barely noticeable
2. Moderate, bothersome
3. Moderately severe, very uncomfortable
4. Most severe or most intense pain ever experienced

This scale is used in rating the subjective pain associated with myocardial insufficiency.
Adapted from American College of Sports Medicine 2006.
From http://www.humankinetics.com/AcuCustom/Sitename/DAM/084/370se_Main.jpg.

TABLE 1–5 Versions of the modified Borg scale used to evaluate dyspnea.

A. Modified Borg Scale—Burdon et al.[a]

0	Nothing at all
0.5	Very, very slight (just noticeable)
1	Very slight
2	Slight
3	Moderate
4	Somewhat severe
5	Severe
6	
7	Very severe
8	
9	Very, very severe (almost maximal)
10	Maximal

B. Modified Borg Scale—Kendrick et al.[b]

0	No breathlessness at all
0.5	Very, very slight (just noticeable)
1	Very slight
2	Slight breathlessness
3	Moderate
4	Somewhat severe
5	Severe breathlessness
6	
7	Very severe breathlessness
8	
9	Very, very severe (almost maximal)
10	Maximal

[a]Reprinted from Burdon JG, Juniper EF, Killian KJ, et al. The perception of breathlessness in asthma. *Am Rev Respir Dis.* 1982;126(5):825-828. Copyright (1982); with permission from American Thoracic Society.

[b]Reprinted from Kendrick KR, Baxi SC, Smith RM, et al. Usefulness of the modified 0–10 Borg scale in assessing the degree of dyspnea in patients with COPD and asthma. *J Emerg Nurs.* 2000;26(3):216-222. Copyright (2000); with permission from Elsevier.

From Proposing a standardized method for evaluating patient report of the intensity of dyspnea during exercise testing in COPD (PDF Download Available). Available from https://www.researchgate.net/publication/228089364_Proposing_a_standardized_method_for_evaluating_patient_report_of_the_intensity_of_dyspnea_during_exercise_testing_in_COPD. Accessed March 15, 2018. Figure 2.

HEART SOUNDS AND LUNG SOUNDS

Heart Sounds

- Patient is in supine position. The diaphragm of the stethoscope is used for high-pitched sounds (S1 and S2); the bell portion is used for lower-pitched sounds (S3 and S4).

- Listen for intensity, quality, and timing during the cardiac cycle. Also listen for additional sounds or abnormal sounds.
- Normal heart sounds:
  - S1 heart sound: "Lub" sound that corresponds to the closure of the AV valves and is the start of ventricular systole.
  - S2 heart sound: "Dub" sound that corresponds to the closure of the aortic and pulmonic SL valves; best heard at Erb's point.
- Gallop heart sounds: Additional sounds heard accompanying S1 and S2. Sounds like the galloping rhythm of horse.
  - S3 heart sound: "Ventricular gallop" is heard after S2 and corresponds with early and rapid filling of the ventricles during diastole. Can be heard in normal conditions or may be abnormal or pathologic.
    - Cadence is like saying "Kentucky"
    - May indicate congestive heart failure (CHF)
  - S4 heart sound: "Atrial gallop" is heard before S1 and corresponds with ventricular filling due to atrial systole ("atrial kick"). It is rarely considered normal and usually indicates pathology.
    - Cadence is like saying "Tennessee"
    - May indicate HTN, CAD, post MI, aortic stenosis, changes in compliance to the heart
- Abnormal findings
  - Systolic murmur: If auscultation reveals AV valve murmur, this could represent regurgitation, as the AV is not closing properly. If auscultation reveals aortic or pulmonary SL valve murmur, this could represent stenosis of the valve because the valve is not opening when needed. Could also indicate mitral valve prolapse. A grading scale for the intensity of systolic murmurs is presented in Table 1–6.
  - Diastolic murmur: If auscultation reveals AV murmur, could represent stenosis, as the AV valve is not opening when needed. If auscultation reveals SL valve murmur, this could represent regurgitation, as the SL valve is not closing properly. Figure 1–16 illustrates the location for auscultating each heart valve.
  - Thrill: Palpable tremor due to movement of blood, and accompanies extra sound or murmur.

TABLE 1–6 Grading systolic murmurs.

Intensity	Description
Grade I/VI	Barely audible
Grade II/VI	Audible, but soft
Grade III/VI	Easily audible
Grade IV/VI	Easily audible and associated with a thrill
Grade V/VI	Easily audible, associated with a thrill, and still heard with the stethoscope only lightly on the chest
Grade VI/VI	Easily audible, associated with a thrill, and still heard with the stethoscope off of the chest

From Grading systolic murmurs. Learn the Heart. https://www.healio.com/cardiology/learn-the-heart/cardiology-review/topic-reviews/grading-systolic-murmurs. Used with permission from SLACK Incorporated.

Lung Sounds

- Normal lung sounds
  - Normal or vesicular: Soft, low-pitched, rustling, wispy sound. Can be heard in most lung fields, especially periphery during inspiration and first part of expiration.
  - Bronchovesicular: Combination of vesicular and bronchial sounds heard in the large central airways over the manubrium, main stem, and segmental bronchi.
  - Bronchial: Harsh, hollow, high-pitched sound. Can be heard during inspiration and expiration and is normally heard over the manubrium and trachea. Figure 1–17 shows the order of auscultating lung sounds.
- Abnormal breath sounds
  - Bronchial: Abnormal to hear over other lung fields and periphery except large central airways. Can indicate atelectasis, pneumonia, consolidation, or lobar collapse.
  - Absent or diminished sounds: Pleural effusion, hemothorax, pneumothorax, obesity.
- Added or adventitious breath sounds
  - **Crackles** (rales): High-pitched or medium- to low-pitched discontinuous sound. Can be indicative of atelectasis, pulmonary fibrosis, or secretions.
  - Wheezes (rhonchi): Mono or polyphonic low-, medium-, or high-pitched sound indicating bronchospasm, asthma, COPD, or secretions in the larger airways.
  - Vocal sounds: Normally sounds are not transmitted in the lungs, and sound is muffled and inaudible.
    - Bronchophony: Can audibly hear patient saying "99."
    - Egophony: The "A" sound is heard when the patient says "E."
    - Whispered pectoriloquy: When auscultating, can distinguish and audibly hear even when patient whispers.

PERIPHERAL CIRCULATION

SKILL KEEPER: PERIPHERAL CIRCULATION

A patient is being evaluated by a physical therapist and during the patient interview, the patient complains of bilateral leg cramping and pain when taking walks, especially when going up the slight hill to his home. What are some possible tests and measures that the therapist might consider using to further assess these symptoms?

- Assess all peripheral pulses of the arms and legs and include carotid artery. Note pulse rate, strength, and auscultate for abnormal sounds.
- Visual inspection for skin color changes (**cyanosis**, redness, pallor), trophic changes (skin is shiny, thin, pale, hairless), presence of skin lesions (ulcers, wounds), changes in the nail bed (bulbous thickening or clubbing at proximal nail bed).
- Doppler/ultrasound flowmetry: Ultrasound frequency can be used to listen to circulation where difficult to palpate or auscultate pulse.
- Edema: Can indicate heart or vascular disease.
  - Can be measured with tape measure or volumetric readings (measure displacement of water).
  - Scale for measuring severity of edema is seen in Table 1–7.

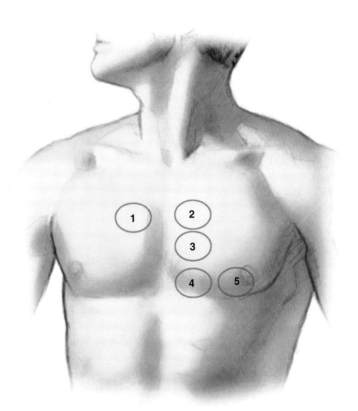

FIGURE 1–16 Areas of auscultation. The five classic areas of cardiac auscultation: (1) aortic (second intercostal space at the right parasternal line), (2) pulmonic (second intercostal space at the left parasternal line), (3) accessory aortic area (third intercostal space at the left parasternal line), (4) tricuspid (fifth intercostal space at the left parasternal), and (5) mitral (over the apical impulse). (From Fuster V, Harrington RA, Narula J, Eapen ZJ. *Hurst's The Heart,* 14e; 2017. Available at: https://accessmedicine.mhmedical.com/content.aspx?bookid=2046& sectionid=176574921 Accessed: September 26, 2018. Copyright © 2018 McGraw-Hill Education. All rights reserved.)

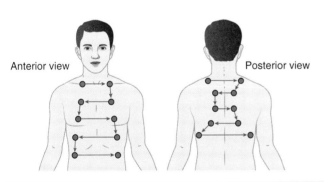

Respiratory patterns	
Normal (eupnea)	Regular and comfortable at 12–20 breaths/minute.
Tachypnea	20 breaths/minute.
Bradypnea	<12 breaths/minute.
Hyperventilation	Repid, deep respiration >20 breaths/minute.
Apneustic	Neurological – sustained inspiratory effort.
Cheyenne-Stokes	Neurological – alternating patterns of depth separated by brief periods of apnea.
Kussmaul's	Rapid, deep, and labored – common in DKA.
Air trapping	Difficulty during expiration – emphysema.

FIGURE 1–17 Order of auscultating lung sounds. (From https://i.pinimg.com/originals/65/99/d5/6599d546afb0b3bb68b10d1ab69bdcdd.jpg.)

Assessment of Peripheral Circulation

- Capillary refill: Pressure applied to distal finger or toe nails. Normally nail will blanch (whiten), then color returns within 3 seconds after release of pressure. Delay can indicate arterial insufficiency.
- Intermittent claudication: Patient may complain of pain in lower extremity (usually in the calf, but can be in the foot, thigh, or buttocks) during ambulation or going up incline or steps.
- Rubor of dependency: Patient is resting in supine position. Then upper extremity (UE) or lower extremity (LE) is elevated to 45 degrees. Changes in skin color are noted. Normally the color remains the same or may blanch slightly. If circulation

TABLE 1–7   Pitting edema scale indentation depth.

Scale	Edema	English Units	Metric Units	Time to Baseline
0	None	0	0	
1+	Trace	0–0.25 inch	<6.5 mm	Rapid
2+	Mild	0.25–0.5 inch	6.5–12.5 mm	6.5–12.5 mm
3+	Moderate	0.5–1 inch	12.5 mm–2.5 cm	1–2 min
4+	Severe	>1 inch	>2.5 cm	2–5 min

From https://clinicalgate.com/wp-content/uploads/2015/03/T000115tabt0020.png.

TABLE 1–8 **Interpretation of ankle brachial index (ABI).**

Generally normal	0.91–1.3	
Mild–moderate disease	0.41–0.90	Pain in the foot, leg, or buttock may occur during exercise due to some narrowing of the arteries
Severe disease	≤0.40	Symptoms may occur even while resting; danger of limb loss
Rigid arteries	>1.3	Calcified vessels: Need an ultrasound test to check for peripheral artery disease instead of an ABI test

Data from Grenon SM et al. *N Engl J Med.* 2009;361:e40 and http://www.educatehealth.ca/media/249760/5-light%20box-dm-investigation%20workup-ankle%20brachial%20index.png.

is compromised, the leg will become pale or grayish in color. Next, the extremity is placed in a dependent position. Normal response is return to normal color or pinkish coloration. If arterial disease is present, the extremity will become bright red (dependent rubor).

- Ankle-brachial index (ABI)
  - Posterior tibial, dorsalis pedis, and brachial artery pulses are palpated. Blood pressure cuff is placed proximally and inflated to occlude pulse.
  - The reading is taken when the pulse returns.
  - Doppler/ultrasound flowmeter can be used for pulses that are difficult to palpate or auscultate.
  - The ratio of LE to UE is calculated. The interpretation of an ABI and the severity of vascular compromise is listed in Table 1–8.

PERCUSSION

- Performed throughout the lungs to assess any possible abnormal findings. Therapist will percuss (tap) one finger over the other and assess the sound produced.
  - Well-ventilated lung tissue will produce a low-pitched resonant sound, like a muffled drum.
  - Dense tissue such as the liver, heart, and visceral organs will have a duller sound.
  - Hollower organs will produce a more resonant or tympanic sound.
  - Higher-pitched, dull "thud" sound could indicate increased density, such as in atelectasis, consolidation, or pleural effusion.
  - Hyper-resonant sound may indicate decreased density, such as a pneumothorax or hyperinflated lung.

RIB CAGE MOVEMENT AND EXCURSION

- Due to the shape of the rib cage, the upper ribs move in a pump handle-like motion, increasing the AP diameter of the chest.

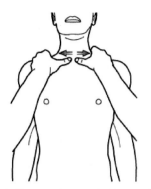

A. Testing of upper thorax

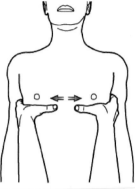

B. Testing of expansion of midthorax

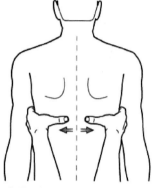

C. Testing of expansion of posterior thorax

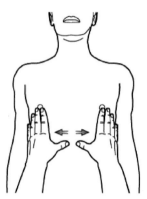

D. Testing movements of costal margins

FIGURE 1–18 Evaluation of chest wall excursion. (From http://accessmedicine.mhmedical.com/data/books/lebl9/lebl9_c008f011.gif.)

- The lower ribs (7th–10th) move in the bucket-handle movement. AP motion is more limited, resulting in ribs swinging out and up, increasing the transverse diameter of the rib.
- Rib cage expansion can be measured with a tape measure at the chest circumference. Patient exhales maximally and measurement is recorded, then patient inhales maximally and measurement is recorded. The difference between the two measurements indicates total chest expansion. Measurements can be taken at the level of the xiphoid process and at the axillary line.
- Upper, middle, and lower lobes are assessed. Movement should be equal, and examiner's thumbs should move apart. Figure 1–18 shows hand positioning to evaluate chest wall excursion.

EXERCISE TESTING

Exercise testing of the cardiopulmonary system can serve several purposes:

- As a diagnostic tool
- To determine severity or involvement of a disease or prognosis
- As objective assessment of disability and to measure progress
- As a part of a treatment or training program

TABLE 1–9 Indications for terminating exercise testing.

Absolute Indications

- Moderate to severe angina
- Increasing nervous system symptoms (eg, ataxia, dizziness, or near syncope)
- Signs of poor perfusion (cyanosis or pallor)
- Technical difficulties in monitoring ECG or systolic blood pressure
- Subject's desire to stop
- Sustained ventricular tachycardia
- ST-segment evaluation (≥1.0 mm) in leads without diagnostic Q waves (other than V or aVR)

Relative Indications

- Drop in systolic blood pressure ≥10 mmHg from baseline blood pressure despite an increase in workload in the absence of other evidence of ischemia
- ST or QRS changes such as excessive ST-segment depression (>2 mm of horizontal or down-sloping ST-segment depression) or marked axis shift
- Arrhythmias other than sustained ventricular tachycardia, including multifocal PVCs, triplets of PVCs, supraventricular tachycardia, heart block, or bradyarrhythmias
- Fatigue, shortness of breath, wheezing, leg cramps, or claudication
- Development of bundle branch block or intraventricular conduction delay that cannot be distinguished from ventricular tachycardia
- Increasing chest pain
- Hypertensive response*

PVC, premature ventricular contraction.

*In the absence of definitive evidence, the committee suggests systolic blood pressure of >250 mmHg and/or a diastolic blood pressure of >115 mmHg.

From https://www.ahcmedia.com/ext/resources/images/ahc/ahcimg_23/emr09012008_table2.gif.

- To improve fitness in healthy individuals as well as those diagnosed with a pathology or disease. With any exercise testing, there are indications for terminating exercise as listed in Table 1–9.

Walking Tests

The 6-minute walk test is one of the standardized walking exercise tests. The patient walks for 6 minutes and the total distance is measured, and symptoms the patient experiences are recorded.

Another test is the 10-meter shuttle walk test, in which the pace is incrementally increased. The patient walks between two cones placed 10 meters apart. The number of shuttles between cones is recorded and an audio tape "beeps" to indicate the time/cadence for the patient to start and stop. At each level, the cadence is increased and the number of completed shuttles increases to progress patient pace.

Step Test

The 3-minute step test involves the patient stepping up and down on a step at a set pace designated by a metronome.

Treadmill Testing

The Bruce protocol is a popular treadmill test used with 12-lead ECG monitoring, though the test can also be adapted to a cycle or step test. The test is progressively more difficult and takes place in 3-minute increments as follows:

- Stage 1 1.7 mph at 10% incline
- Stage 2 2.5 mph at 12% incline
- Stage 3 3.4 mph at 14% incline
- Stage 4 4.2 mph at 16% incline

Other modifications and testing protocols include the modified Bruce, Sheffield, modified Sheffield, Cornell, Northwick Park, and Balke.

Bicycle Ergometry

Bicycle testing has the advantage of making it easier to measure blood pressure, manage ECG leads and lines, and the bicycle takes less space than a treadmill. The disadvantage is that the bicycle relies more heavily on quadriceps muscle action and can limit patient activity if there is fatigue of this muscle group with the test before patient reaches maximum exertion.

ELECTROCARDIOGRAM

SKILL KEEPER: ECG/EKG READINGS

When analyzing an ECG/EKG strip, the physical therapist notes that there is depression of the ST segment. What are possible causes for this? What are other possible changes to the ST segment? What possible changes on an ECG/EKG reading might one expect to see for a patient who is taking calcium channel blockers?

An electrocardiogram (ECG, also called EKG) is a medical device that records the electrical activity of the heart. Physical therapists need to be aware of various heart rhythm disorders for which a patient may have symptoms, and they must also have knowledge of reading ECG strips (Figure 1–19). It is important to follow a systematic approach in order to avoid misreading or missing important key signs of various heart conditions. Various approaches can be utilized. The following is an example of one technique:[4]

- Use the appropriate method to calculate the heart rate.
- What is the rhythm of the pattern? Classification of patterns can include regularly regular, regularly irregular, and irregularly irregular. Observation of the space between R waves indicates regularity of patterns.
- Is there a P wave before each QRS complex? Is there a QRS complex after every P wave? These are indicators of atrial and ventricular activity.
- What is the duration of the PR interval? Increased length of the PR interval may indicate blocks in conduction through the nodal system.

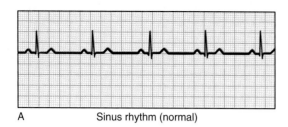

A   Sinus rhythm (normal)

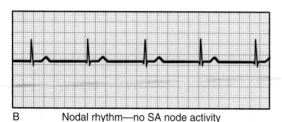

B   Nodal rhythm—no SA node activity

FIGURE 1–19 ECGs: normal and abnormal. (From http://slideplayer.com/slide/7561462/24/images/32/ ECGs:+Normal+and+Abnormal.jpg.)

- What is the size, shape, and duration of the QRS complex?
- Assess the ST segment shape and duration. Is it elevated or depressed? What is the duration?

Determining Heart Rate

Various methods can be used to measure heart rate based on ECG/EKG strip readings.

- **Method 1:** Using the quick-count method, find an R wave that falls on the dark heavy line. Each heavy line after that can be marked and counted down with the following numbers: 300, 150, 100, 75, 60, 50, 43, and 37. The next R wave would be estimated on where it falls either on or between the heavy lines marked. For example, if the next wave fell directly on the fourth heavy line, the heart rate would be estimated at 75 bpm. However, if the next R wave fell directly between the second

and third heavy line, the heart rate would be between 100 and 150 bpm and would be estimated at 125 bpm.[4]
- **Method 2:** Count the number of small boxes between two consecutive R waves. Each small box represents 0.04 seconds. There are 60 seconds in 1 minute. Sixty seconds divided by 0.04 equals 1500. Therefore, divide 1500 by the number of small boxes counted to determine heart rate. For example, if there are 22 small boxes between R waves, 1500/22 = 68 bpm.[4]
- **Method 3:** Some ECG/EKG strips may have a rate-ruler specific to the strip and machine calibration. Instructions on the rate ruler will help determine heart rate.[4]
- **Method 4:** If the EKG has markings that indicate it is a 6-second strip and the rhythm is normal, count the number of RR intervals, then multiply by 10. For example, if there are 7 RR intervals in the 6-second range, the heart rate wold be 70 bpm.[4]

Determining Pattern

Various patterns can be identified in EKG readings (Figure 1–20). They can be categorized based on location, block, or foci that causes the dysrhythmic pattern. A description of the categories and types of patterns follows as well as common EKG readings of the various patterns (Figure 1–21).

- Supraventricular dysrhythmias arise from above the level of the ventricles, and these are further categorized as sinus, atrial, or junctional rhythm.
  - Sinus rhythm
  - Sinus bradycardia
  - Sinus tachycardia
  - Atrial fibrillation
  - Atrial flutter
- Ventricular dysrhythmias arise due to an ectopic pacemaker occurring below the atria.
  - Premature ventricular complex (PVC)
  - Ventricular bigeminy, trigemini, or quadrigeminy (PVC occurs every second, third, or fourth beat)
  - Multifocal PVCs

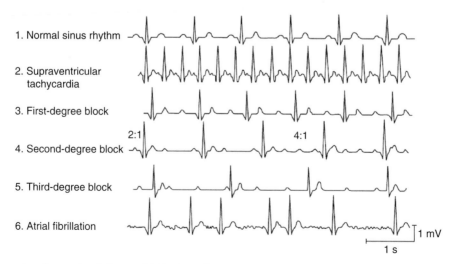

1. Normal sinus rhythm

2. Supraventricular tachycardia

3. First-degree block

4. Second-degree block   2:1   4:1

5. Third-degree block

6. Atrial fibrillation   1 mV   1 s

FIGURE 1–20 Examples of normal and abnormal EKGs. (From http://accessbiomedicalscience.mhmedical.com/data/books/mohr8/ mohr8_c005f001.png.)

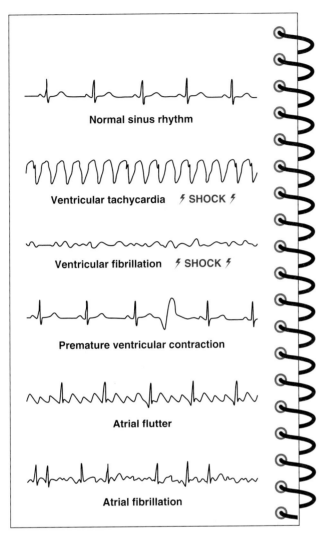

FIGURE 1–21 Common ECG rhythms. (From https://i.pinimg.com/originals/5d/6b/a7/5d6ba7e3fe3afb2d9a8c3ebccf0519fe.jpg.)

- Ventricular tachycardia
- Ventricular fibrillation
- Asystole
- Conduction blocks
  - First-degree AV block: Impairment SA to AV node (delayed conduction)
  - Second-degree AV block: Partial block
    - Type 1 (Mobitz I or Wenckebach): Block high in AV junction
    - Type 2 (Mobitz II): Lower block below bundle of His
  - Third-degree (complete) AV block
- Myocardial ischemia or infarction
  - ST segment elevation. Examples are illustrated in Figure 1–22 (I & J).
  - ST segment depression. Figure 1–22 illustrates depression in examples B & C.

HOLTER MONITORING

Holter monitoring allows for 24-hour noninvasive heart monitoring (Figure 1–23). Patients can also keep a log and match symptoms with daily activities.

PULMONARY FUNCTION TEST

There are various pulmonary function tests (PFTs) that measure inspiration and expiration. Tests can be used to assess lung volumes and capacities, breathing, ventilation and pulmonary mechanics, and diffusion rates. PFTs are used for:

- Diagnosing lung and pulmonary pathologies
- Screening for development of disease processes
- Prognosis for patients diagnosed with lung pathologies
- Measurement of progress before and after treatment intervention

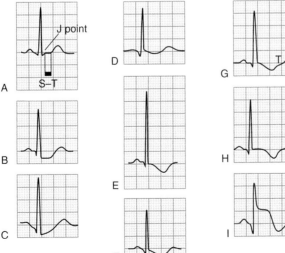
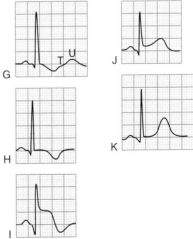

FIGURE 1–22 Normal and abnormal *ST* segments and *T* waves. (From https://image.slidesharecdn.com/ecglecture-110118083934-phpapp01/95/ecg-lecture-34-728.jpg?cb=1295340075.)

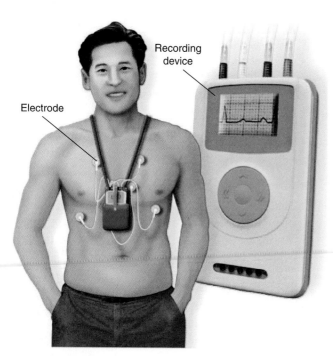

FIGURE 1-23 Holter monitor. (Used with permission of Mayo Foundation for Medical Education and Research. All rights reserved.)

Spirometry

Spirometry measures the amount of air flow and some lung volumes, and in general can indicate obstructive lung pathologies. A patient performs maximal inhalation and exhalation as quickly as possible into a spirometer. This measures the vital capacity (VC). The forced exhalation after maximal inspiration is called the forced vital capacity (FVC), and the amount of expelled air (forced expiratory volume [FEV]) in 1 second is called the FEV_1. A ratio derived from the FEV_1/FVC is also calculated. Together the FVC, FEV_1, and the FEV_1/FVC are the three important measures of spirometry. Spirometry results can be plotted on a graph linearly or in a flow-volume loop. Figure 1–24 demonstrates a spirometric flow diagram showing the flow of air during inhalation and exhalation.

Graphs also demonstrate the peak expiratory flow rate. The steepest slope represents the maximum amount of air expelled. In the presence of disease processes, changes to the peak expiratory flow, lung volumes, and the characteristic flow-volume loop can differentiate obstructive and restrictive lung pathologies. A spirogram for normal lungs, restrictive lung disease, and obstructive lung disease is presented in Figure 1–25. Figure 1–26 shows the flow volume loop and the changes that occur with lung pathologies.

Lung Volume Tests

Lung volume tests measure various lung volumes and capacities, and can effectively indicate restrictive lung diseases. Spirometry testing can measure most lung volumes and capacities; however, residual volume (RV) cannot be captured with these tests, as this is the amount of air that remains in lungs after maximal exhalation.

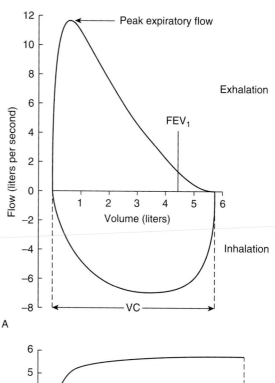

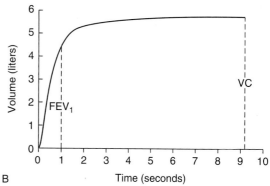

FIGURE 1-24 Spirometric flow diagram. (Used with permission from Crapo RO. Pulmonary-function testing. N Engl J Med 1994; 331:28, Figure 1.)

Therefore, RV is measured using other forms of testing such as gas dilution techniques, body plethosmography, and calculations and extrapolation of RV from chest x-rays or CT scans. RV can then be used to calculate total lung capacity (TLC) and provide a complete picture of the patient's lung volumes and capacities.

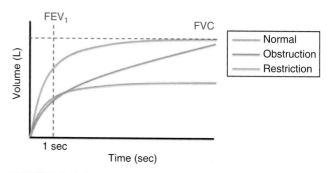

FIGURE 1-25 Comparison of spirograms for normal lungs, restrictive lung disease, and obstructive lung disease. (From http://www.nataliescasebook.com/img/Spirometry/Volume_time.png.)

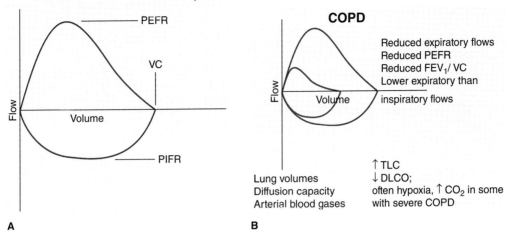

Normal Flow Volume Loop

PEFR

VC

Flow

Volume

PIFR

A

COPD

Flow

Volume

Reduced expiratory flows
Reduced PEFR
Reduced FEV_1/ VC
Lower expiratory than
inspiratory flows

Lung volumes
Diffusion capacity
Arterial blood gases

↑ TLC
↓ DLCO;
often hypoxia, ↑ CO_2 in some
with severe COPD

B

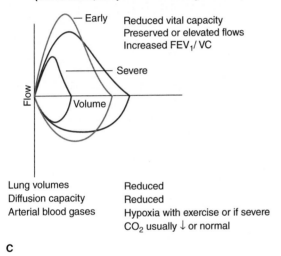

Interstitial Lung Disease
(Sarcoidosis, Idiopathic Pulmonary Fibrosis)

Early

Reduced vital capacity
Preserved or elevated flows
Increased FEV_1/ VC

Severe

Flow

Volume

Lung volumes
Diffusion capacity
Arterial blood gases

Reduced
Reduced
Hypoxia with exercise or if severe
CO_2 usually ↓ or normal

C

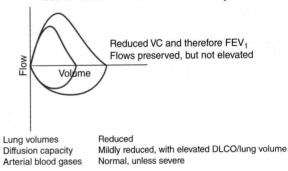

Restrictive Lung Disease
Due to Pleural or Chest Wall Abnormality

Flow

Volume

Reduced VC and therefore FEV_1
Flows preserved, but not elevated

Lung volumes
Diffusion capacity
Arterial blood gases

Reduced
Mildly reduced, with elevated DLCO/lung volume
Normal, unless severe

D

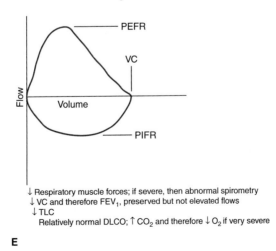

Ventilatory Muscle Weakness

PEFR

VC

Flow

Volume

PIFR

↓ Respiratory muscle forces; if severe, then abnormal spirometry
↓ VC and therefore FEV_1, preserved but not elevated flows
↓ TLC
Relatively normal DLCO; ↑ CO_2 and therefore ↓ O_2 if very severe

E

FIGURE 1–26 Flow-volume loop examples. (**A**) Normal flow-volume loop. (**B**) COPD flow-volume loop. (**C**) Interstitial lung disease flow-volume loop. (**D**) Restrictive lung disease flow-volume loop. (**E**) Ventilatory muscle weakness flow-volume loop. (Used with permission from DeTurk WE, Cahalin LP. *Cardiovascular and Pulmonary Physical Therapy: An Evidence–Based Approach*, 3e; 2017. Available at: https://access physiotherapy.mhmedical.com/content.aspx?bookid=2270&sectionid=176350331. Accessed: September 26, 2018. Copyright © 2018 McGraw-Hill Education. All rights reserved.)

OUTCOME MEASURES, SURVEYS, AND HEALTH QUESTIONNAIRES

Various outcome measures can measure health and fitness, quality of life, overall general health and well-being, and can be specific to respiratory or cardiac disease processes. Some of these outcome measures are listed here.[5]

- Modified AHA/ACSM Health/Fitness Facility Pre-Participation Screening Questionnaire
- Physical Activity Readiness Questionnaire (PAR-Q)
- Short Form 36 (SF-36)
- Sickness Impact Profile (SIP)
- Quality of Well-Being (QWB)
- Duke Health Profile (DUKE)
- Chronic Respiratory Disease Questionnaire (CRQ)
- St. George's Respiratory Questionnaire (SGRQ)
- Seattle Obstructive Lung Disease Questionnaire (SOLDQ)
- Minnesota Living with Heart Failure Questionnaire (LHFQ)
- Chronic Heart Failure Questionnaire (CHQ)
- Kansas City Cardiomyopathy Questionnaire (KCCQ)
- Quality of Life after Myocardial Infarction Questionnaire (QLMI)
- Seattle Angina Questionnaire (SAQ)

■ FOUNDATIONS FOR EVALUATION, DIFFERENTIAL DIAGNOSIS, AND PROGNOSIS

PATHOLOGIES/CONDITIONS OF THE CARDIOVASCULAR SYSTEM

Pathologies and conditions are described here in major categories including (A) ischemic conditions, (B) congestive heart failure, (C) cardiomyopathies, (D) arrhythmic conditions, and (E) heart valve disorders.

A. Ischemic Conditions of the Heart

> **SKILL KEEPER: CORONARY ARTERY DISEASE (CAD)**
>
> *What factors cannot be controlled that contribute to the risk of developing CAD? What factors can be modified for which a physical therapist can make recommendations to reduce the risk of developing CAD? What other members of the healthcare team can contribute to making proper modifications in lifestyle for a patient?*

Coronary artery disease—Coronary artery disease (CAD) results in obstructed blood flow to the heart. CAD is the single greatest cause of death in men and women in the United States, with more than 565,000 new cases of MI each year.[6]

Atherosclerosis—Atherosclerosis is triggered by damage to the innermost layer of the artery. Figure 1–27 shows the various layers of the artery. The risk factors for this include cigarette smoking, high blood pressure, high cholesterol, and sedentary lifestyle. All are modifiable factors that can reduce the risk of atherosclerosis. Non-modifiable contributors to CAD are age, gender, race, and family history.

Atherosclerosis begins with the development of fatty streak deposits because of damage to the inner layer of the artery. Continued fatty or lipid deposits cause a buildup, and atheromas develop. Calcification of the lesion leads to fibrous plaques, and continues to impede blood flow to a point of occlusion. A diagrammatic look at the inside of an atherosclerotic artery is presented in Figure 1–28.

Angina pectoris—Angina pectoris is defined as chest pain related to ischemic conditions of the myocardium due to compromised coronary blood flow to the heart. Angina results when there is greater cardiac demand than available O_2 to the heart or there is insufficient O_2 available to the heart. Pain can be described as substernal pressure, squeezing, tightness, or heaviness. Angina can also present with referred pain patterns, with symptoms appearing at the left shoulder or arm, neck, jaw, and between the shoulder blades. Any pain above the umbilicus should be further examined for possible underlying heart conditions. The four major triggers that can lead to angina are exertion, emotional stress, extreme temperature changes (especially cold), and eating of a large meal. Angina can be classified as stable, unstable, or variant (Prinzmetal angina).

Stable angina—Stable angina, also referred to as chronic angina, can be triggered by increased physical activity or stress. Symptoms may last between 5 and 15 minutes; pain is felt at the substernum and usually does not radiate. The patient's angina does not persist, and cessation from the physical activity or administration of sublingual nitrates alleviates the symptoms.

Variant (Prinzmetal) angina—Variant or Prinzmetal angina is also called atypical angina. Unlike stable angina, it occurs at night or at rest. The affected coronary artery goes into vasospasm, and a high-intensity episode may lead to MI. Compared to unstable angina, variant angina may be less severe, and with low level activity; the symptoms can be relieved (physiological response of vasodilation by coronary artery in response to physical activity). Heart arrhythmias usually accompany this condition.

Unstable angina—Similar to stable angina, unstable angina can be triggered by physical activity, stress, or at rest. However, symptoms are more severe, frequent, and last longer (>15 min). Cessation of activity or administration of sublingual nitrates may not alleviate symptoms. Unstable angina can represent the progression of CHD, and persons are more at risk for MI. Patients may also exhibit changes in cardiac function such as changes in BP or a decline in ability to perform previous levels of activity.

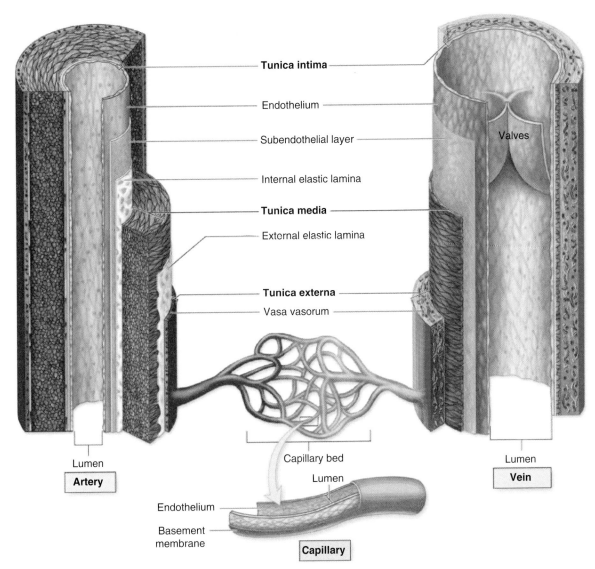

FIGURE 1–27 Layers of the arterial and venous vasculature. (From http://accessmedicinemhmedical.com/data/books/jans1/jans1_c016f004.png.)

Myocardial infarction—MI occurs when there is loss of blood flow to the myocardium for more than 20 minutes, resulting in necrosis of the supplied tissue. The anatomy of the coronary circulation is shown in Figure 1–29. The MI is described and prognosis is determined by the size and extent of the involvement. Transmural (full-wall) involves the endocardium to the epicardium. With nontransmural or intramural infarctions, some involvement may occur at the subendocardial or subepicardial level.

Complications from MI include arrhythmias, cardiogenic shock, pericarditis, congestive heart failure, impaired heart function (decreased SV, contractility, output, and ejection fraction), and sudden death. Clinical manifestations include:

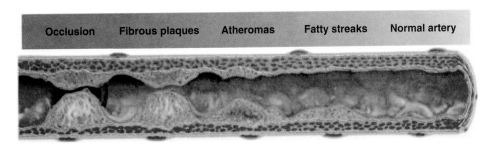

FIGURE 1–28 Pathogenesis of atherosclerosis.

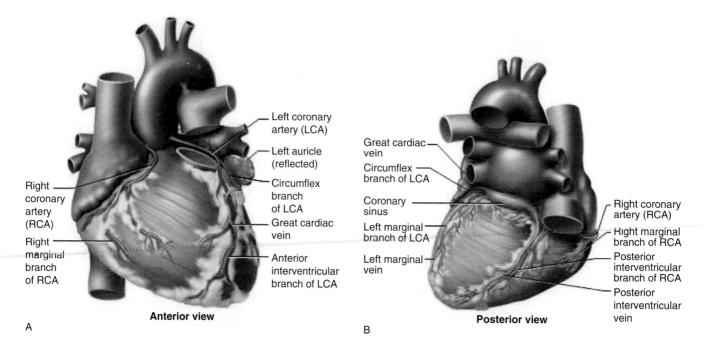

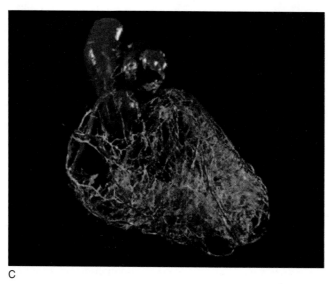

FIGURE 1–29 Anatomy of the coronary circulation. **A.** Anterior view; **B.** Posterior view; **C.** Enhanced 3-D imaging of coronary circulation. (From http://images.slideplayer.com/24/6943673/slides/slide_10.jpg.)

- Severe chest pain, radiating or nonradiating
- Diaphoresis
- Dyspnea
- Nausea and vomiting
- Lightheadedness, dizziness, syncope
- Weakness
- ECG changes such as ST elevation or depression
- Elevation of enzyme levels: troponin, creatine kinase, and phosphokinase

B. Congestive Heart Failure

CHF is a group of clinical manifestations that result in pulmonary congestion from blood that is backed up due to decreased output of the ventricle. The heart is unable to provide adequate cardiac output to meet O_2 demands. CHF can also be described by the side of the heart that is affected. Therefore, because of decreased output, blood is backed up behind the affected side. Ischemia or MI are main causes of CHF.

Adequate cardiac output is a product of SV and heart rate, and is essential in cardiovascular function. Stroke volume can be affected by three factors: the amount of blood in the ventricle after diastole (preload), the amount of pressure the ventricle must overcome to move blood into the systemic circulation (afterload), and the contractile strength of the ventricle. Any effects of these three factors may have a negative impact on SV and also adversely decrease cardiac output.

Right ventricular failure—Right ventricular failure is usually caused by pulmonary hypertension. It can also be caused by mitral valve disease or acute and chronic lung disease such as **cor pulmonale**. When there is decreased action of the right ventricle, blood is backed up to the venous system, causing edema in the extremities. Other clinical manifestations include:

- Dependent edema
- Jugular venous distension
- Weight gain
- Ascites
- Cyanosis
- Hepatomegaly
- Anxiety

Left ventricular failure—Left ventricular failure can be caused by atherosclerotic heart disease, cardiomyopathy, hypertension, valvular disease, arrhythmias, alcohol, and drug toxicity. Because of decreased contractility of the left ventricle, blood is backed up into the pulmonary vasculature of the lungs and causes pulmonary edema. Clinical manifestations include:

- Dyspnea
- Orthopnea
- Dry cough or spasmodic productive cough
- Pulmonary edema
- Pulmonary rales, wheezing ("cardiac asthma")
- Increased respiration

C. Cardiomyopathies

> **SKILL KEEPER: CARDIOMYOPATHIES**
>
> *Compare the various types of cardiomyopathies. What are the effects on ventricular filling, preload, SV, afterload, and cardiac output?*

Cardiomyopathies can be classified based on a functional view and are categorized as dilated, hypertrophic, and restrictive (Figure 1–30).

Dilated cardiomyopathy—Dilated cardiomyopathy (DCM) results in dilation of the ventricle and impaired ventricular muscle function. There is little change in wall thickness; however, ventricular muscle mass does increase. Increase in the ventricular chamber also causes an increased EDV and a decreased SV. The heart is unable to maintain sufficient cardiac output with exercise or increased activity, eventually leading to ventricular failure. Clinical manifestations of DCM include:

- Dyspnea during exertion progressing to dyspnea at rest
- Nocturnal dry cough
- Chest pain during exertion
- S3 to S4 gallop
- Resting tachycardia

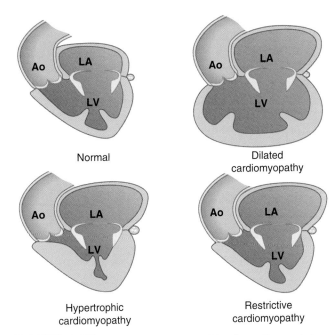

FIGURE 1–30 Types of cardiomyopathies. (From Kumar et al. *Robbins Basic Pathology.* 8e.© Elsevier. www.studentconsult.com.)

- Cardiomegaly
- Systolic murmur from regurgitation of bicuspid or tricuspid valve

Hypertrophic cardiomyopathy—Hypertrophic cardiomyopathy (HCM) results in increased ventricular muscle mass and no dilation of the ventricular chamber. There is decreased ventricular filling (diastolic dysfunction) and decreased compliance impairing ventricular filling. As a result, the ventricle may contract before the chamber is filled, which decreases SV. Clinical manifestations for HCM include:

- Dyspnea
- Angina pectoris
- Fatigue
- Syncope
- Palpitations
- Loud S4 heart sounds

Restrictive cardiomyopathy—Restrictive cardiomyopathy (RCM) is caused by endomyocardial or myocardial disease causing diastolic dysfunction, stiffening of the heart walls, and decreased compliance. Rigidity of the heart walls causes decreased ventricular filling and affects cardiac output. Bicuspid or tricuspid regurgitation as well as pulmonary hypertension accompany RCM. Other clinical manifestations include:

- Exercise intolerance
- Weakness
- Dyspnea
- Edema
- Enlarged liver
- Symptoms of CHF
- Cardiac arrhythmias

D. Arrhythmic Conditions

Cardiac arrhythmic conditions affect heart rate, rhythm, or impulse condition. Classification of cardiac arrhythmias can be based on (a) origin (atria, also called supraventricular or ventricles), (b) type of pattern or rhythm (fibrillation or flutter), and (c) effect on rate or speed (tachycardia or bradycardia). Cardiac arrhythmias can vary in severity from asymptomatic and mild, requiring no intervention, to severe and life-threatening, requiring resuscitation or immediate medical intervention.

Type of pattern or rhythm—Atrial fibrillation is the most common type of supraventricular tachycardia (SVT). The muscles of the atria quiver or flutter instead of producing one coordinated contraction, causing pooling of blood in the atria chamber and decreased filling of the ventricle. This results in decreased O_2 levels and can cause shortness of breath, fatigue, palpitations, and in some instances syncope. Since blood remains in the atria, there is increased risk for thrombus formation and emboli leading to stroke.

Ventricular fibrillation (VF) is caused by electrical disturbances, and there is flutter of the ventricular muscles of the heart causing cessation of cardiac output. VF often leads to cardiac arrest, and immediate medical attention is needed with defibrillation of the heart to end the erratic heart activity and allow for normal electrical conduction to resume.

Heart block is caused by an interruption to the normal conduction pathway in the heart. There are three types of heart block: first-degree, second-degree, and third-degree (complete). Heart block can be caused by CAD, HTN, myocarditis, or overdose of heart medications such as digitalis or beta blockers. Patients may present with dizziness, syncope, lightheadedness, and fatigue. Medication management or placement of a pacemaker are often used to manage these conditions.

Effect on rate or speed—Normal heart rate averages 60 to 100 bpm. The two rate arrhythmias are tachycardia (greater than 100 bpm) and bradycardia (less than 60 bpm). Increased sympathetic stimulation results in tachycardia and can be caused by multiple factors including pain, fear, emotions, exercise, or artificial stimulants (such as caffeine, nicotine, amphetamines). Abnormal conditions may include MI, fever, CHF, infection, and anemia. Bradycardia is normal in well-trained athletes. Patients taking beta blockers also have decreased heart rates.

Signs and symptoms can range from asymptomatic to severe, and may also include:

- No symptoms
- Palpitations or flutter
- Lightheadedness or dizziness
- Syncope
- Chest discomfort
- Weakness or fatigue
- Dyspnea
- Anxiety
- Irregular or weak pulse

E. Heart Valve Disorders

Heart valve disorders are classified as either acquired or congenital. These disorders may lead to cardiac muscle dysfunction due to compensatory mechanisms to increase cardiac output, including ventricular hypertrophy and chamber dilation. They are defined by the following characteristics or causes:

- Atresia: Congenital absence or closure
- Prolapse: Cusp of the heart valve (usually bicuspid/mitral valve) falls back into the atrial chamber
- Regurgitation: Backflow of blood due to incomplete valve closure
- Stenosis: Fibrotic changes and stiffening of the heart valve causing decreased blood flow between chambers

PATHOLOGIES/CONDITIONS OF THE PULMONARY SYSTEM

Injury to the lungs can occur via several means: (a) exposure to toxin or irritants, (b) pathogens, or (c) autoimmune disorders. In response, the lungs initiate acute inflammatory responses with cytokines and inflammatory mediators. The results will either be resolution of the injury, tissue breakdown, tissue destruction, or scarring (fibrosis).

Diseases of the pulmonary system can be classified as (a) acute or chronic, (b) obstructive or restrictive, or (c) infectious or noninfectious. Common conditions of any pulmonary disease include cough or **dyspnea**. Other conditions or symptoms may include chest pain, production of sputum, **cyanosis**, **hemoptysis**, changes in breathing patterns, abnormal lung sounds, respiratory gas changes, and clubbing of the fingers.

Acute Diseases

Pneumonia

- Pneumonia is a state of inflammation of the lung parenchyma
- Viral, bacterial, fungal
  - Viral pneumonia: Influenza virus, adenovirus, measles, herpes, and cytomegalovirus
  - Bacterial pneumonia: Gram-positive pneumococcal pneumonia (streptococcal) is the most common agent; gram-negative organisms such as *Klebsiella*, *Pseudomonas aeruginosa*, and *Haemophilus influenza* are found in compromised individuals such as those with severe illness or those receiving antibiotic therapy
- Inhalation of allergens such as smoke, dust, irritants, and gas
- Aspiration of food, fluids, or vomitus
  - Aspiration pneumonia is present for persons with swallowing disorders caused by neurological or muscular disease, or altered consciousness
  - Pneumonia symptoms are mild and resolve in 1 to 2 weeks
  - Manifestations may include:
    - Productive or nonproductive cough
    - Pleural chest pain
    - Rust- or green-colored sputum
    - Dyspnea and tachypnea
    - Headache, fevers, chills, and generalized aches and fatigue

Pneumocystis carinii Pneumonia (PCP)

- Unknown origin but possibly linked environmentally with transmission by other humans, animals, or other infected host.
- Common in immune-compromised individuals: Immune-suppressing drugs after transplant surgery or post-chemotherapy. Prior increased prevalence for individuals with AIDS. Recent drug advances have limited these incidences.
- Symptoms of PCP may include:
  - Fever
  - Progressive dyspnea
  - Nonproductive cough
  - Fatigue
  - Tachypnea
  - Weight loss

Tuberculosis

- Primary tuberculosis (TB): Exposure to *Mycobacterium tuberculosis*; lasts 10 to 14 days.
- Secondary TB: Occurs at any time after reactivation of the dormant bacteria encapsulated in the lungs. Symptoms do not usually occur during early exposure. Later-onset symptoms (as late as a year post-exposure) may include:
  - Productive cough and hemoptysis
  - Accompanying night sweats
  - Weight loss
  - Fatigue
  - Abnormal lung sounds such as **crackles**/rales and bronchial breath sounds

TB exposure results in positive skin test at initial exposure. Late TB is confirmed by chest x-ray and would show upper lobe involvement with air spaces and segmental lobe consolidation.

Chronic Obstructive Diseases

Chronic Obstructive Pulmonary Disease

Chronic obstructive pulmonary disease (COPD) is characterized by chronic limitations to airflow.
Can be caused by:

- Accumulation of mucus or secretions
- Bronchospasm
- Inflammation of the bronchioles
- Fibrosis of bronchioles

Over time, there is increased compliance of the lungs resulting in air trapping and overstretched alveoli, floppy bronchiole airways, and hyperinflation of the lungs. This causes abnormal pulmonary function tests. Patients may exhibit multiple symptoms or be diagnosed with several of the obstructive lung disease processes. In these instances the general term of COPD is often used.

Asthma

- Reversible obstructive lung disease described by obstruction of the airway from inflammation and increased smooth muscle activity causing bronchospasm

- There are two types of exacerbations or reactions:
  - Extrinsic (allergic)
  - Intrinsic (non-allergic).

Physical findings with asthma may include:

- Inspiratory and expiratory wheezing
- Chest tightness
- Dyspnea
- Anxiety
- Tachycardia
- Tachypnea
- Restlessness
- Increased accessory muscle use
- Nonproductive cough progressing to a productive cough with sputum

Bronchiectasis

- Congenital or acquired disease resulting in abnormal dilation of the bronchi
- Usually caused from bacterial infections
- Loss of elastic and muscle tissues of the bronchi and bronchioles
- Increased sputum production; accumulation of wet secretions and mucus causes bronchospasm, which exacerbates airway obstruction
- Common symptoms may include:
  - Productive cough with purulent sputum
  - Hemoptysis
  - Crackles and wheezing
  - Clubbing of digits
  - Dyspnea
  - Hypoxemia and hypercapnia

Chronic Bronchitis

- Irritation of the airways from smoking, air pollutants, occupational exposure, or infection
- Chronic cough and excessive production of mucus
- Diagnosis: Must have symptoms on most days for at least a 3-month period and for two or more consecutive years
- Term "blue bloaters" is often used to describe patient symptoms
- Other clinical manifestations may include:
  - Smoker's cough progressing to productive cough
  - Dyspnea on exertion
  - Respiratory sensitivity to irritants and cold or damp weather
  - Crackles and wheezing
  - Prolonged expiration

Cystic Fibrosis (CF)

- Genetic disorder with overproduction of mucus from the exocrine glands
- Causes presence of thick mucus, decreased ciliary transport, and poor cough clearance, causing chronic lung infections and tissue damage

Emphysema

- Pathological destruction of the elastic fibers of the lung tissues
- Results in accumulation of air due to destruction of the air spaces distal to the terminal bronchioles
- History of long-term smoking
- Non-smoking cases of alpha antitrypsin deficiency emphysema caused by lack of an enzyme that prevents trypsin, which causes alveolar damage
- Term "pink puffers" is often used to describe patient symptoms
- Other common characteristics include:
  - Barrel chest
  - Marked exertional dyspnea progressing to dyspnea at rest
  - Significant work of breathing
  - Posturing to fix upper extremities to use accessory muscles to aid in breathing
  - Prolonged expiration
  - Wheezing
  - Clubbing
  - Anxiety and distress

Chronic Restrictive Diseases

Encompasses a range of diagnoses in which there is a decreased lung volume or decreased compliance (causing stiffness in lungs). General categories or major classifications include:

- Connective tissue (rheumatoid arthritis, lupus, scleroderma, polymyositis)
- Pulmonary (asbestosis, pneumonia, acute respiratory distress syndrome, pleural effusion)
- Cardiovascular (pulmonary emboli, pulmonary edema)
- Neuromuscular (spinal cord injury, head injury, amyotrophic lateral sclerosis, Guillain–Barre syndrome, muscular dystrophy, polio)
- Musculoskeletal disorders (ankylosing spondylitis, scoliosis, chest injuries, trauma, pectus carinatum/excavatum, chest or abdominal surgery, obesity)

Generalized physical findings for the range of restrictive lung disease may include:

- Dyspnea on exertion
- Decreased exercise tolerance
- Usually nonproductive and dry cough
- Tachypnea
- Decrease in most lung capacity measures
- Weight loss

Specific restrictive lung diseases are described below.

Atelectasis

- Alveolar collapse from pathological or mechanical blockages of the bronchial airway
  - Mucus or tumor
  - Compression from fluid or pneumothorax
  - Lack of surfactant
  - postoperation of the abdomen or thorax

- Neuromuscular diseases causing weakness of the respiratory muscles
- Physical findings more pronounced if large area affected including:
  - Profound dyspnea
  - Hypoxia
  - Tracheal or mediastinal shift toward the affected side
  - Crackles or wheezes

Chest Trauma

- Rib fractures, flail chest, lung contusion.
- Penetration wounds can cause pneumothorax, hemothorax, or pulmonary laceration.
- Flail chest occurs when there are multiple fractures of two or more ribs. Paradoxical movement, or opposite from normal movement, of breathing at the fracture site (inward movement of the flail segment with inspiration and outward movement with expiration) is seen. This can cause significant pain, further compromising breathing.
- Other symptoms include:
  - Chest pain, especially with inspiration
  - Tachypnea
  - Hypoxia and hypercapnia
  - Weak cough
  - Tachycardia

Pneumothorax

- Air or gas in the pleural space that causes collapse of the lung tissue beneath the affected area
- Hemothorax: Entire collapse of the right or left lung
  - Causes increase in thoracic pressure
  - Mediastinal and tracheal shift away from the collapsed area
- Symptoms and findings may also include:
  - Unilateral chest pain
  - Dyspnea
  - Tachycardia
  - Chest x-ray shows dense-appearing lung tissue, absence of lung tissue in the area of the pneumothorax, possible expansion of the rib cage due to lack of negative pleural pressure, flattening of the diaphragm on the side of the affected lung

Pulmonary Effusion

- Excess fluid in the pleural space
- Transudate: Fluid from increased pressure in the lung from CHF, renal disease, or pulmonary embolus
- Exudate: Fluid from infection, malignancy, infarct, toxic drugs, or rheumatoid arthritis
- Physical findings may include:
  - Dyspnea
  - Chest pain from the pleura varying from deep diffuse pain to sharp, stabbing pain
  - Pleural rubbing
  - Fever, chills, and night sweats

Pulmonary Fibrosis (PF)

- Diseases of the lung parenchyma and pleura, also called interstitial lung disease
- Damaged epithelium and chronic inflammation leading to scar formation (fibrosis)
- Asbestosis is a PF disease
- Physical findings may include:
  - Dyspnea
  - Hypoxemia and hypocapnia
  - Crackles
  - Clubbing
  - Dry cough
  - Cyanosis
  - Chest x-rays show increased thickening of the lung pleura due to proliferation of fibroblasts; damage at the alveolar level causes shrinking of the lung and decreased compliance, resulting in the lung becoming stiff

Other Pulmonary Abnormalities

Pulmonary Edema

- Accumulation of fluid in the alveolar spaces from cardiogenic processes with increased pressure, such as in hypertension reflecting back from the heart, causing fluid backup to the pulmonary capillaries
- Other cardiogenic abnormalities: CAD, cardiac valvular disease, and cardiomyopathy
- Noncardiogenic pathologies: Acute lung injury and inflammation causing leakage into the lung tissues, such as in acute respiratory distress syndrome
- Symptoms include:
  - Dyspnea
  - Orthopnea, paroxysmal nocturnal dyspnea (shortness of breath causing awakening at night)
  - Pallor and cyanosis
  - Diaphoresis
  - Tachycardia and heart arrhythmias
  - Anxiety or agitation
  - Chest x-ray shows lung congestion or central infiltrates

Pulmonary Emboli (PE) or Infarction

- Sudden blockage of the pulmonary artery usually from DVT; DVT usually occurs in the lower extremity
- Other causes: PE at right side of heart caused from fat, air, or bone
- PE has a high rate of morbidity and mortality
- Signs and symptoms of DVT or PE can include:
  - Acute dyspnea or tachypnea
  - Chest pain
  - Cough with hemoptysis
  - Tachycardia and weak, feeble pulse
  - Hypotension, lightheadedness, dizziness
  - Syncope

PATHOLOGIES/CONDITIONS OF THE LYMPHATIC SYSTEM[7]

Pathologies of the lymphatic system may be caused from:

Lymphedema

- May occur after surgery (i.e. TKR)
- May also be present prior to surgery usually caused from arthritis
- Edema after surgery is considered part of the normal course of postoperative rehabilitation.

Lymphadenitis

- Inflammation of one or more lymph nodes from infection
- Acute or chronic classification
- Common areas: Cervical region when there is involvement of the teeth or tonsils, and axillary or inguinal regions when the extremities are involved
- Symptoms:
  - Acute lymphadenitis: Warmth, tenderness, and redness of involved area
  - Chronic lymphadenitis: Firmness of the involved lymph node; no warmth or tenderness

Lymphangitis

- Acute subcutaneous inflammation of the lymphatic channels
- Bacterial infection from the infected site toward the lymph node
- Appears as a red streak under the skin and can progress to cellulitis
- Symptoms of throbbing pain, warmth, and edema of involved limb

Lipedema

- Symmetrical swelling of both legs from the hips and down to the ankles with deposits of subcutaneous adipose tissue
- Unknown cause
- Not a pathology of the lymphatic system, but is often confused with lymphedema
- Stage I
  - Skin will be soft and regular, but palpable nodules present
  - Subcutaneous tissues can be described as spongy and soft like a rubber doll
- Stage II
  - Nodules become more firm
  - Large fatty nodules form at the upper thigh and proximal to the medial and lateral malleoli
  - Pitting edema may result at the end of the day; changes in skin color indicate secondary lymphedema and are common in the later stages of lipedema

Lymphadenopathy

- Abnormal enlargement of a lymph node(s).
- Can be caused by:
  - Infection (i.e. TB, Epstein-Barr virus)

- Autoimmune disorders (i.e. rheumatoid arthritis, systemic lupus erythematosus)
- Malignancy (i.e. lymphoma, Hodgkins lymphoma)
- Inflamed nodes may present as enlarged, warm, and tender to touch but remain mobile and soft.
- Malignant nodes are often not tender to touch or mobile and are firm and enlarged.

DIFFERENTIAL DIAGNOSES RELATED TO PATHOLOGIES OF THE CARDIAC, VASCULAR, PULMONARY, AND LYMPHATIC SYSTEMS[6]

Chest Pain/Discomfort

- MI/ischemia
- Pericarditis
- Mitral valve prolapse
- CAD
- Pleurisy
- Pulmonary embolism
- Pneumothorax
- Pulmonary hypertension
- Lung cancer or other pulmonary metastatic disease
- Dissecting aortic aneurysm
- Referred from esophagus; "heartburn"
- Epigastric pain
- Herpes zoster

Cough

- Pulmonary infection
- Pulmonary inflammation
- Tumor, foreign body, aspiration
- Left ventricular failure
- Thoracic aortic aneurysm
- Postnasal drip
- Gastroesophageal: Nonproductive cough at night or after meals; micro-aspiration causing irritation and cough
- Medications such as ACE inhibitors, beta blockers, chemotherapeutic drugs

Dyspnea or Shortness of Breath

- CAD, CHF, dilated cardiomyopathy, valvular disease
- Left ventricular hypertrophy, restrictive cardiomyopathy, constrictive pericarditis
- COPD
- Restrictive lung disease
- Pulmonary edema
- Anemia
- Sepsis
- Peripheral arterial disease
- Deconditioning
- Psychogenic

Edema and Swelling with Weight Gain Greater Than 3 Pounds in 1 Day

- Right ventricular or left and right ventricular failure (CAD, CHF, valvular disease, cardiomyopathy, pulmonary HTN, **cor pulmonale**)
- Fluid overload or kidney failure
- Venous disease (compromised valves in veins, obstruction, thrombophlebitis)
- Lymphatic pathology
- Medication
- Cirrhosis
- Anemia

Fatigue or Weakness

- Left ventricular compromise (CAD, CHF, valvular disease, cardiomyopathy, myocarditis)
- Heart arrhythmic disorders
- Cor pulmonale
- Emotional factors: depression, anxiety, stress
- Sleep disorders or deprivation
- Inadequate nutrition
- Medications such as beta blockers or other antihypertensive medication
- Chemotherapy or radiation treatment
- Chronic fatigue syndrome
- Mitral valve prolapse
- Deconditioning

Hemoptysis

- Pulmonary infections
- TB
- Bronchogenic carcinoma
- Pulmonary infarction
- Mitral stenosis
- Eisenmenger syndrome
- Aortic aneurysm

Leg Pain during Activity

- Peripheral artery disease
- Arthritis of hip, knee
- Stress fractures or other musculoskeletal injuries (meniscal tear, muscle injury)
- Radiculopathy (sciatica, degenerative disk disease, disk herniation or bulge, spinal stenosis)
- Venous insufficiency
- Anterior compartment syndrome
- Neuropathy (neurological disease or diabetes mellitus)

Lightheadedness or Dizziness

- Hypotension
- Impaired cardiac output

- Excess vasodilation which decreases venous return and decreases cardiac output
- Cerebral or vertebral artery insufficiency
- Low blood sugar

Pallor or Cyanosis

- Decreased cardiac output
- Decreased peripheral perfusion
- Hypoxemia
- Pulmonary disease
- Congenital heart disease
- Anemia

Palpitations

- Premature atrial contractions
- PVCs
- Atrial or ventricular tachycardia
- Atrial fibrillation or flutter

Syncope

- Severe compromise of cardiac output
- Cardiac arrhythmias
- LV failure, obstruction, aortic stenosis, obstructive cardiomyopathy
- Aortic dissection
- Orthostatic hypotension, vasovagal reflex, Vasalva maneuver
- Pulmonary embolus
- Pulmonary hypertension
- CVA
- Hyperventilation
- Low blood sugar

DIAGNOSTIC TESTS AND IMAGING OF THE CARDIOVASCULAR/PULMONARY SYSTEM

A. Chest X-Ray (Radiograph)

- Reveals rib cage for possible fractures, size of heart, vessels, and respiratory airways.
- Can look at clarity of lungs and can show evidence of fluid.
- Reveals abnormal tissues, densities, infection, or foreign materials.
- Lung volumes can be analyzed; rib cage expansion can show possible pneumothorax, collapse, hemothorax, or effusion. Overinflation from disease processes can be seen. For comparison, a normal chest x-ray is shown in Figure 1–31.

B. Computed Tomography

- Computed tomography (CT) scans can be used for specific diseases or diagnostic procedures.
- Uses the same ionizing radiation as radiographs, but is more rapid and more detailed. Image slices are created in an axial plane. Figure 1–32 illustrates a CT scan of the chest.

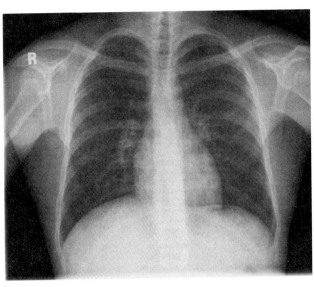

FIGURE 1–31   Normal chest X-ray. (From http://www.chestx-ray.com/index.php/education/normal-cxr-module-train-your-eye#!1.)

- Provides excellent images of lungs, vasculature, and heart.
- Newer software can produce three-dimensional images and can detect small calcification buildup in the coronary arteries (Figure 1–33).

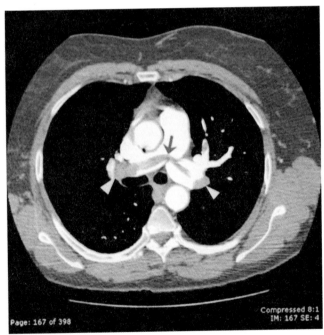

FIGURE 1–32   Example of contrast CT angiogram of chest. Contrast CT angiogram of the chest showing a "saddle" pulmonary embolism (red arrow) as well as filling defects in the left and right pulmonary artery branches (yellow arrowheads) secondary to obstruction by thromboembolic materials. (Used with permission from Lechner AJ, Matuschak GM, Brink DS. *Respiratory: An Integrated Approach to Disease;* 2015. Available at: https://accessmedicine.mhmedical.com/content.aspx?bookid=1623&sectionid=105764262 Accessed September 26, 2018. Copyright © 2018 McGraw-Hill Education. All rights reserved.)

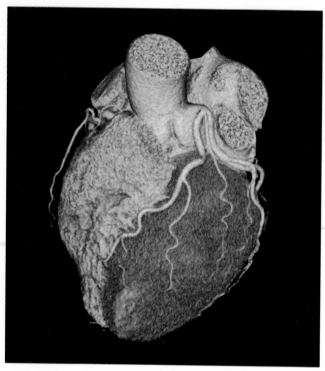

FIGURE 1–33 3D image of the heart. (Courtesy of Philips Healthcare. All rights reserved.)

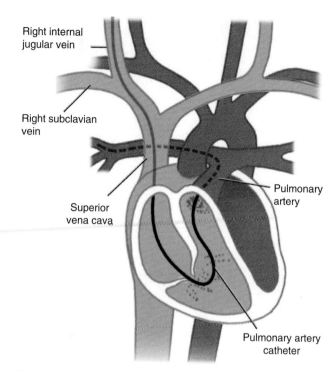

Right internal
jugular vein

Right subclavian
vein

Superior
vena cava

Pulmonary
artery

Pulmonary artery
catheter

FIGURE 1–34 Placement of the Swan-Ganz catheter. (From Reichman EF. *Emergency Medicine Procedures.* 2nd ed. New York, NY: McGraw-Hill; 2013, Figure 53–1, p 345. Used with permission from Eric F. Reichman, MD.)

C. Echocardiogram

- Noninvasive procedure that uses ultrasound to produce images.
- Air affects transmission of ultrasound wave and therefore it is limited in use for the chest; it is primarily used for heart imaging.
- Produces real-time video of heart internal structures, size of heart chambers, valve function, and normal or abnormal heart wall movement.

D. Radionuclide Imaging

- Ventilation-perfusion (V/Q) scanning is used to diagnose pulmonary embolism.
- Radioactive tracers are introduced into the bloodstream and images reveal areas of perfusion. Inert gases are inhaled to show areas of ventilation.
- Images are compared to show where there is a mismatch of V/Q.
- Positron emission tomography (PET) scans are primarily used to detect the spread of lung cancer to the lymph nodes.

E. Cardiac Catheterization

- Hollow tube (catheter) is introduced to the brachial or femoral artery and is guided toward the aorta and heart vessels and then into the coronary arteries.
- Contrast dye is injected into the catheter and x-rays are taken.
- Heart vessels, chambers, walls, and valves can be examined, as well as ejection fraction.

F. Swan–Ganz Catheter

- A central catheter is introduced from the venous system to the right side of the heart (Figure 1–34).
- Pressures can be monitored such as central venous pressure (CVP) and pressures at the pulmonary artery.

G. Magnetic Resonance Imaging

- Used primarily to evaluate soft tissues of the chest cavity. Figure 1–35 shows a gated-3D-MRA image of the chest.
- Advantage of using magnetic energy instead of ionizing radiation.
- Produces higher quality images in various planes (axial and coronal) but takes more time (up to an hour) compared to less than a minute for CT scan.

MEDICAL MANAGEMENT OF THE CARDIOVASCULAR/PULMONARY SYSTEM

Percutaneous Coronary Intervention (PCI)

- Also is known as percutaneous transluminal coronary angioplasty (PTCA).
- Used for increasing blood flow and revascularization in instances of blockage of the coronary arteries.

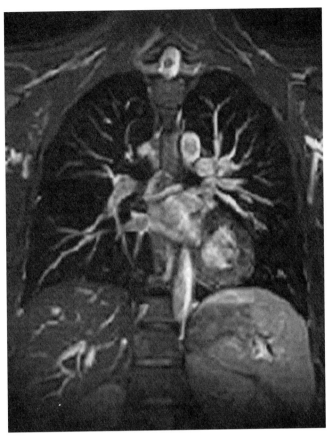

FIGURE 1-35 Gated-3D-FSE MRA image of the chest. (Courtesy of Allen D. Elster, MRIQuestions.com. Used with permission.)

- Balloon-tipped catheter is placed into the heart vessel and is inflated, increasing vessel diameter. Improved blood flow decreases angina, improves effects of CAD with increased coronary blood flow.
- The walls may be reinforced with intravascular stents (wire mesh). Figure 1–36 shows a PCI with a stent inserted into the coronary artery for revascularization of the heart.

Coronary Artery Bypass Graft (CABG)

- Vessels from another site (L or R internal thoracic, radial, or femoral artery) are used to bypass an area of blockage. Figure 1–36 shows an illustration of a CABG that demonstrates revascularization by bypassing an occlusive coronary artery with a vessel.
- Two types of CABG are performed:
  - Traditional CABG
    - Sternotomy is required; patient is placed on a heart-lung machine, and the heart is emptied and stopped.
    - Heart is protected via hypothermia in cardioplegic solution (K^+ with oxygenated blood) at a temperature of 4°C.
  - Mid CABG
    - Sternotomy is not required.
    - Heart-lung machine is not used.
    - Cardioplegia is not used and surgery is performed while the heart is still beating.

Intra-Aortic Balloon Pump (IABP)

- Assists in blood flow from the left ventricle. Essentially creates suction to draw blood from the left ventricle to increase systemic and coronary blood flow. Figure 1–37 presents a diagram

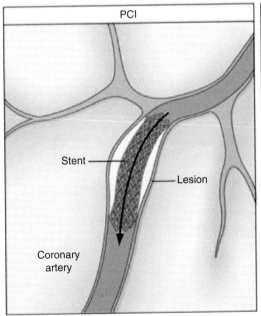

Stent addresses the existing lesion but not future lesions.

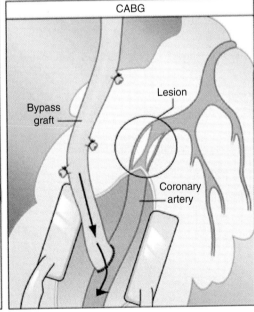

Bypass grafting addresses the existing lesion and also future culprit lesions.

FIGURE 1-36 Coronary revascularization procedures: percutaneous coronary intervention (PCI) and coronary artery bypass graft (CABG). (Reproduced with permission from Gersh BJ, Frye RL. N Engl J Med 352:2235, 2005.)

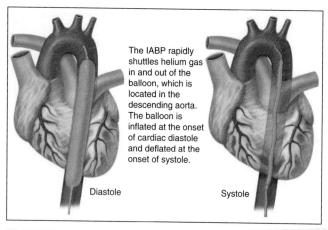

The IABP rapidly shuttles helium gas in and out of the balloon, which is located in the descending aorta. The balloon is inflated at the onset of cardiac diastole and deflated at the onset of systole.

Diastole   Systole

FIGURE 1–37 The ins and outs of the IABP. (From https://vignette.wikia.nocookie.net/bmet/images/9/91/100mmagine_IABP_colori.gif/revision/latest?cb=20090712032858.)

of an IABP with inflation of the balloon during diastole and deflation during systole

Lung Surgeries

- Pneumonectomy: Removal of entire left or right lung
- Lobectomy: Removal of one lobe section of a lung
- Thoracotomy: Incision used to perform lung resections at the fourth intercostal space

Heart and Lung Transplants

- Heart transplant: Utilized in cases of end-stage disease process such as severe damage from MI, valvular disease, or cardiomyopathy. There are two types of heart transplantation surgery:
  - Orthotopic
    - Most common
    - Diseased heart is removed and replaced with donor heart.

- Heteroptic
  - Rarely performed; used in instances of cardiac dysfunction and pulmonary hypertension.
  - Recipient heart is left in place and a donor heart is placed in a "piggyback" procedure in the right chest.
- Midsternotomy incision is utilized by creating an incision down the length of the sternum, and the chest cavity is opened. The sternum is wired after surgery and sternal precautions are observed post-surgery.
- Single-lung or double-lung/bilateral sequential lung transplantation can be performed to replace recipient lung with donor organ.
- Heart and lung transplant can be performed by replacing recipient heart and lung with donor organs.
- Complications from heart and lung transplant are tissue rejection, infection, and compromised immune response due to patient's taking immunosuppressive drugs.

COMMON LABORATORY TESTS AND VALUES

Clinical laboratory studies assist the practitioner in determining the clinical status of a patient. The Tables 1–10, 1–11, and 1–12 provide values for laboratory tests typically used in assessing patients with cardiac dysfunction.

■ INTERVENTIONS

IMPORTANCE OF EARLY MOBILIZATION AND EXERCISE

The negative effects of bedrest within the first 24 to 48 hours is well researched and documented. Changes impact the cardiopulmonary system; fluid shifts and changes in blood volume, impaired O_2 transport, muscle atrophy, loss of bone density, risk for blood clots increase, and many other sequelae can occur.

TABLE 1–10 Critical lab values.

		Lab Values	Critical Values
BMP			
Calcium		8.6–10 mg/dL	≤6 mg/dL, ≥13 mg/dL
Cl⁻		99–109	<80, >115 mEq/L
Glucose		74–106 mg/dL	<40, >450 mg/dL
K⁺		3.5–5.5	<2.8, ≥6.2
Na⁺⁺		132–146 mEq/L	≤120, ≥160 mEq/L
BUN		9–23	≥80 mg/dL
Creatinine	Female	0.5–1.1 mg/dL	>4 mg/dL
	Male	0.7–1/3 mg/dL	

(Continued)

TABLE 1–10 Critical lab values. (*Continued*)

		Lab Values		Critical Values	
Total protein		6.4–8.3 g/L			
Albumin		3.2–4.8 g/L			
CBC					
Hgb		12.0–16.0		≤6.0 g/dL, ≥20 g/dL	
Hct	Female	37–47		≤18%, >60%	
	Male	40–54			
WBC		5.2–12.4		≤2.0, ≥30,000	
RBC	Female	4.2–5.4			
	Male	4.6–6.19			
Platelets		130,000–400,000		≤40,000, ≥999,000	
Ultra-troponin		0.006–0.039		0.040–0.779 (high) >0.78 (critical)	
Serum Drug Levels					
Carbamazepine (Tegretol)		4–10 µg/mL		>15 µg/mL	
Digoxin (Lanoxin)		0.8–2.0 mg/dL		>2.0 mg/dL	
Gentamycin		Peak: 5–10 µg/mL Valley: <2.0 µg/mL		>10 µg /mL	
Phenobarbital		15–40 µg/mL		>40 µg/mL	
Phenytoin (Dilantin)		10–20 µg/mL		>20 µg/mL	
Theophylline (Aminophyllin)		10–20 µg/mL		>20 µg/mL	
Tobramycin		Peak: 5–10 µg/mL Valley: 0.5–2.0 µg/mL		>10 µg/mL	
Valproic acid (Depakene)		50–100 µg/mL		>125 µg/mL	
Vancomycin		Peak: 25–40 µg/mL Valley: 5–15 µg/mL		>30 µg/mL	
Anticoagulant-Related and Clotting					
PT		9.0–11.7 sec		>80 sec	
INR (Coumadin)		0.9–1.2		>6	
PTT (heparin monitoring)		55.0–75.0 sec		>70 sec	
ATTP (therapeutic)		23.3–31.9 sec		**SJH** ≤19 sec, ≥100 **SJE** No low, ≥100	
Fibrinogen level		203–377 mg/dL		≤100.0, ≥600.0 mg/dL	
ABGs —Norms					
pH	7.35–7.45	PO_2	80–100	BE	–2/+2
PCO_2	35–45	HCO_3	22–26	O_2 sat	>95

From https://1l1e3n13v9u93v6zrc1vqx55-wpengine.netdna-ssl.com/wp-content/uploads/2014/06/Critical-Lab-Values.jpg.

TABLE 1–11 Cardiac enzymes.

	Normal Serum Level Values (IU)[a]	Onset of Rise (hours)	Time of Peak Rise (hours)	Return to Normal (days)
CPK	55–71[b]	3–4	33	3
LDH	127[c]	12–24	72	5–14
SGOT	24	12	24	4
Troponin I	<0.1 ng/mL	4–6	12–24	4–7
Troponin T	<0.2 ng/mL	3–4	10–24	10–14

CPK, creatine phosphokinase; LDH, lactic dehydrogenase; SGOT, serum glutamic oxaloacetic transaminase.

[a]1 IU is the amount of enzyme that will catalyze the formation of 1 µmol of substrate per minute under the conditions of the test.

[b]CPK-MB, 0%–3%.

[c]LDH-1, 14%–26%.

From Smith AM, Theirer JA, Huang SH. Serum enzymes in myocardial infarction. *Am J Nurs.* 1973;73(2):277. Used with permission. All rights reserved. Copyright © 1973 The American Journal of Nursing Company.

Physical therapists, as movement specialists, are essential in early mobilization and exercise as early in the rehabilitation process as possible when indicated. Bed exercises, bed mobility, transfers, ambulation, and functional activities significantly help to decrease the deleterious effects of bed rest.

AEROBIC CARDIAC EXERCISE PRESCRIPTION

Adequate Warmup

- Mode: Light intensity aerobic (walking), light calisthenics, and stretching.
- Duration: 5 to 10 minutes.
- Benefits: Gradually increases breathing, BP, and HR; decreases musculoskeletal injury, increases muscle and tissue extensibility, flexibility, and range of motion (ROM). Patients with CV pathology may have decreased exercise response and delayed or impaired heart, lung, or vascular response.

Adequate Cool-Down Period

- Mode: Light aerobic activity such as walking or slow cycling.
- Duration: 5 to 10 minutes.
- Benefits: Return of breathing, HR, and BP to normal levels; prevents venous pooling, decreases lactic acid buildup.

Mode

The type of aerobic activity should be based on what a patient would enjoy and therefore be more motivated to participate in the exercise prescription. Aerobic exercise should incorporate large muscle groups used continuously in a rhythmical pattern.

- Walking, jogging on ground or treadmill
- Cycling (stationary, recumbent, bike path/trail)
- Swimming
- Aerobic equipment (elliptical, stair-stepper, rowing)
- Acute patients in hospital: Walking hospital floor, stationary bike, or treadmill

TABLE 1–12 Normal lipid values.

Lipids	Low Risk (0–1 RF)	Moderate Risk (2 RF)	High Risk
Total cholesterol	<200 mg/dL	<200	<200
LDL	<160 mg/dL	<100 optimal	<100 (optimal <70)
HDL	≥40 mg/dL Male ≥50 mg/dL Female		
VLDL	5–40 mg/dL		
Triglycerides	<150 mg/dL		

HDL, high-density lipoprotein; LDL, low-density lipoprotein; VLDL, very-low-density lipoprotein.

Data from NCEP Expert Panel. Detection, evaluation and treatment of high cholesterol in adults. Adult Treatment Panel III. NIH publication #01-3670 May 2001. Downloaded from http://circahajournals.org/. Accessed August 11, 2015.

- Outpatient or cardiac rehabilitation program: Incorporating multiple modes and varying exercise equipment can provide improved functional gains

Intensity

Commonly use 65% to 80% of maximum heart rate, which is approximately equal to 50% to 70% VO_2 max. Maximum HR is calculated at 220 minus patient age. Intensity can be prescribed in three categories:

- HR
- Rate of perceived exertion (important to use for patients taking beta or Ca^+ channel blockers)
- Metabolic equivalents (METs) of energy expenditure levels: Method that can be used to prescribe exercise and activity. The formula is based on 1 MET equaling the amount of energy used by the body at rest per kilogram of weight per minute. Walking at 3.0 mph is equivalent to 3.3 METs.

Duration

The amount of time engaged in the exercise activity while maintaining the desired intensity.

- Acute and extremely deconditioned individuals may benefit from interval training. Two or three short bouts lasting 3 to 5 minutes with 1 to 2 minutes of rest between. Patients can add 1 to 2 minutes each session. Aim to increase to 10 minutes of continuous activity.
- Sedentary lifestyle: 10 to 20 minutes, adding 1 to 2 minutes per day.
- Goal is to increase to 20 to 30 minutes if moderate intensity and 40 to 60 minutes if low intensity.
- Longer duration and lower intensity effective for patient who has goals to reduce body fat, decrease occurrence of claudication, or manage HTN.

Frequency

- For patients who can tolerate moderate activity, 3 to 5 sessions per week is the goal to improve conditioning
- If exercise is less than 15 to 20 minutes, exercise 2 to 3 times per day
- If greater than 20 minutes, exercise once a day for 3 to 7 days per week depending on intensity

Strength Training

- Light strength training should be incorporated into cardiac rehabilitation.
- Goal of a single set performed 2 times per week to increase strength.
- Light weights or use of resistive bands, incorporated with larger muscle group movement.
- UE exercises have greater demands than LE exercises. For example, arm cycling can increase HR, BP, and O_2 demands. Therefore, patient may have decreased tolerance on rate of perceived exertion (RPE) or onset of angina.

CARDIAC REHABILITATION PROGRAM

Phase I: Acute Phase (Monitoring Phase)[8]

- Postoperation for heart surgery
- Members of the cardiac team include:
  - Physician (cardiac rehabilitation specialist) to oversee patient management and risk factor modification
  - Physical therapist for early mobilization and functional mobility and activities, exercise progression
  - Occupational therapist for self-care and management, activities of daily living, bathing, dressing, grooming, home management, occupational roles
  - Dietician for dietary modifications and risk factor management
- Duration: Hospital stay 3 to 5 days
- Patient is monitored closely 24 hours a day
- Early mobilization (day 1 to 2 postoperation/event)
  - Monitor patient's response, use RPE
  - Decrease risks from bedrest (blood clots, skin breakdown, respiratory illness)
  - Spirometry
  - Bed mobility, sitting at edge of bed, transfers
  - Frequency: Mobilize 2 to 4 times per day as tolerated
- Day 3+
  - Ambulation 2 to 3 times per day
  - Self-care, toileting, hygiene
  - Progress to ambulation of stairs to prepare for discharge
  - Time: Intermittent 3- to 5-minute bouts of activity, 1 to 2 minutes rest
- Sternal precautions
  - No pressure on sternum
  - Encourage use of pillow braced against sternum if coughing
  - No bilateral shoulder flexion and abduction greater than 90 degrees
  - No UE resisted activity
  - Avoid Vasalva
  - No car driving or passenger seat riding for 4 weeks (danger from airbag deployment)
- Care for LE incision site
  - Patient is allowed to be weight bearing as tolerated, and no ROM restrictions if healing normally
  - Patient should avoid crossing legs
  - Patient should wear compression garments and elevate legs

Phase II: Subacute Phase (Conditioning Phase)[8]

- Goals of Phase II
  - Improve exercise ability and endurance safely
  - Continue exercise program and monitor CV response
  - Prepare patient to monitor self and continue at home
  - Educate patient on disease process, rehabilitation process, and on making changes in lifestyle
- Mode: Common aerobic activity of biking or walking.

- Intensity: Interval training at 40% to 60% max HR. If patient showing appropriate CV response, increase target HR by 10 bpm each week.
- Frequency: 5 to 7 sessions of exercise done over a period of 3 weeks.
- Duration: Initial: 10 to 15 minutes of low-level exercise in 2- to 5-minute bouts, working toward 20 to 30 minutes of continuous LE work.
- Discharge criteria
  - Medically stable with no EKG monitor required
  - Patient can self-monitor signs and symptoms
  - Independent and compliant with home exercise program
  - Goal of 9 MET capacity (5 MET needed for self-care at home)
  - Patient passes a maximum symptom-limited exercise test

Phase III: Training and Maintenance Phase (Intensive Rehabilitation) and Phase IV: Disease Prevention Phase (Prevention Programs)[8]

- Patient continues to attend outpatient centers or community centers with cardiac rehabilitation program.
- Patient is screened with exercise stress test, or can also use 6-minute walk test.
- Frequency: 4 to 6 days/week is recommended along with patient's HEP. If MET is less than 4, then multiple brief day sessions recommended.
- Intensity
  - Warmup 5 to 10 minutes
  - Target 40% to 60% VO_2 max with goal to progress to 75% if able
- Mode: Large muscle groups (walking on treadmill or track, cycling).
- Time: Accumulate 30 to 60 minutes of aerobic exercise. Low-functioning patients can use 1:1 ratio of exercise to rest for 3 to 10 minutes.
- Goals
  - Higher level of physical and mental functioning
  - Continue lifelong habits of exercise and risk factor reduction
  - Measure and assess progress and disease stability
  - Enhance quality of life

Special Considerations[8]

Heart Failure

- Patients may not tolerate supine or prone positions due to orthopnea and dyspnea in these positions.
- Exercise can improve impaired blood flow due to vasoconstriction and impaired muscle function.
- Exercise intervals and increasing duration and number of bouts can be effective to improve exercise tolerance.

Pacemakers and Implanted Defibrillators

- Upper extremity exercises are restricted until after 6 weeks of placement or implantation.

- HR should be maintained 10 to 15 bpm below threshold for device to prevent administration of shock due to tachycardia.

Arrhythmias

- Atrial fibrillation (AF) is the most common form of arrhythmia.
- New onset of AF is a contraindication to exercise.
- Ectopic ventricular beats that worsen during exercise is cause for ceasing activity and monitoring the patient.

Diabetes

- Screen patient for vascular complications and symptoms such as retinopathy or peripheral neuropathy.
- It is important to frequently monitor patient's feet and for patient to wear properly fitted footwear.
- Encourage 30 g carbohydrate intake prior to exercise if blood glucose is less than 4 mmol.
- Intensity of 50% to 60% VO_2 max, 3 to 4 times per week for 30 to 60 minutes has shown improved insulin sensitivity and metabolism of carbohydrates.

Pulmonary Rehabilitation and Interventions

Diaphragmatic Breathing

It is important to teach proper techniques if patient is using improper breathing pattern or if patient is in an panic acute episode. Patient can be given cues by therapist placing hand over umbilical area and having patient take a deep, slow breath to expand the abdomen. Patient starts in comfortable supine semi-Fowler position and progresses to sitting, standing, and with ambulation. Patient learns to control breathing and use proper breathing mechanics in all positions and activities.

Postural Drainage

Patient is placed in various positions to optimize gravity-dependent positions and assist in clearing secretions and airway clearance (Figure 1–38).

SKILL KEEPER: ECG/EKG READINGS

What are precautions and contraindications for postural drainage positions where the patient has the head lowered below horizontal? What are precautions and contraindications for percussive techniques?

Percussion

- Used in conjunction with postural drainage.
- Hands are in a cupped position and light percussion is performed over the treated lung segment.

Vibration and Shaking

- Also used in conjunction with postural drainage.
- Different from percussion because vibration and shaking techniques are performed while patient exhales.

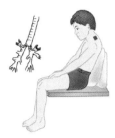

UPPER LOBES Apical segments

Bed or drainage table flat.

Patient leans back on pillow at 30° angle against therapist.

Therapist claps with markedly cupped hand over area between clavicle and top of scapula on each side.

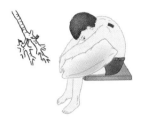

UPPER LOBES Posterior segments

Bed or drainage table flat.

Patient leans over folded pillow at 30° angle.

Therapist stands behind and claps over upper back on both sides.

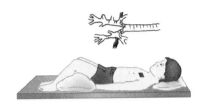

UPPER LOBES Anterior segments

Bed or drainage table flat.

Patient lies on back with pillow under knees.

Therapist claps between clavicle and nipple on each side.

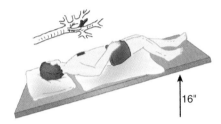

16"

RIGHT MIDDLE LOBE

Foot of table or bed elevated 16 inches.

Patient lies head down on left side and rotates 1/4 turn backward. Pillow may be placed behind from shoulder to hip. Knees should be flexed.

Therapist claps over right nipple area. In females with breast development or tenderness use cupped hand with heel of hand under armpit and fingers extending forward beneath the breast.

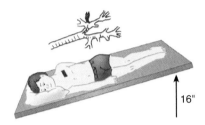

16"

LEFT UPPER LOBE Singular segments

Foot of table or bed elevated 16 inches.

Patient lies head down on right side and rotates 1/4 turn backward. Pillow may be placed behind from shoulder to hip. Knees should be flexed.

Therapist claps with moderately cupped hand over left nipple area. In females with breast development or tenderness use cupped hand with heel of hand under armpit and fingers extending forward beneath the breast.

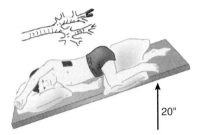

20"

LOWER LOBES Anterior basal segments

Foot of table or bed elevated 20 inches.

Patient lies on side, head down, pillow under knees.

Therapist claps with slightly cupped hand over lower ribs. (Position shown is for drainage of left anterior basal segment. To drain the right anterior basal segment, patient should be on the left side in same posture.)

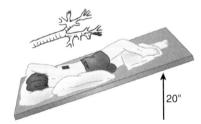

20"

LOWER LOBES Lateral basal segments

Foot of table or bed elevated 20 inches.

Patient lies on abdomen, head down, then rotates 1/4 turn upward. Upper leg is flexed over pillow for support.

Therapist claps over uppermost portion of lower ribs. (Position shown is for drainage of right lateral basal segment. To drain the left lateral basal segment, patient should lie on the right side in the same posture.)

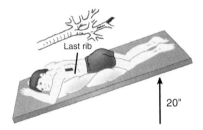

Last rib

20"

LOWER LOBES Posterior basal segments

Foot of table or bed elevated 20 inches.

Patient lies on abdomen, head down, with pillow under hips.

Therapist claps over lower ribs close to spine on each side.

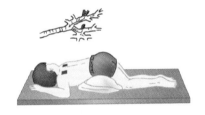

LOWER LOBES Superior segments

Bed of table flat.

Patient lies on abdomen with two pillows under hips.

Therapist claps over middle of back at tip of scapula on either side of spine.

FIGURE 1–38 Positions for postural drainage and bronchial hygiene. (From http://fadavispt.mhmedical.com/data/books/1895/osullrehab6_ch12_f015.png.)

- Mechanically powered devices are available to assist in vibration and shaking force application.
- Vibration
  - Differs from shaking and involves a higher frequency force.
  - Therapist can place both hands on front and back of chest wall, or can place hands on top of one another.
  - Therapist co-contracts all muscles and applies a vibration pressure through the hands and to the chest wall.
- Shaking
  - Force is more rigorous and bouncing action against the chest wall.
  - Produces compression force on the chest wall.

Airway Clearance and Secretion Management

SKILL KEEPER: AIRWAY CLEARANCE AND SECRETION MANAGEMENT

What is the difference between huff and cough? What are the reasons a physical therapist might use one technique over the other?

- Huff
  - Similar to a cough, but glottis remains open.
  - Patient exhales as if trying to produce mist/condensation on a mirror.
  - It is a rapid and forced exhalation without maximal effort.
- Cough
  - Important self-defense mechanism to protect the lungs.
  - Most important component of chest physical therapy.
  - Consists of a voluntary closing of the glottis and the buildup of intrathoracic and intraabdominal pressure behind the glottis. A sudden release of the pressure with glottis opening produces the cough, which causes forceful air pressure to remove secretions or foreign particles.
  - Manually assisted cough
    - Costophrenic assist
    - Heimlich-type assist
    - Anterior chest compression assist
  - Self-assisted cough
    - Prone on elbows
    - Long-sitting
    - Short-sitting
    - Rocking (hands-knees) position

Mechanical Devices and Adjuncts

- Positive expiratory pressure (PEP) devices
  - Provides constant pressure at 10 to 20 cm of H_2O
  - Splints airways open and improves collateral ventilation
- Oscillating PEP devices (Flutter, TherapPep, Acapella)
  - Similar to PEP device and provides positive pressure (10-35 cm of H_2O) that oscillates due to a steel ball contained

Flutter

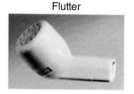

Acapella

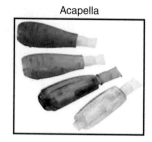

Aerobika oscillating PEP (OPEP)

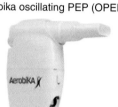

FIGURE 1–39   Mechanical devices for bronchial hygiene therapy. (From http://slideplayer.com/slide/4441549/14/images/27/Devices+for+BHT+Flutter+Acapella+Aerobika+oscillating+PEP+(OPEP).jpg. Used with permission from Clement Clarke International.)

in the device. Figure 1–39 illustrates a variety of oscillating PEP (OPEP) devices for use in airway clearance.
- High-frequency chest compression
  - Inflatable vest is worn that covers the entire chest and is connected to an air-pulse generator.
  - Pressure oscillates at varying duration rates.
  - Cough-like shear force increases mucus stabilization.

Active Cycle of Breathing Technique

The active cycle of breathing technique (ACBT) is a breathing and air clearance technique that a patient can perform independently when properly instructed. The three major components include (a) breathing control (BC), (b) thoracic expansion exercises (TEE), and (c) forced expiratory technique (FET).

- BC
  - Patient focuses on tidal volume breaths and uses diaphragmatic breathing to focus on lower rib cage expansion.
- TEE
  - Patient takes in a maximal inspiration.
  - Patient can hold breath for 3 seconds and can add an additional inhale through nose (encourages collateral ventilation to help re-inflate collapsed alveoli).
  - Therapist can also add vibration or shaking during expiration.
- FET
  - Patient performs huff to assist in movement and removal of secretions followed by breathing control.
  - Patient performs a couple of low- to mid-volume huffs to move secretions in the periphery and from the smaller airways.
  - Patient can then finish with a high-volume huff to clear the secretions in the larger airways and the upper airways.
  - Cycle completes with a high-volume huff or cough.
  - ACBT cycles stop when there is nonproductive cough or patient fatigues.

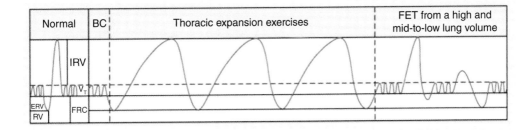

FIGURE 1–40 Active cycle of breathing technique (ACBT). BC = Breathing control; FET = Forced expiration technique. (Used with permission from Savci S, Ince DI, Arikan H: J Cardiopulm Rehabil. 2000;20(1):37-43, Fig 1.)

Depending on which segments are involved, various forms of BC, TEE, and FET are used in combination to clear lower, mid, and upper segments as well as peripheral and central airways. In addition, external devices can be used to aid in secretion clearance. Figure 1–40 presents a diagram illustrating the components of ACBT.

Exercise Prescription for Pulmonary Rehabilitation

Diaphragm Strengthening

- Deep breathing exercises for 10 to 15 minutes several times a day.

- Use of weights on abdomen can give resistance to inspiration and assists in expelling air.

Thoracic Stretching

- Trunk twisting, proprioceptive neuromuscular facilitation (PNF), towel stretches, rib blocking. Figure 1–41 demonstrates a PNF exercise for stretching the thoracic cage.

Exercise Devices for Breathing

- Incentive spirometer (Figure 1–42) or other resistance breathing exercises (Pflex inspiratory muscle trainer; shown in Figure 1–43)

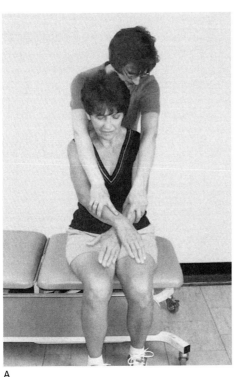
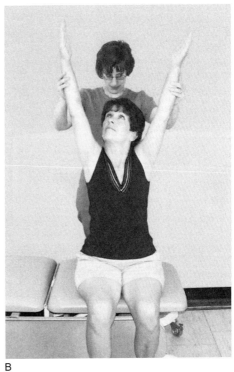

A   B

FIGURE 1–41 Proprioceptive neuromuscular facilitation techniques for thoracic stretching. (From https://fadavispt.mhmedical.com/data/books/1860/osullimprove_ch3_f034.png.)

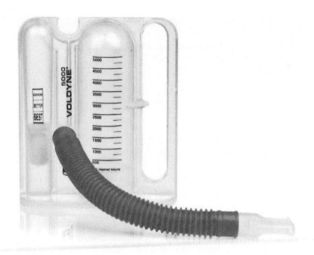

FIGURE 1–42 Incentive spirometer. (From https://www.healthykin.com/images/Product/large/5364.jpg.)

Aerobic Training

- Frequency: Recommended patients participate at least 3 times per week, two of which are supervised to monitor and increase intensity, facilitate compliance, and encourage patient progress.
- Intensity
  - Sixty percent maximum work force for 30 minutes is recommended; however, patients may not tolerate this recommended intensity.
  - Interval training protocols have been developed incorporating high-intensity bouts and recovery periods.
  - Eighty percent average speed achieved on 6-minute walk test or 75% peak speed on shuttle walk test.
  - Sixty percent peak work force on cycle ergometer.
  - Patients should work within a 3 to 5 on the modified (moderate to severe) Borg dyspnea scale.

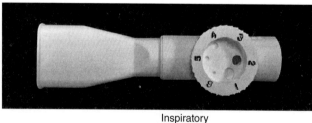

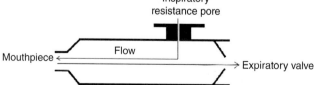

FIGURE 1–43 Respiratory resistance device. (Pflex, Respironics Inc; Pittsburgh, PA). (Used with permission from Wu W, Zhang X, Lin L, et al. Int J Chron Obstruct Pulmon Dis. 2017;12:773-781.)

- Type: Walking exercise on ground surface or treadmill and/or cycling.
- Time: Recommended 20 to 30 minutes.
- Duration: There are greater benefits for a longer-term exercise program of 6 months versus a shorter duration of 12 weeks.

Resistance Training

- Frequency: Recommend 2 to 3 times per week with a day off to allow for recovery and decrease post-exercise muscle soreness
- 50% to 60% of one repetition maximum (RM)
- Type: Large muscle groups of the upper/lower extremity and trunk, starting with the use of light resistance (weights, resistance bands, or machines)
- Progression: Increases of 70% to 85% 1-RM performing 1 to 2 sets with 8 to 12 repetitions

Functional Training, Work Modification, and Energy Conservation

- Teach positions that relieve dyspnea:
  - Sitting leaning forward with elbows supported on thighs, or leaning forward over table
  - Standing and leaning forward over table, or leaning with back against wall
  - Walking and leaning forward with forearms on shopping cart or tall walker
- Use of four-wheel walker or Rollator walker allows patient to lean on walker for support and also provides a chair to sit on when fatigued or short of breath (SOB)
- Overhead activities or overuse of arms can cause increased SOB
- Adapt work for improved ventilation for air movement as well as proper posture for good breathing mechanics
- Relaxation techniques
  - Jacobsen progressive relaxation exercises
  - Biofeedback to control HR, breathing, BP
  - Yoga or meditation
  - Guided imagery or visualization
  - Smart-phone and smart-watch applications for reminders on frequent short-duration relaxation activities

■ SUMMARY

The cardiac, vascular, and pulmonary systems work closely together to maintain adequate blood flow, blood pressure, oxygenation, and removal of waste to ensure that the organs and tissues of the body can maintain functional work and homeostasis. The physical therapist must monitor the effects of activity and exercise on the cardiovascular and pulmonary systems through understanding responses to environmental factors and the use of screening, tests, and measures that include hemodynamic responses. Understanding of physiology, pathology, and the medications to treat abnormalities is a prerequisite to determination of the best treatment interventions, progression, and care.

REFERENCES

1. Moini J. *Anatomy and Physiology for Health Professionals*. 2nd ed. Burlington, MA: Jones and Bartlett Learning; 2016.

2. Trevor AJ, Katzung BG, Kruidering-Hall M. *Katzung and Trevor's Pharmacology: Examination and Board Review*. 11th ed. New York, NY: McGraw-Hill Education; 2015.

3. Hall JE, Guyton AC. *Guyton and Hall Textbook of Medical Physiology*. 12th ed. Philadelphia, PA: Saunders Elsevier; 2011.

4. Frownfelter D, Dean E. *Cardiovascular and Pulmonary Physical Therapy*. 4th ed. St. Louis, MO: Mosby Elsevier; 2006.

5. Pryor JA, Prasad SA. *Physiotherapy for Respiratory and Cardiac problems: Adults and Paediatrics*. 4th ed. London, England: Churchill Livingstone Elsevier; 2008.

6. Watchie J. *Cardiovascular and Pulmonary Physical Therapy: A Clinical Manual*. 2nd ed. St. Louis, MO: Saunders Elsevier; 2010.

7. Goodman CC, Fuller KS. *Pathology: Implications for the Physical Therapist*. 3rd ed. St. Louis, MO: Saunders Elsevier; 2009.

8. Reid DW, Chung F, Hill K. *Cardiopulmonary Physical Therapy: Management and Case Studies*. 2nd ed. Thorofare, NJ: Slack Incorporated; 2014.

QUESTIONS

1. A 72-year-old patient has been diagnosed with atrial flutter and pneumonia and is resting in his room in the inpatient hospital. The physical therapist is going to evaluate the patient and is doing a chart review. In examining the patient's ECG/EKG cardiac strips, which of the following would be indicative of the patient's cardiac diagnosis?
   A. Sawtooth pattern
   B. Prolonged PR interval
   C. Absence of P wave
   D. Elevated ST segment

2. A 65-year-old patient is being seen at a Phase I cardiac rehabilitation program. She is being monitored for exercise response and tolerance. Which of the following symptoms would necessitate ceasing of exercise activity?
   A. RPE of 9 (6–20 scale)
   B. Diastolic BP that remains the same level at rest and with exercise
   C. Persistent dyspnea and diaphoresis
   D. HR increases to 15 bpm over resting rate

3. A physical therapist is conducting a community health education class for patients at risk for developing heart disease. One of the participants raises the question of cholesterol levels on her blood panel lab results and wants to know what the "bad" cholesterol linked to atherosclerosis and CAD is. Which would be the correct response of the physical therapist?
   A. Elevated levels of high-density lipoprotein increase the risk of developing CAD.
   B. Elevated levels of low-density lipoprotein increase the risk of developing CAD.
   C. All cholesterol is bad, and totals should be below 200 mg/dL.
   D. Cholesterol is not an important factor in risk for developing CAD, and the triglycerides should be kept low.

4. The physical therapist is choosing a mode of aerobic activity for an 80-year-old patient who underwent a triple CABG. The patient is 4 weeks in Phase II of her cardiac rehabilitation program. The patient wants to engage in using the arm cycle ergometer for today's session. Which of the following might the physical therapist expect as a response to this exercise intervention?
   A. HR will be higher but SBP would decrease.
   B. Exercise capacity is reduced due to higher SV.
   C. The primary effect would be increased SBP and DBP.
   D. Both the HR and SBP/DBP will be higher.

5. A home health physical therapist is working with an 85-year-old patient who returned home after a transient ischemic attack 3 days ago. The patient also has a diagnosis of HTN, COPD, osteoporosis, and mild dementia. Her husband is helping her at home, but they are confused about her discharge medications. She cannot remember if she took her BP medication earlier in the morning. As her physical therapist, what medication would you educate the family about as the BP medication?
   A. Albuterol
   B. Prednisone
   C. Diltiazem
   D. Amiodarone

6. A physical therapist is performing an examination on a patient who had an MI. The therapist is auscultating for the aortic valve. Which is the best position for the stethoscope to auscultate the aortic valve?
   A. Second right intercostal space at the right sternal border
   B. Fourth intercostal space at the right sternal border
   C. Fourth intercostal space along the lower left sternal border
   D. Fifth intercostal space at the midclavicular line

7. A physical therapist is working with a 20-year-old patient with cystic fibrosis. The therapist wants to use postural drainage techniques for the superior segments of the lower lobe. What is the correct position for this technique?
   A. Sitting, leaning over a folded pillow at a 30-degree angle
   B. Prone with two pillows under the hips
   C. Supine with two pillows under knees
   D. Head down on left side, with ¼ turn from supine

8. A 64-year-old patient developed pulmonary embolism after right total knee replacement surgery. He presented with decreased O_2 saturation and hypoxemia and was admitted to the emergency department for immediate intervention. Which of the following is likely to cause the hypoxemia experienced by the patient?
   A. Retained secretions in the lungs
   B. An ineffective cough
   C. Poor ventilation in the lungs
   D. Poor perfusion in the lungs

9. A 58-year-old gentleman is referred to physical therapy with an excessive cough, sputum production, and SOB. The patient reports that these symptoms have persisted for the past 10 years. The patient's symptoms are most likely indicative of which of the following?
   A. Chronic hypoxia
   B. Chronic bronchitis
   C. Idiopathic hypoventilation
   D. Tuberculosis

10. A physical therapist attempts to prevent alveolar collapse with a patient following thoracic surgery. Which of the breathing techniques would be most beneficial to achieve this goal?
    A. Diaphragmatic breathing and breath control
    B. Pursed-lip breathing
    C. Forced expiratory technique (huff)
    D. Deep breathing exercises with hold of 3 seconds, then sniff through nose

ANSWERS

1. The answer is **A**.
   Rationale:

   - Sawtooth patterns are a hallmark sign of atrial flutter.
   - Prolonged PR interval is indicative of block at the SA or AV node.
   - Absence of a P wave indicates lack of SA activity.
   - Elevated ST segment indicates MI or ventricular involvement.

2. The answer is C.
   Rationale:

   - A patient exhibiting persistent dyspnea (difficulty breathing) and diaphoresis is demonstrating symptoms of not adequately compensating for exercise demands.
   - RPE of 9 represents a "fairly light" exertion perception from the patient.
   - Diastolic BP may remain the same level or may slightly elevate during exercise as a result of vasodilation response due to increased cardiac output, which may maintain diastolic BP, slightly decrease, or slightly increase with increased work.
   - Increase of 15 bpm can be within an expected range of increased HR with exercise.

3. The answer is **B**.
   Rationale: LDL levels are linked to increased risk of developing atherosclerosis and CAD. HDL levels can reduce the risk of developing atherosclerosis and CAD.

4. The answer is **D**.
   Rationale: Use of the arms puts increased strain on the heart, and continuous work of the arms and muscles contracting on the vascular system would increase both SBP and DBP. Patients would have decreased exercise capacity when compared to using a bike for the lower extremities.

5. The answer is **C**.
   Rationale:

   - Diltiazem is a Ca^+ channel blocker that promotes vasodilation.
   - Albuterol is primarily used as bronchodilator.
   - Amiodarone is used to manage heart arrhythmias.
   - Prednisone is a steroid used to alleviate inflammation and allergic response in the lungs.

6. The answer is **A**.
   Rationale: The aortic valve at the second intercostal space is the only structure auscultated on the right side of the sternum. The pulmonic valve, tricuspid, and mitral valve are auscultated on the left side of the sternum.

7. The answer is **B**.
   Rationale: The correct position for the superior segments of the lower lobe is prone with two pillows under the knees. The other positions describe positioning for other segments and lobes of the lungs.

8. The answer is **D**.
   Rationale: Pulmonary embolism involves blockage of blood flow. Blockage would lead to poor perfusion in the lungs. Ventilation would likely be unaffected, as airways are not blocked. Secretions can result from PE; however, the blockage of blood flow has the greatest impact on oxygenation. An ineffective cough affects the ability to clear secretions in the lungs.

9. The answer is **B**.
   Rationale: Chronic bronchitis presents with the symptoms experienced. A patient is diagnosed with chronic bronchitis if the symptoms persist over 2 years. Chronic hypoxia may not lead to development of productive cough but would be compensated in other mechanisms. Idiopathic hypoventilation also would be linked to hypoxia without symptoms of sputum production. TB may have periods of no symptoms after initial exposure.

10. The answer is **D**.
    Rationale: Deep breathing and hold-then-sniff technique increases collateral ventilation of the alveoli. Pursed lip breathing is used for patients who may have COPD and need extra expiration time due to decreased compliance in lungs. Diaphragmatic breathing can inflate alveoli, but the hold-and-sniff technique inflates atelectatic alveoli. Forced huff would promote collapsing of alveoli and airways due to high pressure in the airways.

CHECKLIST

When you complete this chapter you should be able to:

❏ Describe the movement system processes involved in regulating ion flow, conduction of nerve impulses, and pressure changes in cardiac function.

❏ Describe the movement system processes involved in regulating volume changes and movement of gases in the pulmonary system.

❏ Explain the impacts of disease processes and the effects on the cardiovascular, pulmonary, and lymphatic systems.

❏ Explain the impact of various pharmacological agents in mitigating the effects of disease of the cardiac, pulmonary, and vascular systems.

❏ Describe proper assessment tests, measures, and techniques during examination to assess cardiac and pulmonary systems and match with patient presentation and symptoms.

❏ Examine and develop physical therapy diagnoses based on pertinent patient information, clinical findings, and patient presentation and symptoms.

❏ Deploy proper therapeutic interventions for various presentations and pathologies of the cardiac, pulmonary, and vascular systems.

2

Musculoskeletal Physical Therapy

Mark Dutton, Chris Ivey, and Kayla Smith

FOUNDATIONAL SCIENCES

Overview

The musculoskeletal system includes bones, muscles with their related tendons and synovial sheaths, bursa, and joint structures such as cartilage, menisci, capsules, and ligaments. These body tissues are designed to accommodate the stresses of everyday life. An understanding of how these structures are designed and respond to stress is essential for the evidence-based practitioner. Also, it is important to understand the mechanisms behind how energy is provided to the musculoskeletal structures for them to perform optimally. This knowledge helps the clinician perform a thorough examination and establish an accurate diagnosis.

High-Yield Terms to Learn

Collagen	The main structural protein found throughout the various connective tissues.
Elastin	A component of connective tissue that is very good at resisting tensile loads and determines the patterns of distension and recoil in most organs.
Stress-strain curve	A graphical representation of the relationship between the stress and strain that a specific material displays.
Crimp	The first line of response to stress by collagen tissue; occurs in the toe phase of the stress-strain curve. When a load is applied, the fibers line up in the direction of the applied force.
Creep	The gradual rearrangement of collagen fibers, proteoglycans, and water that occurs because of a continuously applied force after the initial lengthening caused by crimp has ceased.
Stress relaxation	A phenomenon in which a stress or force within a deformed structure decreases with time while the deformation is held constant.
Stiffness	The inelasticity of an object and the degree to which the object resists deformation in response to an applied force.
Plastic deformation	Occurs when a tissue remains deformed and does not recover its pre-stress length.
Stress response	The method by which a tissue responds to an applied stress. Exercises may be used to change the physical properties of muscles/tendons and ligaments, as both have demonstrated adaptability to external loads with an increase in strength:weight ratios. The improved strength results from an increase in proteoglycan content and collagen cross-links.
Viscoelasticity	The time-dependent mechanical property of a material to stretch or compress over time and to return to its original shape when the force is removed.
Open (loose)-packed position	The joint position that results in a slackening of the major ligaments of the joint, minimal surface congruity, minimal joint surface contact, maximum joint volume, and minimal stability of the joint.
Close-packed position	The joint position that results in the maximal tautness of the major ligaments, maximal surface congruity, minimal joint volume, and maximum stability of the joint.
Capsular pattern	A capsular pattern of restriction is a limitation of pain and movement in a joint-specific ratio, which is usually present with osteoarthritis or following prolonged immobilization.

High-Yield Terms to Learn (*continued*)

Neutral zone	The zone within a joint's motion in which there is little or no internal resistance offered by the tissues to movement, and the range in which the crimp of the tissue is being taken up.
Elastic zone	The zone in which the first barrier or restriction to movement occurs; takes place at the end of the neutral zone. The elastic zone extends from the crimp area through the physiological barrier (end of the active movement), and toward the anatomic barrier (end of the passive movement).
Plastic zone	The zone in which deformation of the tissue is extended beyond the tissue's elastic recoil and the tissue begins to deform; injury can occur if the deformation is sufficient in time or load.
Concave-convex rule	A concept used with joint mobilizations. If the joint surface is convex relative to the other surface, the slide (arthrokinematic motion) takes place in the opposite direction to the osteokinematic motion. If on the other hand, the joint surface is concave, the slide takes place in the same direction as the osteokinematic motion.

■ SECTION 1: ANATOMY AND BIOMECHANICS

Kinetics is the term applied to define the forces acting on the body. Posture and movement are both governed by the body's ability to control these forces. A wide range of external and internal forces are either generated or resisted by the human body during daily activities. The inherent ability of a tissue to tolerate **load** can be observed experimentally.

STRUCTURES OF THE MUSCULOSKELETAL SYSTEM

Connective Tissue

Connective tissue (CT) is found throughout the body. It provides structural and metabolic support for other tissues and organs of the body including bone, cartilage, tendons, ligaments, and blood tissue. The primary types of CT cells in the blood are macrophages. Macrophages function as phagocytes to clean up debris, mast cells (which release chemicals associated with inflammation), and fibroblasts (which are the principal cells of CT as they produce collagen).[1] Collagenous and elastic fibers are sparse and irregularly arranged in loose CT but are tightly packed in dense CT.[2] The major types of collagen are depicted in Table 2–1.

Various types of connective tissue can be found throughout the musculoskeletal system including the following:

TABLE 2–1 Major types of collagen.

Type	Location
I	Bone, skin, ligament, and tendon
II	Cartilage, nucleus pulposus
III	Blood vessels, gastrointestinal tract
IV	Basement membranes

Fascia

A loose CT that provides support and protection for the joint, and acts as an interconnection between tendons, aponeuroses, ligaments, capsules, nerves, and muscle.

Tendons

Dense regular CT that produces joint motion, stores elastic energy that contributes to movement when stretched, and allows for the optimal distance between the muscle belly and the joint it is acting upon. The main function of tendons is to transmit the load from muscle to bone, and thus they are designed to resist strong tensile loads well, but are not designed to resist shear or compressive forces. Tendons consist of three major sections:

- Bone–tendon junction (enthesis). Functions to absorb and distribute stress and is therefore vulnerable to injury.
- Tendon midsubstance.
- Musculotendinous junction (MTJ). Very susceptible to tensile failure. Common sites of failure include the MTJ of the biceps and triceps brachii, rotator cuff muscles, flexor pollicis longus, fibularis (peroneus) longus, medial head of the gastrocnemius, rectus femoris, adductor longus, iliopsoas, pectoralis major, semimembranosus, and the whole hamstrings group.[3–5]

Ligaments

Ligaments, which are formed from dense CT, serve to connect bones across joints, prevent excessive joint motion/provide stability ("check-reins"), and provide proprioceptive input (Tables 2–2 and 2–3). Except for the ligamentum flavum and the nuchal ligament, a small amount of elastin is found in ligaments. The midportion of a ligament is avascular with a reduced nerve supply, whereas the end portion is highly vascular and more densely innervated.

Cartilage

Cartilage exists in three primary forms: hyaline, elastic, and fibrocartilage.

- Hyaline (articular). Hyaline cartilage is the most abundant cartilage in the body and functions to distribute and dissipate forces. It covers the ends of long bones and permits frictionless motion between the articular surfaces of diarthrodial (synovial)

TABLE 2-2 Major ligaments of the upper quadrant.

Joint	Ligament	Function
Shoulder complex	Coracoclavicular	Fixes the clavicle to the coracoid process
	Costoclavicular	Fixes the clavicle to the costal cartilage of the first rib
Glenohumeral	Coracohumeral	Reinforces the upper portion of the joint capsule
	Glenohumeral ("Z")	Reinforces the anterior and inferior aspect of the joint capsule
	Coracoacromial	Protects the superior aspect of the joint
Elbow	Annular	Maintains the relationship between the head of the radius and the humerus and ulna
	Ulnar (medial) collateral	Provides stability against valgus (medial) stress, particularly in the range of 20°-130° of flexion and extension
	Radial (lateral) collateral	Provides stability against varus (lateral) stresses and functions to maintain the ulnohumeral and radiohumeral joints in a reduced position when the elbow is loaded in supination
Wrist	Extrinsic palmar	Provides the majority of the wrist stability
	Intrinsic	Serve as rotational restraints, binding the proximal carpal row into a unit of rotational stability
	Interosseous	Bind the carpal bones together
Fingers	Volar and collateral interphalangeal	Prevent displacement of the interphalangeal joints

TABLE 2-3 Major ligaments of the spine and lower quadrant.

Joint	Ligament	Function
Spine	Anterior longitudinal ligament	Functions as a minor assistant in limiting anterior translation and vertical separation of the vertebral body
	Posterior longitudinal ligament	Resists vertebral distraction of the vertebral body
		Resists posterior shearing of the vertebral body
		Acts to limit flexion over several segments
		Provides some protection against intervertebral disk protrusions
	Ligamentum flavum	Resists separation of the lamina during flexion
	Interspinous	Resists separation of the spinous processes during flexion
	Iliolumbar (lower lumbar)	Resists flexion, extension, axial rotation, and side bending of L5 on S1
Sacroiliac	Sacrospinous	Creates the greater sciatic foramen
		Resists forward tilting of the sacrum on the ilium during weight-bearing
		Creates the lesser sciatic foramen
	Sacrotuberous	Resists forward tilting (nutation) of the sacrum on the ilium during weight-bearing
	Interosseous	Resists anterior and inferior movement of the sacrum
	Dorsal sacroiliac (long)	Resists backward tilting (counternutation) of the sacrum on the ilium during weight-bearing
Hip	Ligamentum teres	Transports nutrient vessels to the femoral head
	Iliofemoral	Limits hip extension
	Ischiofemoral	Limits anterior displacement of the femoral head
	Pubofemoral	Limits hip extension
Knee	Medial collateral	Stabilizes the medial aspect of the tibiofemoral joint against valgus stress
	Lateral collateral	Stabilizes the lateral aspect of the tibiofemoral joint against varus stress
	Anterior cruciate	Resists anterior translation of the tibia and posterior translation of the femur
	Posterior cruciate	Resists posterior translation of the tibia and anterior translation of the femur
Ankle	Medial collaterals (deltoid)	Provides stability between the medial malleolus, navicular, talus, and calcaneus against eversion
	Lateral collaterals	Static stabilizers of the lateral ankle especially against inversion
Foot	Long plantar	Provides indirect plantar support to the calcaneocuboid joint by limiting the amount of flattening of the lateral longitudinal arch of the foot
	Bifurcate	Supports the medial and lateral aspects of the foot when weight-bearing in a plantarflexed position
	Calcaneocuboid	Provides plantar support to the calcaneocuboid joint and possibly helps to limit flattening of the lateral longitudinal arch

joints. This type of cartilage is avascular and aneural, and its thickness is determined by the degree of peak pressures (the higher the pressure, the thicker the cartilage); the patella has the thickest cartilage in the body.

- Elastic (yellow). Found in the outer ear and larynx.
- Fibrocartilage (white). This type of cartilage, which is avascular, aneural, and alymphatic, primarily functions as a shock absorber. Examples include symphysis pubis, glenoid labrum, hip labrum, triangular fibrocartilage complex (TFCC) of the wrist, the intervertebral disk, and the menisci of the knee.

Bone

Bone, a dynamic tissue that undergoes constant metabolism and remodeling, functions to provide support, enhance leverage, protect vital structures, provide attachments for both tendons and ligaments, and to store minerals, particularly calcium. The general structure of bone and associated conditions are depicted in Table 2–4. Two types of bone are recognized:

- Cortical. Forms the outer shell of a bone
- Cancellous. Forms the epiphyseal and metaphyseal regions of long bones and the interior aspect of short bones

Skeletal structures develop by one of two methods:

- Intramembranous ossification by mesenchymal stem cells (cranium, facial bones, ribs, clavicle, mandible)
- Endochondral ossification (appendicular and axial bones)

The strength of bone is directly related to its density.

Skeletal Muscle

The myofiber (single muscle cell), wrapped in a CT envelope called endomysium, is composed of thousands of myofibrils (Figure 2–1). Bundles of myofibers, which form a whole muscle (fasciculus), are encased in the perimysium. A connective sheath called the epimysium surrounds groups of muscles. Myofibrils are composed of sarcomeres (the contractile machinery of a muscle) arranged in series.

The graded contractions of whole muscles occur because the number of fibers participating in the contraction varies. Increasing the force of movement is achieved by recruiting more cells into cooperative action. Myofilaments, which have a striated appearance, consist primarily of two components:

- Actin (thin). I bands that contain **tropomyosin** and **troponin** that function as the switch for muscle contraction and relaxation (Figure 2–2). In a relaxed state, the tropomyosin physically blocks the cross-bridges from binding to the actin. The tropomyosin must be removed before a contraction can occur.
- Myosin (thick). A bands.

Each muscle fiber is limited by a cell membrane called a **sarcolemma**. The protein *dystrophin* plays an essential role in the mechanical strength and stability of the sarcolemma.[6] Dystrophin is lacking in patients with Duchenne muscular dystrophy. A somatic motor neuron innervates each myofiber. One neuron and the muscle fibers it innervates constitute a motor unit, or functional unit, of the muscle. A skeletal muscle is capable of producing different types of contraction:

- Isometric. Static contraction without change in length.
- Isotonic. Tension within the muscle remains constant as the muscle shortens or lengthens; although in most exercise forms the muscle tension during exercise varies based upon the weight used, joint velocity, muscle length, and type of contraction.
- Concentric. Produces a shortening of the muscle.

TABLE 2–4 General structure of bone.

Site	Comment	Conditions	Result
Epiphysis	Mainly develops under pressure Apophysis forms under traction Forms bone ends Supports articular surface	Epiphyseal dysplasias Joint surface trauma Overuse injury Damaged blood supply	Distorted joints Degenerative changes Fragmented development Avascular necrosis
Physis	Epiphyseal or growth plate Responsive to growth and sex hormones Vulnerable before growth spurt occurs Mechanically weak	Physeal dysplasia Trauma Slipped epiphysis	Short stature Deformed or angulated growth or growth arrest
Metaphysis	Remodeling expanded bone end Cancellous bone heals rapidly Vulnerable to osteomyelitis Affords ligament attachment	Osteomyelitis Tumors Metaphyseal dysplasia	Sequestrum formation Altered bone shape Distorted growth
Diaphysis	Forms shaft of bone Large surface for muscle origin Significant compact cortical bone Strong in compression	Fractures Diaphyseal dysplasias Healing slower than at metaphysis	Able to remodel angulation Cannot remodel rotation Involucrum with infection Dysplasia gives altered density and shape

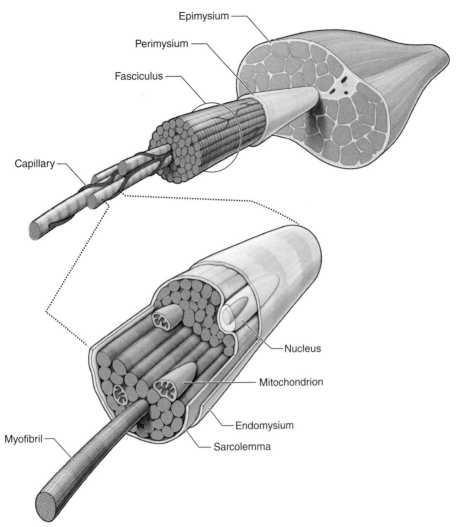

FIGURE 2–1 Microscopic structure of the muscle. (From Dutton M. *Dutton's Orthopaedic Examination, Evaluation and Intervention.* 4th ed. New York, NY: McGraw-Hill, 2017.)

- Eccentric. Muscle lengthens, resulting in maximum lengthening muscle tension. Capable of generating more force than isometric or concentric and is primarily used with activities that require deceleration.
- Isokinetic. Muscle maximally contracts at the same speed throughout the range of its related lever.

Muscle contractions occur at the neuromuscular junction (NMJ), or motor endplate, which is the area of contact between a nerve and the muscle fiber. A contraction occurs in the following manner:

- Acetylcholine (ACh) is released at the NMJ.
- Calcium (Ca^{2+}) is released from the sarcoplasmic reticulum (SR). SR forms a network around the myofibrils, storing and providing Ca^{2+} required for a muscle contraction. As SR is associated with both contraction and relaxation, any change in its ability to release or sequester Ca^{2+} markedly affects both the time course and magnitude of force output by the muscle fiber.
- The Ca^{2+} diffuses into the sarcomeres, binds to troponin, and displaces the tropomyosin, thereby allowing the actin to bind with the myosin cross-bridges. Whenever a somatic motor neuron is activated, all of the muscle fibers that it innervates are stimulated and contract with *all-or-none* twitches.

At the end of the contraction the SR accumulates Ca^{2+} through active transport, requiring degradation of adenosine triphosphate (ATP) to adenosine diphosphate.

A number of muscle fiber types exist (Tables 2–5 and 2–6):

- Type I. Tonic, slow-twitch. Used for endurance (aerobic) and stabilization activities—for example, postural, back, and trunk muscles
- Type II. Phasic fast-twitch. Used for quick, explosive (anaerobic), and dynamic activities

Depending on the type and structure, skeletal muscle can serve a number of roles:

- Prime mover (agonist). Directly responsible for the desired movement
- Antagonist. Produces an action directly opposite the agonist
- Synergist (supporter). Provides cooperative muscle function relative to the agonist

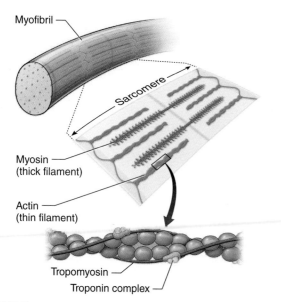

FIGURE 2–2 Troponin and tropomyosin action during a muscle contraction. (From Dutton M. *Dutton's Orthopaedic Examination, Evaluation and Intervention.* 4th ed. New York, NY: McGraw-Hill, 2017.)

The quality of a muscle contraction can be impacted by the effects of velocity:

- Concentric contractions. Inverse relationship (increased speed leads to a decreased force)
- Eccentric. Direct relationship (increased speeds lead to an increased force initially); during slow eccentric muscle actions, the work produced approximates an isometric contraction

The quality of a muscle contraction can also be impacted by its length:

- Active insufficiency. Muscle in shortened or excessively lengthened position, which places the actin/myosin cross-bridges at a disadvantage such that the muscle cannot fully shorten to

TABLE 2–5 Comparison of muscle fiber types.

Characteristics	Type I	Type II A	Type IIx
Size (diameter)	Small	Intermediate	Very large
Resistance to fatigue	High	Fairly high	Low
Capillary density	High	High	Low
Glycogen content	Low	Intermediate	High
Twitch rate	Slow	Fast	Fast
Energy system	Aerobic	Aerobic	Anaerobic
Maximum muscle shortening velocity	Slow	Fast	Fast
Major storage fuel	Triglycerides	Creatine phosphate glycogen	Creatine phosphate glycogen

TABLE 2–6 Functional division of muscle groups.

Movement Group	Stabilization Group
Primarily type II A	Primarily type I
Prone to adaptive shortening	Prone to develop weakness
Prone to develop hypertonicity	Prone to muscle inhibition
Dominate in fatigue and new movement situations	Fatigue easily
Generally cross two joints	Primarily cross one joint
Examples	*Examples*
Gastrocnemius/soleus	Fibularis (peronei)
Tibialis posterior	Tibialis anterior
Short hip adductors	Vastus medialis and lateralis
Hamstrings	Gluteus maximus, medius, and minimus
Rectus femoris	Serratus anterior
Tensor fascia lata	Rhomboids
Erector spinae	Lower portion of trapezius
Quadratus lumborum	Short/deep cervical flexors
Pectoralis major	Upper limb extensors
Upper portion of trapezius	Rectus abdominis
Levator scapulae	
Sternocleidomastoid	
Scalenes	
Upper limb flexors	

Data from Jull GA, Janda V. Muscle and motor control in low back pain. In: Twomey LT, Taylor JR, eds. *Physical Therapy of the Low Back: Clinics in Physical Therapy.* New York, NY: Churchill Livingstone, 1987:258.

produce a full range of motion (ROM). For example, the hamstrings may limit hip flexion when the knee is in full extension.

- Passive insufficiency. Occurs when a two-joint muscle cannot stretch to the extent required for full ROM in the opposite direction at all joints crossed.[7–10] For example, when making a closed fist with the wrist fully flexed, the active shortening of the finger and wrist flexors results in a passive lengthening of the finger extensors.

A muscle functions most efficiently at 38.5°C (101°F). Any increase in temperature with exercise leads to an increase in the speed of nerve and muscle function, higher maximum isometric tension, and a higher maximum velocity of shortening with fewer motor units at any given load.

CT disorders include systemic lupus erythematosus, rheumatoid arthritis, spondyloarthropathies (eg, ankylosing spondylitis, reactive arthritis), polymyalgia rheumatica, polymyositis and dermatomyositis, scleroderma, Sjögren syndrome, crystal-induced arthropathies (eg, gout), and juvenile rheumatoid arthritis.

Joints

A number of major joint types exist:

Synarthrosis

There are two types of synarthrosis:

- Fibrous joints. Formed from dense fibrous CT. Examples include suture (eg, skull), gomphosis (eg, tooth, maxilla, mandible), and syndesmosis (eg, tibiofibular joint, radioulnar joint)

- Cartilaginous. Generally stable joints with little movement (eg, symphysis pubis)

Diarthrosis (Synovial)

Provides greater mobility, unites long bones, joint capsule contains synovial fluid. A number of types exist:

- Simple (uniaxial), or hinge joint. An example is the humeroulnar joint.
- Compound (biaxial), or condyloid. Examples include the metacarpophalangeal (MCP) joint of the finger, and the saddle joint of the thumb-carpometacarpal (CMC).
- Complex (multiaxial). These joints allow movement in and around three planes. They have an intraarticular inclusion within the joint, like a meniscus or disk, which increases the number of joint surfaces. An example is the ball-and-socket joint of the hip.
- Synovial. Synovial joints have some distinguishing characteristics:
  - A joint cavity enclosed by a capsule and which is composed of two layers.
  - Hyaline cartilage that covers the surfaces of the enclosed bones.
  - Synovial fluid, which contains hyaluronan (essential for joint homeostasis) and glycosaminoglycan (GAG). Synovial fluid provides joint lubrication, viscoelastic properties, and anti-inflammatory and antinociceptive properties. In addition to being found within joints, synovial fluid is also found in bursae (enclosed, round, flattened sacs lined with synovium and which function to separate exposed areas of bone from overlapping muscles [deep bursae], or skin and tendons [superficial bursae]).
  - A synovial membrane that lines the inner surface of the capsule.

MOVEMENTS OF BODY SEGMENTS

Movements of the body segments are described using a series of planes and axes. The more common planes of the body include (Figure 2–3):

- Sagittal (anterior-posterior, or median plane). Divides the body vertically into left and right halves of equal size
- Frontal (coronal or lateral plane). Divides the body equally into front and back
- Transverse (horizontal). Divides the body equally into top and bottom halves

The axes of the body, around which movement takes place, are always perpendicular to the plane in which they occur. As with the planes of the body, there are three common types:

- Mediolateral or coronal axis is perpendicular to sagittal plane
- Vertical or longitudinal axis is perpendicular to frontal plane
- Anteroposterior (AP) axis is perpendicular to the transverse plane

Some familiar directional terms are used to describe the relationship of body parts or the location of an external object with

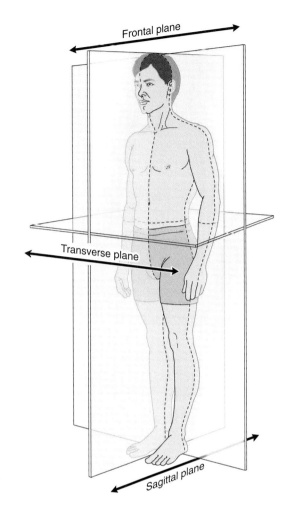

FIGURE 2–3 Planes of the body. (From Dutton M. *Dutton's Orthopaedic Examination, Evaluation and Intervention.* 4th ed. New York, NY: McGraw-Hill, 2017.)

respect to the body.[11] The following are commonly used directional terms:

- Superior or cranial: Closer to the head
- Inferior or caudal: Closer to the feet
- Anterior or ventral: Toward the front of the body
- Posterior or dorsal: Toward the back of the body
- Medial: Toward the midline of the body
- Lateral: Away from the midline of the body
- Proximal: Closer to the trunk
- Distal: Away from the trunk
- Superficial: Toward the surface of the body
- Deep: Away from the surface of the body in the direction of the inside of the body

The center of gravity (COG), or center of mass (COM), of the body, is the point at which all the mass of the object or segment is concentrated; the point at which the line of gravity balances the body (located at the S2 level in a rigid human body).

The base of support (BOS) of the body includes the part of the body in contact with the supporting surface and the intervening area.[12] During static standing, the body's line of gravity is between the individual's feet, which serve as the BOS. Both the COG and BOS are important factors of balance and stability.

The term degrees of freedom (DOF) refers to the number of independent modes of motion at a joint, which in turn correspond to the three dimensions of space:

- 1 DOF. A joint that can only spin or swing in one direction, so joint motion occurs in one plane; for example, proximal interphalangeal (PIP) joint.
- 2 DOF. A joint that can spin and swing in one way only, *or* it can swing in two completely distinct ways, but not spin. Thus, joint motion occurs in two planes; for example, the tibiofemoral joint, temporomandibular joint, proximal and distal radioulnar joints (DRUJs), subtalar joint, and talocalcaneal joint.
- 3 DOF. A joint that can spin and also swing in two distinct directions, so that the joint motion occurs in three planes; for example, a ball-and-socket joint, such as the shoulder or hip.

Joint Kinematics

Kinematics is the study of motion and describes how something is moving without stating the cause. Within the study of joint kinematics, two significant types of motion are commonly described: (1) osteokinematic and (2) arthrokinematic.

- Osteokinematic (bone movement). This includes physiologic movements that can be performed voluntarily, for example, flexion of the shoulder.
- Arthrokinematic (joint movement). This includes the motion of the bone surfaces within a joint. These movements cannot be performed voluntarily and can only occur when resistance to active motion is applied, or when the patient's muscles are completely relaxed. The more common types of joint plane motion include:
  - Roll: The joint motion occurs in the same direction as the swinging bone, and compression of the joint surfaces occurs in the direction of the roll.
  - Slide: Translation of joint surfaces, also referred to as *translatory* motion. The direction of the slide is determined by the shape of the articulating surface. This concept is often referred to as the *concave–convex rule* and is used when applying joint mobilizations:
    - If the joint surface is convex relative to the other surface, the slide occurs in the opposite direction to the osteokinematic motion (Figure 2–4).
    - If the joint surface is concave, the slide takes place in the same direction as the osteokinematic motion (Figure 2–5).
  - Spin: Involves a rotation of one surface on an opposing surface around a vertical axis, for example, rotation of the radial head during forearm pronation and supination.

A wide range of external and internal forces are either generated or resisted by the human body during daily activities.

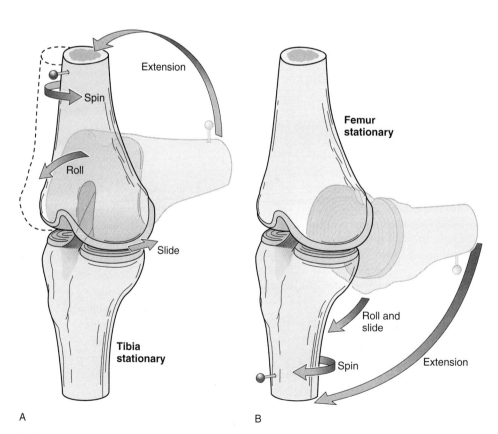

A   B

FIGURE 2–4 Arthrokinematics of motion. (From Dutton M. *Dutton's Orthopaedic Examination, Evaluation and Intervention*. 4th ed. New York, NY: McGraw-Hill, 2017.)

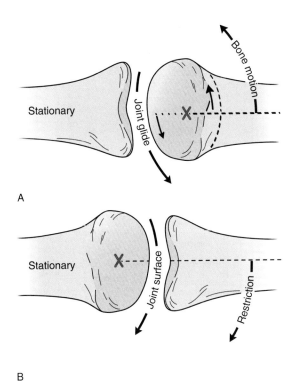

A

B

FIGURE 2–5 Gliding motions according to joint surfaces. (From Dutton M. *Dutton's Orthopaedic Examination, Evaluation and Intervention*. 4th ed. New York, NY: McGraw-Hill, 2017.)

Examples of these external forces include ground reaction forces, gravity, and applied forces through contact. Examples of internal forces include muscle contraction, joint contact, and joint forces including shear, compression, and tension (Figure 2–6).

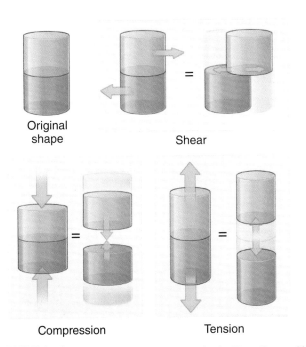

FIGURE 2–6 Internal forces acting on the body. (From Dutton M: *Dutton's Orthopaedic Examination, Evalution and Intervention*, 4th ed. New York, NY: McGraw-Hill, 2017.)

The terms *strain* and *stress* have specific mechanical meanings. Strain is defined as the change in length of a material due to an imposed load, divided by the original length. Stress, or load, is given in units of force per area and is used to describe the type of force applied. As a clinical example, tendons display more elasticity at lower strain rates and more stiffness at higher rates of tensile loading and deform less than ligaments.

The load-deformation curve, or stress-strain curve, of a structure (Figure 2–7) depicts the relationship between the amount of force applied to a structure and the structure's response regarding deformation or acceleration. The horizontal axis (deformation or strain) represents the ratio of the tissue's deformed length to its original length. The vertical axis of the graph (load or stress) denotes the internal resistance generated as a tissue resists deformation, divided by its cross-sectional area. The load-deformation curve is split into four regions, with each region representing a biomechanical property of the tissue (Figure 2–7).

The body uses different types of levers to reduce stress and strain by manipulating the mechanical advantage (MA) (Figure 2–8):

- First class. The fulcrum is located between two forces (eg, cervical flexion/extension). The MA varies depending on the location of the axis of rotation.
- Second class (MA>1). The load (resistance) is located between the fulcrum and the effort, so it takes less force to move the resistance (eg, heel raises).
- Third class (MA<1). The load is located between the fulcrum and the load at the end of the lever and effort. Thus, the effort expended is greater than the load, but the load is moved a greater distance. Most moveable joints in the body use third class levers (eg, flexion of the elbow).

The expression *kinematic chain* is used in rehabilitation to describe the function or activity of an extremity or trunk regarding a series of linked chains. The efficiency of an activity can be dependent on how well these chain links work together. Two types of kinematic chain systems are recognized: *closed kinematic chain* (CKC) and *open kinematic chain* (OKC) systems (Table 2–7).

When referring to the stability of a joint, the two terms close-packed position and open-packed position are commonly used.

Close-packed position (Table 2–8). A joint is said to be in its close-packed position when there is:

- Maximum congruity of joint surfaces
- Maximum tautness of major ligaments
- Minimum joint volume
- Maximum stability

The close-packed position of the joint is often associated with a fall on an outstretched hand (FOOSH) injuries.

Open-packed position (Table 2–9). A joint is said to be in its open-packed position when there is:

- Slackening of the major ligaments
- Minimal joint surface congruity and contact
- Maximum joint volume
- Minimal stability

The open-packed position of the joint is often associated with capsular and ligamentous injuries. Because this position places

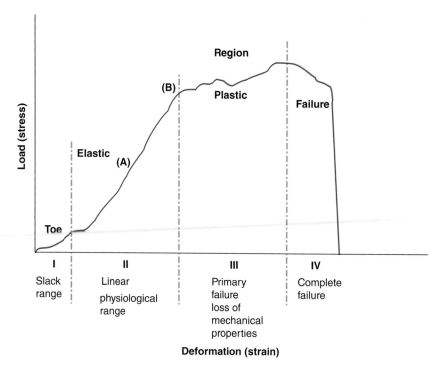

FIGURE 2–7 Stress-strain curve. (From Dutton M. *Dutton's Orthopaedic Examination, Evaluation and Intervention*. 4th ed. New York, NY: McGraw-Hill, 2017.)

the joint in its most relaxed position, the open-packed position is commonly used in joint mobilization interventions.

A **capsular pattern of restriction** (Table 2–10) is a limitation of pain and movement in a joint-specific ratio, which is usually present with arthritis or following prolonged immobilization.[13] Thus, the passive range of motion (PROM) for that joint will be limited in a capsular pattern, and there will be decreased joint play

movement. It is worth remembering that a consistent capsular pattern for a particular joint might not exist, and that these patterns are based on empirical findings and tradition rather than on research.[14,15]

The quality of resistance encountered by the clinician at the end range of passive motion is referred to as the **end feel**. The end feel is evaluated for quality and tenderness, as it can indicate

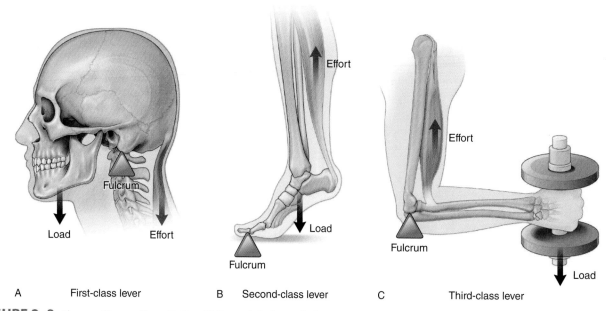

FIGURE 2–8 Classes of levers. (From Dutton M. *Dutton's Orthopaedic Examination, Evaluation and Intervention*. 4th ed. New York, NY: McGraw-Hill, 2017.)

TABLE 2-7   Differential features of OKC and CKC exercises.

Exercise Mode	Characteristics	Advantages	Disadvantages
Open kinematic chain	1. Single muscle group 2. Single axis and plane 3. Emphasizes concentric contraction 4. Non-weightbearing	1. Isolated recruitment 2. Simple movement pattern 3. Minimal joint compression	1. Limited function 2. Limited eccentrics 3. Less proprioception and joint stability with increased joint shear forces
Closed kinematic chain	1. Multiple muscle groups 2. Multiple axes and planes 3. Balance of concentric and eccentric contractions 4. Weight-bearing exercises	1. Functional recruitment 2. Functional movement patterns 3. Functional contractions 4. Increased proprioception and joint stability	1. Difficult to isolate 2. More complex 3. Loss of control of target joint 4. Compressive forces on articular surfaces

Data from Greenfield BH, Tovin BJ. The application of open and closed kinematic chain exercises in rehabilitation of the lower extremity. *J Back Musculoskel Rehabil.* 1992;2:38-51.

TABLE 2-8   Close-packed position of the joints.

Joint	Position
Zygapophyseal (spine)	Extension
Temporomandibular	Teeth clenched
Glenohumeral	Abduction and external rotation
Acromioclavicular	Arm abducted to 90°
Sternoclavicular	Maximum shoulder elevation
Ulnohumeral	Extension
Radiohumeral	Elbow flexed 90°; forearm supinated 5°
Proximal radioulnar	5° of supination
Distal radioulnar	5° of supination
Radiocarpal (wrist)	Extension with radial deviation
Metacarpophalangeal	Full flexion
Carpometacarpal	Full opposition
Interphalangeal	Full extension
Hip	Full extension, internal rotation, and abduction
Tibiofemoral	Full extension and external rotation of tibia
Talocrural (ankle)	Maximum dorsiflexion
Subtalar	Supination
Midtarsal	Supination
Tarsometatarsal	Supination
Metatarsophalangeal	Full extension
Interphalangeal	Full extension

TABLE 2-9   Open-packed (resting) position of the joints.

Joint	Position
Zygapophyseal (spine)	Midway between flexion and extension
Temporomandibular	Mouth slightly open (freeway space)
Glenohumeral	55° of abduction, 30° of horizontal adduction
Acromioclavicular	Arm resting by side
Sternoclavicular	Arm resting by side
Ulnohumeral	70° of flexion, 10° of supination
Radiohumeral	Full extension, full supination
Proximal radioulnar	70° of flexion, 35° of supination
Distal radioulnar	10° of supination
Radiocarpal (wrist)	Neutral with slight ulnar deviation
Carpometacarpal	Midway between abduction-adduction and flexion-extension
Metacarpophalangeal	Slight flexion
Interphalangeal	Slight flexion
Hip	30° of flexion, 30° of abduction, slight lateral rotation
Tibiofemoral	25° of flexion
Talocrural (ankle)	10° of plantar flexion, midway between maximum inversion and eversion
Subtalar	Midway between extremes of range of movement
Midtarsal	Midway between extremes of range of movement
Tarsometatarsal	Midway between extremes of range of movement
Metatarsophalangeal	Neutral
Interphalangeal	Slight flexion

TABLE 2–10 Capsular patterns of restriction.

Joint	Limitation of Motion (Passive Angular Motion)
Glenohumeral	External rotation > abduction > internal rotation (3:2:1)
Acromioclavicular	No true capsular pattern; possible loss of horizontal adduction and pain (and sometimes slight loss of end range) with each motion
Sternoclavicular	See acromioclavicular joint
Humeroulnar	Flexion > extension (±4:1)
Humeroradial	No true capsular pattern; possible equal limitation of pronation and supination
Superior radioulnar	No true capsular pattern; possible equal limitation of pronation and supination with pain at end ranges
Inferior radioulnar	No true capsular pattern; possible equal limitation of pronation and supination with pain at end ranges
Wrist (carpus)	Flexion = extension
Radiocarpal	See wrist (carpus)
Carpometacarpal	Flexion = extension
Midcarpal	Flexion = extension
Carpometacarpal 1	Retroposition
Carpometacarpals 2–5	Fan > fold
Metacarpophalangeal 2–5	Flexion > extension (±2:1)
Interphalangeal 2–5 Proximal (PIP) Distal (DIP)	Flexion > extension (±2:1) Flexion > extension (±2:1)
Hip	Internal rotation > flexion > abduction = extension > other motions
Tibiofemoral	Flexion > extension (±5:1)
Superior tibiofibular	No capsular pattern; pain at end range of translatory movements
Talocrural	Plantar flexion > dorsiflexion
Talocalcaneal (subtalar)	Varus > valgus
Midtarsal	Inversion (plantar flexion, adduction, and supination)
Talonavicular calcaneocuboid	> Dorsiflexion
Metatarsophalangeal 1	Extension > flexion (±2:1)
Metatarsophalangeals 2–5	Flexion ≥ extension
Interphalangeals 2–5 Proximal Distal	Flexion ≥ extension Flexion ≥ extension

Data from Cyriax J. *Textbook of Orthopaedic Medicine, Diagnosis of Soft Tissue Lesions.* 8th ed. London: Bailliere Tindall, 1982.

to the clinician the cause of the motion restriction (Tables 2–11 and 2–12).

The term **arc of pain** is used to describe an occurrence of temporary pain during active or passive motion that disappears before the end of the movement. The presence of a painful arc indicates that some structure is being compressed:

- A painful arc that occurs in association with a positive resistive test (for pain) usually indicates a contractile lesion.
- A painful arc that occurs in association with a negative resistive test (for pain) usually indicates an inert lesion.

TABLE 2–11 **Normal end feels.**

Type	Cause	Characteristics and Examples
Bony	Produced by bone-to-bone approximation	Abrupt and unyielding; gives impression that further forcing will break something *Examples:* Normal: elbow extension Abnormal: cervical rotation (may indicate osteophyte)
Elastic	Produced by muscle–tendon unit; may occur with adaptive shortening	Stretches with elastic recoil and exhibits constant-length phenomenon; further forcing feels as if it will snap something *Examples:* Normal: wrist flexion with finger flexion, the straight-leg raise, and ankle dorsiflexion with the knee extended Abnormal: decreased dorsiflexion of the ankle with the knee flexed
Soft-tissue approximation	Produced by contact of two muscle bulks on either side of a flexing joint where joint range exceeds other restraints	Very forgiving end feel that gives impression that further normal motion is possible if enough force could be applied *Examples:* Normal: knee flexion and elbow flexion in extremely muscular subjects Abnormal: elbow flexion with obese subject
Capsular	Produced by capsule or ligaments	Various degrees of stretch without elasticity; the ability to stretch is dependent on thickness of tissue Strong capsular or extracapsular ligaments produce a hard capsular end feel, whereas a thin capsule produces a softer one Impression given to clinician is that if further force is applied, something will tear *Examples:* Normal: wrist flexion (soft), elbow flexion in supination (medium), and knee extension (hard) Abnormal: inappropriate stretchability for a specific joint; if too hard, may indicate hypomobility due to arthrosis; and if too soft, hypermobility

Data from Meadows JTS. *Manual Therapy: Biomechanical Assessment and Treatment, Advanced Technique.* Calgary: Swodeam Consulting; 1995.

TABLE 2–12 **Abnormal end feels.**

Type	Causes	Characteristics and Examples
Springy	Produced by articular surface rebounding from intra-articular meniscus or disk; impression is that if forced further, something will give way	Rebound sensation as if pushing off from a rubber pad *Examples:* Normal: axial compression of cervical spine Abnormal: knee flexion or extension with displaced meniscus
Boggy	Produced by viscous fluid (blood) within joint	"Squishy" sensation as joint is moved toward its end range; further forcing feels as if it will burst joint *Examples:* Normal: none Abnormal: hemarthrosis at knee
Spasm	Produced by reflex and reactive muscle contraction in response to irritation of nociceptor, predominantly in articular structures and muscle; forcing it further feels as if nothing will give	Abrupt and "twangy" end to movement that is unyielding while the structure is being threatened but disappears when threat is removed (kicks back) With joint inflammation, it occurs early in range, especially toward close-packed position, to prevent further stress With irritable joint hypermobility, it occurs at the end of what should be normal range, as it prevents excessive motion from further stimulating the nociceptor Spasm in grade II muscle tears becomes apparent as muscle is passively lengthened and is accompanied by a painful weakness of that muscle *Note:* Muscle guarding is not a true end feel, as it involves co-contraction *Examples:* Normal: none Abnormal: significant traumatic arthritis, recent traumatic hypermobility, and grade II muscle tears

(Continued)

TABLE 2–12 Abnormal end feels. (*Continued*)

Type	Causes	Characteristics and Examples

Empty	Produced solely by pain; frequently caused by serious and severe pathologic changes that do not affect joint or muscle and so do not produce spasm; demonstration of this end feel is, with the exception of acute subdeltoid bursitis, de facto evidence of serious pathology; further forcing simply increases pain to unacceptable levels	Limitation of motion has no tissue resistance component, and resistance is from patient being unable to tolerate further motion due to severe pain; it is not the same feeling as voluntary guarding, but rather it feels as if patient is both resisting and trying to allow movement simultaneously
		Examples:
		  Normal: none
		  Abnormal: acute subdeltoid bursitis and sign of the buttock

Facilitation	Not truly an end feel, as facilitated hypertonicity does not restrict motion; it can, however, be perceived near end range	Light resistance as from constant light muscle contraction throughout latter half of range that does not prevent end of range being reached; resistance is unaffected by rate of movement
		Examples:
		  Normal: none
		  Abnormal: spinal facilitation at any level

Data from Meadows JTS. *Manual Therapy: Biomechanical Assessment and Treatment, Advanced Technique.* Calgary: Swodeam Consulting; 1995.

A joint can be described as being normal, **hypomobile**, **hypermobile**, or **unstable**.

- *Hypomobile.* A joint that moves less than what is considered normal, or when compared to the same joint on the opposite extremity. A contracture of CT may cause hypomobility. The presence of hypomobility in the absence of contraindications is an indication for joint mobilizations as the intervention of choice.

- *Hypermobile.* A joint that moves more than is considered normal when compared to the same joint on the opposite extremity. May occur as a generalized phenomenon or be localized to just one direction of movement—the result of damaged CT. The presence of hypermobility is a contraindication to joint mobilizations.

- *Unstable.* An unstable joint involves a disruption of the osseous and ligamentous structures of that joint and results in a loss of function. Joint instability is a factor of joint integrity, elastic energy, passive stiffness, and muscle activation.

QUESTIONS

1. Which of the following best describes the characteristics of hyaline cartilage?
   A. Distributes forces, is avascular and aneural, and is located in diarthrotic joints.
   B. Distributes forces, is highly vascular, contains free-nerve endings, and is located in fibrocartilaginous joints.
   C. Resists compressive forces, is highly vascular and aneural, and is located within synovial joints.
   D. Resist compressive forces, is avascular, contains free-nerve endings, and is located in synarthrodial joints.

2. Which type of connective tissue (CT) in the musculoskeletal system is made up of dense CT and provides joint stability and proprioceptive input?
   A. Fascia
   B. Tendons
   C. Ligaments
   D. Cartilage

3. Which of the following joint categories best describes the classification of the intermetatarsal joint?
   A. Spheroid
   B. Trochoid
   C. Planar
   D. Saddle

4. A patient performing a bicep curl with a 10-lb weight in his/her hand is an example of which type of lever?
   A. First-class lever
   B. Second-class lever
   C. Third-class lever
   D. Fourth-class lever

5. After the initial lengthening caused by crimp, what is the term that describes the gradual rearrangement of collagen fibers, proteoglycans, and water that occurs as result of a continuously applied force?
   A. Creep
   B. Tension
   C. Stress-strain curve
   D. Elasticity

6. What is the protein that fibroblasts produce?
   A. Albumin
   B. Collagen
   C. Actin
   D. Myosin

7. The heel raise exercise (rising up on the toes) is an example of this type of lever.
   A. First-class lever
   B. Second-class lever
   C. Third-class lever
   D. Fourth-class lever

ANSWERS

1. The answer is **A**. Hyaline cartilage contains no nerves or blood vessels and is found on the anterior ends of ribs, in the larynx, trachea, and bronchi, and on the articulating surfaces of bones.

2. The answer is **C**. Ligaments function as check-reins to joint motion.

3. The answer is **C**. The intermetatarsal joints, which are a good example of a planar joint, are the articulations between the base of metatarsal bones.

4. The answer is **C**. The third-class lever has the input force between the output force and the fulcrum. The elbow joint is the fulcrum, the 10-lb weight is the resistance/load, and the force is the biceps muscle when the elbow is flexed.

5. The answer is **A**. Creep is the time dependent elongation of a tissue when subjected to a constant stress.

6. The answer is **B**. Fibroblasts are cells within connective tissue that synthesize the extracellular matrix and form collagen.

7. The answer is **B**. A second-class lever has the fulcrum at one end, the effort (which is always less than the load) on the opposite end, and the load in the middle.

■ SECTION 2: TISSUE RESPONSE TO INJURY

Maintaining the health of the various tissues is a delicate balance because insufficient, excessive, or repetitive stresses can prove deleterious. Fortunately, most tissues have an inherent ability to self-heal—a process that is an intricate phenomenon.

TISSUE INJURY

The two major types of tissue injury are as follows:

- Macrotrauma (primary). An acute stress (loading) of a single force that is large enough to cause injury to biological tissues. Can be self-inflicted, caused by another individual or entity, or caused by the environment.[16-19] The acute stress/load is sufficient to cause injury to biological tissues.
- Microtrauma (secondary). This type of injury occurs when repeated or chronic stress over a period of time causes an injury. It is primarily the inflammatory response that occurs with a primary insult.[20] Microtrauma can also result from repetitive stress/loading insufficient to cause damage to the biological tissue itself but can cause an injury over time. Microtraumatic injuries include tendinopathy, tenosynovitis, and bursitis. Can be intrinsic or extrinsic:
  - Intrinsic factors: Physical characteristics that predispose an individual to microtrauma injuries, for example, muscle imbalances, leg length discrepancies, anatomical anomalies.
  - Extrinsic factors: The most common cause of microtrauma. Related to external conditions by which the activity is performed, for example, training errors, type of terrain, environmental temperature, or incorrect use of equipment.

An injury to the musculoskeletal system can be classified as follows:

- Acute. Acute injuries are usually caused by macrotrauma or refer to the early phase of injury and healing, the latter of which typically lasts 4 to 6 days. An acute injury is characterized by:
  - Swelling (due to an increase in the permeability of the venules, plasma proteins, and leukocytes, which leak into the site of injury)
  - Redness
  - Heat
  - Impairment or loss of function

High-Yield Terms to Learn

Macrotrauma	Typically a severity of force sufficient to cause an immediate injury.
Microtrauma	Typically lacks enough force to cause an immediate injury.
Injury classifications	Acute, subacute, chronic, and acute on chronic.
Stages of healing	Coagulation and inflammation (acute), migratory and proliferative (subacute), and remodeling (chronic).
Osteoarthritis	A disease process resulting from the failure of chondrocytes to repair damaged articular cartilage in synovial joints.
Osteoporosis	A disease process in which new bone creation does not keep up with old bone removal.
Sarcopenia	Refers specifically to the universal, involuntary decline in lean body mass that can occur with age, primarily as a result of the loss of skeletal muscle volume.

In the presence of an acute injury, there is typically pain at rest or with active motion, or when specific stress is applied to the injured structure.

- Subacute. A subacute injury typically lasts 10 to 17 days after the acute phase has ended, but it can last for weeks in tissues with limited circulation (ie, tendons). From a clinical perspective, the "active" swelling and local erythema of the inflammatory stage is usually no longer present. However, residual swelling may still be present at this time and resist reabsorption.
- Chronic. The chronic stage of healing has several definitions but usually refers to the final stage of healing, which occurs 26 to 34 days after injury but can last up to 1 year depending on the amount of damage and the type of tissue involved. Because this phase may last several months or even years, it is extremely important to continue applying controlled stresses to the tissue long after healing appears to have occurred.[21]
- Acute on chronic. This is not a normal stage of healing but an acute exacerbation of a chronic condition.

TISSUE HEALING

Some of the factors that can impact healing include:

- Extent of the injury. Macrotears cause more tissue having to be repaired
- Age. The ability to heal decreases with age
- Drugs. Nonsteroidal anti-inflammatory drugs (NSAIDs) and corticosteroids reduce inflammation and swelling, but the latter must be used judiciously
- Edema. Increased pressure can impede nutrition and inhibit neuromuscular control
- Obesity. Oxygen pressure is lower
- Absorbent dressings. The epithelium regenerates twice as quickly in a moist environment
- Hemorrhage. Similar negative effects to edema
- Malnutrition. Need protein and vitamins essential for healing
- Temperature. Hypothermia has an adverse effect on healing
- Poor vascular supply. Inadequate nutrition to healing tissues
- Hormone levels. Affect composition and structure of tissues
- Infection. Inhibits healing processes
- Muscle spasm. Causes tension in already torn tissue; impedes approximation
- Comorbidities. Pre-existing conditions such as diabetes, obesity, congestive heart failure can hinder tissue healing
- Excessive scarring. Can reduce blood flow

Three major stages of healing are recognized in Table 2–13.

SPECIFIC TISSUE BEHAVIOR, INJURY, HEALING, AND TREATMENT

The various musculoskeletal tissues respond and heal based on morphology.

Muscle

Behavior

Muscle behaves in a variety of ways in response to stress/injury, each of which depends on the following:

TABLE 2–13 Stages of wound healing.

Stage	General Characteristics
Coagulation and inflammation (acute)	Area is red, warm, swollen, and painful Pain is present without any motion of involved area Usually lasts 48–72 hours, but can last as long as 7–10 days
Migratory and proliferative (subacute)	Pain usually occurs with activity or motion of involved area Usually lasts 10 days to 6 weeks
Remodeling (chronic)	Pain usually occurs after activity Usually lasts 6 weeks to 12 months

- Age. There is decreased cross-sectional area of muscle, with decreased type II fibers being the most impacted. This loss can be minimized or reversed with exercise. A particular type of muscle fiber atrophy can occur with aging (senescence sarcopenia), resulting in a 20% to 25% loss of skeletal mass and a reduced power output from the muscles.
- Temperature. There is an inverse temperature-elastic modulus relationship whereby increased temperature results in increased elasticity and decreased stiffness.
- Immobilization or disuse. If a muscle is immobilized in a shortened position, it becomes less capable of producing force, and its shorter length makes it more susceptible to a stretching injury. In contrast, if a muscle is immobilized in its lengthened position, it is capable of producing greater force and a more significant change in length is required to cause a tear than in a nonimmobilized muscle.

Injury

Muscle strains are the most common injury in sports. A muscle injury can be classified in a number of ways, based on severity (Table 2–14). Some factors that contribute to muscle injury include the following:

- Inadequate flexibility
- Inadequate strength or endurance
- Dyssynergistic muscle contraction
- Insufficient warmup
- Inadequate rehabilitation from a previous injury

Healing

A muscle tends to heal in three phases:

- Destruction phase. This phase is associated with muscle atrophy, with the amount of atrophy dependent on the usage before the injury and the original function of the muscle. Antigravity muscles (eg, quadriceps) are more prone to atrophy than antagonist muscles (eg, hamstrings). Research has demonstrated that a single bout of exercise can protect against muscle damage, with the effects lasting between 6 and 9 months.
- Repair phase. This phase typically involves three steps: hematoma formation, matrix formation, and collagen formation.

TABLE 2–14 Classification of muscle injury.

Type	Related Factors
Exercise-induced muscle injury (delayed muscle soreness)	Increased activity Unaccustomed activity Excessive eccentric work Viral infections Secondary to muscle cell damage
Strains First degree (mild): minimal structural damage; minimal hemorrhage; early resolution	Onset at 24–48 hours after exercise Sudden overstretch Sudden contraction
Second degree (moderate): partial tear; large spectrum of injury; significant early functional loss	Decelerating limb Insufficient warmup Lack of flexibility
Third degree (severe): complete tear; may require aspiration; may require surgery	Increasing severity of strain associated with greater muscle fiber death, more hemorrhage, and more eventual scarring Steroid use or abuse Previous muscle injury Collagen disease
Contusions Mild, moderate, severe Intramuscular vs. intermuscular	Direct blow, associated with increasing muscle trauma and tearing of fiber proportionate to severity

Data from Reid DC. *Sports Injury Assessment and Rehabilitation*. New York, NY: Churchill Livingstone;1992.

- Remodeling phase. During this phase, the application of controlled mobility and stress is necessary for proper healing.

Treatment

The type of treatment to use for a muscle injury depends on the stage of healing. All or some of the following can be used:

- Prevention and patient education.
- Controlled mobility and activity.
- Medications (pain and anti-inflammatory) and modalities.
- Exercise progression initiated with PROM, then active assisted range of motion (AAROM), then active range of motion (AROM), then submaximal isometrics in protective range, then work throughout range, then maximum isometrics in multiangles, then throughout the whole range, then progressive resisted exercises (PREs).

Tendon

Behavior

Because the collagen fibers are more parallel in tendons than they are in ligaments, the toe-region of the stress-strain curve is smaller in tendons than ligaments since less realignment occurs. The MTJ is the weakest point in the muscle-tendon unit, therefore strain injuries are more common here.

Injury

A number of terms were used for tendon injuries, including tendinosis, and tendinitis. These terms have recently been encompassed into the umbrella term of tendinopathy:

- Tendinopathy. A clinical syndrome characterized by pain, swelling, and impaired performance, often implying overuse of a tendon. The continuum model of tendon pathology, proposed in 2009, synthesized clinical and laboratory-based research to guide treatment choices for the clinical presentations of tendinopathy, but as yet, the identity of a nociceptive driver in tendinopathy remains elusive.[22] In addition, histological evidence consistently demonstrates an absence of prostaglandin-mediated inflammation. Thus, it would appear that tendinopathy is a heterogeneous clinical presentation due to the variable change in the matrix structure, pain, and dysfunction.[23] The most common tendinopathies occur at the patellar and Achilles tendons in the lower extremity, and at the supraspinatus tendon and extensor carpi radialis brevis (ECRB) tendons in the upper extremity. In the presence of a tendinopathy, there is a net loss of collagen that peaks at 24 to 36 hours after exercise, which implies that the need for restitution time interval between exercise bouts is critical for the tissue to adapt and avoid a catabolic situation. In general, tendons become weaker, stiffer, and less yielding with age. In addition, prolonged immobilization of a tendon results in a decrease in tensile strength, increased stiffness, and a reduction in total weight.

Stages of Healing

A tendon heals during a number of stages.

- Inflammatory response (but only if the acute tendon injury disrupts vascular tissues within the tendon). During this phase, a hematoma forms within erythrocytes and platelets, and there is an infiltration of inflammatory cells.
- Repair. Deposition of collagen and tendon matrix components.
- Remodeling. Collagen structure and organization. It is worth noting that an injured tendon never achieves the original histologic or mechanical features it initially had.

Treatment

The treatment approach for tendons has changed over the years. There is no longer an emphasis on anti-inflammatory strategies since studies have consistently shown an absence of inflammatory infiltrates with tendinopathy. The following approach is currently recommended:

- Eccentric exercises. This type of exercise produces about 20% more load on the tendon than concentric training. An incremental load-based rehabilitation program is capable of modifying the balance of excitability and inhibition in muscle control, thus altering the loads transmitted by the tendon.[22]
- Pain control—modalities and isometric exercises. A recent study[24] reported that a single resistance training bout of isometric contractions reduced tendon pain immediately for at least 45 minutes postintervention.
- Addressing the entire kinetic chain.
- Identification and removal of all negative internal and external forces/factors.

- Extracorporeal shockwave therapy, NSAIDs, sclerosing treatments, platelet-rich plasma (PRP), nitric oxide, matrix metalloproteinase inhibitors (aim to decrease the catabolic enzymatic activity in tendinosis lesions).

Ligament

Behavior

A ligament loses mass, stiffness, structural strength, and viscosity with age. In addition, loss of ligament strength and stiffness occurs with low deprivation. In contrast, movement/exercise can maintain and enhance ligament strength and stiffness.

Injury (Sprains)

Ligament injuries typically occur when an applied load is sufficient to deform a taut ligament beyond its elastic (recovery) limit. A ligament injury is characterized by:

- Point tenderness
- Joint effusion
- History of trauma

If sufficient, damage to ligament can result in loss of joint stability. The classification of ligament injuries is outlined in Table 2–15.

Stages of Healing

The process of healing for ligaments is essentially the same as for other vascular tissues. However, intraarticular ligaments (ie, the anterior cruciate ligament [ACL]) do not heal as well as extraarticular ligaments due to the limited blood supply and the presence of synovial fluid, which can hinder the inflammatory process. Normal healing occurs in four phases: hemorrhagic (hematoma fills the tissue gap), inflammatory (influx of macrophages and growth factors), proliferation (fibroblasts to produce collagen and the initial matrix), and remodeling/maturation (organization of matrix). Although the healing tissue matures, it never regains preinjury/normal quality. Total healing can take as long as 3 years—a ligament may reach 50% of its normal tensile strength by 6 months and 80% after 1 year.

Treatment

The treatment of a ligament injury depends on the location and severity but generally follows these guidelines:

- Minimization of immobilization time. A prolonged period of immobilization dramatically compromises the properties of ligaments.
- Controlled mobility. Very low cyclical loads make ligaments stronger and structurally stiffer.
- Transverse friction massage (TFM). TFM appears to improve collagen fiber bundle formation and orientation within the scar region[25] and increase regional perfusion and vascularity in the vicinity of healing[26] more than nontreated ligaments, but may have minimal effect on the outcome of healing.[25]

More invasive techniques include:

- Surgical repair
- Growth factors
- Gene therapy

Articular Cartilage

Behavior

In general, articular cartilage demonstrates low metabolic activity and poor regenerative capacity. The majority of nutrition for articular cartilage occurs through diffusion from synovial fluid.

TABLE 2–15 Ligament injuries.

Grade	Description	Signs and Symptoms	Implications
I (mild)	Some stretching or tearing of the ligamentous fibers	Mild pain Little or no swelling Some joint stiffness Minimal loss of structural integrity No abnormal motion Minimal bruising	Minimal functional loss Early return to training—some protection may be necessary
II (moderate)	Some tearing and separation of the ligamentous fibers	Moderate to severe pain Joint stiffness Significant structural weakening with abnormal motion Often associated hemarthrosis and effusion	Tendency to recurrence Need protection from risk of further injury May need modified immobilization May stretch out further with time
III (complete)	Total rupture of the ligament	Severe pain initially followed by little or no pain (total disruption of nerve fibers) Profuse swelling and bruising Loss of structural integrity with marked abnormal motion	Needs prolonged protection Surgery may be considered Often permanent functional instability

Chondrocyte activity depends on anaerobic metabolism. With increasing age there is a decrease in hydration of matrix and an increase in stiffness, resulting in increased stresses to subchondral bone. In addition, immobilization results in degenerative changes similar to those found in osteoarthritis (OA).

Injury

As articular cartilage is avascular, there is no inflammatory phase of healing. Degradation of articular cartilage occurs because of an imbalance between extracellular matrix (ECM) synthesis and degradation (eg, OA). Stress deprivation (eg, immobilization or bed rest) can have a similar effect. Other causes of articular cartilage damage include:

- Developmental etiologies leading to an abnormal force transmission (eg, hip dysplasia, coxa valgus, genu valgum)
- Joint surface incongruity and instability
- Disease (eg, rheumatoid arthritis [RA])

   Three major types of injury are typically cited:

- Type I: Superficial. Characterized by microscopic damage to chondrocytes and ECM (cell injury).
- Type II: Partial thickness. Characterized by microscopic disruption of the chondral surface (chondral fractures or fissuring). This type has a poorer prognosis due to the lack of penetration of the subchondral bone and therefore no inflammatory response.
- Type III: Full thickness. Characterized by disruption of the articular cartilage with infiltration of the subchondral bone and significant inflammatory response.

Healing

- Limited capacity, dependent on depth of injury
- Type I and II tissues become necrotic and do not repair; progress to degeneration
- Type III tissues undergo repair as result of access to bone blood supply
  - Repaired tissue is different than normal hyaline cartilage; 50% result in fibrillation, fissuring, and extensive degenerative changes
  - Degenerated cartilage in OA does not usually undergo repair but instead progressively degenerates

Treatment

The treatment approach for articular cartilage varies, but typically includes a combination of the following:

- Exhaustion of conservative measures to avoid significant reconstructive surgery. Typical conservative measures include attempts to decrease joint pain and improve function through modalities, patient education, low-impact aerobic exercise, and ROM and strengthening exercises.
- Pharmacological pain control (NSAIDs, opioid analgesics, intraarticular corticosteroid injections)
- Unloading braces to decrease joint stress
- Intraarticular viscosupplementation
- Mesenchymal stem cells
- Surgical management

Bone

Behavior

Bone tissue reacts well to compression but not to tension. The health of bone matrix, which is an organic mineral, and fluid is influenced by diet, hormone levels, and biomechanics. In particular, exercise has been shown to result in increased cortical thickness and mineral content.

Injury

In general, injury to bone tissue involves some form of fracture. The most commonly encountered fracture for the physical therapist is the stress fracture, a fatigue fracture of the bone caused by repeated submaximal stress. Eighty percent to 90% of stress fractures occur in the lower limb, with the tibia being most common site (50%). The diagnostic indicators for stress fractures include:

- X-rays; however, a fracture is often not apparent if x-rays are taken too early in the course
- Bone scan
- Magnetic resonance imaging (MRI)

   Some diseases, including osteoarthritis and osteoporosis, can cause bone (pathological) fractures.

Healing

The healing of bone occurs through repair of the original tissue, and not by scar tissue. Two types of bone healing are recognized:

- Primary (cortical). Cortical healing unites cortex.
- Secondary (callus). Responses occur in the periosteum and external soft tissues with subsequent formation of callus. The majority of fractures heal by secondary fracture healing.

   The stages of bone healing include:

- Hematoma formation (inflammatory) phase
- Soft callus formation (reparative or revascularization) phase
- Hard callus formation (modeling) phase
- Remodeling phase

   The determinants of fracture healing include the following:

- Angiogenesis.
- The amount of movement at the fracture ends. Small degrees of micromotion aid in healing due to stimulation of blood flow, but excessive motion prevents the establishment of intramedullary blood vessel bridging.
- Environment.
- Hormones impact osteoblastic and osteoclastic activities.

   The following techniques are occasionally required to augment healing:

- Pulsed electromagnetic fields (PEMF); stimulates cellular repair
- Pulsed ultrasound
- Direct current
- Demineralized bone matrix (DBM)

Treatment

The treatment for bone fracture depends on the site and level of severity, but typically includes some or all of the following:

- Stabilization of the fracture site through casting. During this period, submaximum isometrics are introduced and progressed to ROM exercises once a clinical union is confirmed.
- Surgery, if indicated. Postsurgical complications can include:
  - Infection
  - Deep vein thrombosis (DVT)
  - Pulmonary embolism (PE)
  - Poor wound healing
  - Scars and adhesions

QUESTIONS

1. The primary cells involved in the proliferation phase of healing are:
   A. Fibroblasts
   B. Macrophages
   C. Leukocytes
   D. Osteoclasts

2. If a patient sustained an injury 18 days ago and progressed appropriately through the phases of healing, what is the expected stage of healing?
   A. Coagulation
   B. Inflammatory
   C. Proliferative
   D. Remodeling

3. Which of the following tissues requires satellite cells to proliferate for proper healing to occur?
   A. Tendon
   B. Ligament
   C. Bone
   D. Muscle

4. Which of the following is an age-associated change in tissue?
   A. Decreased muscle power
   B. Increased number of sarcomeres in series
   C. Increased crimp in a tendon
   D. Decreased stiffness of tendinous tissue

5. Which of the following tissues responds best to very low cyclic loading to promote scar proliferation and material remodeling?
   A. Muscle
   B. Tendon
   C. Ligament
   D. Bone

ANSWERS

1. 1. The answer is **A**. Fibroblasts produce the structural framework for tissues during wound healing.

2. The answer is **C**. The proliferative phase of wound healing, which occurs approximately after 3 days and lasts for 21 days, involves the rebuilding of the wound with new tissue made up of collagen and extracellular matrix.

3. The answer is **D**. Satellite cells are precursors to skeletal muscle cells.

4. The answer is **A**. Decreased muscle power is the only one that occurs from the choices given. The decrease in muscle power can be reduced with strengthening exercises.

5. The answer is **C**. Ligaments require controlled motion to heal effectively.

■ SECTION 3: ENERGY SYSTEMS

Physical activity has been defined as "any bodily movement produced by the contraction of skeletal muscles that results in a substantial increase in resting energy expenditure."[27] When a person undertakes work or exercise, some of the body systems adapt to the demands of the required tasks, particularly the cardiorespiratory and neuromuscular systems.[28]

High-Yield Terms to Learn

Aerobic	Relating to or denoting exercise that improves or is intended to improve the efficiency of the body's cardiovascular system in absorbing and transporting oxygen. Refers to the use of oxygen to adequately meet energy demands during exercise via aerobic metabolism.
Anaerobic	A metabolism that does not depend on oxygen. An aerobic exercise is powered primarily by metabolic pathways that do not use oxygen. Such pathways produce lactic acid, resulting in metabolic acidosis. Examples of anaerobic exercise include sprinting and heavy weight lifting.
Adenosine triphosphate (ATP)	ATP is the energy currency of life. ATP is a high-energy molecule found in every cell. Its job is to store and supply the cell with needed energy.
Phosphocreatine (PCr)	Phosphocreatine, also known as creatine phosphate, is an energy source for muscle contraction naturally present in the skeletal muscle tissue of humans and other vertebrates. It enables the expression of explosive power in the muscles, lasting no longer than 8 to 12 seconds.

TYPES OF ENERGY

- Phosphagen (ATP-PCr) system. Used during anaerobic, ATP-PCr, short-term, high-energy activities; primary energy source first 10 seconds of short, intense activities; active at the start of all exercise; small maximum capacity.
- Glycolytic system. Glycolysis is the metabolic pathway by which glucose is converted into two pyruvates. The pathway involves an anaerobic, carbohydrate breakdown (glycogen in muscle or glucose in the blood) into pyruvate to produce ATP through glycolysis, which is then transformed into lactic acid through anaerobic glycolysis. This system is slower to become fully active than the ATP-PCr system but has a greater capacity to provide energy, so it supplements the ATP-PCr system during maximum exercise.
  - The complete combustion of glucose requires the presence of oxygen and yields 32 ATP for each molecule of glucose.
  - Some energy can be obtained in the absence of oxygen by the pathway that leads to the production of lactic acid. This process results in a net gain of 2 ATP for each glucose molecule (eg, running 400–800 m).
- Oxidative system. An aerobic system that requires O_2, glycogens, fats, and proteins. This is the primary energy source at rest and low-intensity activities. The relative contributions to ATP production for this system are:
  - 0 to 10 seconds: ATP-PCr (phosphagen) system
  - 10 to 30 seconds: ATP-PCr plus anaerobic glycolysis
  - 30 seconds to 2 minutes: Anaerobic glycolysis
  - 2 to 3 minutes: Anaerobic glycolysis plus oxidative
  - >3 minutes: Oxidative

SKILL KEEPER QUESTIONS

1. *A patient is training for a track meet, and he begins to run. Which energy system is predominantly used in the first 10 seconds of his run? Which is used in the next 30 seconds?*

2. *To increase force production, should a patient increase or decrease his speed with an eccentrically-biased exercise or with a concentrically-biased exercise?*

3. *If you are developing an exercise program for a marathon runner with back pain would you want to bias your program toward type I or type II muscle fibers? What about for a sprinter with a quadriceps injury?*

SKILL KEEPER ANSWERS

1. *First 10 seconds: ATP-PCr; next 30 seconds: ATP-PCr + anaerobic glycolysis.*

2. *Increased speed produces more force with an eccentric exercise provided the patient maintains control of the lengthening (ie, they do not allow gravity to lower the weight). With a concentric-biased exercise, the opposite is true; more force production is achieved with slower speeds, partly due to the tendency to use momentum with faster concentric exercises (Figure 2–9). Therefore, eccentric activities will increase force production with increasing speed and concentric activities will increase force production with slower speeds.*

3. *Marathon runner: Type I muscle fibers need to be recruited for the endurance muscles (postural trunk muscles) so the aerobic energy system has to be stimulated. Sprinter: Type II because now training the quadriceps muscles which are dynamic, phasic, will need to work more on the anaerobic energy system required for sprinting.*

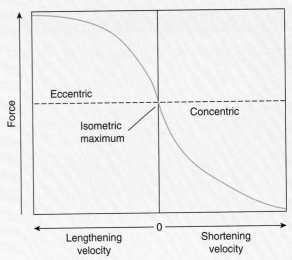

FIGURE 2–9 The force–velocity relationship for muscle tissue. When the resistance (force) is negligible, muscle contracts with maximal velocity. As the load progressively increases, concentric contraction velocity slows to zero at isometric maximum. As the load increases further, the muscle lengthens eccentrically. (From Hall SJ. *Basic Biomechanics*. 7th ed. New York, NY: McGraw-Hill Education, 2015.)

■ SECTION 4: FUNCTIONAL ANATOMY AND BIOMECHANICS OF SPECIFIC JOINTS

An understanding of the functional anatomy and biomechanics of the various joint complexes is essential for every examination and intervention.

SHOULDER COMPLEX

The shoulder complex (Figure 2–10) is composed of four articulations:

- The glenohumeral (G-H) joint
- The acromioclavicular (A-C) joint
- The sternoclavicular (S-C) joint
- The scapulothoracic pseudoarticulation

A fifth "articulation"—the subacromial articulation between the coracoacromial arch (a rigid structure above the humeral head and rotator cuff tendons) and the rotator cuff tendons—is included by some authors.[29]

The blood supply to the shoulder complex comes from a number of arteries (Figure 2–11), but primarily from the anterior and posterior circumflex humeral arteries and the suprascapular artery.

The shoulder complex is embryologically derived from C5 to C8, except the A-C joint, which is derived from C4.[30-32] The sympathetic nerve supply to the shoulder originates primarily in the thoracic region from T2 down as far as T8.[33]

Glenohumeral Joint

- The convex humeral head articulates with the concave glenoid fossa of the scapula. The humeral head is retroverted 20° to 30°. The longitudinal axis of the head is 135° from the axis of the neck.
- The glenoid is retroverted approximately 7°. It faces anteriorly at an angle of approximately 45° to the coronal plane, as it sits on the chest wall. The depth of the glenoid fossa is enhanced by the glenoid labrum, which can contribute up to 50% of the fossa's depth.

High-Yield Terms to Learn

Open and closed kinetic chain	The expression *kinematic chain* is used in rehabilitation to describe the function or activity of an extremity or trunk regarding a series of linked chains.
Scaption	The forward elevation of the arm in the scapular plane.
Scapulohumeral rhythm	During elevation of the arm overhead, approximately one-third of the motion occurs at the scapulothoracic joint and two-thirds occurs at the glenohumeral joint. The scapula rotates upwardly, externally rotates, and tilts posteriorly.
Scapular dyskinesia	Also referred to abnormal scapulohumeral rhythm, scapular winging, and scapular dysrhythmia; describes abnormal or atypical movement of the scapula during normal active motion tasks. The finding is common in patients with an unstable glenohumeral joint and in patients with impingement syndrome. A scapular dyskinesia may occur primary or secondary to shoulder impingement and instability.
Snapping scapula	Attributed to friction between the mobile scapula and its attached soft tissues and the relatively stable thoracic wall. Anatomic explanations for snapping scapula include thickened bursa, bone spurs on the scapula or a rib, and osteochondroma.
Hill-Sachs lesion	A compression fracture of the posterolateral aspect of the humeral head, which results from impact on the anteroinferior rim of the glenoid during an anterior dislocation of the shoulder.
Reverse Hill-Sachs lesion	Also referred to as a McLaughlin lesion, is defined as an impaction fracture of anteromedial aspect of the humeral head following a posterior dislocation of the humerus.
Bankart lesion	An avulsion or detachment of the anterior portion of the inferior glenohumeral ligament complex and glenoid labrum of the anterior rim of the glenoid. Bankart lesions can contribute to recurrent instability.
Superior labrum anterior and posterior (SLAP)	An injury to the glenoid labrum associated with overhead and throwing activities.
Myotome	A muscle or group of muscles served by a single nerve root. *Key muscle* is a better, more accurate term, as the muscles tested are the most representative of the supply from a particular segment.
Cubital tunnel	A fibroosseous canal through which the ulnar nerve passes. The volume of the cubital tunnel is greatest with the elbow held in extension, and the least in full elbow flexion.
The triangular space	Formed by the long head of the triceps laterally, the teres minor superiorly, and the teres major inferiorly. Through it passes the circumflex scapular artery, a branch of the scapular artery.
The quadrangular space	Formed by the shaft of the humerus laterally, the long head of the triceps medially, the teres minor muscle superiorly, and the teres major muscle inferiorly. Through it pass the axillary nerve and the posterior humeral circumflex artery.

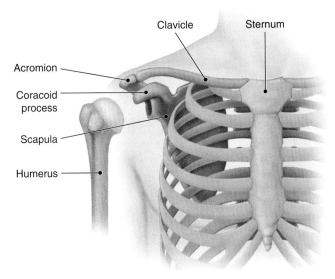

FIGURE 2–10 Skeletal structures of the shoulder complex.

- The scapula is a flat triangular bone, situated over the second through seventh ribs. The glenoid fossa is located on the lateral angle of the scapula and faces anterior, laterally and superiorly. This orientation places true abduction at 30° anterior to the frontal plane.
- An important bony landmark in the shoulder is the coracoid process, medial and lateral to which run the major blood vessels and brachial plexus. The coracoid serves as a muscular attachment for the pectoralis minor, the short head of the biceps, and the coracobrachialis.
- The ligaments of the shoulder complex (Table 2–16) function as static stabilizers during motion of the arm to reciprocally

TABLE 2–16 Major ligaments of the shoulder.

Joint	Ligament	Function
Shoulder complex	Coracoclavicular	Fixes the clavicle to the coracoid process.
	Costoclavicular	Fixes the clavicle to the costal cartilage of the first rib.
Glenohumeral	Coracohumeral	Reinforces the upper portion of the joint capsule.
	Glenohumeral ("Z")	Reinforces the anterior and inferior aspect of the joint capsule.
		• Inferior glenohumeral ligament (IGHL): A complex—parts include the anterior band, axillary pouch, and the posterior band. The IGHL provides anterior stabilization, especially during abduction of the arm.
		• Middle glenohumeral ligament: Strongest of the glenohumeral ligaments and provides anterior stabilization during the combined motion of external rotation and 45° of abduction.
		• Superior glenohumeral ligament: Runs from glenoid rim to anatomical neck and works in conjunction with the coracohumeral ligament to provide inferior stabilization during adduction.
	Coracoacromial	Protects the superior aspect of the joint.

tighten and loosen, thereby limiting translation and rotation of the joint surfaces in a load-sharing fashion.
- The bursae (small fluid-filled sacs) of the shoulder (Table 2–17) serve to decrease friction and aid mobility.

A number of dysfunctions are associated with the shoulder complex (Table 2–18).

TABLE 2–17 Major bursae of the shoulder.

Bursa	Location
Subacromial-subdeltoid	Located between the rotator cuff muscles and the deltoid muscle. As the humerus elevates, this bursa permits the rotator cuff to slide easily beneath the deltoid muscle.
Subcoracoid	Located between the joint capsule and the coracoid process of the scapula
Subscapular (subtendinous bursa of the scapularis)	Located between the capsule and the tendon of the subscapularis muscle
Coracobrachial	Located between the subscapularis muscle and the tendon of the coracobrachialis muscle

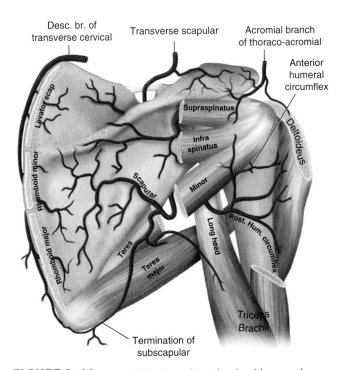

FIGURE 2–11 Arterial blood supply to the shoulder complex.

TABLE 2–18 Differential diagnosis for common causes of shoulder pain.

Condition	Patient's Age (Approximate)	Mechanism of Injury	Area of Symptoms	Symptoms Aggravated by	Observation	AROM	PROM	End Feel	Pain with Resisted	Tenderness Palpation
Rotator cuff tendinitis										
Acute	20–40	Microtrauma/macrotrauma	Anterior and lateral shoulder	Overhead motions	Swelling—anterior shoulder	Limited abduction	Limited abduction	ER	Abduction	Pain below anterior acromial rim
Chronic	30–70	Microtrauma/macrotrauma	Anterior and lateral shoulder	Overhead motions Atrophy of shoulder area	Atrophy of scapular area	Limited abduction and flexion	Pain on IR and ER at 90° abduction	ER IR	Abduction Pain below anterior acromial rim	Anterior shoulder
Bicipital tendinitis	20–45	Microtrauma	Anterior shoulder	Overhead motions	Possible swelling—anterior shoulder	Limited ER when arm at 90° abduction	Pain on combined extension of shoulder and elbow	Speed test painful, Yergason test occasionally painful	Elbow flexion	Of biceps tendon over bicipital groove
				May see signs of concomitant rotator cuff pathology	Pain on full flexion from full extension	Biceps stability test may be abnormal (if tendon unstable)				
Rotator cuff rupture	40+	Macrotrauma	Posterior/superior shoulder	Arm elevation	Atrophy of scapular area	Limited abduction Pain with or without restriction	Full and pain free	ER	Abduction	Pain below anterolateral acromial rim
Adhesive capsulitis	35–70	Microtrauma/macrotrauma	Shoulder and upper arm—poorly localized	All motions	Atrophy of shoulder area	All motions limited especially ER and abduction	All motions limited especially ER and abduction	Capsular	Most/all	Varies
A-C joint sprain	Varies	Macrotrauma	Point of shoulder	Horizontal adduction	Step/bump at point of shoulder	Limited abduction	Limited abduction	Flexion	ER	Point of shoulder
						Limited horizontal adduction	Pain with horizontal adduction	Flexion	Soft tissue thickening at point of shoulder	

	Age	Mechanism	Location of pain	Aggravating activities	Observation	Range of motion	Pain	End feel	Strength	Palpation
Subacromial bursitis	Varies	Microtrauma	Anterior and lateral shoulder	Overhead motions	Often unremarkable	Limited abduction and IR; May have full range but pain in midrange of flexion/abduction	Pain on IR at 90° abduction; Pain only in midrange abduction and flexion		Most/all	Pain below anterolateral acromial rim
Gleno-humeral arthritis	50+	Gradual onset, but can be traumatic	Poorly localized	Arm activity	Possible posterior positioning of humeral head	Capsular pattern (ER>abduction>IR)	Pain	Capsular	Weakness of rotator cuff, rather than pain	Poorly localized
SICK Scapula	20–40	Microtrauma	Anterior/superior shoulder; Postero-superior scapular; Arm, forearm, hand	Overhead activities	Scapular malposition; Inferior medial border prominence; Dyskinesia of Scapular movement	Decreased forward flexion which diminishes when clinician manually repositions the scapula into retraction and posterior tilt	Normal		Weakness rather than pain	Medial coracoid; Superomedial angle of scapula
Cervical radiculopathy	Varies	Typically none but can be traumatic	Upper back, below shoulder	Cervical extension, cervical side bending and rotation to ipsilateral side, full arm elevation	May have lateral deviation of head away from painful side	Decreased cervical flexion, cervical side bending and rotation to ipsilateral side; decreased arm elevation on involved side	Painful into restricted active range of motions; Positive Spurling's test	Empty	Weakness rather than pain; Other neurological changes	Varies; may have numbness over dermatomal area

The G-H joint is relatively unstable:

- Static stability for the joint is provided by the previously mentioned labrum, and a variety of ligaments (Table 2–16). The joint capsule is reinforced by the G-H ligaments, which are distinct capsular thickenings that limit excessive rotation and translation of the humeral head by reinforcing the connection between the glenoid fossa and the humerus.
- Dynamic stability for the joint is afforded by the muscular dynamic stabilizers, in particular the rotator cuff, the biceps tendon, and the muscles of scapular motion (Table 2–19). Normal strength ratios for the shoulder are:

- Internal and external rotation 3:2
- Adduction and abduction 2:1
- Extension and flexion 5:4

Available ranges of motion of the shoulder complex, end feels, and potential causes of pain are listed in Table 2–20.

TABLE 2–19 Muscles of the shoulder complex according to their actions on the scapula and at the glenohumeral joint.

Action	Nerve Supply	Blood Supply
Scapular Abductors		*Shoulder complex*: Primarily provided by branches of the axillary artery, a continuation of the subclavian artery. The axillary artery meets the brachial plexus in the neck, and here they are encased in the axillary sheath, together with the axillary vein.
Trapezius	Accessory nerve (motor), cervical spinal nerves C3 and C4 (motor and sensation)	
Serratus anterior (upper fibers)	Long thoracic nerve (C5–7)	
Scapular Adductors		*G-H joint*: Receives its blood supply from the anterior and posterior circumflex humeral (Figure 2–11) as well as the suprascapular and circumflex scapular vessels.
Levator scapulae	Posterior (dorsal) scapular nerve (C3–5)	
Rhomboids	Posterior (dorsal) scapular nerve (C4–5)	
Scapular Flexors		*Labrum*: Vascular supply arises mostly from its peripheral attachment to the capsule and is from a combination of the suprascapular circumflex scapular branch of the subscapular and posterior humeral circumflex arteries.
Serratus anterior (lower fibers)	Long thoracic nerve (C5–7)	
Scapular Extensors		
Pectoralis minor	Medial pectoral nerve (C6–8)	
Scapular External Rotators		*Rotator cuff*: Consists of three main sources: the thoracoacromial, suprahumeral, and subscapular arteries.
Trapezius	Accessory nerve (motor), cervical spinal nerves C3 and C4 (motor and sensation)	
Rhomboids	Posterior (dorsal) scapular nerve (C4–5)	*Brachial artery*: Provides the dominant arterial supply to each of the two heads of the biceps brachii. The artery travels in the medial intermuscular septum and is bordered by the biceps muscle anteriorly, the brachialis muscle medially, and the medial head of the triceps muscle posteriorly.
Shoulder Flexors		
Coracobrachialis	Musculocutaneous nerve (C5–7)	
Short and long head of biceps	Musculocutaneous nerve (C5–7)	
Pectoralis major	Medial (lower fibers) pectoral nerves (C8–T1); Lateral (upper fibers) pectoral nerves (C5–7)	
Anterior deltoid	Axillary (C5–6)	
Shoulder Extensors		
Triceps	Radial (C6–8) and axillary nerve[34]	
Posterior deltoid	Axillary (C5–6)	
Teres minor	Axillary (C5–6)	
Teres major	Lower subscapular nerve (C5–6)	
Latissimus dorsi	Lower subscapular nerve (C5–6)	
Shoulder Abductors		
Supraspinatus	Suprascapular nerve (C5–6)	
Deltoid	Axillary (C5–6)	
Shoulder Adductors		
Subscapularis	Upper and lower subscapular nerve (C5–6)	
Pectoralis major	Medial (lower fibers) pectoral nerves (C8–T1); Lateral (upper fibers) pectoral nerves (C5–7)	
Latissimus dorsi	Lower subscapular nerve (C5–6)	
Teres major	Lower subscapular nerve (C5–6)	
Teres minor	Axillary (C5–6)	

(Continued)

TABLE 2–19 Muscles of the shoulder complex according to their actions on the scapula and at the glenohumeral joint. (*Continued*)

Action	Nerve Supply	Blood Supply
Shoulder Internal Rotators		
Pectoralis major and minor	(see above)	
Serratus anterior	Long thoracic nerve (C5–7)	
Subscapularis	Upper and lower subscapular nerve (C5–6)	
Pectoralis major	Medial (lower fibers) pectoral nerves (C8–T1); Lateral (upper fibers) pectoral nerves (C5–7)	
Latissimus dorsi	Lower subscapular nerve (C5–6)	
Teres major	Lower subscapular nerve (C5–6)	
Shoulder External Rotators		
Infraspinatus	Suprascapular nerve (C5–6)	
Supraspinatus	Suprascapular nerve (C5–6)	
Deltoid	Axillary (C5–6)	
Teres minor	Axillary (C5–6)	

TABLE 2–20 Movements of the shoulder complex, normal ranges, end feels, and potential causes of pain.

Motion	Range Norms (Degrees)	End Feel	Potential Source of Pain
Elevation-flexion (sagittal plane—spin) Muscles performing motion: Pectoralis major (clavicular portion), deltoid (anterior fibers), coracobrachialis, biceps brachii Peripheral nerves involved: Lateral and medial pectoral, axillary, musculocutaneous	0–180	Tissue stretch Motion limited by: Posterior band of the coracohumeral ligament, inferoposterior joint capsule	Suprahumeral impingement Stretching of glenohumeral, acromioclavicular, sternoclavicular joint capsule Triceps tendon if elbow flexed
Extension (sagittal plane—spin) Muscles performing motion: Deltoid (posterior fibers), teres major, latissimus dorsi, pectoralis major (sternocostal portion) Peripheral nerves involved: Axillary, lower subscapularis, thoracodorsal, lateral and medial pectoral	0–60	Tissue stretch Motion limited by: Coracohumeral ligament, anterior joint capsule.	Stretching of glenohumeral joint capsule Severe suprahumeral impingement Biceps tendon if elbow extended
Elevation-Abduction (frontal plane—humerus rolls superiorly, glides inferiorly) Muscles performing motion: Deltoid, supraspinatus Peripheral nerves involved: Axillary, suprascapular	0–180	Tissue stretch Motion limited by: Inferior joint capsule, glenohumeral ligament, approximation of grated tuberosity and glenoid labrum	Suprahumeral impingement Acromioclavicular arthritis at terminal abduction
External rotation (transverse plane—humerus rolls posteriorly, glides anteriorly) Muscles performing motion: Infraspinatus, deltoid (posterior fibers), teres minor Peripheral nerves involved: Lateral and medial pectoral, axillary, thoracodorsal, lower subscapularis, upper and lower subscapularis	0–85	Tissue stretch Motion limited by: Anterior capsule, glenohumeral ligament	Anterior glenohumeral instability
Internal rotation (transverse plane—humerus rolls anteriorly, glides posteriorly) Muscles performing motion: Pectoralis major, deltoid (anterior fibers), teres major, subscapularis Peripheral nerves involved: Suprascapular, axillary	0–95	Tissue stretch Motion limited by: Posterior capsule	Suprahumeral impingement Posterior glenohumeral instability

TABLE 2–21 Movements of the acromioclavicular and sternoclavicular complex.

Motion of the Proximal Clavicle at the A-C Joint	Range of Motion	Motion Limited By
Protraction: The concave surface of the proximal clavicle moves on the convex sternum, producing an anterior glide of the clavicle and an anterior rotation of the distal clavicle *Muscles performing motion*: Serratus anterior, pectoralis minor *Peripheral nerves involved*: Long thoracic, lateral and medial pectoral	The distal clavicle (at the S-C joint) moves approximately 10 cm	Anterior S-C ligament, costoclavicular ligament (posterior portion), anterior capsule of the S-C joint
Retraction: The proximal clavicle articulates with a flat surface and tilts or swings, causing an anterolateral gapping, and a posterior rotation at the distal end *Muscles performing motion*: Trapezius, rhomboids *Peripheral nerves involved*: Spinal accessory, dorsal scapular	The distal clavicle (at the S-C joint) moves approximately 3 cm	Posterior S-C ligament, costoclavicular ligament (anterior portion), posterior capsule of the S-C joint
Elevation: The clavicle rotates upward on the manubrium and produces an inferior glide to maintain joint contact; only slight angular motion of the clavicle *Muscles performing motion*: Upper trapezius, levator scapulae *Peripheral nerves involved*: Spinal accessory, directly via C3–4 and dorsal scapular	The distal clavicle (at the S-C joint) moves approximately 10 cm	Costoclavicular ligament, inferior capsule of the S-C joint
Depression: The clavicle rotates downward on the manubrium and produces an superior glide to maintain joint contact; only slight angular motion of the clavicle *Muscles performing motion*: Serratus anterior (lower portion), pectoralis minor *Peripheral nerves involved*: Long thoracic, lateral and medial pectoral	The distal clavicle (at the S-C joint) moves approximately 3 cm	Interclavicular ligament, S-C ligament, articular disk of S-C joint, superior capsule of S-C joint
Rotation: The clavicle rotates passively as the scapula rotates *Muscles performing motion*: Upper trapezius, serratus anterior (lower portion) *Peripheral nerves involved*: Spinal accessory, long thoracic	30° occurs at A-C joint, then 30° at the S-C joint	S-C: Anterior and posterior sternoclavicular ligament, interclavicular ligament, costoclavicular ligament A-C: A-C ligament, coracoclavicular ligament (conoid [limits backward rotation], trapezoid [limits forward rotation])

Sternoclavicular Joint

The S-C joint, a saddle joint, is the only joint that directly attaches the upper extremity to the thorax. This saddle joint allows elevation and depression, protraction and retraction, and rotation. The biomechanics of the S-C and A-C joints are discussed in Table 2–21.

Acromioclavicular Joints

A plane joint, but also described as diarthrodial, with fibrocartilage surfaces—a convex clavicle and a concave acromion. The joint contains an intra-articular fibrocartilaginous disk, which degenerates during the third and fourth decades of life.

ELBOW COMPLEX

The elbow complex (Figure 2–12) is composed of four articulations:

• The humeroulnar joint
• The humeroradial joint
• The proximal and distal radioulnar joints

The elbow is a very congruous joint, and hence inherently very stable. Much of this stability is due to a number of ligaments (Figure 2–13) (Tables 2–22 and 2–23).

Dynamic stability and motion for the joint is also afforded by numerous muscles (Table 2–24).

The bursae of the elbow (Table 2–25) serve to decrease friction and aid mobility.

The cubital fossa represents the triangular space, or depression, which is located over the anterior surface of the elbow joint, and which serves as an "entrance" to the forearm, or antebrachium. The boundaries of the fossa are:

• Lateral—brachioradialis and extensor carpi radialis longus (ECRL) muscles
• Medial—pronator teres muscle
• Proximal—an imaginary line that passes through the humeral condyles
• Floor—brachialis muscle

The contents of the fossa are as follows:

• The tendon of the biceps brachii lies as the central structure in the fossa.
• The median nerve runs along the lateral edge of the pronator teres muscle.

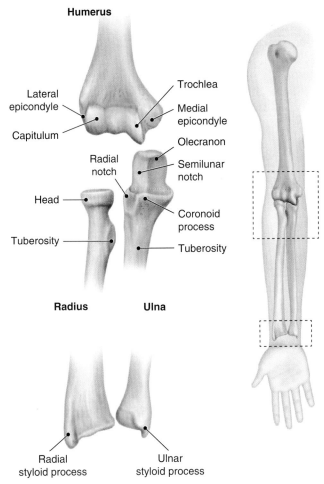

FIGURE 2-12 Skeletal structures of the elbow, forearm, and wrist.

- The brachial artery enters the fossa just lateral to the median nerve and just medial to the biceps brachii tendon.
- The radial nerve runs along the medial edge of the brachioradialis and ECRL muscles, and is vulnerable to injury here.

TABLE 2-22 Major ligaments of the elbow.

	Function
Annular	Maintains the relationship between the head of the radius and the humerus and ulna
Ulnar (medial) collateral	Primary stabilizer against valgus (medial) stress, particularly in the range of 20°-130° of flexion and extension
Radial (lateral) collateral	Provides stability against varus (lateral) stress and functions to maintain the ulnohumeral and radiohumeral joints in a reduced position when the elbow is loaded in supination

- The median cubital or intermediate cubital cutaneous vein crosses the surface of the fossa.
- The elbow complex receives its blood supply from the brachial artery, anterior ulnar recurrent artery, posterior ulnar recurrent artery, radial recurrent artery, and middle collateral branch of the arteria profunda brachii.

Humeroulnar Joint

The motions that occur at the humeroulnar joint involve impure flexion and extension, which are primarily the result of rotation of the ulna about the trochlea. The range of flexion-extension is from 0° to 150°, with about 10° of hyperextension being available. Full active extension in the normal elbow is some 5° to 10° short of that obtainable by forced extension, due to passive muscular restraints (biceps, brachialis, and supinator).[35,36]

- Passive extension is limited by the impact of the olecranon process on the olecranon fossa and tension on the ulnar collateral ligament and anterior capsule.[37]
- Passive flexion is limited by bony structures (the head of the radius against the radial fossa, and the coronoid process against the coronoid fossa), tension of the posterior capsular ligament, and passive tension in the triceps.[37]

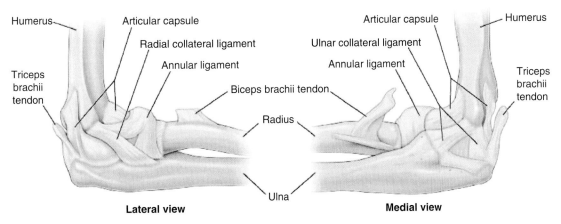

FIGURE 2-13 Ligaments of the lateral and medial aspects of the elbow.

TABLE 2–23 Articular and ligamentous contributions to elbow stability.

Stabilization	Elbow Extended	Elbow Flexed 90°
Valgus stability	Anterior capsule UCL and bony articular (proximal half of sigmoid notch) *equally divided*	UCL proves 55% 0% anterior capsule and bony articulation (proximal half of sigmoid notch)
Varus stability	Anterior capsule (32%) Joint articulation (55%) RCL (14%)	Joint articulation (75%) Anterior capsule (13%) RCL (9%)
Anterior displacement	Anterior oblique ligament Anterior joint capsule Trochlea-olecranon articulation (minimal)	
Posterior displacement	Anterior capsule Radial head against the capitellum Coracoid against the trochlea	
Distraction	Anterior capsule (85%) RCL (5%) UCL (5%) Triceps, biceps, brachialis, brachioradialis, and forearm muscles	RCL 10% UCL 78% Capsule 8%

UCL, ulnar collateral ligament; RCL, radial collateral ligament.

Data from Sobel J, Nirschl RP. Elbow injuries. In: Zachazewski JE, Magee DJ, Quillen WS, eds. *Athletic Injuries and Rehabilitation*. Philadelphia, PA: WB Saunders; 1996:543-583.

- The normal carrying angle of the elbow varies with flexion and extension, ranging from 6° of varus with full flexion to 11° of valgus in full extension. Women tend to have a larger carrying angle.

Humeroradial Joint

The motions occurring at this joint include flexion and extension of the elbow. Some supination and pronation also occur at this joint due to a spinning of the radial head.

Proximal Radioulnar Joint

At the proximal radioulnar joint, one DOF exists, permitting pronation and supination. Pronation and supination involve the articulations at the elbow as well as the DRUJ and the radiocarpal articulation.

Motion at the elbow is primarily gliding for both flexion and extension. Rolling occurs in the final 5° to 10° of ROM for both flexion and extension.

TABLE 2–24 Muscles of the elbow and forearm: their actions, nerve supply, and nerve root derivation.

Action	Muscles Acting	Peripheral Nerve Supply	Nerve Root Deviation	Blood Supply
Elbow flexion	Brachialis	Musculocutaneous	C5–C6 (C7)	The vascular supply to the elbow includes the brachial artery, the radial and ulnar arteries, the middle and radial collateral artery laterally, and the superior and inferior ulnar collateral arteries.
	Biceps brachii	Musculocutaneous	C5–C6	
	Brachioradialis	Radial	C5–C6, (C7)	
	Pronator teres	Median	C6–C7	
	Flexor carpi ulnaris	Ulnar	C7–C8	
Elbow extension	Triceps	Radial	C7–C8	
	Anconeus	Radial	C7–C8, (T1)	
Forearm supination	Supinator	Posterior interosseous (radial)	C5–C6	
	Biceps brachii	Musculocutaneous	C5–C6	
Forearm pronation	Pronator quadratus	Anterior interosseous (median)	C8, T1	
	Pronator teres	Median	C6–C7	
	Flexor carpi radialis	Median	C6–C7	

TABLE 2-25 Major bursae of the elbow.

Bursa	Location
Olecranon	Located posteriorly between the skin and the olecranon process; the main bursa of the elbow joint complex
Deep intratendinous and deep subtendinous	Located between the triceps tendon and olecranon
Bicipitoradial	Separates the biceps tendon from the radial tuberosity
Coracobrachial	Located between the subscapularis muscle and the tendon of the coracobrachialis muscle

FOREARM, WRIST, AND HAND

The wrist and hand joint complex (Figure 2–14) is comprised of:

- The distal radioulnar joint (DRUJ)
- Eight carpal bones
- The bases of five metacarpals
- More than 20 radiocarpal, intercarpal, and CMC joints

While these structures can be differentiated anatomically, they are functionally interrelated, with movement in one joint having an effect on the motion of neighboring joints. The hand accounts for about 90% of upper limb function.[38] The thumb, which is involved in 40% to 50% of hand function, is the more functionally important of the digits.[38] The index and middle fingers are each involved in about 20% of hand function, and are the second

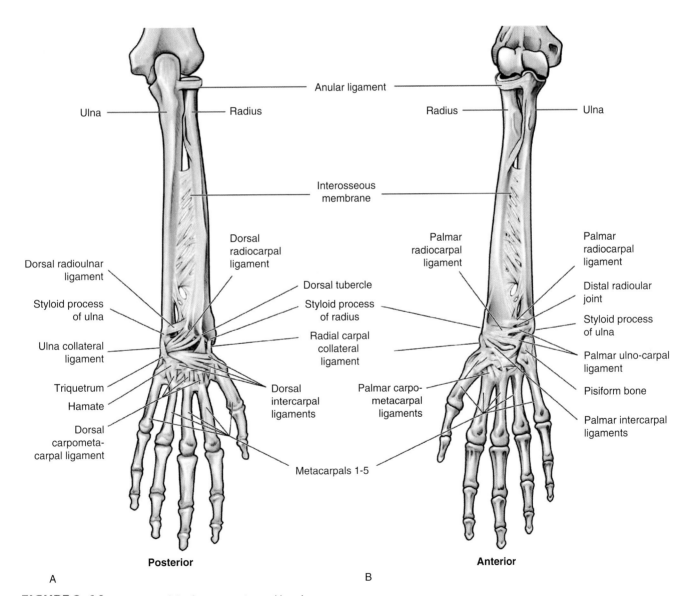

FIGURE 2-14 Ligaments of the forearm, wrist, and hand.

TABLE 2–26 Major Ligaments of the wrist and hand.

Wrist	Extrinsic palmar	Provides the majority of the wrist stability
	Intrinsic	Serves as rotational restraint, binding the proximal carpal row into a unit of rotational stability
	Interosseous	Binds the carpal bones together
Fingers	Volar and collateral interphalangeal	Prevent displacement of the interphalangeal joints

most important, with the ring finger being the least important. The middle finger is the strongest finger and is important for both precision and power functions.[38] The major ligaments of the wrist and hand are described in Table 2–26.

The muscle compartments of the forearm are described in Table 2–27. The muscles of the wrist and hand are described in Table 2–28. The AROM norms for the forearm, wrist, and hand are described in Table 2–29.

Distal Radioulnar Joint

The DRUJ is a double-pivot joint that unites the distal radius and ulna and an articular disk. The articular disk, known as the triangular fibrocartilaginous complex (TFCC), assists in binding the distal radius and is the main stabilizer of the DRUJ, as it improves joint congruency and cushions against compressive forces. The proximal and distal radial ulnar joints are intimately related biomechanically, with the function and stability of both joints dependent on the configuration of, and distance between, the two bones. Supination tightens the anterior capsule, while

TABLE 2–27 Muscle compartments of the forearm.

Compartment	Principal Muscles
Anterior	Pronator teres
	Flexor carpi radialis
	Palmaris longus
	Flexor digitorum superficialis
	Flexor digitorum profundus
	Flexor pollicis longus
	Flexor carpi ulnaris
	Pronator quadratus
Posterior	Abductor pollicis longus
	Extensor pollicis brevis
	Extensor pollicis longus
	Extensor digitorum communis
	Extensor digitorum proprius
	Extensor digiti quinti
	Extensor carpi ulnaris
Mobile wad	Brachioradialis
	Extensor carpi radialis longus
	Extensor carpi radialis brevis

pronation tightens the posterior part, adding to the overall stability of the wrist.

The Wrist

The carpals

The carpal bones lie in two transverse rows (Figure 2–15).

The proximal row contains (from radial to ulnar) the scaphoid (navicular), lunate, triquetrum, and pisiform. The distal row holds (radial to ulnar) the trapezium, trapezoid, capitate, and hamate. Various instabilities can occur in the carpal joints (Table 2–30).

Midcarpal joints

The midcarpal joint lies between the two rows of carpals. It is referred to as a "compound" articulation because each row has both concave and convex segments. Wrist movements occur around a combination of three functional axes: longitudinal, transverse, and anterior-posterior. In a neutral wrist position, the scaphoid contacts the radius and the lunate contacts the radius and disk. Due to the morphology of the wrist, movement at this joint complex involves a coordinated interaction between a number of articulations including the radiocarpal joint, the proximal row of carpals, and the distal row of the carpals.[39] The movements of flexion and extension of the wrist are shared between the radiocarpal articulation and the intercarpal articulation in varying proportions.

Wrist flexion, extension, and radial deviation are mainly midcarpal joint motions. Approximately 60%:40% (proximal carpal row on distal radius/ulna:midcarpal joint) motion occurs with wrist extension and 60%:40% (midcarpal joint:proximal carpal row on distal radius/ulna) occurs with wrist flexion.[40,41]

Each carpal in the proximal row is convex on its lateral surface and concave on its medial surface. At their distal aspect:

- The scaphoid and lunate present with a concave surface to the distal row of carpals.
- The triquetrum presents with a convex surface to the distal row of carpals.

The wrist also allows relatively extensive traction and gliding accessory movements. There is a physiological ulnar deviation at rest. The amount of deviation is approximately 40° of ulnar deviation and 15° of radial deviation.

The position of the wrist in flexion or extension influences the tension of the long, or "extrinsic," muscles of the digits. Neither the flexors nor the extensors of the fingers are long enough to allow maximal ROM at the wrist and the fingers simultaneously.

Carpal ligaments—Migration of the carpal bones is prevented by strong ligaments and by the ulnar support provided by the TFCC. The major ligaments of the wrist include the palmar intrinsic ligaments, the volar extrinsic, and the dorsal extrinsic and intrinsic ligaments.

Radiocarpal Joint

The radiocarpal joint is formed by the large articular concave surface of the distal end of the radius, the scaphoid and lunate of the proximal carpal row, and the TFCC.

TABLE 2–28 Muscles of the wrist and hand.

Action	Muscles	Nerve Supply
Wrist extension	Extensor carpi radialis longus	Radial C6,7
	Extensor carpi radialis brevis	Posterior interosseous C6,7
	Extensor carpi ulnaris	Posterior interosseous C7,8
Wrist flexion	Flexor carpi radialis	Median C6,7
	Flexor carpi ulnaris	Ulnar C8,T1
Ulnar deviation of wrist	Flexor carpi ulnaris	Ulnar C8,T1
	Extensor carpi ulnaris	Posterior interosseous C7,8
Radial deviation of wrist	Flexor carpi radialis	Median C6,7
	Extensor carpi radialis longus	Radial C6,7
	Abductor pollicis longus	Posterior interosseous C7,8
	Extensor pollicis brevis	Posterior interosseous C7,8
Finger extension	Extensor digitorum communis	Posterior interosseous C6,7,8
	Extensor indicis	Posterior interosseous C7,8
	Extensor digiti minimi	Posterior interosseous C7,8
Finger flexion	Flexor digitorum profundus	Anterior interosseous, lateral two digits C8,T1
		Ulnar, medial two digits C8,T1
	Flexor digitorum superficialis	Median C7,8,T1
	Lumbricals	First and second: median C8,T1
		Third and fourth: ulnar C8,T1
	Interossei	Ulnar C8,T1
	Flexor digiti minimi	Ulnar C8,T1
Abduction of fingers	Dorsal interossei	Ulnar C8,T1
	Abductor digiti minimi	Ulnar C8,T1
Adduction of fingers	Palmar interossei	Ulnar C8,T1
Thumb extension	Extensor pollicis longus	Posterior interosseous C7,8
	Extensor pollicis brevis	Posterior interosseous C7,8
	Abductor pollicis longus	Posterior interosseous C7,8
Thumb flexion	Flexor pollicis brevis	Superficial head: median C8,T1
		Deep head: ulnar C8, T1
	Flexor pollicis longus	Anterior interosseous C8,T1
	Opponens pollicis	Median C8,T1
Abduction of thumb	Abductor pollicis longus	Posterior interosseous C7,8
	Abductor pollicis brevis	Median C8,T1
Adduction of thumb	Adductor pollicis	Ulnar C8,T1
Opposition of thumb and little finger	Opponens pollicis	Median C8,T1
	Flexor pollicis brevis	Superficial head: median C8,T1
	Abductor pollicis brevis	Median C8,T1
	Opponens digiti minimi	Ulnar C8,T1

TABLE 2–29 Active range of motion norms for the forearm, wrist, and hand.

Motion	Degrees
Forearm pronation	85–90
Forearm supination	85–90
Radial deviation	15
Ulnar deviation	30–45
Wrist flexion	80–90
Wrist extension	70–90
Finger flexion	MCP: 85–90; PIP: 100–115; DIP: 80–90
Finger extension	MCP: 30–45; PIP: 0; DIP: 20
Finger abduction	20–30
Finger adduction	0
Thumb flexion	CMC: 45–50; MCP: 50–55; IP: 85–90
Thumb extension	MCP: 0; IP: 0–5
Thumb adduction	30
Thumb abduction	60–70

TABLE 2–30 Common wrist dysfunctions.

Dysfunction	Cause
Dorsal intercalated segment instability (DISI)	Results from disruption between the scaphoid and lunate, allowing the scaphoid to rotate into volar flexion. The remaining components of the proximal row rotate into dorsiflexion because of loss of connection to the scaphoid.
Volar intercalated segment instability (VISI)	Results from disruption of the ligamentous support to the triquetrum and lunate and leads to volar rotation of the lunate and extension of the triquetrum.
Scapholunate dissociation	A complete tear of the scapholunate ligaments that may result from a hyperextension injury. The lunate and triquetrum extend abnormally, supinate, and deviate radially, while the scaphoid tilts into flexion, pronation, and ulnar deviation (see Watson test).
Triangular fibrocartilaginous complex (TFCC) tear	This injury typically occurs following a fall on the supinated outstretched wrist or as the result of chronic repetitive rotational loading. Patients complain of medial wrist pain just distal to the ulna, which is increased with end-range forearm pronation/supination and with forceful gripping. TFCC tears can be a cause of distal radioulnar joint/wrist instability.

Antebrachial Fascia

The antebrachial fascia is a dense connective tissue "bracelet" that encases the forearm and maintains the relationships of the tendons that cross the wrist.

Extensor Retinaculum

Where the tendons cross the wrist, a retinaculum serves to prevent the tendons from "bow-stringing" when the tendons turn a corner at the wrist.[42] The tunnel-like structures formed by the retinaculum and the underlying bones are called fibroosseous compartments. There are six fibroosseous compartments, or tunnels, on the dorsum of the wrist. The compartments, from lateral to medial, contain the tendons of:

1. Abductor pollicis longus (APL) and extensor pollicis brevis (EPB)
2. ECRL and ECRB
3. Extensor pollicis longus (EPL)
4. Extensor digitorum and indicis
5. Extensor digiti minimi
6. Extensor carpi ulnaris

The mnemonic 2 2 1 2 1 1 can be used to remember the number of tendons in each compartment.

Flexor Retinaculum

The flexor retinaculum (transverse carpal ligament) spans the area between the pisiform, hamate, scaphoid, and trapezium. It transforms the carpal arch into a tunnel, through which pass the median nerve and some of the tendons of the hand. Proximally, the retinaculum attaches to the tubercle of the scaphoid and the pisiform. Distally it

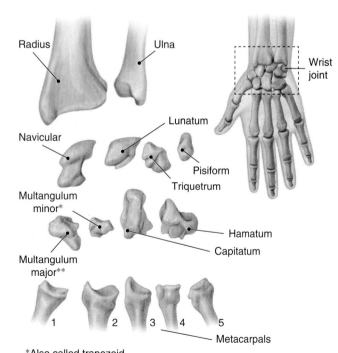

*Also called trapezoid.
**Also called trapezium.

FIGURE 2–15 The carpal bones of the hand and their relationship with the bones of the wrist and fingers.

attaches to the hook of the hamate and the tubercle of the trapezium. The tendons that pass *deep* to the flexor retinaculum include:

- Flexor digitorum superficialis (FDS)
- Flexor digitorum profundus (FDP)
- Flexor pollicis longus (FPL)
- Flexor carpi radialis (FCR)

Structures that pass *superficial* to the flexor retinaculum include:

- Ulnar nerve and artery
- Tendon of the palmaris longus
- Sensory branch (palmar branch) of the median nerve

Most hand surgeons use the Verdan[43] classification to refer to the area of the hand represented by the distal crease in the palm and the middle crease in the finger as "no-man's land," or zone II (Figure 2–16). This is because the area is one of complex anatomy and one that has demonstrated a poor level of healing due to an increased chance of adhesion formation.

Carpal Tunnel

The carpal tunnel serves as a conduit for the median nerve and nine flexor tendons (the eight tendons of the FDS and FDP, and the FDP).

- The palmar radiocarpal ligament and the palmar ligament complex form the floor of the canal.
- The roof of the tunnel is formed by the flexor retinaculum (transverse carpal ligament).
- The ulnar and radial borders are formed by carpal bones (hook of hamate and trapezium, respectively).

Within the tunnel, the median nerve divides into a motor branch and distal sensory branches.

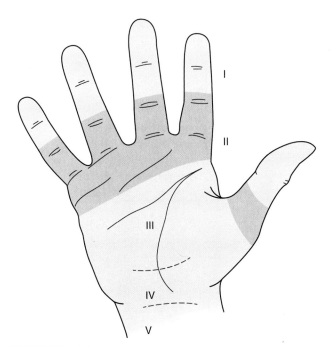

FIGURE 2–16 Zone II of the flexor tendon zones—the surgical no man's land of the hand.

Tunnel of Guyon

The tunnel of Guyon is a depression superficial to the flexor retinaculum, located between the hook of the hamate and the pisiform bones. From radial to ulnar, the ulnar artery and ulnar nerve pass through the canal. The flexor carpi ulnaris tendon is most ulnar but lies outside the tunnel.

Phalanges

The 14 phalanges each consist of a base, shaft, and head. Two shallow depressions, which correspond to the pulley-shaped heads of the adjacent phalanges, mark the concave proximal bases. Motion thus follows the concave-on-convex rule.

Metacarpophalangeal Joints of the Second to Fifth Fingers

The second to fifth metacarpals articulate with the respective proximal phalanges in biaxial joints. The MCP joints allow flexion-extension and medial-lateral deviation associated with a slight degree of axial rotation. Motions at these joints follow the concave-on-convex rule.

- Approximately 90° of flexion is available at the second MCP. The amount of available flexion progressively increases toward the fifth MCP.
- Active extension at these joints is 25° to 30°, while 90° is obtainable passively.
- Approximately 20° of abduction/adduction can occur in either direction, with more being available in extension than in flexion.
- Abduction-adduction movements of the MCP joints are restricted in flexion and freer in extension.[39]

The joint capsule of these joints is relatively lax and redundant, endowed with collateral ligaments. Although lax in extension, these collateral ligaments become taut in approximately 70° to 90° of flexion of the MCP joint.

Carpometacarpal Joints

The distal borders of the distal carpal row bones articulate with the bases of the metacarpals thereby forming the CMC joints. The CMC joints progress in mobility from the second to the fifth.

The palmar and dorsal CMC and intermetacarpal ligaments provide stability for the CMC joints. While the trapezoid articulates with only one metacarpal, all of the other members of the distal carpal row combine one carpal bone with two or more metacarpals.

First Carpometacarpal Joint

The thumb is the most important digit of the hand, and the sellar (saddle-shaped) CMC joint is the most important joint of the thumb. Motions that can occur at this joint include flexion/extension, adduction/abduction, and opposition (which includes varying amounts of flexion, internal rotation, and palmar adduction). Although sellar surfaces follow the same rules as ovid surfaces, because of the nature of the curvature of their joint surfaces, a swing in one direction involves movement of a male surface, and a swing in a direction at 90° to the first swing involves movement of a female surface. For example, at the first CMC joint, the following biomechanics are involved:

- Flexion/extension of metacarpal occurs around an anterior-posterior axis in the frontal plane that is perpendicular to the sagittal plane of finger flexion and extension: the metacarpal surface is concave, and the trapezium surface is convex.
  - The swing of the bone occurs in an anteromedial/posterolateral direction.
  - The base glides and rolls in an anteromedial/posterolateral direction.
  - Flexion occurs with a conjunct rotation of internal rotation of the metacarpal. Extension occurs with a conjunct rotation of external rotation of the metacarpal.
- Abduction/adduction of metacarpal occurs around a medial-lateral axis in the sagittal plane, which is perpendicular to the frontal plane of finger abduction and adduction: the convex metacarpal surface moves on the concave trapezium.
  - The swing of the bone occurs in an anterolateral/posteromedial direction.
  - The base glides in the opposite direction of the swing, and rolls in the same direction as the swing.
- Abduction occurs with a conjunct rotation of internal rotation. Adduction occurs with a conjunct rotation of external rotation.
- Opposition of the thumb involves a wide arc motion comprised of sequential palmar adduction, and flexion from the anatomic position accompanied by internal rotation of the thumb. Retroposition of the thumb returns the thumb to the anatomic position, a motion that incorporates elements of abduction with extension and external rotation of the metacarpal.

Metacarpophalangeal Joint of the Thumb

The MCP joint of the thumb is a hinge joint. Its bony configuration, which resembles the interphalangeal (IP) joints, provides it with some inherent stability. In addition, palmar and collateral ligaments provide support for the joint. Approximately 75° to 80° of flexion is available at this joint. The extension movements as well as the abduction and adduction motions are negligible. Traction, gliding, and rotatory accessory movement are also present. Motions follow the concave-on-convex rule.

Interphalangeal Joints

Adjacent phalanges articulate in hinge joints that allow motion in only one plane. The congruency of the IP joint surfaces contributes greatly to finger joint stability. Motion follows the concave-on-convex rule.

Proximal interphalangeal joint—The PIP joint is a hinged joint capable of flexion and extension and is stable in all positions. The supporting ligaments and tendons provide the bulk of the static and dynamic stability of this joint. The motions available at these joints consist of approximately 110° of flexion at the PIP joints and 90° at the thumb IP joint. Extension reaches 0° at the PIP joints and 25° at the thumb IP joint. Traction, gliding, and accessory movement also occur at the IP joints.

Distal interphalangeal joints—The distal interphalangeal (DIP) joint has similar structures but less stability and allows some

hyperextension. The motions available at these joints consist of approximately 80° of active flexion and 25° of passive extension. Traction, gliding, and accessory movements also occur at the DIP joints.

Palmar Aponeurosis

The palmar aponeurosis is located just deep to the subcutaneous tissue. It is a dense fibrous structure continuous with the palmaris longus tendon and fascia covering the thenar and hypothenar muscles.

Extensor Hood

At the level of the MCP joint, the tendon of the extensor digitorum (ED) fans out to cover or shroud the dorsal aspect of the joint in a hood-like structure. A complex tendon that covers the dorsal aspect of each digit is formed from a combination of the tendons of insertion of the ED, extensor indicis, and extensor digiti minimi. The distal portion of the hood receives the tendons of the lumbricales and interossei over the proximal phalanx. The tendons of the intrinsic muscles pass palmar to the MCP joint axes but dorsal to the PIP and DIP joint axes. Between the MCP and PIP joints, the complete, complex ED tendon (after all contributions have been received) splits into three parts—a central slip and two lateral bands:

- Central slip. This band inserts into the proximal dorsal edge of the middle phalanx.
- Lateral bands. The lateral bands rejoin over the middle phalanx into a terminal tendon, which inserts into the proximal dorsal edge of the distal phalanx. Rupture of the tendon insertion into the distal phalanx produces a "mallet" finger (see Common Orthopedic Conditions section, later)

The arrangement of the muscles and tendons in this expansion hood creates a "cable" system that provides a mechanism for *extending* the MCP and IP joints, and allows the lumbrical, and possibly interosseous muscles, to assist in the *flexion* of the MCP joints and extension of the IP joints.

Synovial Sheaths

Synovial sheaths can be thought of as long narrow balloons filled with synovial fluid, which wrap around a tendon so that one part of the balloon wall (the visceral layer) is directly on the tendon, while the other part of the balloon wall (the parietal layer) is separate.[42] During wrist motions, the sheaths move longitudinally, reducing friction.

At the wrist, the tendons of both the FDS and FDP are essentially covered by a synovial sheath and pass deep to the flexor retinaculum. The FDP tendons are deeper than those of the FDS.

In the palm, the FDS and FDP tendons are covered for a variable distance by a synovial sheath.

At the base of the digits, both sets of tendons enter a "fibro-osseous tunnel" formed by the bones of the digit (head of the metatarsals and phalanges) and a fibrous digital tendon sheath on the palmar surface of the digits.

Flexor Pulleys

Annular (A) and cruciate (C) pulleys restrain the flexor tendons to the metacarpals and phalanges and contribute to fibroosseous tunnels through which the tendons travel, allowing the muscles to move the wrist and hand.

Anatomical Snuff Box

The anatomical snuff box is represented by a depression on the dorsal surface of the hand at the base of the thumb, just distal to the radius. The tendons of the APL and EPB form the radial border of the snuff box, while the tendon of the EPL forms the ulnar border. Along the floor of the snuff box are the deep branch of the radial artery and the tendinous insertion of the ECRL. Underneath these structures, the scaphoid and trapezium bones are found. Tenderness with palpation in the anatomical snuff box suggests a scaphoid fracture, but also can present in minor wrist injuries or other conditions.

Nerve Supply

The three peripheral nerves that supply the skin and muscles of the wrist and hand include the median, ulnar, and radial nerve. The following areas of the hand typically have autonomous innervation:

- The dorsal thumb-index webspace (radial nerve)
- The distal tip of the little finger (ulnar nerve)
- The volar tip of the index finger (median nerve)

Blood Supply

The brachial artery bifurcates at the elbow into radial and ulnar branches, which are the main arterial branches to the hand. Kienböck's disease is in avascular necrosis of the lunate, usually as a result of distant trauma. It has also been associated with relative shortening of the ulna (negative ulnar variance) compared with the radius bone. The four stages of the disease are sclerosis, fragmentation, collapse, and arthritis.

HIP

Anatomy

The hip joint is classified as an unmodified ovoid (ball and socket) joint. The acetabulum is made up of three bones: the ilium, ischium, and pubis (Figure 2–17).

The acetabular labrum deepens the acetabulum and increases articular congruence. A number of muscles act across the hip (Table 2–31).

The femur is largely held in the acetabulum by three ligaments (Figure 2–18) (Table 2–32).

Vascular Supply

The proximal shaft of the femur and the femoral neck has a plentiful blood supply from the medial circumflex femoral artery and its branches. The femoral head, on the other hand, has an extremely tenuous blood supply from a small branch of the obturator artery that passes within the femoral ligament.

Biomechanics

Motion at the hip occurs in three planes: sagittal (flexion and extension around a transverse axis), frontal (abduction and adduction around an anterior-posterior axis), and transverse (internal and external rotation around a vertical axis). All three of these axes pass through the center of the femoral head. Motions about the hip joint can occur independently; however, the extremes of motion require motion at the pelvis.[44] For example, end-range hip flexion is associated with a posterior rotation of the ilium bone. The end range of hip extension is associated with an anterior rotation of the ilium. Hip abduction and adduction are associated with a lateral tilt of the pelvis.

In the anatomic position, the orientation of the femoral head causes the contact force between the femur and acetabulum to be high in the anterior-superior region of the joint.[45] Because the anterior aspect of the femoral head is somewhat exposed in this position, the joint has more flexibility in flexion than extension.[46]

The angle between the femoral shaft and the neck is called the **collum/inclination** angle. This angle is approximately 125°-135° (according to source),[47] but can vary with body types. In a tall person, the collum *angle* is larger (valga). The opposite is true with a shorter individual.

The collum angle has an important influence on the hips. An increase in the collum angle causes the femoral head to be directed more superiorly in the acetabulum, and is known as **coxa valga**. Coxa valga has the following effects at the hip joint:

- It changes the orientation of the joint reaction force from the normal vertical direction to one that is almost parallel to the femoral shaft.[48,49] This lateral displacement of the joint reaction force reduces the weight-bearing surface, resulting in an increase in stress applied across joint surfaces not specialized to sustain such loads.
- It shortens the moment arm of the hip abductors, placing them in a position of mechanical disadvantage.[49] This causes the abductors to contract more vigorously to stabilize the pelvis, producing an increase in the joint reaction force.[46]
- It increases the overall length of the lower extremity, affecting other components in the kinetic chain. Coxa valga, which is associated with genu varum, decreases the normal physiological angle at the knee. This places an increased mechanical stress on the medial aspect of the knee joint and more tensile stress on the lateral aspect of the joint.

If the collum angle is reduced, it is known as **coxa vara**. The mechanical effects of coxa vara are, for the most part, the opposite of those found in coxa valga, although they appear to be less deleterious than those of coxa valga.[50] Coxa vara is associated with genu valgum.

Femoral alignment in the transverse plane also influences the mechanics of the hip joint.

Anteversion is defined as the anterior position of the axis through the femoral condyles.[51,52] **Retroversion** is defined as a femoral neck axis that is parallel or posterior to the condylar axis.[46] The normal range for femoral alignment in the transverse plane in adults is 12° to 15° of anteversion.[52,53] Subjects with excessive anteversion usually have more hip internal rotation ROM than

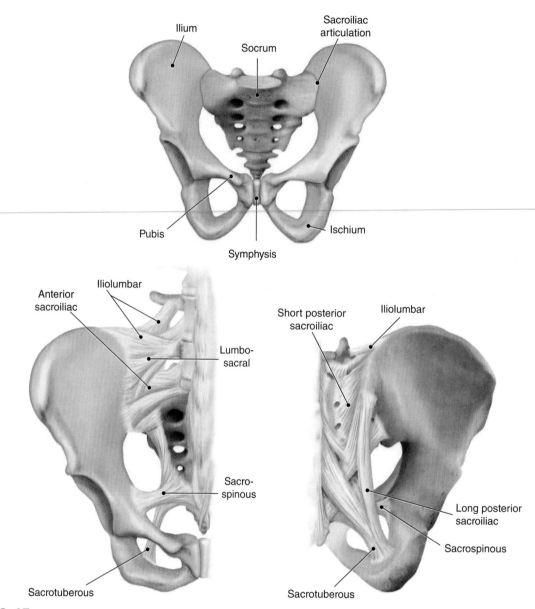

FIGURE 2–17 Bony and ligament structures of the pelvis.

external rotation, and gravitate to the typical "frog-sitting" posture as a position of comfort. There is also associated in-toeing while weight-bearing.[46] The degree of anteversion is clinically measured with the Craig test.

Excessive anteversion directs the femoral head toward the anterior aspect of the acetabulum when the femoral condyles are aligned in their normal orientation; excessive anteversion is considered a value greater than 15° with the Craig test measurement of hip internal rotation (IR).

The degree of pelvic tilt, known as the angle of inclination and which is measured as the angle between the horizontal plane and a line connecting the ASIS with the PSIS, varies from 5° to 12° in normal individuals.[54] Angles less than this can be associated with

posterior pelvic tilt, and angles greater may be associated with anterior pelvic tilt.

The most stable position of the hip is the normal standing position: hip extension, slight abduction, and slight internal rotation.[55-57]

KNEE JOINT COMPLEX

The knee is the largest and most complex joint in the body. It is considered a "physiological" joint because it requires the normal functioning of all its parts (ie, bony, ligamentous, and muscular) to simultaneously provide smooth motion, stability in stance, and

TABLE 2-31 Muscles acting across the hip joint and major actions.

Muscle	Origin	Insertion	Innervation
Adductors			
Adductor brevis	External aspect of the body and inferior ramus of the pubis	By an aponeurosis to the line from the greater trochanter of the linea aspera of the femur	Obturator nerve, L3
Adductor longus	Pubic crest and symphysis	By an aponeurosis to the middle third of the linea aspera of the femur	Obturator nerve, L3
Adductor magnus	Inferior ramus of pubis, ramus of ischium, and inferolateral aspect of the ischial tuberosity	By an aponeurosis to the linea aspera and adductor tubercle of the femur	Obturator nerve and tibial portion of the sciatic nerve, L2–L4
Pectineus	Pecten pubis	Along a line leading from the lesser trochanter to the linea aspera	Femoral or obturator or accessory obturator nerves, L2
Gracilis	The body and inferior ramus of the pubis	The anterior-medial aspect of the shaft of the proximal tibia, just proximal to the tendon of the semitendinosus	Obturator nerve, L2
Hip Extensors			
Biceps femoris (long head)	Arises from the sacrotuberous ligament and posterior aspect of the ischial tuberosity	By way of a tendon, on the lateral aspect of the head of the fibula, the lateral condyle of the tibial tuberosity, the lateral collateral ligament, and the deep fascia of the leg	Tibial portion of the sciatic nerve, S1
Semimembranosus	Ischial tuberosity	The posterior-medial aspect of the medial condyle of the tibia	Tibial nerve, L5-S1
Semitendinosus	Ischial tuberosity	Upper part of the medial surface of the tibia behind the attachment of the sartonus and below that of the gracilis	Tibial nerve, L5–S1
Gluteus maximus	Posterior gluteal line of the ilium, iliac crest, aponeurosis of the erector spinae, dorsal surface of the lower part of the sacrum, side of the coccyx, sacrotuberous ligament, and intermuscular fascia	Iliotibial tract of the fascia lata, gluteal tuberosity of the femur	Inferior gluteal nerve, S1–S2
Hip Abductors			
Gluteus medius	Outer surface of the ilium between the iliac crest and the posterior gluteal line, anterior gluteal line and fascia	Lateral surface of the greater trochanter	Superior gluteal nerve, L5
Tensor fasciae latae	Outer lip of the iliac crest and the lateral surface of the anterior superior iliac spine	Iliotibial tract	Superior gluteal nerve, L4–L5
Gluteus minimus	Outer surface of the ilium between the anterior and inferior gluteal lines and the margin of the greater sciatic notch	A ridge laterally situated on the anterior surface of the greater trochanter	Superior gluteal nerve, L5
Hip Flexors			
Iliacus	Super two-thirds of the iliac fossa, upper surface of the lateral part of the sacrum	Fibers converge with tendon of the psoas major to lesser trochanter	Femoral nerve, L2
Psoas major	Transverse processes of all the lumbar vertebrae, bodies, and intervertebral discs of the lumbar vertebrae	Lesser trochanter of the femur	Lumbar plexus, L2–L3

(Continued)

TABLE 2–31 Muscles acting across the hip joint and major actions. (*Continued*)

Muscle	Origin	Insertion	Innervation
Rectus femoris	By two heads, from the anterior inferior iliac spine, and a reflected head from the groove above the acetabulum	Base of the patella	Femoral nerve, L3–L4
Sartorius	Anterior superior iliac spine and notch below it	Upper part of the medial surface of the tibia in front of the gracilis	Femoral nerve, L2–L3
External Rotators			
Gemelli (superior and inferior)	Superior-dorsal surface of the spine of the ischium, inferior-upper part of the tuberosity of the ischium	Superior and inferior-medial surface of the greater trochanter	Sacral plexus, L5–S1
Quadratus femoris	Ischial body next to the ischial tuberosity	Quadrate tubercle on femur	Nerve to quadratus femoris
Obturator internus	Internal surface of the anterolateral wall of the pelvis, and obturator membrane	Medial surface of the greater trochanter	Sacral plexus, S1
Piriformis	Front of the sacrum, gluteal surface of the ilium, capsule of the sacroiliac joint, and sacrotuberous ligament	Upper border of the greater trochanter of femur	Sacral plexus, S1
Obturator externus	Rami of the pubis, ramus of the ischium, medial two-thirds of the outer surface of the obturator membrane	Trochanteric fossa of the femur	Obturator nerve, L4

protection against deterioration over time.[58,59] The knee joint complex includes three articulating surfaces, which form two distinct joints contained within a single joint capsule: the patellofemoral and tibiofemoral joint (Figure 2–19).

Despite its proximity to the tibiofemoral joint, the patellofemoral joint can be considered as its own entity in much the same way as the craniovertebral joints are when compared to the rest of the cervical spine. The muscles that impact the knee joint complex are described in Table 2–33.

Tibiofemoral Joint

The tibiofemoral joint, or knee joint, is a ginglymoid, or modified hinge joint, which has 6° of freedom. The bony configuration of the knee joint complex is geometrically incongruous and lends little inherent stability to the joint. Joint stability is therefore dependent upon the static restraints of the joint capsule, ligaments, and menisci (Figure 2–19) and (Table 2–34), and the dynamic restraints of the quadriceps, hamstrings, and gastrocnemius.

Patellofemoral Joint

The quadriceps tendon (extensor mechanism) represents the confluence of the four muscle tendon units (rectus femoris, vastus lateralis, vastus intermedius, and vastus medialis) and inserts on the superior pole of the patella.

- Laterally, the iliotibial band (ITB) supports the extensor mechanism and is an important lateral stabilizer of the patellofemoral joint. It originates above the hip joint as a wide fascial band, originating from the gluteal muscles, tensor fascia lata, and vastus lateralis.
- Distally, the ITB consists of two tracts. The iliotibial tract inserts on the Gerdy tubercle of the lateral tibial plateau.

The patellar retinaculum is an important soft tissue stabilizer of the patellofemoral joint. The thicker lateral retinaculum comprises a distinct thick, deep layer and a thin superficial layer.

The patella, the largest sesamoid bone in the body, possesses the thickest articular cartilage. The articular surface, which can have a variable contour, articulates with the trochlear groove of the femur.

The patellar tendon, occasionally termed the patellar ligament, originates at the inferior pole of the patella and inserts onto the tibial tuberosity.

Biomechanics

Tibiofemoral Joint

The motions that occur about the knee consist of flexion and extension, coupled with other motions such as varus and valgus motions and external and internal rotation. All of the motions

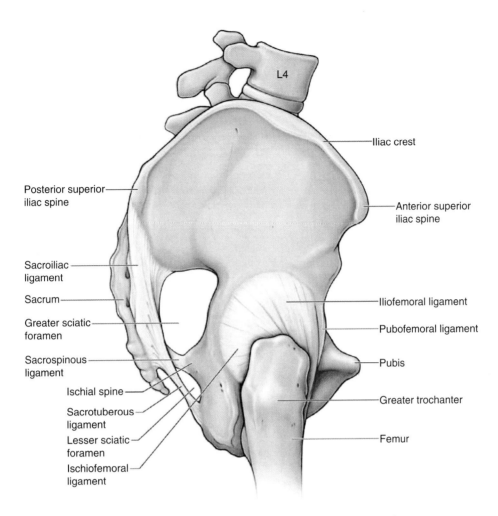

FIGURE 2–18 Ligament structures of the hip and the relationship of the hip joint to the lateral pelvis.

TABLE 2–32 Ligaments of the hip.

Ligament	Origin	Insertion	Action
Iliofemoral (Y ligament of Bigelow) Consists of two parts: an inferior (medial) portion and a superior (lateral) portion, making it resemble an inverted Y	The anterior inferior iliac spine at its apex	Medial portion inserts into the inferior aspect of the trochanteric line, while the lateral portion inserts onto the superior aspect of the trochanteric line	Exhibits the greater stiffness and prevents anterior translation during extension and external rotation, in both flexion and extension Hip adduction tightens the superior portion of the iliofemoral ligament
Pubofemoral	Blends with the inferior band of the iliofemoral, and with the pectineus muscle	Attaches medially to the iliopectineal eminence, the superior pubic ramus, and the obturator crest and membrane, and laterally to the anterior surface of the trochanteric line	Its fibers tighten in extension, and also tighten in external rotation
Ischiofemoral	Posterior thickening of the joint capsule	The anterior aspect of the femur	Tightens with internal rotation of the hip in flexion and extension, as well as adduction of the flexed hip More commonly injured than the other hip ligaments

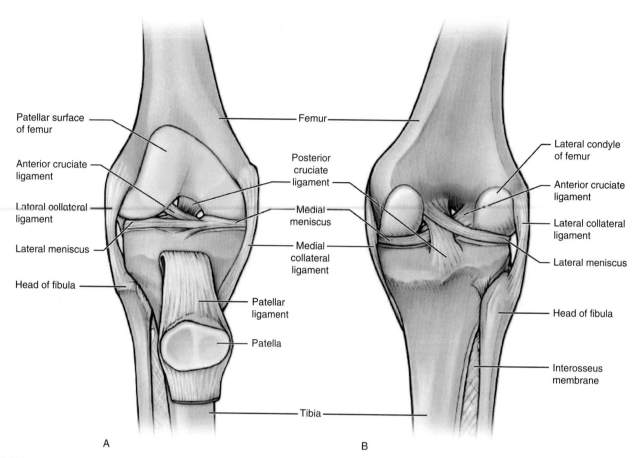

FIGURE 2–19 Ligaments and menisci of the (A) anterior and (B) posterior knee.

TABLE 2–33 **Muscles of the knee: actions, nerve supply, and nerve root derivation.**

Action	Primary Muscles	Peripheral Nerve Supply	Nerve Root Derivation
Flexion of knee	Biceps femoris	Sciatic	L5, S1–2
	Semimembranosus	Sciatic	L5, S2–2
	Semitendinosus	Sciatic	L5, S1–2
	Gracilis	Obturator	L2–3
	Sartorius	Femoral	L2–3
	Popliteus	Tibial	L4–5, S1
	Gastrocnemius	Tibial	S1–2
	Tensor fascia latae	Superior gluteal	L4–5
Extension of knee	Rectus femoris	Femoral	L2–4
	Vastus medialis	Femoral	L2–4
	Vastus intermedius	Femoral	L2–4
	Vastus lateralis	Femoral	L2–4
	Tensor fascia latae	Superior gluteal	L4–5
Internal rotation of flexed leg (non-weightbearing)	Popliteus	Tibial	L4–5
	Semimembranosus	Sciatic	L5, S1–2
	Semitendinosus	Sciatic	L5, S1–2
	Sartorius	Femoral	L2–3
	Gracilis	Obturator	L2–3
External rotation of flexed leg (non-weightbearing)	Biceps femoris	Sciatic	L5, S1–2

Data from Magee DJ. *Orthopaedic Physical Assessment*. 2nd ed. Philadelphia, PA: WB Saunders; 1992.

TABLE 2–34 Common ligamentous and meniscal injuries.

	Mechanism of Injury	Subjective Complaints
MCL	Most commonly involves external valgus or rotational force while leg is firmly planted; often associated with ACL injury	Localized swelling and tenderness over injured area
ACL	Commonly involves noncontact pivoting/twisting mechanism while foot is planted; noncontact hyperextension; sudden deceleration; forced internal rotation; sudden valgus impact	Reports of being unable to continue activity; hearing "pop" in the knee; extreme pain at time of injury; acute knee swelling (within 1–2 hours of injury)
Meniscus	Usually caused by noncontact injury; rotational/torsional force applied to flexed knee with foot firmly planted	Reports of swelling developing within 12 hours of injury; localized swelling and tenderness over injured area, history of popping, clicking, or locking with knee motions

about the tibiofemoral joint consist of a rolling, gliding, and rotation between the femoral condyles and the tibial plateaus. This rolling, gliding, and rotation occur almost simultaneously, albeit in different directions. For flexion to be initiated from a position of full extension, the knee joint must first be "unlocked." The service of locksmith is provided by the popliteus muscle, which acts to internally rotate the tibia with respect to the femur, enabling the flexion to occur.

During flexion of the knee, the femur rolls posteriorly and glides anteriorly, with the opposite occurring with extension of the knee. This arrangement resembles a twin wheel rolling on a central rail. In the last 30° to 5° of weight-bearing knee extension, the lateral condyle of the femur and the lateral meniscus (LM) become congruent, moving the axis of movement more laterally. The tibial glide now becomes much greater on the medial side, which produces internal rotation of the femur, and the ligaments, both extrinsic and intrinsic, start to tighten near terminal extension. At this point, the cruciates become crossed and are tightened.

In the last 5° of extension, rotation is the only movement accompanying the extension. This rotation is referred to as the *screw home mechanism*, and is a characteristic motion in the normal knee in which the tibia externally rotates and the femur internally rotates as the knee approaches extension. Zero degrees to 15° of knee hyperextension is usually available.[60] During knee hyperextension, the femur does not continue to roll anteriorly but instead tilts forward. This creates anterior compression between the femur and tibia.[61] In the normal knee, hyperextension is checked by the soft tissue structures. When the knee hyperextends, the axis of the thigh runs obliquely inferiorly and posteriorly, which tends to place the ground reaction force anterior to the knee. In this position, the posterior structures are placed in tension, which helps to stabilize the knee joint, negating the need for quadriceps muscle activity.[62]

Patellofemoral Joint

The patella is a passive component of the knee extensor mechanism, where the static and dynamic relationships of the underlying tibia and femur determine the patellar-tracking pattern. To assist in the control of the forces around the patellofemoral joint, there are a number of static and dynamic restraints. The static restraints include:

- The medial retinaculum. This is the primary static restraint to lateral patellar displacement at 20° of knee flexion, contributing 60% of the total restraining force.[63]
- Bony configuration of the trochlea. The patellofemoral joint is intrinsically unstable because the tibial tubercle lies lateral to the long axis of the femur and the quadriceps muscle, and the patella is therefore subject to a laterally-directed force.
- The medial patellomeniscal ligament and the lateral retinaculum contribute 13% and 10% of the restraint to lateral translation of the patella, respectively.

The passive restraints to medial translation of the patella are provided by the structures that form the superficial and deep lateral retinaculum.

The primary dynamic restraints to patellar motion are the quadriceps muscles, particularly the vastus medialis oblique (VMO). However, the muscle vector of the VMO is more vertical than normal when a patella malalignment is present, making it less effective as a dynamic stabilizer.[64,65] The timing of the VMO contractions relative to the other quadriceps muscles, especially the vastus lateralis, has been found to be abnormal with patellar malalignment, and the VMO is vulnerable to inhibition when swelling is present.

The Quadriceps Angle

The quadriceps ("Q") angle can be described as the angle formed by the bisection of two lines, one line drawn from the anterior superior iliac spine (ASIS) to the center of the patella, and the other from the center of the patella to the tibial tubercle. Various normal values for the Q-angle have been reported in the literature. The most common ranges cited are 8° to 14° for males and 15° to 17° for females.[66,67] The discrepancy between males and females is supposedly due to the wider pelvis of the female, although this has yet to be proven.

The Q-angle can vary significantly with the degree of foot pronation and supination, and when compared with measurements made in the supine position.[66,67]

Patella-Femur Contact and Loading

The amount of contact between the patella and the femur appears to vary according to a number of factors including (1) the angle of knee flexion, (2) the location of contact, (3) the surface area of contact, and (4) the patellofemoral joint reaction force.[68] Each of these factors is discussed separately.

Angle of knee flexion—As knee flexion proceeds, the stress on the patella increases significantly.[69]

Location of contact—In the normal knee, as the knee flexes from 10° to 90°, the contact area shifts gradually from the distal to the proximal pole of the patella.

- At full extension, the patella is not in contact with the femur, but rests on the supratrochlear fat pad.[70]
- From full extension to 10° of flexion, the tibia internally rotates, allowing the patella to move into the trochlea.[68] This brings the inferior third of the patellar into contact with the femur.
- From 10° to 20° of flexion, the patella contacts the lateral surface of the femur on the inferior patellar surface.[71,72]
- The middle surfaces of the inferior aspect of the patellar come into contact with the femur at around 30° to 60° of flexion, at which point the patella is well seated in the groove.[71,72]
- As the knee continues to flex to 90° the patella moves laterally, and the area of patella contact moves proximally.[68] At 90° of knee flexion, the entire articular surface of the patella (except the odd facet) is in contact with the femur.[71,72]
- Beyond 90°, the patella rides down into the intercondylar notch. At this point, the medial and lateral surfaces of the patella are in contact with the femur and the quadriceps tendon articulates with the trochlear groove of the femur.[68]
- At approximately 120° of knee flexion, there is no contact between the patella and the medial femoral condyle. At 135° of knee flexion, the odd facet of the patella makes contact with the medial femoral condyle.

Surface area of contact[73]—From 0° to 60° of flexion, the magnitude of the patellofemoral contact area increases as flexion proceeds. Between 30° and 60° of flexion, the patella moves medially to become centered in the trochlear groove. Contact between the quadriceps tendon and the femur begins at more than 70° of flexion.[73] When the knee is flexed beyond 90°, the patella tilts so that its medial facet articulates with the medial femoral condyle.[68] As knee flexion approaches 120°, the contact area moves back toward the center of the patella. This is the point of maximum contact area between the patella and the femur.[74]

Patellofemoral joint reaction force—The patellofemoral joint reaction force (PJRF) causes compression of the patellofemoral joint. The PJRF is due to the increase in patellar and quadriceps tendon tension and the increase in the acuity of the Q-angle that occurs during knee flexion. Maximum force in the quadriceps muscle and patellar tendon is generated at 60° of flexion.

Patellar Tracking

In the normal knee, the patella glides in a sinuous path inferiorly and superiorly during flexion and extension respectively, covering a distance of 5 to 7 cm with respect to the femur.[75] The patella produces a concave lateral C-shaped curve as it moves from a knee flexion of approximately 120° toward approximately 30° of knee extension. Further extension of the knee (between 30° and 0°) produces a lateral glide of the patella in the frontal plane and a lateral tilt in the sagittal plane.

Open and Closed Kinetic Chain Activities

A closed-chain motion at the knee joint complex occurs when the knee bends or straightens, while the lower extremity is weight-bearing, or when the foot is in contact with any firm surface. An open-chain motion occurs when the knee bends or straightens when the foot is not in contact with any stable surface.

Whether the motion occurring at the knee joint complex occurs as a closed or open kinetic chain has implications on the biomechanics and the joint compressive forces induced.

Closed-chain motion

TIBIOFEMORAL JOINT   During closed-chain knee flexion, the femoral condyles roll backward and glide forward on the tibia. During closed-chain knee extension, the femoral condyles roll forward and slide backward. During closed-chain knee flexion, as the femur rolls posteriorly, the distance between the tibial and femoral insertions of the ACL increases. Since the ACL cannot lengthen, it guides the femoral condyles anteriorly.[60] In contrast, during closed-chain extension of the knee, the distance between the femoral and tibial insertions of the posterior cruciate ligament (PCL) increases. Since the PCL cannot lengthen, the ligament guides the femoral condyles posteriorly as the knee extends.[60]

Some studies have demonstrated that CKC exercises at greater than 30° of knee flexion can exacerbate patellofemoral problems.[76,77]

PATELLOFEMORAL JOINT   During closed kinetic exercises, the flexion moment arm increases as the angle of knee flexion increases. Also, the joint-reaction force increases proportionately more during knee flexion than the magnitude of the contact area.[65] Thus, the articular pressure gradually increases as the knee flexes from 0° to 90°,[65] with maximum values occurring at 90° of flexion.[74] However, because this increasing force is distributed over a larger patellofemoral contact area, the contact stress per unit area is minimized.

From 90° to 120° of flexion, the articular pressure remains essentially unchanged because the quadriceps tendon is in contact with the trochlea, which effectively increases the contact area.[78]

Due to the effect of joint reaction forces, CKC exercises involving the patellofemoral joint are performed in the 0° to 45° range of flexion, with caution used when exercising between 90° and 50° of knee flexion, where the patellofemoral joint reaction forces can be significantly greater.[78]

Open-chain motion

TIBIOFEMORAL JOINT   During open-chain flexion, the tibia rolls and glides posteriorly on the femur, while during extension the opposite occurs. Open-chain knee extension involves a conjunct external rotation of the tibia, while open-chain knee flexion involves a conjunct internal rotation of the tibia.

Open-chain activities produce shear forces at the tibiofemoral joint in the direction of tibial movement.

Open-chain knee flexion, resulting from an isolated contraction of the hamstrings, reduces ACL strain throughout the ROM[79] but increases the strain on the PCL as flexion increases from 30° to 90°.[80]

PATELLOFEMORAL JOINT In an open-chain activity, the forces across the patella are their lowest at 90° of flexion. As the knee extends from this position, the flexion moment arm (contact stress/unit) for the knee increases, peaking between 35° and 40° of flexion, while the patella contact area decreases.[76,81] This produces an increase in the PJRF at a point when the contact area is very small. At 0° of flexion (full knee extension), the quadriceps force is high but the contact stress/unit is low.

Due to the effect of joint reaction forces, OKC exercises for the patellofemoral joint should be performed from 25° to 90° of flexion (60°-90° if there are distal patellar lesions), or at 0° of extension (or hyperextension) from a point of view of cartilage stress.[78] OKC exercises are not recommended for the patellofemoral joint between 0° and 45° of knee flexion, especially if there are proximal patellar lesions, as the PJRFs are significantly greater.[78]

HIP INFLUENCES Some recent studies have suggested that proximal factors may play a contributory role concerning knee injuries.[82] These studies indicate that impaired muscular control of the hip, pelvis, and trunk can affect multiple planes of tibiofemoral and patellofemoral joint kinematics and kinetics, resulting in such injuries as anterior cruciate ligament tears, ITB syndrome, and patellofemoral joint pain.[82]

ANKLE AND FOOT JOINT COMPLEX

The majority of the support provided to the ankle and foot joints come by way of the arrangement of the ankle mortise and the numerous ligaments found here (Table 2–35).

Further stabilization is afforded by an abundant number of short and long tendons that cross this joint complex (Tables 2–36 and 2–37). These tendons are also involved in producing foot and ankle movements and are held in place by retinaculae.

Even with this remarkable level of protection, the foot and ankle complex is at the mercy of truly impressive forces that act upon it during normal and athletic activities. As elsewhere, injuries to this area can be either microtraumatic or macrotraumatic.

Biomechanics

Terminology

Motions of the leg, foot, and ankle consist of single-plane and multiplane movements.

The single-plane motions include:

- The frontal plane motions of inversion and eversion
- The sagittal plane motions of dorsiflexion and plantarflexion
- The horizontal plane motions of adduction and abduction

Triplanar motions occur at the talocrural, subtalar, and midtarsal joints and at the first and fifth rays. Pronation and supination are considered triplanar motions.

- The three body plane motions in pronation are abduction in the transverse plane, dorsiflexion in the sagittal plane, and eversion in the frontal plane.
- The three body plane motions in supination are a combined movement of adduction, plantarflexion, and inversion.

In pronation, the forefoot is rotated big toe downward and little toe upward, whereas in supination the reverse occurs.

Distal Tibiofibular Joint

The two tibiofibular joints (proximal and distal) are described as individual articulations, but in fact they function as a pair. The movements that occur at these joints are primarily a result of the ankle's influence.

The ligaments of the distal tibiofibular joint are more commonly injured than the anterior talofibular ligament. Injuries to the ankle syndesmosis most often occur as a result of forced external rotation of the foot or during internal rotation of the tibia on a planted foot. Hyperdorsiflexion may also be a contributing mechanism.

Talocrural Joint

The primary motions at this joint are dorsiflexion and plantar flexion, with a total range of 70° to 80°. The orientation of the talocrural joint axis is oriented on average 20° to 30° posterior to the frontal plane as it passes posteriorly from the medial malleolus to the lateral malleolus. Although talocrural motion occurs primarily in the sagittal plane, an appreciable amount of horizontal motion appears to occur in the horizontal plane, especially during internal rotation of the tibia or pronation of the foot.

The tibia follows the talus during weight-bearing so that the talocrural joint externally rotates with supination and internally rotates with pronation.[83] Therefore the tibia internally rotates during pronation and externally rotates during supination.[84]

Stability for this joint in weight-bearing is provided by the articular surfaces, while in non-weightbearing, the ligaments appear to provide the majority of stability.

Subtalar Joint

The subtalar joint is responsible for inversion and eversion of the hindfoot (Figure 2–20). Approximately 50% of apparent ankle inversion observed actually comes from the subtalar joint. The axis of motion for the subtalar joint is approximately 45° from horizontal and 20° medial to the midsagittal plane.

This axis, which moves during subtalar joint motion, allows the subtalar joint to produce a triplanar (pronation/supination) and varies according to whether the joint is weight-bearing (close chain) or non-weightbearing (open chain).[85]

- During weight-bearing activities, pronation involves a combination of calcaneal eversion, adduction and plantarflexion of the talus, and internal rotation of the tibia, whereas supination involves a combination of calcaneal inversion, abduction and dorsiflexion of the talus, and external rotation of the tibia.
- During non-weightbearing activities, pronation involves a combination of calcaneal eversion and abduction and dorsiflexion of the talus, whereas supination involves a combination of calcaneal inversion and adduction and plantarflexion of the talus.

TABLE 2–35 Ankle and foot joints and associated ligaments.

Joint	Associated Ligament	Fiber Direction	Motions Limited
Distal tibiofibular	Anterior tibiofibular	Distolateral	Distal glide of fibula
	Posterior tibiofibular	Distolateral	Plantar flexion
	Interosseous		Distal glide of fibular
			Plantar flexion
			Separation of tibia and fibula
Ankle	Deltoid (medial collateral)		
	Superficial		
	Tibionavicular	Plantar-anterior	Plantar flexion, abduction
	Tibiocalcaneal	Plantar, plantar-posterior	Eversion, abduction
	Posterior tibiotalar	Plantar-posterior	Dorsiflexion, abduction
	Deep		Eversion, abduction, plantar flexion
	Anterior tibiotalar		Plantar flexion
	Lateral or fibular collateral		
	Anterior talofibular	Anterior	Inversion
			Anterior displacement of foot
	Calcaneofibular	Anterior-medial	Inversion
			Dorsiflexion
	Posterior talofibular	Posterior-medial	Dorsiflexion
			Posterior displacement of foot
	Lateral talocalcaneal	Horizontal (lateral)	Inversion
			Dorsiflexion
	Anterior capsule	Posterior-medial	Plantar flexion
	Posterior capsule		Dorsiflexion
Subtalar	Interosseous talocalcaneal		
	Anterior band	Proximal-anterior-lateral	Inversion
	Posterior band	Proximal-posterior-lateral	Joint separation
	Lateral talocalcaneal		Inversion
	Deltoid	(See ankle)	Joint separation
	Lateral collateral	(See ankle)	Dorsiflexion
	Posterior talocalcaneal	(See ankle)	Eversion
	Medial talocalcaneal	Vertical	
	Anterior talocalcaneal (cervical ligaments)	Plantar-anterior Plantar-posterior-lateral	Inversion
Main ligamentous support of longitudinal arches	Long plantar	Anterior, slightly medial	Eversion
	Short plantar	Anterior	Eversion
	Plantar calcaneonavicular	Dorsal-anterior-medial	Eversion
	Plantar aponeurosis	Anterior	Eversion
Midtarsal or transverse	Bifurcated		Joint separation
	Medial band	Longitudinal	Plantar flexion
	Lateral band	Horizontal	Inversion
	Dorsal talonavicular	Longitudinal	Plantar flexion of talus on navicular
	Dorsal calcaneocuboid ligaments supporting the arches	Longitudinal	Inversion, plantar flexion
Intertarsal	Numerous ligaments named by two interconnected bones (dorsal and plantar ligaments)		Joint motion in direction causing ligament tightening
	Interosseous ligaments connecting cuneiforms, cuboid, and navicular ligaments supporting arches		Flattening of transverse arch
Tarsometatarsal	Dorsal, plantar, and interosseous		Joint separation

(Continued)

TABLE 2-35 Ankle and foot joints and associated ligaments. (*Continued*)

Joint	Associated Ligament	Fiber Direction	Motions Limited
Intermetatarsal	Dorsal, plantar, and interosseous		Joint separation
	Deep transverse metatarsal		Joint separation
			Flattening of transverse arch
Metatarsophalangeal	Fibrous capsule		Flexion
	Dorsally, thin—separated from extensor tendons by bursae		Extension
	Inseparable from deep surface of plantar and collateral ligaments		
	Collateral	Plantar-anterior	Flexion, abduction, or adduction in flexion
	Plantar, grooved for flexor tendons		Extension
Interphalangeal	Collateral		Flexion, abduction, or adduction in flexion
	Plantar		Extension
	Extensor hood replaces dorsal ligaments		Flexion

TABLE 2-36 Intrinsic muscles of the foot.

Muscle	Attachments	Action	Innervation
Extensor digitorum brevis	Proximal: Superior surface of calcaneus Distal: Dorsal surface of second through fourth toes, base of proximal phalanx	Extends digits 2 through 4	Deep peroneal S1 and S2
Abductor hallucis	Proximal: Tuberosity of calcaneus and plantar aponeurosis Distal: Base of proximal phalanx, medial side	Abducts hallux	Medial plantar L5 and S1 (L4)
Adductor hallucis	Proximal: Base of second, third, and fourth metatarsals and deep plantar ligaments Distal: Proximal phalanx of first digit lateral side	Adducts hallux	Medial and lateral plantar S1 and S2
Lumbricals	Proximal: Medial and adjacent sides of flexor digitorum longus tendon to each lateral digit Distal: Medial side of proximal phalanx and extensor hood	Flex metatarso-phalangeal joints; extend interphalangeal joints	Medial and lateral plantar L5, S1, and S2 (L4)
Plantar interossei		Adduct toes	Medial and lateral plantar S1 and S2
First	Proximal: Base and medial side of third metatarsal Distal: Base of proximal phalanx and extensor hood of third digit		
Second	Proximal: Base and medial side of fourth metatarsal Distal: Base of proximal phalanx and extensor hood of fourth digit		
Third	Proximal: Base and medial side of fifth metatarsal Distal: Base of proximal phalanx and extensor hood of fifth digit		
Dorsal interossei		Abduct toes	Medial and lateral plantar S1 and S2
First	Proximal: First and second metatarsal bones Distal: Proximal phalanx and extensor hood of second digit medially		
Second	Proximal: Second and third metatarsal bones Distal: Proximal phalanx and extensor hood of second digit laterally		
Third	Proximal: Third and fourth metatarsal bones Distal: Proximal phalanx and extensor hood of third digit laterally		
Fourth	Proximal: Fourth and fifth metatarsal bones Distal: Proximal phalanx and extensor hood of fourth digit laterally		
Abductor digiti minimi	Proximal: Lateral side of fifth metatarsal bone Distal: Proximal phalanx of fifth digit	Flexion and abduction of the fifth toe	Lateral plantar S1 and S2

TABLE 2–37 Extrinsic muscle attachments and innervation.

Muscle	Attachments	Action	Innervation
Gastrocnemius	Proximal: Medial and lateral condyle of femur Distal: Posterior surface of calcaneus through Achilles tendon	Plantarflexes foot flexes knee	Tibial S2 (S1)
Plantaris	Proximal: Lateral supracondylar line of femur Distal: Posterior surface of calcaneus through Achilles tendon	Plantarflexes foot and flexes knee	Tibial S2 (S1)
Soleus	Proximal: Head of fibula, proximal third of shaft, soleal line and midshaft of posterior tibia Distal: Posterior surface of calcaneus through Achilles tendon	Plantarflexes foot	Tibial S2 (S1)
Tibialis anterior	Proximal: Distal to lateral tibial condyle, proximal half of lateral tibial shaft, and interosseous membrane Distal: First cuneiform bone, medial and plantar surfaces and base of first metatarsal	Dorsiflexion and inversion of the foot	Deep fibular (peroneal) L4 (L5)
Tibialis posterior	Proximal: Posterior surface of tibia, proximal two thirds posterior of fibula, and interosseous membrane Distal: Tuberosity of navicular bone, tendinous expansion to other tarsals and metatarsals	Plantar flexion and inversion of the foot	Tibial L4 and L5
Fibularis (peroneus) longus	Proximal: Lateral condyle of tibia, head and proximal two-thirds of fibula Distal: Base of first metatarsal and first cuneiform, lateral side	Plantarflexion, eversion of the foot	Superficial fibular (peroneal) L5 and S1 (S2)
Fibularis (peroneus) brevis	Proximal: Distal two-thirds of lateral fibular shaft Distal: Tuberosity of fifth metatarsal	Plantarflexion, eversion of the foot	Superficial fibular (peroneal) L5 and S1 (S2)
Fibularis (peroneus) tertius	Proximal: Lateral slip from extensor digitorum longus Distal: Tuberosity of fifth metatarsal	Dorsiflexion and eversion of the foot	Deep fibular (peroneal) L5 and S1
Flexor hallucis brevis	Proximal: Plantar surface of cuboid and third cuneiform bones Distal: Base of proximal phalanx of great toe	Flexion of the hallux	Medial plantar S3 (S2)
Flexor hallucis longus	Proximal: Posterior distal two-thirds fibula Distal: Base of distal phalanx of great toe	Flexion of all joints of the big toe; plantar flexion of the ankle joint	Tibial S2 (S3)
Flexor digitorum brevis	Proximal: Tuberosity of calcaneus Distal: One tendon slips into base of middle phalanx of each of the lateral four toes	Flexion of the lateral four digits	Medial and lateral plantar S3 (S2)
Flexor digitorum longus	Proximal: Middle three-fifths of posterior tibia Distal: Base of distal phalanx of lateral four toes	Flexion of the four smaller digits	Tibial S2 (S3)
Extensor hallucis longus	Proximal: Middle half of anterior shaft of fibula Distal: Base of distal phalanx of great toe	Extension of the big toe and assists in dorsiflexion of the foot at the ankle Also a weak evertor/invertor	Deep fibular (peroneal) L5 and S1
Extensor hallucis brevis	Proximal: Distal superior and lateral surfaces of calcaneus Distal: Dorsal surface of proximal phalanx	Extends the hallux	Deep fibular (peroneal) S1 and S2
Extensor digitorum longus	Proximal: Lateral condyle of tibia proximal anterior surface of shaft of fibula Distal: One tendon to each lateral four toes, to middle phalanx and extending to distal phalanges	Extension of toes and dorsiflexion of ankle	Deep fibular (peroneal) L5 and S1

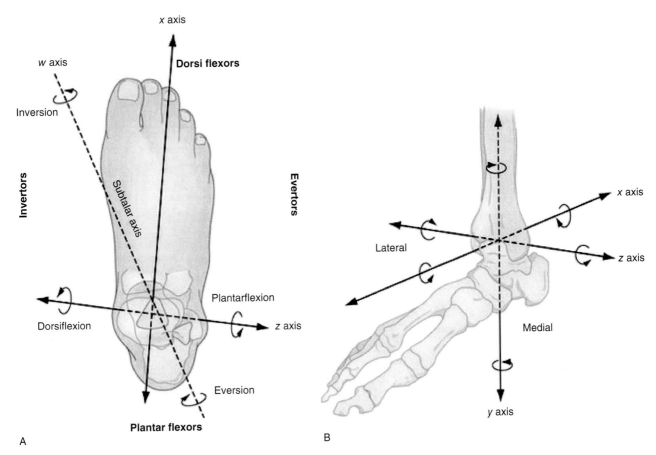

FIGURE 2-20 Biomechanical axes of the foot-ankle complex.

The subtalar joint controls supination and pronation in close conjunction with the transverse tarsal joints of the mid foot. In normal individuals, there is an eversion to inversion ratio of 2:3 to 1:3, which amounts to approximately 20° of inversion and 10° of eversion. For normal gait, a minimum of 4° to 6° of eversion and 8° to 12° of inversion are required.[86]

Stability for the subtalar joint is provided by the calcaneofibular ligament (CFL), the cervical ligament, the interosseous ligament, the lateral talocalcaneal ligament, the fibulotalocalcaneal ligament (ligament of Rouviere), and the extensor retinaculum.

Midtarsal (Transverse Tarsal) Joint Complex

The function of the midtarsal joint complex is to provide the foot with an additional mechanism for raising and lowering the arch, and to absorb some of the horizontal plane tibial motion that is transmitted to the foot during stance.[83,87] The joints of the foot and ankle have varying degrees of freedom (Table 2–38).

The function of the great toe is to provide stability to the medial aspect of the foot and to provide for normal propulsion during gait. Normal alignment of the first metatarsophalangeal (MTP) joint varies between 5° varus and 15° valgus.

The great toe is characterized by having a remarkable discrepancy between active and passive motion. Approximately 30° of active plantar flexion is present and at least 50° of active extension, the latter of which can be frequently increased passively to between 70° to 90°.

CRANIOVERTEBRAL JOINTS

The craniovertebral (CV) junction is a collective term that refers to the region of the cervical spine where the skull and vertebral column articulate. It comprises the bony structures of the foramen magnum, occiput, atlas, and axis, and their supporting ligaments.

TABLE 2–38 Degrees of freedom for ankle and foot joints.

Joint	Degrees of Freedom	Motions Available
Talocalcaneal	2	Plantar/dorsiflexion, inversion/eversion
Cuneonavicular	2	Plantar/dorsiflexion, inversion/eversion
Intercuneiform and cuneocuboid	1	Inversion/eversion
Metatarsophalangeal	2	Flexion/extension, abduction/adduction
First metatarsophalangeal	2	Flexion/extension, abduction/adduction
Interphalangeal (IP)	1	Flexion/extension

The posterior portion of the foramen magnum houses the brainstem-spinal cord junction.

Occipito-Atlantal Joint

The occipito-atlantal (O-A) joint is formed between the occipital condyles and the superior articular facets of the atlas (C1). The paired occipital condyles are ovoid structures with their long axis situated in a posterolateral-to-anteromedial orientation.

Atlantoaxial Joint

This is a relatively complex articulation, which consists of:

- Two lateral synovial zygapophyseal joints between the articular surfaces of the inferior articular processes of the atlas and the superior processes of the axis.
- Two medial synovial joints: One between the anterior surface of the dens of the axis and the anterior surface of the atlas, and the other between the posterior surface of the dens and the anterior hyalinated surface of the transverse ligament.

Craniovertebral Ligaments

The craniovertebral ligaments (Figure 2–21) are outlined in Table 2–39.

Craniovertebral Muscles

The muscles of the craniovertebral region are outlined in Table 2–40.

Craniovertebral Nerves

The dorsal ramus of spinal nerve C1 is larger than the ventral ramus, and supplies most of the muscles that form that triangle. It usually has no cutaneous distribution.

The dorsal ramus of spinal nerve C2, also known as the greater occipital nerve, supplies most of the posterior aspect of the scalp, extending anteriorly to a line across the scalp that extends from one external auditory meatus to the other.

Blood Supply

The cervical cord is supplied by two arterial systems, central and peripheral, which overlap but are discrete. The first is dependent entirely on the single anterior spinal artery (ASA). The second, without clearcut boundaries, receives supplies from the ASA and both posterior spinal arteries.[94]

Biomechanics

The upper cervical spine is responsible for approximately 50% of the motion that occurs in the entire cervical spine. Motion at

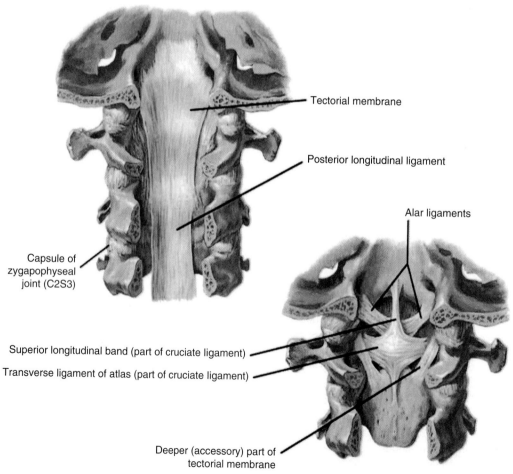

Tectorial membrane

Posterior longitudinal ligament

Alar ligaments

Capsule of zygapophyseal joint (C2S3)

Superior longitudinal band (part of cruciate ligament)

Transverse ligament of atlas (part of cruciate ligament)

Deeper (accessory) part of tectorial membrane

FIGURE 2–21 Ligaments of the upper cervical spine.

TABLE 2–39 Craniovertebral ligaments.

Ligament	Description
Capsule and accessory capsular	These ligaments are quite lax, to permit maximal motion, so they provide only moderate support to the joints during contralateral head rotation.
Apical	Extends from the apex of the dens to the anterior rim of the foramen magnum. The ligament appears to be only a moderate stabilizer against posterior translation of the dens relative to both the atlas and the occipital bone.
Vertical and transverse bands of the cruciform	The transverse portion stretches between tubercles on the medial aspects of the lateral masses of the atlas. The major responsibility of the transverse portion is to counteract anterior translation of the atlas relative to the axis, thereby maintaining the position of the dens relative to the anterior arch of the atlas. The transverse ligament also limits the amount of flexion between the atlas and axis.[88] These limiting functions are of extreme importance because excessive movement of either type could result in the dens compressing the spinal cord, epipharynx, vertebral artery, or superior cervical ganglion.
Alar and accessory alar	Connect the superior part of the dens to fossae on the medial aspect of the occipital condyles, although they can also attach to the lateral masses of the atlas. The function of the ligament is to resist flexion, contralateral side bending, and rotation.[89] Due to the connections of the ligament, side bending of the head produces a contralateral rotation of the C2 vertebra.[90]
Anterior occipito-atlantal membrane	Thought to be the superior continuation of the anterior longitudinal ligament. It extends from the anterior arch of vertebra C1 to the anterior aspect of the foramen magnum.
Posterior occipito-atlantal membrane	A continuation of the ligamentum flavum. This ligament interconnects the posterior arch of the atlas and the posterior aspect of the foramen magnum.
Tectorial membrane	Interconnects the occipital bone and the axis. This ligament is the superior continuation of the posterior longitudinal ligament, and connects the body of vertebra C2 to the anterior rim of the foramen magnum. This bridging ligament is an important limiter of upper cervical flexion.

the atlantoaxial (A-A) joint occurs relatively independently, while below C2, normal motion is a combination of motion occurring at other levels.

Occipito-Atlantal Joint

The primary motion that occurs at this joint is flexion and extension, although side-bending and rotation also occur. It is generally agreed that rotation and side-bending at this joint occur to opposite sides when they are combined.

Occipital rotation, and to some degree anterior-posterior translation of the occiput on C1, is thought to be limited by the alar ligaments.

Atlantoaxial Joint

The major motion that occurs at all three of the A-A articulations is axial rotation, totaling approximately 40° to 47° to each side. This large amount of rotation has the potential to cause compression of the vertebral artery if it becomes excessive. As the atlas rotates, the ipsilateral facet moves posteriorly and inferiorly while the contralateral facet moves anteriorly and inferiorly, so that each facet of the atlas slides along the convex surface of the axial facet, telescoping the head downward.

Flexion and extension movements of the A-A joint amount to a combined range of 10° to 15°: 10° of flexion, and 5° of extension.

TABLE 2–40 Muscles of the craniovertebral region.

Region	Specific Muscle	Function	Nerve Supply
Anterior suboccipital	Rectus capitis anterior	Aids in flexion of the head and the neck.	C1, C2
	Rectus capitis lateralis	Aids in side flexion. Also stabilizes the occipito-atlantal joint.	C1, C2
Posterior suboccipital	Rectus capitis posterior major Rectus capitis posterior minor Obliquus capitis superior Obliquus capitis inferior	These muscles function in the control of segmental sliding between C1 and C2,[91] and may have an important role in proprioception, having more muscle spindles than any other muscle for their size.[91] All of the posterior suboccipital muscles are innervated by the posterior ramus of C1, and are also strongly linked with the trigeminal nerve.[92,93] The suboccipitals receive their blood supply from the vertebral artery.	Suboccipital nerve

CERVICAL SPINE

The cervical spine is made up of seven vertebrae, C1 to C7. Eight pairs of cervical spinal nerves exit bilaterally through the intervertebral foramina. Each spinal nerve is named for the vertebra above which it exits; for example, the C6 nerve exits above the C6 vertebra. This naming changes at the C7-T1 segment. The C8 nerve exits at the C7-T1 segment. All of the spinal nerves inferior to this segment are named for the vertebra beneath; for example, the T1 nerve exits at T1-2 segment.

With stability being sacrificed for mobility, the cervical spine is rendered more vulnerable to both direct and indirect trauma. The cervical spine can be the source of many pain syndromes, including neck, upper thoracic and periscapular syndromes, cervical radiculopathy, and shoulder and elbow syndromes.

Biomechanics

At the zygapophyseal joints, significant flexion occurs at C5–C6, and extension around C6–C7.

The only significant arthrokinematic motion available to the zygapophyseal joint is an inferior, medial glide of the inferior articular process of the superior facet during extension and a superior, lateral glide during flexion. Segmental side-bending is therefore extension of the ipsilateral joint and flexion of the contralateral joint. Rotation, coupled with ipsilateral side bending, involves extension of the ipsilateral joint and flexion of the contralateral.

Muscle Control

The muscle groups of the cervical region may be divided into those that produce global movements and those local muscles that sustain postures or stabilize the segments.[95-97]

- The global muscles of the neck are thought to be the sternocleidomastoid (ventrally) and the semispinalis capitis and splenius capitis (dorsally).
- The local system is thought to comprise the longus capitis and longus colli[98] and semispinalis cervicis and multifidus.[99]

TEMPOROMANDIBULAR JOINT

Three bony components make up the masticatory system: the maxilla and the mandible, which support the teeth, and the temporal bone, which supports the mandible at its articulation with the skull. The temporomandibular joint (TMJ) is a synovial, compound modified ovoid bicondylar joint formed between the articular eminence of the temporal bone, the intra-articular disk, and the head of the mandible. The TMJ is unique in that, even though the joint is synovial, the articulating surfaces of the bones are covered, not by hyaline cartilage, but by fibrocartilage. The development of fibrocartilage over the load-bearing surface of the TMJ indicates that the joint is designed to withstand large and repeated stresses, and that this area of the joint surface has a greater capacity to repair itself than would hyaline cartilage.

Located between the articulating surface of the temporal bone and the mandibular condyle is a fibrocartilaginous disk (sometimes incorrectly referred to as "meniscus"). The shape of the condyle and the articulating fossa determines the biconcave shape of the disk.

The disk is usually located on top of the condyle in the 12 o'clock to 1 o'clock position on the mandibular head when the jaw is closed. Because the only firm attachment of the disk to the condyle occurs medially and laterally, the disk can move somewhat independently of the condyle.

The disk effectively divides the TMJ into a lower and upper joint cavity.

Muscles of the TMJ Region

The muscles of this region are described in Table 2–41.

Working in combinations, the muscles of the TMJ are involved as follows:

- Mouth opening—bilateral action of the lateral pterygoid and digastric muscles
- Mouth closing—bilateral action of the temporalis, masseter, and medial pterygoid muscles
- Lateral deviation—action of the ipsilateral masseter and contralateral medial pterygoid muscles
- Protrusion—bilateral action of the lateral pterygoid, medial pterygoid, and anterior fibers of the temporalis muscles
- Retrusion—bilateral action of the posterior fibers of the temporalis muscle and the digastric, stylohyoid, geniohyoid, and mylohyoid muscles.

Supporting Structures

The supporting structures of the TMJ are outlined in Table 2–42.

Nerve Supply

The TMJ is primarily supplied from three nerves that are part of the mandibular division of the fifth cranial (trigeminal) nerve.

Biomechanics

The movements that occur at the TMJ are extremely complex. The TMJ has three degrees of freedom, with each of the degrees of freedom associated with a separate axis of rotation.[100] Two primary arthrokinematic movements (rotation and anterior translation) occur at this joint around three planes: sagittal, horizontal, and frontal.

- Mouth opening, contralateral deviation, and protrusion all involve an anterior osteokinematic rotation of the mandible and an anterior, inferior, and lateral glide of the mandibular head and disk.
- Mouth closing, ipsilateral deviation, and retrusion all involve a posterior osteokinematic rotation of the mandible and a posterior, inferior, and lateral glide of the mandibular head and disk.

Occlusal Positions

Occlusal positions are functional positions of the TMJ. The occlusal position is defined as the point at which contact between some or all of the teeth occur. Under normal circumstances, the upper molars rest directly on the lower molars and the upper

TABLE 2–41 Muscles of the face, mouth, and pharynx.

	Anatomy	Action	Innervation
Muscles of the Face			
Levator anguli oris	Arises from the canine fossa of the maxilla and inserts into the upper and lower lips	Contraction results in drawing the corner of the mouth up and medially	Superior buccal branches of CN VII
Zygomatic major (zygomaticus)	Arises lateral to the zygomatic minor on the zygomatic bone Courses obliquely and inserts into the corner of the orbicularis oris	Elevates and retracts the angle of the mouth (smiling)	
Depressor labii inferioris	Originates form the mandible and courses up and in to insert into the lower lip	Dilation of the orifice of the mouth; pulls the lips down and out; counterpart to the levator triad	Mandibular marginal branches of VII
Depressor anguli oris (triangularis)	Originates along the lateral margins of the mandible Fanlike fibers converge on the orbicularis oris and upper lip at the corner	Depresses the corners of the mouth and compresses the upper lip against the lower lip	
Mentalis	Arises from the region of the incisive fossa of the mandible and inserts into the skin of the chin	Contraction elevates and wrinkles the chin and pulls the lower lip out	Innervated by the mandibular marginal branch of the facial nerve
Platysma (also considered a neck muscle)	Arises from the fascia overlying the pectoralis major and deltoid Courses up and inserts into the corner of the mouth below the symphysis mente, the lower margin of the mandible, and then into the skin near the masseter	Appears to assist in depression of the mandible	The cervical branch of CN VII
Muscles of the Mouth			
Orbicularis oris	Considered a single muscle encircling the mouth opening as well as paired upper and lower muscles (obicularis oris superior, obicularis oris inferior)	Serves as a point of insertion for other muscles	Branches of the VII facial nerve
Risorius	Superficial to the buccinators, originates from the posterior region of the face along the fascia of the masseter muscle; courses forward and inserts into the corners of the mouth	Retracts the lips at the corners (smiling)	Cranial nerve VII (facial nerve)
Buccinator	Deep to the risorius; originates on the pterygomandibular ligament and the posterior alveolar portion of the mandible and maxillae; courses forward to insert into the upper and lower orbicularis oris	Involved in mastication; also constricts the oropharynx	Cranial nerve VII (facial nerve)
Levator triad (a group of three muscles)	1. Levator labii superioris alaeque nasi (most medial)—courses vertically along the lateral margin of the nose, arising from the frontal process of maxilla; inserts into the wing of the nostril and UL (flares the nares) 2. Levator labii superioris (intermediate)—originates from the infraorbital margin of the maxilla; courses down and into the upper lip 3. Zygomatic minor (lateral)—originates at the facial surface of the zygomatic bone and courses downward into the upper lip	Dominant muscles for lip elevation and also dilate oral opening	Buccal branches of CN VII

(Continued)

TABLE 2–41 Muscles of the face, mouth, and pharynx. (*Continued*)

	Anatomy	Action	Innervation
Intrinsic Muscles of the Tongue			
Median fibrous septum	Divides right and left halves of the tongue—originates on the body of the hyoid bone via the hyoglossal membrane; courses the length of the tongue	Serves as the point of origin for transverse muscle of the tongue Forms tongue attachment with the hyoid	
Longitudinal muscle (superior lingualis)	Thin layer of oblique and longitudinal muscle fibers lying just deep to the mucous membrane of the dorsum Fibers arise from the submucous fibrous tissue near the epiglottis, hyoid, and the median fibrous septum Fibers fan forward and outward then insert into the lateral margins of the tongue	Bilateral contraction will elevate the tongue tip Unilateral contraction will pull the tongue toward the side of contraction	
Inferior longitudinal muscle (inferior lingualis)	A bundle of muscle fibers located on the undersurface of the tongue (absent in the medial tongue base) Originates at the root of the tongue and corpus hyoid Courses between the genioglossus and hyoglossus muscles and to the apex of the tongue Longitudinal muscle fibers interdigitate with them	Bilateral contraction will pull the tip of the tongue downward and assist in retraction of the tongue if co-contracted with the superior longitudinal Unilateral contraction will cause the tongue to turn toward the contracted side and downward	
Transverse muscle (transverse lingualis)	Fibers originate at the median fibrous septum Course laterally to insert into the submucous tissue at the lateral margins of the tongue Some fibers continue as the palatopharyngeus muscle	Contraction pulls the edges of the tongue toward midline, narrowing and elongating the tongue	
Vertical muscles (vertical lingualis)	Originate from the mucous membrane of the dorsum Course vertically downward and somewhat laterally Fibers of the transverse and vertical muscles interweave Insert into the sides and inferior surface of the tongue	Contraction flattens the tongue	
Extrinsic Tongue Muscles			
Genioglossus	Flat, triangular muscle located close to the median plane Arises from the inner mandibular surface at the symphysis Lower fibers course to the hyoid bone and attach by a thin aponeurosis to the upper part of the body Remainder of fibers radiate fanlike to the dorsum of the tongue inserting into the submucous fibrous tissues	The prime mover of the tongue (strongest and largest of the extrinsic muscles) Contraction of the anterior fibers results in retraction of the tongue Contraction of the posterior fibers draws the tongue forward to aid protrusion of the apex Contraction of both anterior and posterior fibers will draw the middle portion of the tongue down into the floor of the mouth (cupping the tongue)	
Hyoglossus	Arises from the length of the greater cornu and lateral body of the hyoid Courses upward and inserts into the lateral portions of the tongue	Contraction pulls the sides of the tongue down Antagonist to the palatoglossus	

(*Continued*)

TABLE 2-41 Muscles of the face, mouth, and pharynx. (*Continued*)

	Anatomy	Action	Innervation
Styloglossus	Originates from the anterolateral margin of styloid process Courses forward and down to insert into the inferior sides of the tongue Divides into two portions: One interdigitates with the inferior longitudinal muscle and the other with the hyoglossus	Bilateral contraction draws the tongue back and up	
Chondroglossus	Also considered to be a part of the hyoglossus Arises from the lesser cornu of the hyoid Courses up to interdigitate with the intrinsic muscles of the tongue medial to the point of insertion of the hyoglossus	Contraction depresses the tongue	
Palatoglossus	Can be considered a muscle of the tongue or the velum	Serves a dual purpose—depresses the soft palate, and elevates the back of the tongue	
Mandibular Elevators			
Masseter	Most superficial of the mastication muscles Originates on the lateral, inferior, and medial surfaces of the zygomatic arch External fibers insert into the ramus Internal (deep) fibers terminate on the coronoid process	Places maximum force on the molars Contraction elevates the mandible, closing the jaw Clenching the teeth will make the muscular belly visible	Innervated by CN V-trigeminal nerve
Temporalis	Deep to the masseter Arises from the temporal fossa (a region of the temporal and parietal bones) The broad, thin, fan-shaped muscle converges as it courses down and forward Terminal tendon passes through the zygomatic arch and inserts in the coronoid process and ramus	Contraction elevates the mandible and draws it back if protruded	Innervated by CN V-trigeminal
Medial pterygoid (internal pterygoid muscle, internal masseter)	Originates primarily in the vertically directed pterygoid fossa and from the medial surface of the lateral pterygoid plate Fibers course down and back inserting into the ramus	Contraction elevates the mandible in conjunction with the masseter	Innervated by CN V
Mandibular Protrusors			
Lateral pterygoid	Arises from the sphenoid bone Two heads—lateral pterygoid plate; greater wing of the sphenoid bone Fibers course back to insert into the pterygoid fossa (fovea) of the mandible (a depression on the anterior neck of the condyle of the mandible) and to the anterior margin of the articular disc of the temporomandibular articulation	Contraction protrudes the mandible, causing the condyle to slide down and forward on the articular eminence Unilateral contraction moves the jaw in a grinding motion	
Mandibular Depressors			
Digastricus	Anterior and posterior	When infrahyoid musculature is fixed, contraction of anterior digastricus will depress the mandible Bilaterally, the digastrics assist in forced mouth opening by stabilizing the hyoid The posterior bellies are especially active during coughing and swallowing	

(Continued)

TABLE 2–41   Muscles of the face, mouth, and pharynx. (*Continued*)

	Anatomy	Action	Innervation
Mandibular Depressors (*Continued*)			
Mylohyoid	Forms floor of the mouth	When hyoid is in fixed position, contraction will depress the mandible	
		Stabilizes or elevates the tongue during swallowing, and elevates the floor of the mouth in the first stage of deglutition	
Geniohyoid	A narrow muscle situated under the mylohyoid muscle	Contraction depresses the mandible if the hyoid is fixed; elevates the hyoid bone if mandible is fixed	
Platysma	Also considered a muscle of the face	Contraction depresses the mandible	
Hyoid Muscles			
Sternohyoid	A strap-like muscle	Functions to depress the hyoid as well as assist in speech and mastication	C1–C3 by a branch of ansa cervicalis (cervical loop)
Omohyoid	Situated lateral to the sternohyoid; consists of two bellies	Functions to depress the hyoid	
Sternothyroid and thyrohyoid	Located deep to the sternohyoid muscle	The sternothyroid muscle is involved in drawing the larynx downward, while the thyrohyoid depresses the hyoid and elevates the larynx	
Stylohyoid		Elevates the hyoid and base of the tongue and has an undetermined role in speech, mastication and swallowing	
Pharyngeal Constrictors			
Superior pharyngeal constrictor Middle pharyngeal constrictor Inferior pharyngeal constrictor Cricopharyngeus muscle Thyropharyngeus muscle	The constrictors, innervated by the vagus nerve, work to convey a food bolus downward into the esophagus. Superior pharyngeal constrictor is a quadrilateral muscle in the pharynx that is the highest located muscle of the three constrictors. Middle pharyngeal constrictor is a fanshaped muscle, which is the smallest of the three constrictors. Inferior pharyngeal constrictor is the thickest of the three constrictors. The upper esophageal sphincter (UES) is a musculoskeletal valve composed of the cricopharyngeus muscle, the lower part of the inferior pharyngeal constrictor, and the cricoid cartilage, to which these muscles attach.		

TABLE 2–42   Supporting structures of TMJ.

Structure	Description
Joint capsule or capsular ligament	Surrounds the entire joint; is thought to provide proprioceptive feedback regarding joint position and movement.
Temporomandibular (or lateral) ligament	The capsule of the temporomandibular joint is reinforced laterally by an outer oblique portion and an inner horizontal portion of the temporomandibular ligament, which function as a suspensory mechanism for the mandible during moderate opening movements. The ligament also functions to resist rotation and posterior displacement of the mandible.
Stylomandibular ligament	This ligament becomes taut and acts as a guiding mechanism for the mandible, keeping the condyle, disk, and temporal bone firmly opposed.
Sphenomandibular ligament	This ligament acts to check the angle of the mandible from sliding as far forward as the condyles during the translatory cycle, and serves as a suspensory ligament of the mandible during wide opening.

incisors slightly override the lower incisors. The ideal position provides mutual protection of anterior and posterior teeth, comfortable and painless mandibular function, and stability.[101]

Resting Position

The resting position, or "freeway space," corresponds to the position where the residual tension of the muscles are at rest and no contact occurs between maxillary and mandibular teeth. In this position, the tongue is against the palate of the mouth with its most anterior-superior tip in the area against the palate, just posterior to the rear of the upper central incisors.

THORACIC SPINE AND RIB CAGE

In the thoracic spine, protection and function of the thoracic viscera take precedence over segmental spinal mobility. Each thoracic segment includes twelve articulations, ten of which are synovial. In addition the posterior thoracic muscles, spinous processes, anterior and posterior longitudinal ligaments, vertebral bodies, zygapophyseal and costotransverse joints, inferior and superior articular processes, pars interarticularis, intervertebral disk, nerve root, joint meniscus, and dura mater are all capable of producing pain in this region.

Biomechanics

The thoracic spinal segments possess the potential for a unique array of movements. The load bearing capacity of the spine has been found to be up to three times greater with an intact rib cage.[102,103] There is very little agreement in the literature with regard to the biomechanics of the thoracic spine.

Respiration

During inspiration, in the upper ribs an anterior elevation (pump handle) occurs, and in the middle and lower ribs (excluding the free ribs) a lateral elevation (bucket handle) occurs (Figure 2–22).

The former movement increases the anterior-posterior diameter of the thoracic cavity, and the latter increases the transverse diameter. The reverse occurs with expiration.

Both kinds of rib motion are produced by the action of the diaphragm. The seventh through tenth ribs act to increase the abdominal cavity free space to afford space for the descending diaphragm.

LUMBAR SPINE

The spinous process is primarily horizontal in orientation. The region between the superior articular process and the lamina is the pars interarticularis.

The primary ligamentous support for the lumbar spine includes the anterior longitudinal ligament, the posterior longitudinal ligament, the attachments of the annulus fibrosis, the facet joints, and the interosseous ligaments between the spinous processes.

Biomechanics

Motions at the lumbar spine joints can occur in three cardinal planes: sagittal (flexion and extension), frontal (side bending), and transverse (rotation). Six degrees of freedom are available at the lumbar spine.

The amount of segmental motion at each vertebral level varies. Most of the flexion and extension of the lumbar spine occurs in the lower segmental levels, whereas most of the side bending of the lumbar spine occurs in the mid-lumbar area. Rotation, which occurs with side bending as a coupled motion, is minimal and occurs most at the lumbosacral junction. The amount of range available in the lumbar spine decreases with age.

Different trunk muscles play differing roles in the provision of dynamic stability to the spine. These muscles can be classified functionally as either *global* or *local*.

The Global Muscle System

This system consists of muscles whose origins are on the pelvis and whose insertions are on the thoracic cage. These muscles include:

- The rectus abdominis
- The external obliques
- The lateral fibers of the quadratus lumborum
- The thoracic part of the lumbar iliocostalis

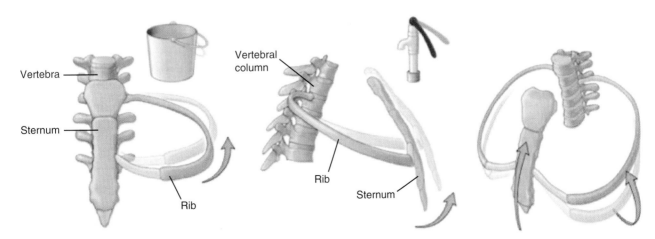

FIGURE 2–22 Artistic impression of the two main rib motions during breathing–bucket handle (right) and pump handle (left).

The global muscle system acts on the trunk and spine without being directly attached to it. These muscles appear to provide general trunk stabilization but are not capable of having a direct segmental influence on the spine.

The Local Muscle System

The local muscle system consists of muscles that have insertions and/or origins at the lumbar vertebra or pelvis and which are responsible for providing segmental stability and directly controlling the lumbar segments and sacroiliac joint. These muscles include:

- The lumbar portions of the iliocostalis and longissimus thoracis muscles
- The medial fibers of the quadratus lumborum
- The diaphragm
- The lumbar multifidus—considered to have the greatest potential to provide dynamic control to the motion segment, particularly in its neutral zone
- The pelvic floor muscles
- The transversus abdominis—primarily active in providing rotational and lateral control to the spine while maintaining adequate levels of intra-abdominal pressure and imparting tension to the thoracolumbar fascia
- The posterior fibers of the internal oblique that attach to the tensor fascia latae
- The local muscle system is important for the provision of segmental control to the spine, and provides an important stiffening effect on the lumbar spine, thereby enhancing its dynamic stability

SACROILIAC JOINT

The sacroiliac joint (SIJ) is a true diarthrodial joint that joins the sacrum to the pelvis. In this joint, hyaline cartilage on the sacral side moves against fibrocartilage on the iliac side. The joint is generally C-shaped with two lever arms that interlock at the second sacral level. The SIJ contains numerous ridges and depressions, indicating its function for stability more than motion. However, studies have documented that motion does occur at the joint; therefore, slightly subluxed and even locked positions can occur.

Stability at the SIJ is provided not just by the ridges present in the joint, but also by the presence of generously sized ligaments. The ligamentous structures offer resistance to shear and loading. The deep anterior, posterior, and interosseous ligaments resist the load of the sacrum relative to the ilium. More superficial ligaments (eg, sacrotuberous ligament) react to dynamic motions (eg, straight-leg raising during physical motion). The long dorsal sacroiliac ligament can become stretched in periods of reduced lumbar lordosis (eg, pregnancy).

Many large and small muscles have relationships with these ligaments and the SIJ. These include the piriformis, biceps femoris, gluteus maximus and minimus, erector spinae, latissimus dorsi, thoracolumbar fascia, and iliacus. Any of these muscles can be involved with a painful SIJ. As a true joint, the SIJ is a pain-sensitive structure richly innervated by a combination of unmyelinated free nerve endings and posterior primary rami of L2–S3.

Biomechanics

There is very little agreement, either among disciplines or within disciplines, about the biomechanics of the pelvic complex. The results from the numerous studies on mobility of the SIJ have led to a variety of different hypotheses and models of pelvic mechanics over the years.

■ SECTION 5: EXAMINATION OF THE MUSCULOSKELETAL SYSTEM

The International Classification of Functioning, Disability, and Health (IFC) is used in the physical therapy assessment to establish a common language between practitioners to communicate about the impairments and limitations of patients.[104] The ICF includes domains of body structure and function at the physiological systems level, activity limitations at the individual level, and participation restriction at the societal level. The ICF model proposes that the patient will have primary impairments due to the dysfunction in any of the three domains as well as secondary impairments that are the result of the primary impairment and can further limit the patient or increase that patient's level of dysfunction. Physical therapy treatment and patient management can be centered on the ICF domains to improve the patient's physiological systems, individual activities, and societal roles.[104]

An example for cervical spine disorders using the ICF classification system is provided in Table 2–43. An example for lumbar spine disorders using the ICF classification system is provided in Table 2–44.

PATIENT HISTORY AND SYSTEMS REVIEW

It is estimated that 80% of the necessary information to explain the presenting patient problem can be provided by a thorough history.[105] Differential diagnosis involves the ability to quickly differentiate problems of a serious nature from those that are not, using the history and physical examination. Problems of a serious nature include, but are not limited to, visceral diseases, cancer, infections, fractures, and vascular disorders. Some key points are noted below.[106]

High-Yield Terms to Learn

Referred pain	Used to describe those symptoms that have their origin at a site other than where the patient feels the pain.
Patient history	Information gained by a clinician by asking specific questions, either of the patient or of other people who know the patient.
Systems review	A questioning technique used to elicit those aspects of a medical history from a patient that could preclude the patient from receiving physical therapy.
Special test	A clinical test designed to help confirm a working hypothesis/diagnosis.
Accessory joint motion	A motion that occurs at joint surfaces to allow motion to occur. Accessory motion is assessed using joint mobility testing.
Differential diagnosis	A process by which a particular disease or condition is differentiated from others that present with similar clinical features.

Neutral questions should be used whenever possible. These questions are structured in such a way so as not to lead the patient into giving a particular response. "Leading" questions, such as "does it hurt more when you walk?" should be avoided. A more neutral question would be "Tell me what activities make your symptoms worse."

The frequency and duration of the patient's symptoms can help the clinician to classify the injury according to its stage of healing: acute (inflammatory), subacute (migratory and proliferative), and chronic (remodeling). Of particular importance are the patient's chief complaint and the relationship of that complaint to specific aggravating activities or postures. It must be remembered that the location of symptoms for many musculoskeletal conditions is quite separate from the source, especially in those peripheral joints that are more proximal, such as the shoulder and the hip.

The clinician must determine whether pain is the only symptom or whether there are other symptoms that accompany the pain, such as dizziness, bowel and bladder changes, tingling (paresthesia), radicular pain/numbness, weakness, and increased sweating.

The systems review is the critical part of the examination that identifies possible health problems, or red flags (Table 2–45) that require consultation with, or referral to, another health care provider.[107] The systems review is based on the clinician's knowledge of body system physiology so that malfunctions of the various systems can be detected through comprehensive questioning.

Red flags specific to the cervical and lumbar spine are outlined in Table 2–46 and Table 2–47, respectively.

The Cyriax scanning (screening) examination traditionally follows the history and is often incorporated as part of the systems review, especially if:

- There are symptoms when no history of trauma is present.
- There is no history to explain the signs and symptoms.
- The signs and symptoms are unexplainable.

The scanning examination should be carried out until the clinician is confident that there is no serious pathology present, and is routinely carried out unless there is some good reason for postponing it (eg, recent trauma, in which case a modified differential diagnostic examination is used).[108] The upper quarter scanning examination (Table 2–48) is appropriate for upper thoracic, upper extremity, and cervical problems, whereas the lower quarter scanning examination (Table 2–49) is typically used for thoracic, lower extremity, and lumbosacral problems.

TESTS AND MEASURES

The tests and measures component of the examination serves as an adjunct to the history and systems review. The physical examination may be modified based on the history—the examination of an acutely injured patient differs greatly from that of a patient in less discomfort or distress. In addition, the examination of a child differs in some respects to that of an adult. An overview of the examination of each of the major joints is provided in Tables 2-50 through 2-58.

Observation

The patient's general posture and ability to perform functional tasks provides information about the severity of symptoms, willingness to move, ROM, and muscle strength.[109]

The following should be noted during palpation:

- Myofascial mobility
- Skin temperature
- Areas of localized tenderness
- Skin and soft tissue density and extensibility
- Peripheral pulses as indicated
- Areas of edema

Range of Motion

Active and passive motion are commonly measured, but for differing reasons.

TABLE 2–43 Classification of cervical spine disorders using ICF classification.

Classification	Symptoms	2017 CPG-Recommended Assessments	Impairments	Interventions
Cervical hypomobility ICF: Neck Pain with Mobility Deficits	• Neck pain • Neck motion limitations • Possible referred UE pain	• Cervical AROM • Cervical flexion-rotation test • Cervical and thoracic segmental mobility test	• Limited ROM • Neck pain reproduced at end of range active and passive motions • Restricted cervical and thoracic segmental mobility • Provocation testing reproduces cervical and/or related UE symptoms	• Mobilization/manipulation of cervical and/or thoracic spine • Stretching and mobility exercises • Coordination, strengthening, and endurance exercises
Cervical hypermobility/ clinical instability ICF: Neck Pain with Movement Coordination Impairments (including WAD)	• Neck pain linked to history of trauma or whiplash • Associated UE or shoulder girdle referred pain • Dizziness, nausea, headache, confusion, concentration or memory difficulties; hypersensitivity to mechanical, thermal, acoustic, odor, or light stimuli; heightened affective distress	• (+) Cranial cervical flexion test • (+) Neck flexor muscle endurance tests • (+) Pressure algometry • Strength/endurance deficits of neck muscles • Neck pain with mid-range motion that worsens end–ranges • Possible myofascial trigger points • Sensorimotor impairment may include altered muscle activation patterns, proprioceptive deficit, postural balance or control • Neck and referred pain with provocation	• Limited/guarded AROM • Hypermobility with segmental testing • Strength, endurance, and coordination deficits of deep cervical spine flexor and extensor muscles • Aberrant motion with AROM • Supine AROM > seated AROM (Non-WB > WB) • Neck and referred pain with provocation	• Coordination, endurance, strengthening exercises • Stretching exercises • Mobilization/manipulation above and below hypermobilities • Ergonomic correction • Gentle AROM pain-free and progressed with supervision • Activity modification • Physical modalities (ice, heat TENS) • Minimize collar use (acute) • Reassurance, encouragement, pain management • Functional training using cognitive therapy principles, eye-neck coordination, and neuromuscular coordination elements

Cervical radiculopathy ICF: Neck Pain with Radiating Pain	• Neck pain with associated radiating pain in UE
	• UE paresthesia, numbness, and weakness may be present
		• Neurodynamic testing
		• Spurling test
		• Distraction test
		• Valsalva test
			• Neck and radiating pain reproduced with:
			  (+) Spurling A test
			  (+) ULTT 1
			• Pain relieved with cervical distraction
			• May have sensory, strength, or reflex deficits associated with involved nerves
				• Nerve mobilization
				• Traction
				• Craniocervical flexion exercises
				• Postural exercises
				• Thoracic mobilization/manipulation

Cervicogenic headaches ICF: Neck Pain with Headaches	• Noncontinuous unilateral neck pain and associated headache (referred) • Unilateral headache precipitated or aggravated by neck movements or sustained positions/postures	• Cervical AROM • Cervical flexion-rotation test • Upper cervical segmental mobility testing	• Headache elicited by pressure on posterior neck, especially at one of three upper cervical joints • Limited cervical ROM, C1-2 mobility deficit noted with cervical flexion-rotation test • Strength and endurance deficits of deep neck flexor muscles	• Cervical and thoracic mobilization/manipulation including C1-2 self-SNAG • Strengthening, endurance, and coordination exercises • Postural education

AROM, active range of motion; CPG, clinical practice guidelines; ICF, International Classification of Function; ROM, range of motion; UE, upper extremity; ULTT 1, upper limb tension test 1 (median nerve bias); WAD, whiplash-associated disorders; WB, weight-bearing.

Olson, KA, *Manual Physical Therapy of the Spine.* 2nd ed. St Louis, MO: Saunders/Elsevier; 2015; Blanpied PR, Gross AR, Elliott JM, et al. Neck Pain: Revision 2017. *J Othop Sports Phys Ther.* 2017;47(7):A1-A83.

TABLE 2–44 Classification of low back pain disorders using ICF classification.

Classification	Symptoms	Recommended Assessments	Impairments	Interventions
McKenzie-based directional preference depending on centralization and peripheralization of symptoms; LBP that centralizes ICF: Low Back Pain with Related (Referred) Lower Extremity Pain	*Extension Syndrome:* • LBP and leg pain that may travel beyond the knee • Centralization with BB • Peripheralization with FB *Flexion Syndrome:* • Centralization with FB • Peripheralization with BB	• Repeated motions to determine directional preference	• Lateral shift or kyphotic posture • Limited/guarded AROM • Mobility restrictions possible	• Repeated movement exercises into directional preference (symptoms centralize, pain decreases, ROM improves) • Non-thrust mobilizations • Patient education on positions of centralization and modification of those that peripheralize symptoms • General conditioning • Mobility and stabilization programs
Lumbar spinal stenosis (flexion syndrome) ICF: LBP with Related Lower Extremity Pain	*Flexion Syndrome:* • Centralization with FB • Peripheralization with BB • Often associated with leg pain • Neurogenic claudication symptoms: pain, paresthesia and cramping brought on by walking, relieved by sitting • Deficits in mobility, flexibility, and strength	• Treadmill test • Hip mobility, flexibility (commonly hip flexor tightness), and strength (commonly gluteus medius weakness) assessment • Gait and balance assessment	• Deficits in mobility, flexibility, and strength and endurance • Possible adverse neural tension • Gait dysfunction	• Flexion-based exercise program • Manual therapy to hip, lumbopelvic, and thoracic spine • Unweighted treadmill walking program • Strengthening exercises for LEs and core • Patient education Aerobic conditioning • Nerve mobilization • Balance training exercises as indicated
Lumbar radiculopathy that does not centralize (traction) ICF: LBP with Radiating Pain	• LBP with LE pain tends to travel below knee • Lumbar movements do not centralize symptoms Lumbar BB peripheralizes symptoms • No directional preference noted • (+) SLR <45° • (+) Crossed SLR <45° • (+) LE neurologic signs: strength, sensory and/or reflex changes • Poor tolerance to WB postures (sitting or standing) • Traction centralizes/relieves symptoms	• Neurovascular screen (dermatomes, myotomes, reflexes, neural tension tests) • Spinal mobility • Surrounding joints and tissue mobility and strength	• Deficits in mobility, flexibility, and strength and endurance • Possible adverse neural tension • Gait dysfunction	• Lumbar manual or mechanical traction (but **not** indicated for patients with acute or subacute nonradicular LBP or in patients with CLBP) • Positional distraction • Nerve mobility exercises (subacute and chromic patients) • Manual therapy to adjacent articulations or soft tissues
Lumbar spine instability ICF: LBP with Movement Coordination Impairments	• LBP and/or low back–related LE pain that worsens with sustained positions • Tenderness of lumbar region • Referred pain into buttock or thigh • Paraspinal muscle guarding • Hypermobility with passive segmental mobility testing	• Hypermobility with PA and segmental mobility testing • (+) Prone instability test • Trunk and pelvic strength testing • Neuromuscular control and endurance assessment • Trendelenberg and ASLR testing • Palpation of ligaments • Imbalance between global and local muscles	• Motor control deficits • Muscle imbalance between global and local muscles • Decreased trunk and pelvic muscle strength, endurance, and neuromuscular control • Poor quality of motions/aberrant motions	• Neuromuscular re-education to facilitate strength, motor control, and coordination of the local stabilizers and inhibit the overactive global muscles • Manual therapy • Work-specific and sport-specific training dynamic stabilization training including lifting training and balance/agility training • Consider external device temporarily to support lumbopelvic region • Self-care home strategies for pelvic neutral and maintaining active lifestyle

(Continued)

TABLE 2–44 Classification of low back pain disorders using ICF classification. (*Continued*)

Classification	Symptoms	Recommended Assessments	Impairments	Interventions
Chronic LBP ICF: Chronic LBP with Related Generalized Pain	• LBP and/or low back–related LE pain >3 months • Generalized pain not consistent with impairment-based classification • Presence of depression, fear-avoidance beliefs, or pain catastrophizing • Movement impairments (ie, hypomobility of thoracic, lumbopelvic, hip joints with poor neuromuscular control and coordination of spinal motions)	• FABQ, PCS • Four-Item Patient Health Questionnaire (PHQ-4) • May develop central sensitization, depression, anxiety • Examination of AROM, PROM, segmental mobility, strength of lumbopelvic and hip musculature, movement analysis	One or more of the following: • Two positive responses to Primary Care Evaluation of Mental Disorders screen, and affect consistent with an individual who is depressed • High scores on the FABQ and behavioral processes consistent with an individual who has excessive anxiety and fear • High scores on the PCS, and cognitive process consistent with rumination, pessimism, or helplessness	• Interventions for secondary impairments (mobilization/manipulation, soft tissue mobilization, mobility and motor control exercises) • Stabilization (motor control) program • Hip and thoracic mobility • Myofascial techniques for trunk and LE • Psychologically informed pain management physical therapy approach • FAM including encouraging patients to confront and overcome fears and unhelpful beliefs by performing previously avoided activities • Patient education on neurophysiology of pain • Graded activity/exercise and exposure • Cognitive behavioral therapy • Low-intensity prolonged aerobic exercise
ICF: Acute or Subacute LBP with Related Cognitive or Affective Tendencies	• Acute or subacute LBP and/or related LE pain • High scores on FABQ and behavioral processes consistent with individual with excessive fear or anxiety	One or more of the following: • Two positive responses to Primary Care Evaluation of Mental Disorders screen and affect consistent with an individual who is depressed • High scores on the FABQ and behavioral processes consistent with an individual who has excessive anxiety or fear • High scores on the PCS and cognitive process consistent with rumination, pessimism, or helplessness	• AROM lumbopelvic • PROM lumbopelvic • Passive segmental mobility • Soft tissue quality and quantity • Psychosocial assessment (FABQ)	• Patient education and counseling to address specific classification exhibited by the patient (ie, depression, fear avoidance, pain catastrophizing)
Lumbar hypomobility ICF: LBP with Mobility Deficits	• LBP with or without LE pain above knee	• AROM lumbopelvic • PROM lumbopelvic • Passive segmental mobility • Soft tissue quality and quantity • Psychosocial assessment (FABQ)	• Limited active lumbar spine mobility • Hypomobility with passive segmental mobility testing • Myofascial restrictions with muscle guarding • (+) Pain provocation with passive accessory testing	• Spinal manipulation thrust and non-thrust • Hip mobilization • Mobility and stretching exercises • Soft tissue mobilization • HEP

(Continued)

TABLE 2–44 Classification of low back pain disorders using ICF classification. (*Continued*)

Classification	Symptoms	Recommended Assessments	Impairments	Interventions
Sacroiliac joint dysfunctions (pelvic girdle pain) ICF: LBP with Movement Coordination Impairments/Sacroiliac Joint Hypermobility	• Dull ache with fixed postures and pelvic girdle pain with possible referral LE above knee	• (+) Pain provocation tests • (+) Pain palpation tests • No centralization or peripheralization of pain with repeated BB • ASLR test • Segmental mobility test; (+) hypermobility • Soft tissue tone/mobility assessment	• SIJ joint and ligament impairments • Pubic symphysis joint and ligament impairment • Impaired motor function of lumbopelvic/hip muscles • Hypertonicity of ipsilateral thoracolumbar erector spinae muscles • Hypermobility with passive mobility assessments • (+) ASLR	• Stabilization exercises • SIJ belt • Activity modification and rest • Manual therapy and exercise of surrounding dysfunctions including hip • Pelvic floor muscle function assessment and treatment
Sacroiliac joint dysfunctions (pelvic girdle pain) ICF: LBP with Mobility Deficits/Sacroiliac Joint Displacement	• Asymmetrical iliac crest heights • Restricted passive motion • Provocations testing • Limited mobility assessment	• Cluster of SIJ tests for position, mobility, and provocation • ASLR	• (+) Hypomobility SIJ joint • Possible hip and/or lumbar mobility dysfunctions	• Manipulation to reduce displacement • Treatment then as per hypermobile SIJ above

AROM, active range of motion; ASLR, active straight leg raise test; BB, backward bend; FAM, Fear-Avoidance Model; FABQ, Fear Avoidance Belief Questionnaire; FB, forward bend; HEP, home exercise program; ICF, International Classification of Function; LE, lower extremity; PCS, pain catastrophizing scale; PROM, passive range of motion; ROM, range of motion; SIJ, sacroiliac joint; WB, weight-bearing; (+), positive test finding.

Olson, KA, Manual Physical Therapy of the Spine. 2nd ed. St Louis, MO: Saunders/Elsevier, 2015; Delitto A, George S, Van Dillen L, et al. Low Back Pain Clinical Practice Guidelines Linked to the International Classification of Functioning, Disability, and Health from the Orthopaedic Section of the American Physical Therapy Association. *J Othop Sports Phys Ther.* 2012;42(4): A1-A57.

Active Range of Motion

The pattern of motion restriction (capsular/noncapsular). AROM testing may be deferred if small and unguarded motions provoke intense pain, as this may indicate a high degree of joint irritability. The normal AROM for each of the joints is depicted in Table 2–59.

Full and pain-free AROM suggests normalcy for that movement, although it is important to remember that normal *range of motion* is not synonymous with normal motion.[110] Normal motion implies that the control of motion must also be present.

Dynamic and static testing in the cardinal planes follows if the single motions do not provoke symptoms. Dynamic testing involves repeated movements in specific directions. Repeated movements can give the clinician some valuable insight into the patient's condition:[111]

• Internal derangements tend to worsen with repeated motions.
• The symptoms of a postural dysfunction remain unchanged with repeated motions.
• Pain that is increased with tissue loading, but ceases at rest indicates a contractile tissue at fault.
• Repeated motions can indicate the irritability of the condition.

• Repeated motions can indicate to the clinician the direction of motion to be used as part of the intervention. If pain increases during repeated motion in a particular direction, exercising in that direction is not indicated. If pain only worsens in part of the range, repeated motion exercises can be used for that part of the range that is pain-free, or which does not worsen the symptoms.
• Pain that is increased after the repeated motions may indicate a re-triggering of the inflammatory response, and repeated motions in the opposite direction should be explored.
• Sustained static positions may be used to help detect symptoms that are provoked with certain postural positions or habits.[111]

Combined motion testing may be used when the symptoms are not reproduced with the cardinal plane motion tests. Combined motions, as their name suggests, use single-plane motions with other motions superimposed. For example, at the elbow, the single-plane motion of elbow flexion is tested together with forearm supination and then forearm pronation. As with the single-plane tests, the combined motions are testing statically and then dynamically in an effort to reproduce the patient's symptoms.

The AROM will be found to be either abnormal or normal. Abnormal motion is typically described as being reduced. It must

TABLE 2–45   Red-flag findings.

History	Possible Condition
Constant and severe pain, especially at night	Neoplasm and acute neuromusculoskeletal injury
Unexplained weight loss	Neoplasm
Loss of appetite	Neoplasm
Unusual fatigue	Neoplasm and thyroid dysfunction
Visual disturbances (blurriness or loss of vision)	Neoplasm
Frequent or severe headaches	Neoplasm
Arm pain lasting >2–3 month	Neoplasm or neurologic dysfunction
Persistent root pain	Neoplasm or neurologic dysfunction
Radicular pain with coughing	Neoplasm or neurologic dysfunction
Pain worsening after 1 month	Neoplasm
Paralysis	Neoplasm or neurologic dysfunction
Trunk and limb paresthesia	Neoplasm or neurologic dysfunction
Bilateral nerve root signs and symptoms	Neoplasm, spinal cord compression, and vertebrobasilar ischemia
Signs worse than symptoms	Neoplasm
Difficulty with balance and coordination	Spinal cord or CNS lesion
Fever or night sweats	Common findings in systemic infection and many diseases
Frequent nausea or vomiting	Common findings in many diseases, particularly of the gastrointestinal system
Dizziness	Upper cervical impairment, vertebrobasilar ischemia, craniovertebral ligament tear, inner ear dysfunction, CNS involvement, and cardiovascular dysfunction
Shortness of breath	Cardiovascular and/or pulmonary dysfunction and asthma
Quadrilateral paresthesia	Spinal cord compression (cervical myelopathy) and vertebrobasilar ischemia

CNS, central nervous system.

Data from Meadows J. *A Rationale and Complete Approach to the Sub-Acute Post-MVA Cervical Patient.* Calgary, AB: Swodeam Consulting; 1995.

TABLE 2–46   Red flags for the cervical spine.

Condition	History and Physical Examination Data
Tumor/ neoplastic conditions	Constant pain not affected by position or activity; worse at night
	Age >50 years old
	History of cancer
	Unexplained weight loss
	No relief with bed rest
Cervical myelopathy	Sensory disturbance of hand
	Muscle wasting of hand intrinsic muscles
	Unsteady gait
	Hoffmann reflex
	Inverted supinator sign
	Babinski sign
	Hyperreflexia
	Bowel and bladder disturbances
	Multisegmental weakness or sensory changes
	Age >45 years
Inflammatory or systemic disease	Fever
	Blood pressure >160/95 mmHg
	Resting pulse >100 bpm
	Resting respiration >25 bpm
	Fatigue
Compression fracture	History of trauma, fall, direct blow
	Age >50 years
	Prolonged use of corticosteroids
	Point tenderness over fracture site
	Increased pain with weight-bearing
	History of osteoporosis
Upper cervical ligamentous instability	Occipital headache and numbness
	Severe limitation during neck active range of motion in all directions
	Signs of myelopathy
Vertebral or internal carotid vascular insufficiency	Drop attacks
	Dizziness
	Dysphasia
	Dysarthria
	Diplopia
	Numbness/paresthesia
	Nystagmus
	Nausea
	Cranial nerve signs

Data from Olson KA. *Manual Physical Therapy of the Spine.* 2nd ed. St Louis, MO: Saunders/Elsevier; 2015. Clinical practice guidelines linked to the International Classification of Functioning, Disability and Health from the Orthopaedic Section of the American Physical Therapy Association. *J Orthop Sports Phys Ther.* 2017;47(7):A1-A83.

be remembered, though, that abnormal motion may also be excessive. Excessive motion is often missed and is erroneously classified as normal motion. To help determine whether the motion is normal or excessive, PROM, in the form of passive overpressure, and the end feel are assessed.

Passive Range of Motion

PROM testing gives the clinician information about the integrity of the contractile and inert tissues, and the *end feel*. It is important to perform gentle PROM and overpressure at the end of the active range in order to fully test the motion. The passive overpressure

TABLE 2–47 Red flags for the lumbar spine.

Condition	History and Physical Examination Data
Tumor	Constant pain not affected by position or activity; worse with weight-bearing; worse at night Age >50 years old History of cancer Failure of conservative intervention (failure to improve within 30 days) Unexplained weight loss No relief with bed rest
Cauda equine syndrome	Urine retention Fecal incontinence Saddle anesthesia
Infection	Recent infection, intravenous drug user/abuser Concurrent immunosuppressive disorder Deep, constant pain, increases with weight-bearing Fever, malaise, and swelling Spine rigidity; accessory mobility may be limited
Compression fracture	History of trauma, fall, direct blow Age >50 years Prolonged use of corticosteroids Point tenderness over fracture site Increased pain with weight-bearing History of osteoporosis
Abdominal aneurysm	Back, abdominal, or groin pain Presence of PVD or CAD and associated risk factors (age >50 years, smoker, hypertension, DM) Non-Caucasian Symptoms not related to movement Presence of bruit in central epigastric area with auscultation Palpation of abdominal aortic pulse

PVD, peripheral vascular disease; CAD; coronary artery disease; DM; Diabetes mellitus.

Data from Olson, KA. *Manual Physical Therapy of the Spine*. 2nd ed. St Louis, MO: Saunders/Elsevier; 2015.

Delitto A, George S, Van Dillen L, et al. Low Back Pain Clinical Practice Guidelines linked to the International Classification of Functioning, Disability, and Health from the Orthopaedic Section of the American Physical Therapy Association. *J Othop Sports Phys Ther*. 2012;42(4): A1-A57.

TABLE 2–48 Upper-quarter-quadrant scanning motor examination.

Muscle Action	Muscle Tested	Root Level	Peripheral Nerve
Shoulder abduction	Deltoid	Primarily C5	Axillary
Elbow flexion	Biceps brachii	Primarily C6	Musculocutaneous
Elbow extension	Triceps brachii	Primarily C7	Radial
Wrist extension	Extensor carpi radialis longus, brevis, and extensor carpi ulnaris	Primarily C6	Radial
Wrist flexion	Flexor carpi radialis and flexor carpi ulnaris	Primarily C7	Median nerve for radialis and ulnar nerve for ulnaris
Finger flexion	Flexor digitorum superficialis, flexor digitorum profundus, and lumbricales	Primarily C8	Median nerve for superficialis and both median and ulnar nerves for profundus and lumbricales
Finger abduction	Posterior (dorsal) interossei	Primarily T1	Ulnar

TABLE 2–49 Lower-quarter-quadrant scanning motor examination.

Muscle Action	Muscle Tested	Root Level	Peripheral Nerve
Hip flexion	Iliopsoas	L1–2	Femoral to iliacus and lumbar plexus to psoas
Knee extension	Quadriceps	L2–4	Femoral
Hamstrings	Biceps femoris, semimembranosus, and semitendinosus	L4–S3	Sciatic
Dorsiflexion with inversion	Tibialis anterior	Primarily L4	Deep fibular (peroneal)
Great toe extension	Extensor hallucis longus	Primarily L5	Deep fibular (peroneal)
Ankle eversion	Fibularis (peroneus) longus and brevis	Primarily S1	Superficial fibular (peroneal) nerve
Ankle plantarflexion	Gastrocnemius and soleus	Primarily S1	Tibial
Hip extension	Gluteus maximus	L5–S2	Inferior gluteal nerve

TABLE 2–50 Examination of the cervical spine.

Observation and Inspection	
Upper quarter and peripheral joint scan	Temporomandibular joint, shoulder complex, elbow, forearm, and wrist and hand
	Dermatomes, and key muscle tests as appropriate
Examination of movements	Flexion, extension, side-bending (right and left), rotation (right and left)
Active range of motion with passive overpressure (except extension, and rotation)	Combined movements as appropriate
	Repetitive movements as appropriate
	Sustained positions as appropriate
	Craniovertebral joint movement testing
Resisted isometric movements	All active range of motion directions
Palpation	
Neurological tests as appropriate	Reflexes, key muscle tests, sensory scan, peripheral nerve assessment
	Neurodynamic mobility tests (upper limb tension tests, slump test)
Joint mobility tests	a. Side glides
	b. Anterior and posterior glides
	c. Traction and compression
Special tests (refer to Special Tests section)	As indicated
Diagnostic imaging	As appropriate

TABLE 2–51 Examination of the lumbar spine.

Observation and Inspection	
Lower quarter and peripheral joint scan	Hip, knee, ankle, and foot
	Dermatomes, and key muscle tests as appropriate
Examination of movements	Flexion, extension, side-bending (right and left), rotation (right and left)
Active range of motion with passive overpressure	Combined movements as appropriate
	Repetitive movements as appropriate
	Sustained positions as appropriate
	Sacroiliac joint movement testing
Resisted isometric movements	All active range of motion directions
	Rectus abdominis, internal and external obliques, quadratus lumborum, back and hip extensors
Palpation	
Neurological tests as appropriate	Reflexes, key muscle tests, sensory scan, peripheral nerve assessment
	Neurodynamic mobility tests (straight leg raise, slump test, prone knee flexion)
Joint mobility tests	a. Side glides
	b. Anterior and posterior glides
	c. Traction and compression
Special tests (refer to Special Tests section).	As indicated
Diagnostic imaging	As appropriate

TABLE 2–52 Examination of the thoracic spine.

Observation and Inspection	
Upper quarter and peripheral joint scan	Temporomandibular joint, shoulder complex, elbow, forearm, and wrist and hand
	Dermatomes, and key muscle tests as appropriate
Examination of movements	Flexion, extension, side-bending (right and left), rotation (right and left)
Active range of motion with passive overpressure	Bucket handle and pump handle rib motions
	Combined movements as appropriate
	Repetitive movements as appropriate
	Sustained positions as appropriate
Resisted isometric movements	All active range of motion directions
	Rectus abdominis, internal and external obliques, quadratus lumborum, back and hip extensors

Palpation	
Neurological tests as appropriate	Reflexes, key muscle tests, sensory scan, peripheral nerve assessment
	Neurodynamic mobility tests (straight leg raise, slump test) as appropriate
Joint mobility tests	a. Distraction and compression
	b. Flexion and extension of the zygapophyseal joints
	c. Rib springing
	d. Posteroanterior unilateral vertebral pressure
Special tests (refer to Special Tests section).	As indicated
Diagnostic imaging	As appropriate

TABLE 2–53 Examination of the shoulder.

I.	History
II.	Observation and inspection
III.	Upper quarter scan as appropriate
IV.	Examination of movements; active range of motion with passive overpressure of the following movements:
	Elevation (forward flexion, abduction, scaption)—painful arc
	Adduction, extension horizontal adduction and abduction, circumduction, external rotation, and internal rotation
	Scapulohumeral range of abduction—scapulohumeral rhythm
V.	Resisted isometric movements
	Elevation (forward flexion, abduction, scaption)
	Extension
	Adduction
	Abduction
	External rotation
	Internal rotation
	Elbow flexion
	Elbow extension
VI.	Palpation
VII.	Neurological tests as appropriate (reflexes, sensory scan, peripheral nerve assessment)
VIII.	Joint mobility tests
	Glenohumeral joint
	Distraction
	Inferior glide of the humeral head
	Posterior glide of the humeral head
	Anterior glide of the humeral head
	Sternoclavicular joint
	Superior glide of the clavicle on the sternum
	Inferior glide of the clavicle on the sternum
	Posterior glide of the clavicle on the sternum
	Anterior glide of the clavicle
	Acromioclavicular joint
	Compression/distraction
	Anterior glide of the clavicle on the acromion
	Posterior glide of the clavicle
	Scapulothoracic joint
	Rotation of the scapula on the thoracic wall
	Elevation of the scapula on the thoracic wall
	Depression of the scapula on the thoracic wall
	Retraction of the scapula on the thoracic wall
	Protraction of the scapula on the thoracic wall
	Distraction of the scapula from the thoracic wall
IX.	Special tests (refer to Special Tests section)
X.	Diagnostic imaging

should be applied carefully in the presence of pain. The barrier to active motion should occur earlier in the range than the barrier to passive motion. Pain that occurs at the end-range of active and passive movement is suggestive of hypermobility or instability, a capsular contraction, scar tissue that has not been adequately remodeled, on an inflamed inert structure such as a bursa or fat pad.[111]

• If active and passive motions are limited/painful in the same direction, the injured tissue is likely inert in nature.

• If active and passive motions are limited/painful in the opposite direction, the injured tissue is likely contractile in nature.

The exception to this generalization occurs with tenosynovitis. Cyriax[112] introduced the concept of the end feel, which is the quality of resistance at end range. The end feel can indicate to the clinician the cause of the motion restriction. The common end feels, both normal and abnormal, are described in Tables 2–10 and Table 2–11.[113]

The planned intervention and its intensity are based on the type of tissue resistance to movement demonstrated by the end feel, and the acuteness of the condition (Table 2–60).[112]

Manual Muscle Testing

The Guide to Physical Therapist Practice[107] lists both manual muscle testing (MMT) and dynamometry as appropriate measures of muscle strength.

• MMT is a procedure for the evaluation of the function and strength of individual muscles and muscle groups based on the effective performance of a movement in relation to the forces of gravity and manual resistance.[114]

TABLE 2–54 Examination of the elbow, forearm, wrist, and hand.

History

Observation and inspection

Upper quarter scan as appropriate

Examination of movements; active range of motion with passive overpressure of the following movements:

    Flexion and extension of the elbow

    Pronation and supination of the forearm

    Wrist flexion and extension

    Radial deviation and ulnar deviation of the wrist

    Finger flexion, finger extension (MCP, PIP, and DIP joints)

    Finger abduction and adduction

    Thumb flexion, extension, abduction, adduction

    Opposition of the thumb and little finger

Resisted isometric movements:

    Elbow flexion and extension

    Pronation and supination of the forearm

    Wrist flexion and extension

    Radial deviation and ulnar deviation of the wrist

    Finger flexion, finger extension (MCP, PIP, and DIP joints)

    Finger abduction and adduction

    Thumb flexion, extension, abduction, adduction

    Opposition of the thumb and little finger

    Palpation

Neurological tests as appropriate (reflexes, sensory scan, peripheral nerve assessment)

Joint mobility tests:

    Distraction/compression of the ulnohumeral joint

    Medial and lateral glide of the ulnohumeral joint

    Distraction of the radiohumeral joint

    Anterior and posterior glide of the radial head

    Anterior and posterior glide of the proximal radioulnar joint

    Anterior and posterior glide of the distal radioulnar joint

    Long-axis extension at the wrist and fingers (MCP, PIP, and DIP joints)

    Anteroposterior glide at the wrist and fingers (MCP, PIP, and DIP joints)

    Side glide at the wrist and fingers (MCP, PIP, and DIP joints)

    Anteroposterior glides of the intermetacarpal joints

    Rotation of the MCP, PIP, and DIP joints

    Individual carpal bone mobility

Special tests, including functional testing (refer to Special Tests section)

Diagnostic imaging

TABLE 2–55 Examination of the sacroiliac joint.

History

Observation and inspection

Upper quarter scan as appropriate

Examination of movements; active range of motion with passive overpressure of the following movements:

    Lumbar spine flexion, extension, side-bending (right and left), rotation (right and left)

    Hip flexion, extension, abduction, adduction, internal rotation, external rotation

    Weight-bearing kinetic tests (ipsilateral and contralateral)

Resisted isometric movements:

    Lumbar spine flexion

    Hip flexion, extension, abduction, adduction, internal rotation, external rotation

    Palpation

Neurological tests as appropriate (reflexes, sensory scan, peripheral nerve assessment)

Joint mobility tests:

    Anterior and posterior joint distraction

    Anterior posterior joint compression

    Short-and long-arm tests

Special tests, including ligament stress tests (refer to Special Tests section)

Diagnostic imaging

TABLE 2–56 Examination of the knee joint complex.

History

Observation and inspection

Upper quarter scan as appropriate

Examination of movements; active range of motion with passive overpressure of the following movements:

    Hip flexion, extension, abduction, adduction, internal rotation, external rotation.

    Knee flexion, extension

    Ankle dorsiflexion, plantar flexion

    Internal rotation of the tibia on the femur, external rotation of the tibia on the femur

Resisted isometric movements:

    Hip flexion, extension, abduction, adduction, internal rotation, external rotation

    Knee flexion, extension

    Ankle dorsiflexion, plantar flexion

Ligament stability tests:

    One plane medial instability

    One plane lateral instability

    One plane anterior and posterior instability

    Anteromedial and anterolateral rotary instability

    Posteromedial and posterolateral rotary instability

Palpation

Neurological tests as appropriate (reflexes, sensory scan, peripheral nerve assessment)

Joint mobility tests:

    Anterior and posterior glides of the tibia on the femur

    Medial and lateral translation of the tibia on the femur

    Patellar glides

    Anteroposterior glides of the proximal tibiofibular joint

Special tests (refer to Special Tests section) and diagnostic imaging as appropriate

- Dynamometry is a method of strength testing using sophisticated strength measuring devices (eg, hand-grip, hand-held, fixed, and isokinetic dynamometry).

Valuable information can be gleaned from these tests, including:

- The amount of force the muscle is capable of producing and whether the amount of force produced varies with the joint angle.

- The endurance of the muscle, and how much substitution occurs during the test.

- Whether any pain or weakness is produced with the contraction (Table 2–61).

TABLE 2-57 Examination of the lower leg, ankle, and foot.

History

Observation and inspection

Upper quarter scan as appropriate

Examination of movements; active range of motion with passive over-pressure of the following movements:

Plantar flexion, dorsiflexion in weight-bearing and non-weightbearing

Supination, pronation in weight-bearing and non-weightbearing

Toe extension, flexion in weight-bearing and non-weightbearing

Resisted isometric movements:

Knee flexion, extension

Plantar flexion, dorsiflexion

Supination, pronation

Toe extension, flexion

Palpation

Neurological tests as appropriate (reflexes, sensory scan, peripheral nerve assessment)

Joint mobility tests:

Inversion and eversion at the subtalar joint

Adduction and abduction at the midtarsal joints

Anteroposterior glide at the talocrural joint

Tarsal bone mobility

Special tests (refer to Special Tests section)

Diagnostic imaging

TABLE 2-58 Examination of the temporomandibular joint.

History

Observation and inspection

Upper quarter scan as appropriate

Examination of movements; active range of motion with passive over-pressure of the following movements:

Cervical flexion, extension, side-bending (right and left), rotation (right and left)

Mouth opening, closing (occlusion), protrusion, retrusion, lateral deviation (left and right)

Resisted isometric movements:

Mouth opening, closing (occlusion), lateral deviation

Palpation

Neurological tests as appropriate (reflexes, sensory scan, cranial nerve assessment)

Joint mobility tests:

Distraction and anterior glide of the mandible

Lateral glide of the mandible

Medial glide of the mandible

Posterior glide of the mandible

Special tests (refer to Special Tests section)

Diagnostic imaging

TABLE 2-59 Active ranges of the major joints.

Joint	Action	Degrees of motion
Shoulder	Flexion	0–180
	Extension	0–40
	Abduction	0–180
	Internal rotation	0–80
	External rotation	0–90
Elbow	Flexion	0–150
Forearm	Pronation	0–80
	Supination	0–80
Wrist	Flexion	0–60
	Extension	0–60
	Radial deviation	0–20
	Ulnar deviation	0–30
Finger flexion	Flexion	MCP: 85–90
		PIP: 100–115
		DIP: 80–90
Hip	Flexion	0–100
	Extension	0–30
	Abduction	0–40
	Adduction	0–20
	Internal rotation	0–40
	External rotation	0–50
Knee	Flexion	0–150
Ankle	Plantarflexion	0–40
	Dorsiflexion	0–20
Foot	Inversion	0–30
	Eversion	0–20
Toe	Flexion	Great toe: MTP, 45 IP, 90 Lateral four toes: MTP, 40 PIP, 35 DIP, 60
	Extension	Great toe: MTP, 70 IP, 0 Lateral four toes: MTP, 40 PIP, 0 DIP, 30

TABLE 2–60 Appropriate technique based on barrier to motion and end feel.

Barrier	End Feel	Technique
Pain	Empty	None
Pain	Spasm	None
Pain	Capsular	Oscillations
Joint adhesions	Early capsular	Passive articular motion stretch
Muscle adhesions	Early elastic	Passive physiologic motion stretch
Hypertonicity	Facilitation	Hold-relax
Bone	Bony	None

MMT is an ordinal level of measurement[115] and has been found to have both interrater and intrarater reliability, especially when the scale is expanded to include plus or minus a half or a full grade.[116-118] Examples of common grading scales used with MMT are depicted in Table 2–62.

Choosing a particular grading system is based on the skill level of the clinician while ensuring consistency for each patient, so that coworkers who may be re-examining the patient are using the same testing methods.

To be a valid test, strength testing must elicit a maximum contraction of the muscle being tested. Five strategies ensure this:

- Placing the joint that the muscle to be tested crosses in, or close to, its open packed position.
- Placing the muscle to be tested in a shortened position. This puts the muscle in an ineffective physiological position and has the effect of increasing motor neuron activity.
- Having the patient perform an eccentric muscle contraction by using the command "Don't let me move you." As the tension at each cross-bridge and the number of active cross-bridges is greater during an eccentric contraction, the maximum eccentric muscle tension developed is greater with an eccentric contraction than a concentric one.

TABLE 2–61 Findings from muscle testing.

Finding	Possible Explanation
Strong and painless contraction	Normal finding
Strong and painful contraction	Grade I contractile lesion
Weak and painless contraction	Palsy (nerve compression, neuropathy) Complete rupture of the muscle-tendon unit/avulsion
Weak and painful contraction	Serious pathology such as significant muscle tear, fracture, tumor, etc.

- Breaking the contraction. It is important to break the patient's muscle contraction in order to ensure that the patient is making a maximal effort and that the full power of the muscle is being tested.
- Holding the contraction for at least 5 seconds. Weakness due to nerve palsy has a distinct fatigability. If a muscle appears to be weaker than normal, further investigation is required.

The test is repeated three times. Muscle weakness resulting from disuse will be consistently weak and should not get weaker with several repeated contractions.

Another muscle that shares the same innervation (spinal nerve or peripheral nerve) is tested. Knowledge of both spinal nerve and peripheral nerve innervation will aid the clinician in determining which muscle to select (Tables 2–63, 2–64, and 2–65).

Substitutions by other muscle groups during testing indicates the presence of weakness. It does not, however, tell the clinician the cause of the weakness. Whenever possible, the same muscle is tested on the opposite side, using the same testing procedure, and a comparison is made.

Interpretation of Findings

Cyriax reasoned that if you isolate and then apply tension to a structure, you could make a conclusion as to the integrity of that structure.[112] According to Cyriax, pain with a contraction generally indicates an injury to the muscle, tendon, or tendon attachment to bone.[112] This can be confirmed by combining the findings from the isometric test with the findings of the passive motion and the joint distraction and compression.

Cyriax also introduced the concept of tissue reactivity. Tissue reactivity is the manner in which different stresses and movements can alter the clinical signs and symptoms. This knowledge can be used to gauge any subtle changes to the patient's condition.[122]

- Pain that occurs consistently with resistance, at whatever the length of the muscle, may indicate a tear of the muscle belly. Pain with muscle testing may indicate a muscle injury, a joint injury due to compressive forces across the joint with the muscle contraction, or a combination of both.
- Pain that does not occur during the test but occurs upon the release of the contraction is thought to have an articular source, produced by the joint glide that occurs following the release of tension.

The degree of significance with the findings in resisted testing depends on the position of the muscle and the force applied. For example, pain reproduced with a minimal contraction in the rest position for the muscle is more strongly suggestive of a contractile lesion than pain reproduced with a maximal contraction in the lengthened position for the muscle.

Accessory Joint Motion

A variety of measurement scales have been proposed for judging the amount of accessory joint motion present between two joint surfaces, most of which are based on a comparison with a comparable contralateral joint using manually applied forces in a logical

TABLE 2-62 Comparison of MMT grades.[119]

Medical Research Council[120]	Daniels and Worthingham[121]	Kendall and McCreary[61]	Explanation
5	Normal (N)	100%	Holds test position against maximal resistance
4+	Good + (G+)		Holds test position against moderate to strong pressure
4	Good (G)	80%	Holds test position against moderate resistance
4–	Good – (G–)		Holds test position against slight to moderate pressure
3+	Fair + (F+)		Holds test position against slight resistance
3	Fair (F)	50%	Holds test position against gravity
3–	Fair – (F–)		Gradual release from test position
2+	Poor + (P+)		Moves through partial ROM against gravity OR Moves through complete ROM gravity eliminated and holds against pressure
2	Poor (P)	20%	Able to move through full ROM gravity eliminated
2–	Poor – (P–)		Moves through partial ROM gravity eliminated
1	Trace (T)	5%	No visible movement; palpable or observable tendon prominence/flicker contraction
0	0	0%	No palpable or observable muscle contraction
Grades of 0, 1, and 2 are tested in the gravity-minimized position (contraction is perpendicular to the gravitational force) All other grades are tested in the anti-gravity position	The more functional of the three grading systems because it tests a motion that utilizes all of the agonists and synergists involved in the motion[119]	Designed to test a specific muscle rather than the motion, and requires both selective recruitment of a muscle by the patient and a sound knowledge of anatomy and kinesiology on the part of the clinician to determine the correct alignment of the muscle fibers[119]	

and precise manner.[123] Using these techniques to assess the joint glide (arthrokinematic), joint motion is described as hypomobile (restricted), normal (unrestricted but not excessive), or hypermobile (excessive). The joint glides are tested in the loose (open) pack position of a peripheral joint and at the end of available range in the spinal joints to avoid soft tissue tension affecting the results. The information gathered from these tests will help determine the integrity of the inert structures:

- The joint glide is unrestricted. An unrestricted joint glide indicates two differing conclusions:
  - The integrity of both the joint surface and the periarticular tissue is good. If this is the case, the patient's loss of motion

must be due to a contractile tissue. With this scenario, the intervention should emphasize soft tissue mobilization techniques designed to change the length of a contractile tissue.

- The joint glide is both unrestricted and excessive. Stress tests are then used to assess the integrity of the inert tissues, particularly the ligaments, and to determine whether instability exists at the joint. Instability at a joint may occur if the joint has undergone significant degenerative changes or trauma. The intervention for excessive motion that is impeding function focuses on stabilizing techniques designed to give secondary support to the joint through muscle action.

- The joint glide is restricted. If the joint glide is restricted, the joint surface and periarticular tissues are implicated as the cause

TABLE 2-63 Peripheral nerves of the upper quadrant.

Nerves	Nerve Root	Muscles	Action
Musculocutaneous	C5–6	Biceps, brachialis Coracobrachialis	Flexion of elbow Shoulder flexion
Lateral brachial cutaneous nerve of the arm	C5–6	Sensory only	
Median	C5–T1	Flexor carpi radialis Flexor digitorum sublimis Flexor digitorum profundus (lateral half) Pronator teres, pronator quadratus Abductor pollicis brevis Opponens pollicis brevis Flexor pollicis longus Flexor pollicis brevis	Radial flexion of wrist Flexion of middle phalanges (digiti II–V) Flexion of distal phalanges (digiti II, III) Pronation of forearm Abduction of thumb Opposition of thumb Flexion of distal phalanx of thumb Flexion of proximal phalanx of thumb
Axillary	C5–6	Deltoid Teres minor	Shoulder abduction
Radial	C5–T1	Triceps Brachioradialis Extensor carpi radialis/ulnaris Supinator Extensor pollicis brevis Extensor pollicis longus Extensor indicis proprius Extensor digiti proprius Extensor digiti communis	Extension at elbow Flexion of forearm Extension at wrist with radial/ulnar deviation Supination of forearm Extension of thumb (proximal) Extension of thumb (distal) Extension of index (proximal) Extension of little finger (proximal) Extension of digits (II–V, proximal)
Medial (dorsal) cutaneous (antebrachial) nerve of the forearm	C6–T1	Sensory only	
Lateral cutaneous (antebrachial) nerve of the forearm	C5–6	Sensory only	
Ulnar	C8–T1	Flexor carpi ulnaris Flexor digitorum profundus (medial half) Abductor digiti minimi All other intrinsics of hand	Ulnar flexion of wrist Flexion of distal phalanges (digiti IV, V) Abduction of digiti V Finger abduction/adduction

for the patient's loss of motion; however, as mentioned above, the contractile tissues cannot definitively be ruled out. The intervention for this type of finding initially involves a specific joint mobilization to restore the glide. Once the joint glide is restored following these mobilizations, the osteokinematic motion can be assessed again. If it is still reduced, the surrounding tissues have likely adaptively shortened. Distraction and compression can be used to help differentiate the cause of the restriction.

- Distraction. Traction is a force imparted passively by the clinician that results in a distraction of the joint surfaces.
  - If the distraction is limited, a contracture of connective tissue should be suspected.
  - If the distraction increases the pain, it may indicate a tear of connective tissue, and may be associated with increased range.
  - If the distraction eases the pain, it may indicate an involvement of the joint surface.
- Compression. Compression is the opposite force to distraction, and involves an approximation of joint surfaces.
  - If the compression increases the pain, a loose body or internal derangement of the joint may be present.
  - If the compression decreases the pain, it may implicate the joint capsule.

Neurological Testing

The evaluation of the transmission capability of the nervous system is performed to detect the presence of either upper motor neuron (UMN) lesion or lower motor neuron (LMN) lesion (Table 2–66). In addition, the neurological examination can often determine the exact site of the lesion.

TABLE 2-64 Peripheral nerves of the lumbar plexus.

Nerves	Nerve Root	Muscles	Action
The iliohypogastric nerve	T12, L1	Sensory	The lateral (iliac) branch supplies the skin of the upper lateral part of the thigh The anterior (hypogastric) branch supplies the skin over the symphysis
The ilioinguinal nerve	L1	Sensory	Supplies the skin of the upper medial part of the thigh and the root of the penis and scrotum or mons pubis and labium majores
The genitofemoral nerve	L1, 2	Sensory	The genital branch supplies the cremasteric muscle and the skin of the scrotum or labia The femoral branch supplies the skin of the middle upper part of the thigh and the femoral artery
Femoral	L2-4	Iliopsoas Quadriceps	Flexion of hip Extension of knee
Saphenous	L3-4		
Obturator	L2-4	Adductor longus, adductor brevis, adductor magnus	Adduction of hip
Lateral cutaneous (femoral) nerve of the thigh	L2-3	Sensory	
Posterior cutaneous nerve of the thigh	L2-3	Sensory	
Anterior cutaneous (femoral) nerve of the thigh	L2-3	Sensory	

TABLE 2-65 Nerves of the sacral plexus.

Nerves	Nerve Root	Muscles	Action
Superior gluteal	L4, L5, S1	Gluteus medius Gluteus minimus Tensor of the fascia latae	Abduction of hip
Inferior gluteal	L5-S2	Gluteus maximus	Extension of the hip
Sciatic	L4-S3	Biceps femoris, semitendinosus, semimembranosus	Flexion of leg at knee
Sciatic branches: Deep fibular (peroneal)	L4-S2	Tibialis anterior Extensor digitorum longus Extensor hallucis longus	Dorsiflexion of foot Extension of toes Extension of great toe
Sciatic branches: Superficial fibular (peroneal)	L4-S1	Fibularis (peroneus) muscles	Eversion of foot
Sciatic branches: Tibial	L4-S3	Gastrocnemius, soleus Flexor digitorum longus Flexor hallucis longus Flexor digitorum brevis Flexor hallucis brevis	Plantar flexion of foot Flexion of distal phalanges (II–IV) Flexion of distal phalanges (I) Flexion of middle phalanges (II–V) Flexion of middle phalanges (I)
Lateral cutaneous nerve of the leg	L4-S2	Sensory	
Medial plantar	L4-5		
Sural	S1-2		
Lateral plantar	S1-2		

TABLE 2–66 Major Differences between UMN and LMN lesion signs and symptoms.

	Upper Motor Neuron Lesion	Lower Motor Neuron Lesion
Location/structures	Central nervous system—cortex, brainstem, corticospinal tracts, spinal cord	Cranial nerve nuclei/nerves and anterior horn cell, spinal roots, peripheral nerve
Pathology	Cerebrovascular accident (CVA), traumatic brain injury (TBI), spinal cord injury (SCI), myelopathy	Peripheral nerve neuropathy, radiculopathy, polio, Guillain-Barre
Tone	Increased: Hypertonia, velocity dependent	Decreased or absent: Hypotonia, flaccidity, non-velocity–dependent
Reflexes	Increased: Hyperreflexia, clonus, exaggerated cutaneous and autonomic reflexes, + pathological reflexes (Babinski, Hoffman, inverted supinator)	Decreased or absent: Hyporeflexia, cutaneous reflexes decreased/absent
Involuntary movements	Muscle spasms: Flexor or extensor	Fasciculations: With denervation
Voluntary movements	Impaired or absent: Dyssynergic patterns, mass synergies	Weak or absent (if nerve integrity interrupted)
Strength	Weakness or paralysis: Ipsilateral (stroke) or bilateral (SCI) Corticospinal: Contralateral if above decussation in medulla; ipsilateral if below Distribution: Never focal	Ipsilateral weakness or paralysis in limited distribution: Segmental/focal/root pattern
Muscle appearance	Disuse atrophy: Variable, widespread distribution, especially of antigravity muscles	Neurogenic atrophy

Special Tests of the Upper Extremity

Special Tests of the Shoulder Complex

The special tests for the shoulder are divided into diagnostic categories. Selection for their use is at the discretion of the clinician and is based on a complete patient history.

Subacromial impingement tests—Patients with subacromial impingement syndrome usually perceive pain when a compressing force is applied on the greater tuberosity and rotator cuff region.[124] Pain may also be elicited with shoulder abduction in internal or external rotation.[124]

NEER IMPINGEMENT TEST Post and Cohen[125] found the Neer test to have a sensitivity of 93% in the confirmation of subacromial impingement.

HAWKINS-KENNEDY IMPINGEMENT TEST Ure and colleagues[126] found the sensitivity of the Hawkins-Kennedy test to be 62% for diagnosing subacromial impingement.

YOCUM TEST A study[127] comparing the Neer, Hawkins-Kennedy, and Yocum tests found all three to demonstrate a high sensitivity for diagnosing subacromial impingement.

ROTATOR CUFF RUPTURE TESTS

DROP ARM TEST If at any point in the descent, the patient's arm drops, this is indicative of a full thickness tear.

BICEPS AND SUPERIOR LABRAL TEARS

CLUNK TEST The clunk test is the traditional test for diagnosing labral tears. A clunk-like sensation may be felt if a free labral fragment is caught in the joint.[128]

CRANK TEST A positive test is indicated by the reproduction of a painful click in the shoulder during the maneuver.

SPEED TEST The Speed test suggests a superior labral tear when resisted forward flexion of the shoulder causes bicipital groove pain. The Speed test is also used to detect bicipital tendinopathy (see Yergason test).

YERGASON TEST[129] Speed and Yergason tests are better at discriminating between the different bicipital tendon disorders.[124] However, irritation and edema may occur in the long head of biceps, in any stage of subacromial impingement syndrome.

O'BRIEN TEST Pain with this maneuver into internal rotation and decreased pain with external rotation is typical in patients with superior labral tears. The test is also used to assess the integrity of the A-C joint.

ANTERIOR SLIDE TEST The anterior slide test[130] is another clinical test designed to stress the superior labrum.[128] The test is considered positive if pain is localized to the anterior-superior aspect of the shoulder, if there is a pop or a click in the anterior-superior region, or if the maneuver reproduces the symptoms.

The remaining tests are reserved for when the clinician needs to differentiate the structure causing the symptoms, when the provocation of symptoms during the examination has been minimal, or to rule out the possibility of instability.

ACROMIOCLAVICULAR TESTS

ACROMIOCLAVICULAR SHEAR TEST The patient is seated. The clinician cups his or her hands over the patient's deltoid muscle with one hand on the clavicle and the other on the spine of the scapula. The clinician then squeezes the heels of the hand together. Abnormal movement is a positive test.

STABILITY TESTING It is important to remember that there is no correlation between the amount of joint laxity/mobility and joint instability at the shoulder. Joint stability is more likely a function of connective tissue support and an intact neuromuscular system.

The reproduction of symptoms is important because laxity alone does not indicate instability. Pain and muscle spasm can make the examination challenging.

GLENOHUMERAL—LOAD AND SHIFT TEST
The normal motion anteriorly is half of the distance of the humeral head.

APPREHENSION TEST Patient apprehension from this maneuver, rather than pain, is considered a positive test for anterior instability. Pain with this maneuver, but without apprehension, may indicate pathology other than instability, such as posterior impingement of the rotator cuff.

JOBE SUBLUXATION/RELOCATION TEST This test is similar to the apprehension test, except that manual pressure is applied anteriorly by the clinician in an attempt to provoke a subluxation before using manual pressure in the opposite direction to relocate the subluxation. Pain and apprehension from the patient indicate a positive test for laxity and possibly a superior labral tear (relocation part of the test). Reduction of pain and apprehension further substantiates the clinical finding of anterior instability and may indicate a positive test.

ANTERIOR RELEASE TEST A positive test produces an increase or reproduction in the patient's symptoms upon release of the posteriorly directed force on the humerus.

SULCUS SIGN FOR INFERIOR INSTABILITY[131] The sulcus sign is used to detect inferior instability due to a laxity of the superior G-H and coracohumeral ligaments. A positive test results in the presence of a sulcus sign (a depression greater than a finger-width between the lateral acromion and the head of the humerus) when longitudinal traction is applied to the dependent arm in more than one position.

The sulcus sign can be graded by measuring the distance from the inferior margin of the acromion to the humeral head. A distance of less than 1 cm is graded as 1+ sulcus, 1 to 2 cm as a 2+ sulcus, and greater than 2 cm as a grade 3+ sulcus.

ROCKWOOD TEST FOR ANTERIOR INSTABILITY[132] A positive test is indicated when apprehension is noted in the latter three positions (45°, 90°, and 120°).

Special Tests of the Elbow Complex
- Tennis elbow. A number of tests exist for tennis elbow (lateral epicondylitis).
  - Cozen's test: A reproduction of pain in the area of the lateral epicondyle indicates a positive test.
  - Mill's Test: A reproduction of pain in the area of the lateral epicondyle indicates a positive test.
- Golfer's elbow (medial epicondylitis). A reproduction of pain in the area of the medial epicondyle indicates a positive test.
- Elbow flexion test for cubital tunnel syndrome. Tingling or paresthesia in the ulnar distribution of the forearm and hand indicates a positive test.

- Pressure provocative test for cubital tunnel syndrome. Tingling or paresthesia in the ulnar distribution of the forearm and hand indicates a positive test.
- Tinel sign (at the elbow). A positive sign is indicated by a tingling sensation in the ulnar distribution of the forearm and hand distal to the tapping point.

Special Tests of the Wrist and Hand
A number of tests can be used to document the neurovascular status of the wrist and hand.

Neurological and autonomic tests—

TINEL SIGN AT CARPAL TUNNEL Positive test causes tingling or paresthesia into thumb, index, middle, and lateral half of ring finger (median nerve distribution), indicating carpal tunnel syndrome.

PHALEN (WRIST FLEXION) TEST Positive test causes tingling or paresthesia into thumb, index, middle, and lateral half of ring finger (median nerve distribution), indicating carpal tunnel syndrome.

REVERSE PHALEN (PRAYER TEST) A positive test produces same symptoms as seen in Phalen test and indicates median nerve pathology.

CARPAL COMPRESSION TEST The test is considered positive if there is an onset of median nerve symptoms within 15 to 30 seconds.

FROMENT SIGN The terminal phalanx of the patient's thumb flexes because of paralysis of the adductor pollicis muscle, indicating a positive test. If, at same time, the MCP of the patient's thumb hyperextends, the hyperextension is noted as a positive Jeanne sign. If both tests are positive it indicates the presence of an ulnar nerve palsy.

EGAWA SIGN The patient flexes the middle digit and then alternately deviates the finger radially and ulnarly. If the patient is unable to perform this maneuver, the interossei are affected, indicating a positive sign for an ulnar nerve palsy.

WRINKLE (SHRIVEL) TEST The patient's finger is placed in warm water for 5 to 20 minutes. The finger is then removed and observed as to whether the skin over the pulp is wrinkled. Normally, the skin should wrinkle, but in the presence of denervation it will not. This test is only valid in first few months after injury.

WEBER'S (MOBERG'S) TWO-POINT DISCRIMINATION TEST Normal discrimination is less than 6 mm. Fair = 6–10 mm. Poor = 11–15 mm. Protective = 1 point perceived. Winding a watch = 6 mm. Sewing = 6–8 mm. Handling precision tools = 12 mm. Gross tool handling >15 mm.

"O" OR "OK" TEST The inability to make the "O" is caused by paralysis of flexor pollicis longus, pronator quadratus, and FDP to index finger, implicating anterior interosseous nerve involvement.

Vascular tests

ALLEN TEST If it flushes slowly, the artery is partially or completely occluded.

Ligament, capsule, and joint instability tests
LIGAMENTOUS INSTABILITY TESTS FOR THE FINGERS

MP COLLATERAL LIGAMENT TEST The absence of a firm end feel accompanied by associated sensations of pain or instability indicate an ulnar collateral ligament sprain. This same test may then be reversed by distracting the proximal phalanx ulnarly to stress the radial collateral ligament.

PIP COLLATERAL LIGAMENT TEST   The absence of a firm end feel accompanied by associated sensations of pain or instability indicates a radial collateral ligament sprain.

DIP COLLATERAL LIGAMENT TEST   The PIP tests may be repeated in similar fashions to assess the collateral stability of the DIP joints.

TEST FOR TIGHT RETINACULAR LIGAMENTS (RETINACULAR OR BUNNEL-LITTLER TEST)   The Bunnel-Littler test helps identify the source of PIP tension or flexion motion limitation by evaluating the intrinsic muscle or capsular tightness in the affected digit.

LUNATOTRIQUETRAL BALLOTEMENT (REAGAN) TEST   A positive test for lunatotriquetral instability.

MURPHY SIGN   The patient is asked to make a fist. If the head of the third metacarpal is level with the second and fourth metacarpals, this is a positive sign, indicating lunate dislocation.

WATSON (SCAPHOID SHIFT) TEST   If the scaphoid (and lunate) are unstable, the dorsal pole of the scaphoid subluxes over the dorsal rim of the radius and patient complains of pain, indicating a positive test for scapholunate dissociation.

SCAPHOID STRESS TEST   If there is excessive laxity, there is a resulting clunk and pain, indicating a positive test for scaphoid instability. This is an active modification of the Watson test.

"PIANO KEYS" TEST   A positive test is indicated by a difference in mobility and production of pain/tenderness, indicating DRUJ instability.

AXIAL LOAD TEST   Pain and/or crepitation indicates a positive test for a fracture of metacarpal or adjacent carpal bones or joint arthrosis. May also be done for the fingers.

PIVOT SHIFT TEST OF THE MIDCARPAL JOINT   The test is positive if the capitate "shifts" away from lunate, indicating injury to anterior capsule and interosseous ligaments.

GRIND TEST   If pain is elicited, the test is positive, and indicates degenerative joint disease (DJD) in the MCP or metacarpotrapezial joint.

TABLETOP TEST   This test is used to highlight the presence of a Dupuytren contracture. If the patient is unable to completely place the palm of the hand flat on the surface, the test is considered positive.

Tests for tendons and muscles—

FINKELSTEIN TEST   The Finkelstein test is used to determine the presence of de Quervain's or Hoffman's disease, tenosynovitis in the APL and the EPB tendons of the thumb, respectively. This maneuver will cause a stretching in these tendons which is painful if tenosynovitis is present.

FLEXOR DIGITORUM PROFUNDUS   Test for jersey (sweater) finger sign—The patient is asked to make a fist. Inability to flex or close distal phalanx indicates that the FDP is ruptured.

FLEXOR DIGITORUM SUPERFICIALIS TEST   Inability to flex or close the middle phalanx indicates a rupture of the FDS.

TEST FOR EXTENSOR HOOD RUPTURE   A positive test, indicating a torn central extensor hood, is demonstrated by a lack of pressure from the middle phalanx while the distal phalanx is extending.

LINBURG SIGN   If limited index finger extension and pain are noted, the test is positive for tendinitis at the interconnection between the FPL and flexor indicis (seen in 10%–15% of hands).

MALLET FINGER TEST   Inability to actively extend distal phalanx indicates an extensor tendon rupture or avulsion of the distal phalanx.

Special Tests of the Lower Extremity

Special Tests of the Hip

Quadrant (scour) test—The quadrant or scour test is a dynamic test of the inner quadrant and outer quadrant of the hip joint surface. The position of flexion and adduction of the hip has the potential to compress or stress a number of structures including:

- The articular surfaces of the hip joint
- The insertion of the tensor fascia latae and the sartorius
- The iliopsoas muscle
- The iliopsoas bursa and neurovascular bundle
- The insertion of the pectineus
- The insertion of the adductor longus
- The femoral neck

Care must be taken when interpreting the results from this test. At the end range of flexion and adduction, a compression force is applied at the knee along the longitudinal axis of the femur. From this point, the clinician moves the hip into a position of flexion and abduction to examine the outer quadrant. Throughout the entire movement, the femur is held midway between internal and external rotation, and the movement at the hip joint should follow the smooth arc of a circle. An abnormal finding is pain or resistance felt anywhere during the arc. The resistance may be caused by capsular tightness, an adhesion, a myofascial restriction, or a loss of joint congruity.

FABER or Patrick test—The flexion, abduction, and external rotation (FABER) test is a screening test for hip, lumbar or sacroiliac joint dysfunction, or an iliopsoas spasm. A positive test results in pain and/or loss of motion as compared with the uninvolved side.

Having the patient demonstrate where the pain is with this test may assist with the interpretation.

SI provocation tests—A number of simple stress or provocative tests can be used to examine the sacroiliac joint. In addition to the provocative tests, the passive motions of the hip can be examined with the innominate stabilized. The hip motions and their respective innominate motions in parenthesis are outlined in Table 2–67.

Craig test—The Craig test is used to assess femoral anteversion/retroversion. If the angle is greater than 8° to 15° in the direction

TABLE 2-67 Hip motions and their associated innominate motions.

Flexion (posterior rotation)
Extension (anterior rotation)
Abduction (upward)
Adduction (downward)
Internal rotation (IR)
External rotation (ER)

of internal rotation when measured from the vertical and long axis of the tibia, the femur is considered to be in anteversion.

Flexion-adduction test—This test is used as a screening test for early hip pathology. The resultant end feel, restriction, and discomfort or pain is noted and compared with the normal side.

Trendelenburg sign—The Trendelenburg sign indicates weakness of the gluteus medius muscle during unilateral weight-bearing. This position produces a strong contraction of the gluteus medius, which is powerfully assisted by the gluteus minimus and tensor fascia latae in order to keep the pelvis horizontal. For example, when the body weight is supported by the right foot, the right hip abductors contract isometrically and eccentrically to prevent the left side of the pelvis from being pulled downward.

If the hip remains level, the test is negative. A positive Trendelenburg sign is indicated when, during unilateral weight-bearing, the pelvis drops toward the unsupported limb. A number of dysfunctions can produce the Trendelenburg sign. These include superior gluteal nerve palsy, a lumbar disk herniation, weakness of the gluteus medius, and pain inhibition with advanced degeneration of the hip.

Pelvic drop test—[133]On lowering the leg there should be no arm abduction, anterior or pelvic motion, or trunk flexion, nor should there be any hip adduction or internal rotation of the weight-bearing hip. These compensations are indications of an unstable hip or weak external rotators.

Sign of the buttock—The sign of the buttock, devised by Cyriax, actually consists of seven signs. If all of the following tests are positive, the sign of the buttock is present:

- Buttock large and swollen and tender to touch
- Straight leg raise (SLR) limited and painful
- Limited trunk flexion
- Hip flexion with knee flexion limited and painful
- Empty end feel on hip flexion
- Noncapsular pattern of restriction at hip
- Resisted hip movements painful and weak (particularly hip extension)

If the hip flexion does not increase when the knee is flexed, it is a positive sign of the buttock test. If the sign of the buttock is encountered, the patient must be immediately returned to the physician for further investigation, as a positive sign indicates the presence of serious pathology such as osteomyelitis or neoplasm of the upper femur, sacral fracture, septic sacroiliitis, ischiorectal abscess, or septic gluteal bursitis.

Muscle length tests

THOMAS TEST AND MODIFIED THOMAS TEST The original Thomas test was designed to test the flexibility of the iliopsoas complex, but has since been modified and expanded to assess a number of other soft tissue structures.

If the thigh is raised off the surface of the treatment table, the test is positive. A positive test indicates a decrease in flexibility in the rectus femoris or iliopsoas muscles or both.

A modified version to this test is commonly used. In this position, the thigh should be parallel with the bed, in neutral rotation, and neither abducted nor adducted, with the lower leg perpendicular to the thigh and in neutral rotation. Approximately 80° of knee flexion should be present with the thigh in full contact with the table.

If the thigh is raised off the treatment table, a decrease in the flexibility of the iliopsoas muscle complex should be suspected. If the rectus femoris is adaptively shortened, the amount of knee extension should increase with the application of overpressure into hip extension. If the decrease in flexibility lies with the iliopsoas, attempts to correct the hip position should result in an increase in the external rotation of the thigh.

The application of overpressure into knee flexion can also be used. If the knee flexion produces an increase in hip flexion (the thigh rises higher off the bed), the rectus femoris is implicated, whereas if the overpressure produces no change in the degree of hip flexion, the iliopsoas is implicated.

This test can also be used to assess the flexibility of the tensor fascia latae, if the hip of the tested leg is maximally adducted while monitoring the ipsilateral ASIS for motion. Twenty degrees of hip adduction should be available.

Two things must be kept in mind when interpreting the results of this test:

- The criteria are arbitrary and have been shown to vary between genders, limb dominance, and depend on the types and the levels of activity undertaken by the individual.
- The apparent tightness might simply be normal tissue tension producing a deviation of the leg due to an increased flexibility of the antagonists.

As always, the cause of the asymmetry must be found (or at least looked for) and addressed.

ELY TEST This is a test to assess the flexibility of the rectus femoris. If the rectus is tight, the pelvis is observed to anteriorly rotate early in the range of knee flexion, and the hip flexes.

OBER'S TEST Ober's test is used to evaluate tightness of the ITB and tensor fascia lata (see Thomas test also). The test is considered positive when the leg fails to lower past neutral horizontal.

STRAIGHT LEG RAISE TEST FOR HAMSTRING LENGTH The hamstrings are considered shortened if a straight leg cannot be raised to an angle of 80° from the horizontal while the other leg is straight. Any limitation of flexion is interpreted as being caused by contracted hamstring muscles.

This SLR test may also be used as a screen for adverse neural tension, particularly of the sciatic nerve.

90-90 STRAIGHT LEG RAISE   The hamstring length can also be assessed with the patient positioned in supine and the tested leg flexed at the hip and knee to 90°. Davis et al.[134] found the normal values of the popliteal angle (180° minus the knee extension angle) in a population of healthy college students to be 71.6° for men and 77.7° for women, with a mean of 74.6°.

PIRIFORMIS   The patient is positioned in supine. The clinician flexes the involved hip to 60°. After stabilizing the patient's pelvis, the clinician applies a downward pressure through the femur, and maximally adducts the involved hip. From this position, the hip is moved into internal rotation and then external rotation. Internal rotation stresses the superior fibers, while external rotation stresses the inferior fibers. Normal ROM should be 45° into either rotation.

HIP ADDUCTORS   Maintaining the tested knee in extension, the clinician passively abducts the tested leg. The normal range is 40°. When the full range is reached, the knee of the tested leg is passively flexed and the leg abducted further. If the maximum range does not increase when the knee is flexed, the one-joint adductors (pectineus, adductor magnus, adductor longus, adductor brevis) are shortened. If the range does increase with the knee passively flexed, the two-joint adductors (gracilis, biceps femoris [long head], semimembranosus, and semitendinosus) are shortened.

Leg length discrepancy—There are two types of leg length discrepancy described in the literature: functional or *apparent*, and anatomical or *true*. With the former, the leg length is the same but the apparent difference is caused by a structural problem elsewhere such as a spinal scoliosis or pelvic asymmetry. With the latter, there is an actual measurable skeletal difference in the shape and length of the femur, tibia, or fibula. The test for a leg length discrepancy is best performed radiographically. However, clinically, two tests are commonly used, with the patient positioned in supine to highlight the more significant discrepancies. An apparent leg length can be measured from the umbilicus to the medial malleoli of the ankle using a tape measure. A more direct measurement can be performed using a tape measure to measure the "true" leg length by measuring from the ASIS to the medial malleolus.

Fulcrum test—A positive test is when the patient reports sharp pain or expresses apprehension when the fulcrum arm is placed under the fracture site.

Special Tests of the Knee Complex

Stress testing—Stress tests are used to determine the integrity of the joint, ligaments, and menisci. Serious functional instability of the knee appears to occur unpredictably. The reasons for such discrepancies are unknown, but they may be due to the following:

- Varying definitions of instability
- Varying degrees of damage of the ACL
- Different combinations of injuries
- Different mechanisms of compensation for the loss of the ACL
- Differences in rehabilitation

- The diverse physical demands and expectations of different populations

ONE-PLANE MEDIAL INSTABILITY

ABDUCTION VALGUS STRESS   Normally, there is little or no valgus movement in the knee, and if present should be less than the amount of varus motion, with a firm end feel. With degeneration of the medial or lateral compartments varus and valgus motions may be increased, while the end feels will be normal.

With the knee tested in full extension, any demonstrable instability is usually very significant. Pain with this maneuver is caused by an increase in tension of the medial collateral structures, or the connection of these structures with the medial meniscus (MM). If pain or an excessive amount of motion is detected compared with the other extremity, a hypermobility or instability should be suspected. The following structures may be implicated:

- Superficial and deep fibers of the medial collateral ligament (MCL)
- Posterior oblique ligament
- Posterior-medial capsule
- Medial capsular ligament
- ACL
- PCL

The test is then repeated at 10° to 30° of flexion to further assess the MCL, the posterior oblique ligament, and the PCL. One-plane valgus instability in 30° of flexion usually denotes a tearing, of at least a second degree, of the middle third of the capsular ligament and the parallel fibers of the MCL.

The posterior fibers of the MCL can be isolated by placing the knee in 90° of flexion with full external rotation of the tibia. Under normal conditions, the end feel is firm after slight movement.

If this test is positive for pain or excessive motion as compared with the other extremity, the following structures may be implicated:

- Lateral collateral ligament (LCL)
- Lateral capsular ligament
- Arcuate-popliteus complex
- ACL
- PCL

If the instability is gross, one or both cruciate ligaments may be involved as well as, occasionally, the biceps femoris tendon and the ITB, leading to a rotary instability, if not in the short term, certainly over a period of time.

The test is then repeated at 10° to 30° of flexion and the tibia in full external rotation to further assess the LCL, the posterior-lateral capsule, and the arcuate-popliteus complex.

ONE-PLANE ANTERIOR INSTABILITY   A number of tests have been advocated for testing the integrity of the ACL. Two of the more commonly used ones are the Lachman test and the anterior drawer test.

THE STABLE LACHMAN TEST   If the tibia moves forward and the concavity of the patellar tendon/ligament becomes convex, the test is considered positive.

Grading of knee instability is as follows:[135-137]

- 1+ (mild): 5 mm or less
- 2+ (moderate): 5-10 mm
- 3+ (serious): more than 10 mm

False negatives with this test can occur. False negatives may be caused by a significant hemarthrosis, protective hamstring spasm, or a tear of the posterior horn of the MM.

ANTERIOR DRAWER TEST   This test is positive when an abnormal anterior movement of the tibia occurs compared with the other extremity.

ONE-PLANE POSTERIOR INSTABILITY   The PCL is very strong and is rarely completely torn. It is typically injured in a dashboard injury, or in knee flexion activities (kneeling on the patella). A number of tests have been advocated to test the integrity of the PCL.

GRAVITY (GODFREY) SIGN   If there is a rupture (partial) of the PCL, the tibial tuberosity on the involved side will be less visible than on the noninvolved side. This is caused by an abnormal posterior translation, resulting from a rupture of the PCL.

POSTERIOR DRAWER   A positive test is excessive posterior tibial translation.

ROTARY INSTABILITIES   Rotary or complex instabilities occur when the abnormal or pathological movement is present in two or more planes. The ligamentous laxities present at the knee joint in these situations allow motion to take place around the sagittal, coronal, and horizontal axes.

POSTERIOR-LATERAL INSTABILITY   This type of instability is relatively rare, as it requires complete posterior cruciate laxity. It occurs when the lateral tibial plateau subluxes posteriorly on the femur, with the axis shifting posteriorly and medially to the medial joint area. With a hyperextension test, this posterior displacement is obvious, and has been labeled the external rotation recurvatum sign.

ACTIVE POSTEROLATERAL DRAWER TEST[138]   A positive result for the test is a posterior subluxation of the lateral tibial plateau.

HUGHSTON POSTERIOR-LATERAL DRAWER TEST[136,137]   If the tibia translates posteriorly and laterally during the test, the test is positive for posterior-lateral instability and indicates that the following structures may have been injured:

- PCL
- Arcuate-popliteus complex
- LCL
- Posterior-lateral capsule

The one-plane medial and lateral stability tests can be used to help differentiate further which lateral and posterior-lateral structures are affected.

HUGHSTON EXTERNAL ROTATIONAL RECURVATUM TEST   This test is used to detect an abnormal relationship between the femur and tibia in knee extension. In the presence of a posterior-lateral rotary instability, the knee moves into relative hyperextension at the lateral side of the knee, and the tibia externally rotates.

POSTERIOR-MEDIAL ROTARY INSTABILITY
HUGHSTON POSTERIOR-MEDIAL DRAWER TEST   The patient is positioned in supine with the involved leg flexed at the hip to 45°, the knee flexed to 80° to 90°, and the lower leg in slight internal rotation. The clinician pushes the lower leg posteriorly. If the tibia translates posteriorly and laterally during the test, the test is positive for posterior-medial instability and indicates that the following structures may have been injured:

- PCL
- Posterior oblique ligament
- MCL
- Posterior-medial capsule
- ACL

The one-plane medial and lateral stability tests can be used to help differentiate further which medial and posterior-medial structures are affected.

ANTERIOR-LATERAL ROTARY INSTABILITY   The pathology for this condition almost certainly involves the PCL and clinically, the instability allows the medial tibial condyle to sublux posteriorly, as the axis of motion has moved to the lateral joint compartment.

The diagnosis of anterior-lateral instability is based on the demonstration of a forward subluxation of the lateral tibial plateau as the knee approaches extension and the spontaneous reduction of the subluxation during flexion, in the lateral pivot shift test.

PIVOT SHIFT TEST   The pivot shift is the anterior subluxation of the lateral tibial plateau that occurs when the lower leg is stabilized in (almost) full extension, whereby further flexion produces a palpable "spring-like" reduction. The pivot shift is the most widely recognized dynamic instability of the knee, and it has been shown to correlate with reduced sports activity, degeneration of the cartilage, reinjury, meniscal damage, joint arthritis, and a history of instability symptoms.

Since the majority of patients with an ACL rupture complain of a "giving-way" sensation, the pivot shift test is regarded in current literature as capable of identifying rotational instability.

There are two main types of clinical tests to determine the presence of the pivot shift: the reduction test and the subluxation test.

- In the reduction test, the knee is flexed from full extension under a valgus moment. A sudden reduction of the anteriorly subluxed lateral tibial plateau is seen as the pivot shift.
- The subluxation test is effectively the reverse of the reduction test. However, only 35% to 75% of patients whose knees pivot while the patient is under anesthesia will experience such pivot when awake. The test begins with patient's knee extended. The clinician internally rotates the patient's tibia with one hand and applies a valgus stress to the patient's knee joint with the other. As the clinician gradually flexes the patient's ACL-deficient knee joint, the patient's subluxated anterior tibia snaps back into normal alignment at 20° to 40° of flexion.

There is little agreement in the literature with regard to the sensitivity of the pivot shift test, which varies between 0% and 98%.

The pivot shift can be positive with an isolated ACL injury or a tear or stretching of the lateral capsule, although an injury to the MCL reduces the likelihood of a pivot shift even with ACL injury.

MACINTOSH (TRUE PIVOT SHIFT)   The MacIntosh test is the most frequently used test to detect anterior-lateral instability, although

Hughston, Slocum, and Losee have all described variations. The clinician picks up the relaxed leg by grasping the ankle, and flexes the leg by placing the heel of the other hand over the lateral head of the gastrocnemius. The knee is then extended and a slight valgus stress is applied to its lateral aspect to support the tibia. Under the influence of gravity, the femur falls backwards, and as the knee approaches extension, the tibial plateau subluxes forward. This subluxation can be accentuated by gently internally rotating the tibia with the hand that is cradling the foot and ankle. At this point, a strong valgus force is placed on the knee by the upper hand, thereby impinging the subluxed tibial plateau against the lateral femoral condyle by jamming the two joint surfaces together. This will prevent easy reduction as the tibia is then flexed on the femur. At approximately 30° to 40° of flexion, the displaced tibial plateau will suddenly reduce, often in a dramatic fashion.

ANTERIOR-MEDIAL INSTABILITY   Patients who demonstrate excessive anterior medial tibial condylar displacement during the anterior drawer test are exhibiting anterior-medial instability, as the axis of motion has moved to the lateral joint compartment. The pathology involves the ACL, the MCL, and the posterior medial capsule which, along with its reinforcing fibers, is termed the posterior oblique ligament.

SLOCUM TEST   The Slocum test is designed to assess for both rotary and anterior instabilities. A positive test results from movement occurring primarily on the lateral side of the knee, and indicates a lesion to one or more of the following structures:

- ACL
- Posterior-lateral capsule
- Arcuate popliteus complex
- LCL
- PCL

If this test is positive, the second part of the test, which assesses anterior-medial rotary instability, is less reliable.

Movement occurring primarily on the medial side of the knee during testing is a positive result, and indicates a lesion to one or more of the following structures:

- MCL
- Posterior oblique ligament
- Posterior-medial capsule
- ACL

Patellar stability tests—If these tests are positive for laxity, further testing is needed by applying medial and lateral patellar glides, tilts, and rotations with the knee in relaxed extension, and noting any limitations of motion or excessive excursion.

- Glide. The glide component determines the amount of lateral deviation of the patella in the frontal plane. A 5-mm lateral displacement of the patella causes a 50% decrease in VMO tension. In the normal knee when fully extended and relaxed, the patella can be passively displaced medially and laterally approximately 1 cm in each direction, or approximately 25% to 50% of the width of the patella. Displacement of more than half the patella over the medial or lateral aspect is considered abnormal. If the patient is apprehensive as this is being done, the problem is likely to be one of poor patellar engagement. A decreased medial glide of the patella has been found to be related to ITB or lateral retinaculum tightness.
- Tilt. The degree of patella tilt is assessed by comparing the height of the medial patellar border with the height of the lateral border, which helps to determine the degree of tightness in the deep retinacular fibers. A slight lateral tilt of patella is normal. An increased lateral tilt results from a tight lateral retinaculum. If the passive lateral structures are too tight, the patella will tilt so that the medial border is higher than the lateral border, making the posterior edge of the lateral border difficult to palpate. Conversely, an increased medial tilt results from a tight medial retinaculum. Also, an inferior or superior tilt around an A-P axis may result in fat pad irritation.
- Rotation. The rotation component determines if there is any deviation of the long axis of the patella from the long axis of the femur. If the inferior pole is sitting lateral to the long axis of the femur, the patient has an externally rotated patella, whereas if the inferior pole is sitting medial to the long axis, the patient has an internally rotated patella.

A patient may have one or more of these components present, but the clinician needs to determine which of them is abnormal.

Meniscal lesion tests—No single test provides predictive results for diagnosing meniscal tears. A combination of several positive results is highly predictive of meniscal tears.

MODIFIED MCMURRAY TEST[139]   This test is positive when a palpable click or audible thump is elicited that is also painful. It is thought that pain with passive external rotation implicates lesions of the posterior horn of the lateral meniscus, while pain with passive internal rotation implicates a lesion of the posterior horn of the MM, although false-positives are common.

When the test is positive, the lesion can be in the posterior horn, but could also be elsewhere in the MM. In addition, a lesion of the LM can also provoke pain during this test.

If the test is negative, there still may be a meniscus lesion. One after the other, a similar maneuver can be repeated with valgus pressure and external rotation, then with varus pressure and external rotation, and finally with varus pressure and internal rotation.

APLEY TEST[140]   Pain with this maneuver may indicate a meniscal lesion.

O'DONAHUE TEST   Pain is a positive sign for capsular irritation or a meniscal tear.

BOEHLER TEST   Valgus stress results in pain with LM tears. Varus stress results in pain with MM tears.

THESSALY TEST   The test is considered positive for a meniscus tear if the patient experiences medial or lateral joint-line discomfort, or a sense of locking or catching in the knee during the test.

Special tests for specific diagnoses

PLICAL IRRITATION   Plical irritation has a characteristic pattern of presentation. The anterior pain in the knee is episodic and associated with painful clicking, giving-way, and the feeling of something catching in the knee. Careful palpation of the patellar retinaculum and fat pad, with the knee extended and then flexed, can be used to detect tender plicae and for the differentiation of tenderness within the fat pad from tenderness over the anterior horn of the menisci.

- The patella bowstring test can be used to test for plical irritation. The patient is positioned in side lying, tested side up. Using the heel of the cranial hand, the clinician pushes the patella medially and maintains it there. While the patella is maintained in this position, the clinician flexes the knee and internally rotates the tibia with the other hand. The knee is then extended from the flexed position while the clinician palpates for any clunks.
- Medial shift at about 30° of knee flexion (Mital-Hayden test). If a painful click is elicited during this test, there is likely to be a symptomatic mediopatellar synovial plica.

SUPRA/INFRAPATELLAR TENDONITIS   The patient is positioned in supine with the lower extremity extended.

- Infrapatellar. The clinician pushes down on the suprapatellar aspect, palpates under the inferior pole of the patella, and checks for tenderness, which may indicate infrapatellar tendinopathy.
- Suprapatellar. The clinician pushes on the infrapatellar aspect of the patella, palpates under the superior pole of the patella, and checks for tenderness, which may indicate suprapatellar tendinopathy.

INTEGRITY OF PATELLOFEMORAL ARTICULATING SURFACES   These tests involve the application of manual compression to the patella in an attempt to elicit pain.

MCCONNELL TEST   This test involves manual compression to the patella with the palm of the hand at various angles of knee flexion to compress the articulating facets. While the findings have little bearing on the overall intervention, they can guide the clinician as to which knee flexion angles to avoid during exercise.

- 20° flexion: inferior facet
- 45° flexion: middle facet
- 90° flexion: all facets except odd facet
- Full flexion: odd facet (medial) and lateral facet

ZOHLER (PATELLAR GRIND) TEST   If this test is painful, there is likely to be a symptomatic patellar chondromalacia, although this test may be positive in a large proportion of asymptomatic individuals.

CLARKE TEST   This test is similar to the one above, except that the clinician applies an increasing compressive force to the base of the patella while the patient actively contracts the quadriceps. Like the Zohler test, this test may also be positive in a large proportion of asymptomatic individuals.

WALDRON TEST   The patient is positioned in standing. While the patient performs a series of slow deep knee bends, the clinician palpates the patella for crepitus and its occurrence relative to the range.

PATELLAR MOBILITY AND RETINACULUM TESTS   Patella glides can be used to examine for retinacular mobility. The patella should be able to translate at least 25% of its width both medially and laterally. Inability to do this indicates tightness of the retinacula. Hypermobility can be suspected if the patella glides greater than two quadrants or greater than 50% of its width.

The lateral retinaculum is assessed by way of a patellar tilt and a medial-lateral displacement (glide). A number of patient positions can be used to assess the flexibility of the retinacular tissue.

FAIRBANKS APPREHENSION TEST FOR PATELLAR INSTABILITY   Positive test is patient apprehension with a laterally directed force to the patella.

WILSON TEST FOR OSTEOCHONDRITIS DISSECANS   The following accessory test can be performed when osteochondritis dissecans of the knee is suspected. The clinician flexes the patient's hip and knee to 90°. Axial compression is exerted at the knee by pushing proximally, in line with the tibia, with the distal hand. The lower leg is held in internal rotation while the knee is slowly extended, while the axial compression is maintained. In many cases of osteochondritis dissecans, the patient experiences pain because the pressure on the medial cartilaginous surfaces is increased significantly.

HAMSTRING FLEXIBILITY   The popliteal angle is the most popular method reported in the literature for assessing hamstring tightness, especially in the presence of a knee flexion contracture. The popliteal angle is at the maximum of 180° from birth to age 2 years. This angle then decreases to average 155° by age 6 years and remains steady thereafter. An angle <125° suggests significant hamstring tightness.

ILIOTIBIAL BAND FLEXIBILITY   The cardinal sign for iliotibial contracture is that in the supine patient an abduction contracture is present when the hip and knee are extended, but is eliminated by flexion of the hip and knee.

RENNE CREAK TEST[141]   The patient stands on the affected leg. As the patient flexes the knee to 30° to 40°, a positive test is indicated when a palpable "creak" is produced, as the maneuver brings the ITB into tight contact with the lateral femoral condyle.

NOBLE'S COMPRESSION TEST[142]   A positive test is indicated when pain is reproduced at 30° to 40° of knee flexion.

Special Tests of the Ankle and Foot

Ligamentous stress tests—The examination of the ligamentous structures in the ankle and foot is essential, not only because of their vast array, but also because of the amount of stability that they provide. Positive results for the ligamentous stability tests include excessive movement as compared with the same test on the uninvolved extremity, pain, depending on the severity, or apprehension.

MORTISE/SYNDESMOSIS

CLUNK (COTTON) TEST   A clunk can be felt as the talus hits the tibia and fibula if there has been significant mortise widening.

Alternatively, the patient can be positioned in supine with their knee flexed to the point where the ankle is in full dorsiflexion. The clinician applies overpressure into further dorsiflexion by grasping the femoral condyles with one hand and leaning down into the table. The clinician uses the other hand to pull the tibia (crura) anteriorly. Because the ankle is in its closed packed position, no movement should be felt.

POSTERIOR DRAWER TEST   Used to test for the presence of instability at the inferior tibiofibular joint. If the inferior tibiofibular joint is stable, there will be no drawer available, but if there is instability, there will be a drawer.

SQUEEZE (DISTAL TIBIOFIBULAR COMPRESSION) TEST   In the squeeze test, the clinician squeezes the upper to middle third of the leg at a point about 6 to 8 inches below the knee. Pain felt in the distal third of the leg may indicate a compromised syndesmosis if the presence of a tibia and/or fibula fracture, calf contusion, or compartment syndrome have been ruled out.

LATERAL COLLATERALS   The lateral collaterals resist inversion and consist of the anterior talofibular, calcaneofibular, and posterior talofibular. An additional function of the lateral ligaments of the ankle is to prevent excessive varus movement, especially during plantar flexion. In extreme plantar flexion, the mortice no longer stabilizes the broader anterior part of the talus, and varus movement of the ankle is then possible.

ANTERIOR TALOFIBULAR LIGAMENT (ATFL)   Pain on the lateral aspect of the ankle with this test, and/or displacement depending on severity, may indicate a sprain of the ligament.

ANTERIOR DRAWER TEST   The anterior drawer stress test is performed to estimate the stability of the ATFL. If the test is positive, the talus, and with it the foot, rotates anteriorly out of the ankle mortice, around the intact deltoid ligament, which serves as the center of rotation.

DIMPLE SIGN   Another positive sign for a rupture of the ATFL, if pain and spasm are minimal, is the presence of a "dimple" located just in front of the tip of the lateral malleolus, during the anterior drawer test. This results from a negative pressure created by the forward movement of the talus, which draws the skin inward at the site of ligament rupture. This dimple sign is also seen with a combined rupture of the ATFL and CFLs. However, the sign is only present within the first 48 hours of injury.

CALCANEOFIBULAR LIGAMENT   The inversion stress maneuver is a test that attempts to assess CFL integrity. Pain on the lateral aspect of the ankle with this test, and/or displacement depending on severity, may indicate a sprain of the ligament.

POSTERIOR TALOFIBULAR   Pain on the lateral aspect of the ankle with this test, and/or displacement, depending on severity, may indicate a sprain of the ligament.

MEDIAL COLLATERALS (DELTOID COMPLEX)   The medial collaterals function to resist eversion. Given their strength, these ligaments are only usually injured as the result of major trauma.

KLEIGER (EXTERNAL ROTATION) TEST   This is a general test to assess the integrity of the deltoid ligament complex, but can also implicate the syndesmosis if pain is produced over the anterior or posterior tibiofibular ligaments and the interosseous membrane. If this test is positive, further testing is necessary to determine the source of the symptoms.

Pain on the medial and lateral aspect of the ankle and/or displacement of the talus from the medial malleolus, depending on severity, with this test may indicate a tear of the deltoid ligament.

THOMPSON TEST FOR ACHILLES TENDON RUPTURE   An absence of plantarflexion indicates a complete rupture of the Achilles tendon.

ARC SIGN FOR ACHILLES TENDINOPATHY   The arc sign is performed with the patient in prone, with instructions to actively plantarflex and dorsiflex the ankle. The clinician notes the localized swelling, and if this area moves proximal and distal during the active ankle movements, the sign is positive.[143]

THE ROYAL LONDON HOSPITAL TEST FOR ACHILLES TENDINOPATHY   The test is performed in prone. The area of tenderness is located, and the patient is asked to actively dorsiflex. A positive test is indicated by a decreased pain response to palpation in the dorsiflextion position.[143]

PATLA TEST FOR TIBIALIS POSTERIOR LENGTH[144]   The patient is positioned in prone, with the knee flexed to 90°. The clinician stabilizes the calcaneus in eversion and the ankle in dorsiflexion with one hand. With the other hand, the clinician contacts the plantar surface of the bases of the second, third, and fourth metatarsals with the thumb, while the index and middle fingers contact the plantar surface of the navicular. The clinician then pushes the navicular and metatarsal heads dorsally and compares the end feel and patient response with the uninvolved side. A positive test is indicated with reproduction of the patient's symptoms.

FEISS LINE TEST   The Feiss line test is used to assess the height of the medial arch, using the navicular position. With the patient non-weightbearing, the clinician marks the apex of the medial malleolus and the plantar aspect of the first MTP joint, and a line is drawn between the two points. The navicular is palpated on the medial aspect of the foot, and an assessment is made as to the position of the navicular relative to the imaginary line. The patient is then asked to stand with their feet about 3 to 6 inches apart. In weight-bearing, the navicular normally lies on or very close to the line. If the navicular falls one-third of the distance to the floor, it represents a first-degree flatfoot; if it falls two-thirds of the distance, it represents a second-degree flatfoot, and if it rests on the floor, it represents a third-degree flatfoot.

"TOO MANY TOES" SIGN   The patient is asked to stand in a normal relaxed position while the clinician views the patient from behind. If the heel is in valgus, the forefoot abducted, or the tibia externally rotated more than normal, the clinician will observe more toes on the involved side than on the normal side.

Articular stability tests

NAVICULAR DROP TEST   The navicular drop test is a method by which to assess the degree to which the talus plantarflexes in space on a calcaneus that has been stabilized by the ground, during subtalar joint pronation.

The clinician attempts to quantify inferior displacement of the navicular tubercle as the patient assumes 50% weight-bearing on the tested foot. A navicular drop greater than 10 mm from the neutral position to the relaxed standing position suggests excessive medial longitudinal arch collapse of abnormal pronation.

TALAR ROCK   A positive test result is a "clunk" felt at the end of each of the movements.

Neurovascular status

HOMAN SIGN   Pain in the calf with this maneuver may indicate a positive Homan sign for deep vein thrombophlebitis, especially if there are associated signs including pallor and swelling in the leg and a loss of the dorsal pedis pulse.

BUERGER TEST   The patient is positioned in supine with the knee extended. The clinician elevates the patient's leg to about 45° and maintains it there for at least 3 minutes. Blanching of the foot is positive for poor arterial circulation, especially if, when the patient sits with the legs over the end of the bed, it takes 1 to 2 minutes for the limb color to be restored.

MORTON TEST The reproduction of pain with this maneuver indicates the presence of a neuroma or a stress fracture.

DUCHENNE TEST The patient is positioned in supine with their legs straight. The clinician pushes through the sole on the first metatarsal head, and pushes the foot into dorsiflexion. The patient is asked to plantarflex the foot. If the medial border dorsiflexes and offers no resistance while the lateral border plantarflexes, a lesion of the superficial peroneal nerve, or a lesion of the L4, L5, and S1 nerve root is indicated.

TINEL SIGN There are two locations around the ankle from where the Tinel sign can be elicited. The anterior tibial branch of the deep peroneal nerve can be tapped on the anterior aspect of the ankle, or the posterior tibial nerve may be tapped behind the medial malleolus. Tingling or paresthesia with this test is considered a positive finding.

DORSAL PEDIS PULSE The dorsal pedis pulse can be palpated just lateral to the tendon of the extensor hallucis longus over the dorsum of the foot.

Windlass (plantar fasciitis) test—This is used to detect the presence of fascial and ligamentous impairments of the foot. There are two parts to the test.

- Part 1: A positive test is considered if the passive extension of the MTP elicits reproduction of the patient's symptoms.
- Part 2: The patient stands on a stool with the metatarsal heads just over the edge of the stool. The patient is instructed to place equal weight on both feet. The clinician passively extends the first phalange while allowing the IP to flex. A positive test is considered if the passive MTP extension is continued and reproduces patient's symptoms.

Special Tests of the Spine and Sacroiliac Joint

Special Tests of the Upper Cervical Spine
Cervical arterial dysfunction (CAD) tests

VERTEBRAL ARTERY TESTS A positive vertebral artery test includes the onset or reproduction of the following signs and/or symptoms with testing: diplopia, dysphagia, dysarthria, drop attacks, dizziness, numbness, paresthesias, nystagmus, and nausea.

INITIAL TEST It is widely recognized that passive therapeutic maneuvers applied to the cervical spine carry a small risk of developing iatrogenic stroke. In those cases in which the clinician is to perform cervical mobilizations of grade I to IV rather than a grade V thrust technique, the Australian Physiotherapy Association's Protocol for Premanipulative Testing of the Cervical Spine continues to be recommended, although this cannot be viewed as a prescriptive guideline.[145] The protocol recommends that the clinician should maintain the immediate premobilization position for a minimum of 10 to 30 seconds to test the patency of the vertebrobasilar

system. Others recommend assessing the patient's responses for a further 20 to 30 seconds to note any latent response.[146,147] The clinician should note any symptoms of dizziness or headache, or any signs of nystagmus, slurred speech, or loss of consciousness either before, during, or after the tests. Following a positive vertebral artery test or positive responses in the history, the patient must be handled very carefully, and further intervention, particularly manipulation of the cervical spine, should not be delivered. The patient should not, under any circumstance, be allowed to leave the clinic until his or her physician has been contacted, and until the necessary arrangements have been made for the safe transport of the patient to an appropriate facility.

MUSCLE COMPRESSION TEST The initial test consists of having the patient rotate the head to each side while in supine or sitting position. The longus colli and scalene muscles rotate the cervical spine and can squeeze the vertebral artery on the side contralateral to the rotation.[148] The presence of muscular compression of the artery can be further tested by combining cervical flexion with rotation to place the inferior oblique capitis on stretch.[148]

BARRE TEST The Barre test can be used to test for vertebral artery insufficiency, especially if the patient is unable to lie supine.

The patient is seated with the arms outstretched, forearms supinated. The patient is asked to close their eyes and move their head and neck into maximum extension and rotation. A positive test is one in which one of the outstretched arms sinks toward the floor and pronates, indicating the side of the compromise.

HAUTARD (HAUTANT, HAUTART, OR HAUTARTH) TEST[108,149] As with the Barre test, proprioceptive loss rather than dizziness is sought in the Hautard test. The test has two parts. The patient is seated. Both arms are actively flexed to 90° at the shoulders. The eyes are then closed for a few seconds while the clinician observes for any loss of position of one or both arms. If the arms move, the proprioception loss has a nonvascular cause. If the first part of the test is negative, the patient is asked to extend and rotate the neck. Because the second part of the test is performed to elicit a vascular cause for the dizziness, the eyes can be open or closed. Having the eyes open allows the clinician to observe for nystagmus and changes in pupil size. Each position is held for 10 to 30 seconds. If wavering of the arms occurs with the second part of the test, a vascular cause for the symptoms is suspected.

CERVICAL QUADRANT TEST[106] Although the cervical quadrant test can be used to detect for other cervical dysfunctions (eg, nerve root irritation or impingement, or facet joint irritation or sprain), it can also be used to help detect vertebrobasilar insufficiency. A positive test is one in which referring symptoms are produced if the opposite artery is involved.

A variety of other tests exist, some of which include cervical rotation only while others combine cervical side flexion and extension and/or traction.

Cervical ligamentous integrity tests

MODIFIED SHARP-PURSER TEST This test was originally designed to test the sagittal stability of the A-A segment in rheumatoid arthritic patients, as a number of pathological conditions can affect the stability of the osseoligamentous ring of the median joints of this segment in this patient population. These changes result in degeneration and thinning of the articular cartilage between the odontoid process and the anterior arch of atlas, or the dens can become softened.

The aim of the test was to determine whether the instability was significant enough to provoke central nervous system signs and/or symptoms. A positive test includes onset or reproduction of UMN signs or symptoms or a "clunk." Local symptoms such as soreness, etc. are ignored for the purposes of evaluating the test. The clinician stabilizes C2 with one hand, and applies a posteriorly oriented force to the head.

In the presence of a positive test, a provisional assumption is made that the symptoms are caused by excessive translation of the atlas compromising one or more of the sensitive structures listed above. The test is considered positive and the physical examination is terminated. No intervention should be attempted other than the issuing of a cervical collar to prevent craniovertebral flexion, and an immediate referral to their physician.

Other upper-cervical ligament integrity tests include the alar ligament test, the tectorial membrane test, and the direct transverse ligament test.

Special Tests of the Cervical Spine and Temporomandibular joint

Temporomandibular joint screen—As the temporomandibular joint can refer pain to this region, the clinician is well advised to rule out this joint as the cause for the patient's symptoms. The patient is asked to open and close the mouth, and to laterally deviate the jaw as the clinician observes the quality and quantity of motion, and notes any reproduction of symptoms.

Lhermitte symptom or "phenomenon"—This is not so much a test as a symptom, described as an electric shock–like sensation that radiates down the spinal column into the upper or lower limbs when flexing the neck. It can also be precipitated by extending the head, coughing, sneezing, or bending forward, or by moving the limbs.[150] Lhermitte's symptom and abnormalities in the posterior part of the cervical spinal cord on MRI are strongly associated.[151]

Brachial plexus tests

STRETCH TEST   This test is similar to the SLR for the lower extremity, as it stretches the brachial plexus. The patient is positioned in sitting. The patient is asked to side bend the head to the uninvolved side and to extend the shoulder and elbow on the involved side. Pain and paresthesia along the involved arm is indicative of a brachial plexus irritation.

COMPRESSION TEST   The patient is positioned in sitting. The patient is asked to side bend the head to the uninvolved side. The clinician applies firm pressure to the brachial plexus by squeezing the plexus between the thumb and fingers. Reproduction of shoulder or upper arm pain is positive for mechanical cervical lesions.[152]

TINEL SIGN   The patient is positioned in sitting. The patient is asked to side bend the head to the uninvolved side. The clinician taps along the trunks of the brachial plexus using the fingertips. Local pain indicates a cervical plexus lesion. A tingling sensation in the distribution of one of the trunks may indicate a compression or neuroma of one or more trunks of the brachial plexus.[153]

Thoracic outlet tests—The thoracic outlet is the anatomical space bordered by the first thoracic rib, the clavicle, and the superior border of the scapula through which the great vessels and nerves of the upper extremity pass. The outlet passage is further defined by the interscalene interval, a triangle with its apex directed superiorly. This triangle is bordered anteriorly by the anterior scalene muscle, posteriorly by the middle scalene muscle, and inferiorly by the first rib. The lowest trunk of the brachial plexus, which is made up of rami from the C8 and T1 nerve roots, is the most commonly compressed neural structure in thoracic outlet syndrome. These nerve roots provide sensation to the fourth and fifth fingers of the hand and motor innervation to the hand intrinsic muscles. There may be multiple points of compression of the peripheral nerves between the cervical spine and hand, in addition to the thoracic outlet.

Thoracic outlet syndrome (TOS) is a clinical syndrome characterized by symptoms attributable to compression of the neural or vascular structures that pass through the thoracic outlet. The other names used for TOS are based on descriptions of the potential sources for its compression. These names include cervical rib syndrome, scalenus anticus syndrome, hyperabduction syndrome, costoclavicular syndrome, pectoralis minor syndrome, and first thoracic rib syndrome. Despite their widespread use, no studies documenting the reliability of the common thoracic outlet maneuvers of Adson, Allen, or the costoclavicular maneuver have been performed.[118]

When performing thoracic outlet syndrome tests, evaluation for either the diminution or disappearance of pulse or reproduction of neurological symptoms indicates a positive test. However, the aim of the tests should be to reproduce the patient's symptoms rather than to obliterate the radial pulse, as more than 50% of normal, asymptomatic people will exhibit obliteration of the radial pulse during classic provocative testing.[154]

A baseline pulse should be established first, before performing the respective test maneuvers.

ADSON VASCULAR TEST   The patient extends their neck, turns their head toward the side being examined, and takes a deep breath. This test, if positive, tends to implicate the scalenes, because the test increases the tension of the anterior and middle scalenes and compromises the interscalene triangle.[155]

ALLEN PECTORALIS MINOR TEST   The Allen test increases the tone of the pectoralis minor muscle. This test, if positive, tends to implicate pectoralis tightness as the cause for the symptoms.

COSTOCLAVICULAR TEST   During this test, the shoulders are drawn back and downward in an exaggerated military position to reduce the volume of the costoclavicular space.

HALLSTEAD MANEUVER   A positive test for TOS is indicated if there is an absence or diminishing of the pulse.

ROOS TEST[156]   The radial pulse may be reduced or obliterated during this maneuver, and an infraclavicular bruit may be heard. If the patient is unable to maintain the arms in the start position for

3 minutes or reports pain, heaviness, or numbness and tingling, the test is considered positive for TOS on the involved side. This test is also referred to as the *hands-up* test or the *elevated arm stress test* (EAST).

OVERHEAD TEST   The overhead exercise test is useful to detect thoracic outlet arterial compression. A positive test is achieved if the patient experiences heaviness, fatigue, numbness, tingling, blanching, or discoloration of a limb within 20 seconds.[155]

HYPERABDUCTION MANEUVER (WRIGHT TEST)[157]   This test is considered by many to be the best provocative test for thoracic outlet compression caused by compression in the costoclavicular space.

PASSIVE SHOULDER SHRUG   This simple but effective test is used with patients who present with TOS symptoms to help rule out thoracic outlet syndrome. Any changes in the patient's symptoms are noted. The maneuver has the effect of slackening the soft tissues and the plexus.

The aim of all of the thoracic outlet tests is to reproduce the patient's symptoms. The most common symptoms are diffuse arm and shoulder pain, especially when the arm is elevated beyond 90°, pain localized in the neck, face, head, upper extremity, chest, shoulder, or axilla; and upper extremity paresthesias, numbness, weakness, heaviness, fatigability, swelling, discoloration, ulceration, or Raynaud phenomenon.[158] Neural compression symptoms occur more commonly than vascular symptoms.[159]

Upper Limb Tension Tests
Special tests of the lumbar spine and SIJ

NEURODYNAMIC MOBILITY TESTING

STRAIGHT LEG RAISE TEST   The SLR test should be a routine test during the examination of the lumbar spine among patients with sciatica or pseudoclaudication. However, the test is often negative in patients with spinal stenosis.[160] A leg elevation of less than 60° is abnormal, suggesting compression or irritation of the nerve roots. A positive test reproduces the symptoms of sciatica, with pain that radiates below the knee, not merely back or hamstring pain.[160] Ipsilateral straight-leg raising has sensitivity but not specificity for a herniated intervertebral disk (IVD), whereas crossed straight-leg raising is insensitive but highly specific. The clinician must remember that the SLR test stresses a number of structures including:

- The lumbosacral nerve roots
- The hamstrings
- The hip joint
- The sacroiliac joint

The following guidelines can be used to interpret the results from the test:[161]

- Symptoms reproduced in the 0° to 30° range may indicate hip pathology or a severely inflamed nerve root.
- Symptoms reproduced in the 30° to 50° range may indicate sciatic nerve root involvement.
- Symptoms reproduced in the 50° to 70° range may indicate hamstring involvement.
- Symptoms reproduced in the 70° to 90° range may indicate involvement of the SIJ.

PHEASANT TEST   The Pheasant test introduces an anterior pelvic tilt/increase in lordosis through the pull of the rectus femoris. Once motion occurs at the pelvis, the clinician determines whether the low back symptoms have been reproduced.[162] A pulling sensation on the anterior aspect of the thighs is a normal finding. Patients who test positive for this maneuver tend to have the following subjective complaints:

- Pain with supine lying with the legs straight, unless the rectus and hip flexors are especially flexible
- Pain with prone lying
- Pain with sitting erect
- Pain with prolonged standing

The cause of the pain is thought to be due to the passive stretching or compression of pain-sensitive structures. These structures include the zygapophyseal joints, the segmental ligaments, and the anterior aspect of the IVD.

ANTERIOR SI JOINT STRESS (GAPPING) TEST   The procedure stresses the ventral ligament and compresses the posterior aspect of the joint. A positive test is one in which the patient's groin and/or SIJ pain is reproduced anteriorly, posteriorly, unilaterally, or bilaterally.[163]

The anterior gapping test and its posterior counterpart (see later) are believed to be sensitive for severe arthritis or anterior ligament tears,[112] although they have been shown to be poorly reproducible.[164]

POSTERIOR SACROILIAC JOINT STRESS (ANTERIOR COMPRESSION) TEST   The procedure creates a medial force that tends to gap the posterior aspect of the joint while compressing its anterior aspect. The reproduction of pain over one or both of the SIJs is considered positive.

FADE POSITIONAL TEST[165]   The setup for the flexion, adduction, extension (FADE) test is similar to that of the FABER test, except that the start position involves moving the patient's hip into flexion and adduction. From that position, the clinician moves the patient's hip into extension and slight adduction. A positive test is indicated by pain or loss of motion as compared with the uninvolved side.

POSTERIOR-ANTERIOR PRESSURES   Posterior-anterior (P-A) pressures, advocated by Maitland,[106] are applied over the spinous, mammillary, and transverse processes of this region. As a screening tool, the P-A pressures have their uses, and help detect the presence of excessive motion, and/or spasm.

BICYCLE TEST OF VAN GELDEREN   This is a test that is used to help differentiate between neurogenic and vascular claudication. The patient is positioned appropriately on a bicycle and asked to pedal against resistance until the onset of leg symptoms, with the onset of symptoms time recorded. The patient is then asked to repeat the test but this time in a slouched position, and the time of symptom onset is recorded.

- A patient with lateral spinal stenosis tolerates this position well and can ride further before onset of symptoms due to increased spinal foramen and posterior column space.
- A patient with intermittent claudication of the lower extremities typically experiences an increase in symptoms with continued exercise, regardless of the position of the spine, as the

requirement of oxygen demand is not met due to vascular dysfunction.

- A patient with intermittent cauda equina compression typically has an increase of symptoms with an increase in lumbar lordosis.

- A patient with a disk herniation usually fares well if the lumbar spine remains extended, but would be worse in flexion due to the increase in disk pressure posteriorly with the slouched/flexed seated posture.

■ SECTION 6: COMMON ORTHOPEDIC CONDITIONS

Frequently encountered orthopedic conditions are described here. The intervention strategies for many of these conditions are described in the Intervention Principles for Musculoskeletal Injuries section. Treatments specific to certain conditions are included with the descriptions.

OSTEOARTHRITIS

OA, or degenerative joint disease, occurs when the joint cartilage deteriorates to a point when pain and/or dysfunction occur. Due to its avascularity, articular cartilage has low metabolic activity and poor regenerative capacity.[166] Nutrition of the articular cartilage occurs by diffusion from the synovial fluid.

Clinical Significance

OA is the most common chronic condition of the joints, affecting approximately 27 million Americans, most commonly in people over the age of 50. Primary OA is an idiopathic phenomenon, occurring in previously intact joints, that is related to the aging process and typically occurs in older individuals. Primary OA occurs most commonly in the hands, particularly in the DIP, PIP, and first CMC joints. Secondary OA is a degenerative disease of the synovial joints that results from some predisposing condition, usually trauma that has adversely altered the articular cartilage and/or subchondral bone of the affected joints. Secondary OA often occurs in relatively young individuals.

Injuries to the articular cartilage can be divided into three distinct types:

- Type I injuries (superficial) involve microscopic damage to the chondrocytes and ECM (cell injury).
- Type II injuries (partial thickness) involve microscopic disruption of the articular cartilage surface (chondral fractures or fissuring).[167] This type of injury has traditionally had an extremely poor prognosis because the injury does not penetrate the subchondral bone and therefore does not provoke an inflammatory response.[167]
- Type III injuries (full-thickness) involve disruption of the articular cartilage with penetration into the subchondral bone, which produces a significant inflammatory process.[167] This inflammatory process, OA, is a significant health problem worldwide, affecting approximately 10% of men and 18% of women over 60 years of age.[168] OA typically affects weight-bearing joints and is a major cause of morbidity, disability, and pain.[169] The onset of OA increases with age, and up to half of people over 50 years of age report symptomatic OA.[141]

High-Yield Terms to Learn	
Osteoarthritis	Degeneration of joint cartilage and the underlying bone, most common from middle age onward. It causes pain and stiffness, especially in the hip, knee, and thumb joints.
Osteoporosis	A medical condition in which the bones become brittle and fragile from loss of tissue, typically as a result of hormonal changes or deficiency of calcium or vitamin D.
Autoimmune disease	A disease in which the body produces antibodies that attack its own tissues, leading to the deterioration and in some cases the destruction of such tissue.
Red flags	Signs or symptoms indicating a more serious problem.
Neurogenic claudication	Group of symptoms commonly associated with spinal stenosis, which is the narrowing of the spinal canal. This condition commonly develops in the lumbar (lower) region of the spine with the symptoms of pain, numbness, and tingling.
Vascular claudication	Pain caused by too little blood flow, usually during exercise. Sometimes called intermittent claudication, this condition generally affects the blood vessels in the legs, but claudication can also affect the arms.
Sprain	Stretch or tearing of ligaments.
Strain	Stretch or tearing of muscle or tendon.

Data from *The American Heritage® New Dictionary of Cultural Literacy*. 3rd ed. Copyright © 2005 by Houghton Mifflin Company.

Tests and Measures and Response

Signs and symptoms include:

- Swelling: Variable from minimum to severe
- Warmth
- Pain with weight-bearing activities and potentially at rest
- Capsular pattern of motion limitation common
- Diagnosis confirmed through radiograph/diagnostic tests

Clinical Findings, Secondary Effects, or Complications

Impaired mobility, impaired muscle performance, impaired balance, and activity limitations and participation restrictions. Deep, achy joint pain exacerbated by extensive use is the primary symptom. Also, reduced ROM and crepitus are frequently present. Joint malalignment may be visible. Heberden nodes, which represent palpable osteophytes in the DIP joints, are characteristic in women but not men. (Heberden nodes are features of OA, not rheumatoid arthritis, and they have no known association with G-H disease or inguinal lymphadenopathy.) Inflammatory changes are typically absent or at least not pronounced.

Comorbidities such as obesity and cardiovascular disease can negatively impact the clinical course.

Diagnostic Tests

The diagnostic tests used to help confirm a diagnosis of OA include joint aspiration, x-rays, or MRI (in the early stages of the disease).

Common findings on radiograph with OA:

- Joint space narrowing
- Sclerosis
- Osteophytes
- Lucent cysts
- Swelling

Interventions/Treatment

Medical—The extent of the medical intervention depends on the severity of the disease and can range from a conservative course to a variety of surgical procedures. A typical medical intervention includes:

- NSAIDs
- Corticosteroid injections
- Topical analgesics

Surgical procedures that can be used in advanced cases of OA include:

- Total or partial joint replacement
- Osteotomy to change a bony alignment

Pharmacological—NSAIDs and acetaminophen (Tylenol).

Physical therapy—The goals of a physical therapy intervention include:

- Reduction of pain and muscle spasm through the use of modalities and relaxation training

- Improvement of balance and ambulation
- Maintenance or improvement of ROM
- Correction of muscle imbalances in both strength and flexibility

Physical therapy interventions to meet these goals are:

- Strengthening exercises
- Flexibility exercises
- Balance and neuromuscular training
- Functional training
- Assistive devices as needed (canes, walkers, orthotics, reachers, etc.)
- Aerobic conditioning using low- to nonimpact exercises (walking program, pool exercises)
- Patient education and empowerment:
  - Joint protection strategies
  - Energy conservation techniques
  - Activities to avoid
  - Promotion of healthy lifestyle, for example, weight reduction

Differential Diagnosis

The differential diagnosis of OA depends largely on the location but generally include crystalline arthropathies (eg, gout and pseudogout), seronegative spondyloarthropathies (eg, psoriatic arthritis and reactive arthritis), and inflammatory arthritis (eg, rheumatoid arthritis).

BURSITIS

Bursitis is defined as inflammation of a bursa, and occurs when the synovial fluid becomes infected by bacteria or irritated because of too much friction. When inflamed, the synovial cells increase in thickness and may show villous hyperplasia.

Clinical Significance

Common forms of bursitis include:

- Subacromial (subdeltoid) bursitis. Repetitive activities with an elevated arm most frequently cause inflammation of this bursa. Difficulty in G-H abduction may occur, specifically from 70° to 100°.
- Olecranon bursitis. Because of its superficial location, this bursa is easily traumatized from acute blows or chronic stress. Trauma of the skin and surrounding tissues makes the olecranon a frequent location for infectious bursitis.
- Iliopsoas bursitis. This type of bursitis is often associated with hip pathology (eg, rheumatoid arthritis, OA) or recreational injury (eg, running). Pain from iliopsoas bursitis radiates down the anteromedial side of the thigh to the knee and is increased on extension, adduction, and internal rotation of the hip.
- Trochanteric bursitis. Although the trochanteric bursa can become inflamed, it is now thought that the more common cause for lateral hip pain is gluteal tendinopathy. The bursae can become inflamed through either friction or direct trauma, such as a fall on the side of the hip. Palpable tenderness, and the reproduction of the pain when the ITB is stretched across the trochanter with hip adduction, or the extremes of internal or external hip rotation, indicate either gluteal tendinopathy

or trochanteric bursitis.[171] Resisted abduction, extension, or external rotation of the hip are also painful.

- Ischial bursitis. Inflammation of this bursa commonly arises as a result of trauma, prolonged sitting on a hard surface (weaver bottom), or prolonged sitting in the same position (spinal cord injury).
- Prepatellar bursitis. Inflammation arises secondary to trauma or constant friction between the skin and the patella, most commonly when frequent forward kneeling is performed.
- Infrapatellar bursitis. The symptoms from this bursitis, which is often caused by frequent kneeling in an upright position, are located more distally than those of prepatellar bursitis.
- Pes anserine bursitis. This type of bursitis can result from an abnormal pull of any of the three tendons (sartorius, gracilis, and semitendinosus) or can be due to repetitive friction from a dysfunctional gait. Patients with pes anserine bursitis are commonly obese, older females with a history of OA of the knees.

Tests and Measures and Response

There are no specific clinical tests to diagnose bursitis. The diagnosis is made through the patient's history (complaints of aching muscle stiffness, pain with pressure on the affected area) and the presenting signs (red and swollen area), and tenderness on palpation.

Clinical Findings, Secondary Effects, or Complications

- Inflammation/edema
- Localized tenderness
- Warmth
- Erythema
- Loss of function

Diagnostic Tests

Although not commonly used, the physician may prescribe a series of x-rays to rule out bone spurs/arthritis, or an aspiration of the bursa to examine the fluid and rule out such conditions as gout or infection.

Interventions/Treatment

Pharmacological—NSAIDs to help control pain and inflammation.

Physical therapy

- Modalities to reduce swelling and pain
- Patient education on activity modification
- Therapeutic exercise to progress back to full ROM and strength
- Functional training

Differential Diagnosis

Tendinopathy, cellulitis, septic arthritis, gout and pseudogout, fracture, ligamentous injury, and OA.

RHEUMATIC DISEASES

There are more than 100 rheumatic diseases. Rheumatic diseases are a series of pathologies that affect both joints and muscles, that can also be classified as autoimmune diseases. Some of the more common ones are presented here.

Rheumatoid Arthritis

Rheumatoid arthritis (RA) is a disease that affects the entire body and the whole person. It is an autoimmune systemic disease in which the immune system attacks the synovium. The cycle of stretching, healing, and scarring that occurs as a result of the inflammatory process seen in rheumatoid arthritis causes significant damage to the soft tissues and periarticular structures, often resulting in joint destruction and laxity.[172]

Clinical Significance

RA is the most common type of autoimmune arthritis. It is now well accepted that early treatment of RA helps prevent joint damage, increases muscle strength, and provides better long-term results.

Tests and Measures and Response

The diagnosis of RA is made radiographically, through blood-work, or through joint aspiration.

Clinical Findings, Secondary Effects, or Complications

- Systemic manifestations: Morning stiffness lasting for more than 30 minutes, anorexia, weight loss, and fatigue.
- Arthritis of three or more joint areas: The 14 more commonly involved joints include the right or left PIP, MCP, wrists, elbow, knee, ankle, and MTP joints. In the hand, many common deformities can be seen, such as ulnar deviation of the MCP joints, radial deviation of the CMC block, boutonnière deformity, and swan neck deformities of the digits.
- Muscle atrophy and myositis.
- Tenosynovitis.
- Positive laboratory tests: Elevated erythrocyte sedimentation rate (ESR) or C-reactive protein; synovial fluid analysis.
- Radiographic findings.

Diagnostic Tests

The physical therapy examination of the patient with suspected RA involves:[172]

- Measurement of joint ROM. Goniometric measurement of PROM is indicated at all affected joints following a gross ROM screening.
- Measurement of strength. Application of standard manual muscle tests to determine strength and pain at various points in the range.
- Measurement of independence with functional activities. Functional measures may include activities of daily living (ADL), work, and leisure activities. The choice of a functional instrument is influenced by several factors, including the characteristics and needs of the individual patient, the level and depth of information required, and its predictive value in gauging the efficacy of treatment.
- Measurement of joint stability. The ligamentous laxity of any affected joint should be fully investigated.
- Measurement of mobility and gait.

- Measurement of sensory integrity.
- Measurement of psychological status.
- Determination of level of impairment including deconditioning, pain, weakness, cardiopulmonary complications, neurological manifestations, environmental barriers, and fatigue.

Interventions/Treatment

Medical—The medical interventions for RA, usually by a rheumatologist, depend on the acuity and severity, but almost all interventions include some form of drug therapy.

Pharmacological—While there is no cure for RA, the use of disease-modifying antirheumatic drugs (DMARDs) help to relieve symptoms and slow the progression of the joint damage. Patients with more advanced cases of the disease may be prescribed biologic response modifiers.

Physical therapy—Based on the pathomechanics of the rheumatoid process, the following concepts form the foundation of any intervention to manage RA:[172]

- Decrease pain.
- Control the inflammation.
- Increase or maintain the ROM of all joints sufficient for functional activities. Focus on joint systems rather than isolated joints.
- Increase or maintain muscle strength sufficient for functional activities.
- Increase joint stability and decrease mechanical stress on all affected joints. The clinician should target functional activities that require specific techniques of joint protection.
- Increase endurance for or functional activities.
- Promote independence in all ADLs, including bed mobility and transfers.
- Improve efficiency and safety of gait pattern.
- Establish patterns of adequate physical activity or exercise to maintain or improve musculoskeletal and cardiovascular fitness and general health.
- Educate the patient, family, and other personnel to promote the individual's capacity for self-management.
- Consider the type of rheumatoid disease:
  - The type in which scarring outweighs the articular damage. Patients with stiff joints because of scarring do poorly after soft tissue surgery. Patients in this group require aggressive and sustained therapy, often for 3 to 4 months.
  - The type in which joint laxity and tissue laxity become difficult to stabilize after soft tissue procedures. The patients in this group require careful treatment and control of the ROM and the direction of motion by the use of splints for many months after surgery. Also, extreme caution should be taken in the treatment of upper cervical issues with RA patients, as these individuals often have subcranial laxity at the A-A joint, and at the transverse ligament and dens articulations.

Differential Diagnosis

The differential diagnosis for RA includes all of the pathologies with similar clinical features, particularly psoriatic arthritis, systemic lupus erythematosus (SLE), polyarticular gout, acute viral polyarthritis, or calcium pyrophosphate deposition disease.

Gout

Gout (known as podagra when it involves the big toe) is caused by an altered purine metabolism that leads to hyperuricemia and the accumulation of uric acid crystals in synovial joints.

Clinical Significance

Gout is the most common form of inflammatory arthritis in men older than 40 years of age, and appears to be on the increase.[173] Arthritis caused by gout (ie, gouty arthritis) accounts for millions of outpatient visits annually. The rising prevalence of gout is thought to stem from dietary changes, environmental factors, increasing longevity, subclinical renal impairment, and the increased use of drugs causing hyperuricemia, particularly diuretics.[174]

Tests and Measures and Response

There are no specific physical therapy tests to diagnose gout, but the following signs and symptoms usually highlight its presence: sudden attacks of pain, erythema, and swelling of one or a few joints in the lower extremities.

Clinical Findings, Secondary Effects, or Complications

Gout can present in a number of ways, although the most usual is a gouty arthritis attack of acute inflammatory arthritis (red, tender, hot, swollen) of the involved joint.

Diagnostic Tests

Diagnosis is confirmed clinically by the visualization of the characteristic crystals in joint fluid.

Interventions/Treatment

Medical—Modifiable risk factors (eg, diuretic therapy, high-purine diet, alcohol use, and obesity) are typically addressed.

Pharmacological—NSAIDs or corticosteroids are usually the first drugs to be used, depending on comorbidities. Colchicine is prescribed in the more recalcitrant cases.

Physical therapy—During any acute exacerbation, physical therapy is focused on pain management and splinting, orthotics, or other assistive devices to protect the affected joint(s). If the patient is not experiencing an acute exacerbation, the intervention is focused on maintenance of ROM, strength, and function, a suitable home exercise program, and patient education about weight control.

Differential Diagnosis

The differential diagnosis includes, but is not limited to, pseudogout (another form of arthritis), rheumatoid arthritis, septic/infectious arthritis, neoplasm, acute fracture, and acute rheumatic fever.

Ankylosing Spondylitis

Ankylosing spondylitis (AS; also known as Bekhterev's or Marie-Strümpell disease) is an autoimmune systemic inflammatory disease that impacts the enthesitis, or attachment sites, of tendons and ligaments to bone.

Clinical Significance

Thoracic involvement in AS occurs almost universally. The patient is usually between 15 and 40 years of age.[175] Although males are affected more frequently than females, mild courses of AS are more common in the latter.[176] The disease includes involvement of the anterior longitudinal ligament and ossification of the disk, thoracic zygapophyseal joint joints, costovertebral joints, and manubriosternal joint and SIJ. This multijoint involvement makes the checking of chest expansion measurements a required test in this region. In time, AS progresses to involve the whole spine and results in spinal deformities, including flattening of the lumbar lordosis, kyphosis of the thoracic spine, and hyperextension of the cervical spine. These changes in turn result in flexion contractures of the hips and knees, with significant morbidity and disability.[176]

Tests and Measures and Response

Inspection usually reveals a flat lumbar spine and gross limitation of side bending in both directions. Mobility loss tends to be bilateral and symmetric. There is loss of spinal elongation on flexion (Schober test), although this can occur in patients with chronic low back pain or spinal tumors and is thus not specific for inflammatory spondylopathies.[177] The patient may relate a history of costochondritis, and upon examination, rib springing may give a hard end feel. Basal rib expansion often is decreased. The glides of the costotransverse joints and distraction of the sternoclavicular joints are decreased, and the lumbar spine exhibits a capsular pattern.

As the disease progresses, the pain and stiffness can spread up the entire spine, pulling it into forward flexion, so that the patient adopts the typical stooped-over position. The patient gazes downward, the entire back is rounded, the hips and knees are semiflexed, and the arms cannot be raised beyond a limited amount at the shoulders.[178]

Exercise is particularly important for these patients to maintain mobility of the spine and involved joints for as long as possible, and to prevent the spine from stiffening in an unacceptable kyphotic position.

Clinical Findings, Secondary Effects, or Complications

The most characteristic feature of the back pain associated with AS is pain at night, as the SIJ is often the first symptomatic joint, especially in females.[179] Patients often awaken in the early morning (between 2:00 and 5:00 am) with back pain and stiffness, and usually either take a shower or exercise before returning to sleep.[176] Backache during the day is typically intermittent irrespective of exertion or rest.[176] Although not as common, ankylosing spondylitis can also cause peripheral joint pain, particularly in the hips, knees, ankles, and shoulders and neck. If peripheral arthritis occurs, it is usually late in the course of the arthritis.[180] The arthritis usually occurs in the lower extremities in an asymmetric distribution, with involvement of the "axial" joints, including shoulders and hips, more common than involvement of more distal joints.[176,181]

Diagnostic Tests

Calin and colleagues[182] describe five screening questions for AS:

1. Is there morning stiffness?
2. Is there improvement in discomfort with exercise?
3. Was the onset of back pain before age 40 years?
4. Did the problem begin slowly?
5. Has the pain persisted for at least 3 months?

Using at least four positive answers to define a "positive" result, the sensitivity of these questions was 0.95, and specificity 0.85.[182] A human leukocyte antigen (HLA) haplotype association (HLA-B27) has been found with ankylosing spondylitis and remains one of the strongest known associations of disease with HLA-B27, but other diseases are also associated with the antigen.[176]

The diagnosis of AS is generally confirmed with radiographs, which typically show the characteristic finding of "bamboo spine."

Interventions/Treatment

Physical therapy—Much of the physical therapy intervention involves patient education and instruction. The patient is taught a strict regimen of daily exercises, which include positioning and spinal extension exercises, breathing exercises, and exercises for the peripheral joints.[183] Several times a day, patients should lie prone for 5 minutes, and they should be encouraged to sleep on a hard mattress and avoid the side-lying position. Swimming is the best routine sport.

Differential Diagnosis

The differential diagnosis includes, but is not limited to, any of the systemic rheumatic disease processes, such as psoriasis, or reactive arthritis, nonspecific low back pain, degenerative disk disease, lumbar spinal stenosis, and Reiter syndrome. Peripheral involvement may present with an insidious onset of bilateral inflammatory processes such as bilateral Achilles tendonitis or plantar fascititis.

Systemic Lupus Erythematosus

SLE, sometimes referred to as lupus, is a chronic inflammatory autoimmune disorder that can affect any organ or system of the body. More than 90% of cases of SLE occur in women, often starting at childbearing age.

Clinical Significance

The seronegative arthropathies include ankylosing spondylitis, Reiter syndrome (the classic triad of arthritis, conjunctivitis, and urethritis), psoriatic arthritis, and arthritis associated with inflammatory bowel disease.

Tests and Measures and Response

SLE can affect almost any organ system; thus, its presentation and course are highly variable. The classic triad of fever, joint pain, and rash in a woman of childbearing age should prompt exploration into the diagnosis of SLE.

Clinical Findings, Secondary Effects, or Complications

Clinical manifestations for the physical therapist to note include:

- Musculoskeletal involvement: Arthralgias and arthritis constitute the most common presenting manifestations of SLE.
- Cardiopulmonary signs: Pleuritis, pericarditis, and dyspnea.
- Neurologic involvement: Headaches, depression, seizures, peripheral neuropathy (Raynaud phenomenon).
- Kidney dysfunction or failure.

    Physical therapy goals include:

- Patient education on how to control and restrict activities—energy conservation.
- Careful observation for signs of a renal failure such as weight gain, edema, or hypertension.
- If Raynaud phenomenon is present, patient education on how to warm and protect the hands and feet.

Diagnostic Tests

The diagnosis of SLE is based on a combination of clinical findings and laboratory results. According to the American College of Rheumatology (ACR), a person is considered to have SLE if 4 of the following 11 criteria, conveniently put into a mnemonic of SOAP BRAIN MD, are present:

- Serositis
- Oral ulcers
- Arthritis—nonerosive arthritis of two or more peripheral joints characterized by tenderness, swelling, or effusion
- Photosensitivity
- Blood disorders—hemolytic anemia, leukopenia, leukopenia, or thrombocytopenia
- Renal involvement
- Antinuclear antibodies—abnormal titer
- Immunologic phenomena (eg, dsDNA; anti-Smith [Sm] antibodies)
- Neurologic disorder
- Malar rash
- Discoid rash

Interventions/Treatment

Medical—The medical management of SLE typically depends on the individual's disease severity and manifestations.

Pharmacological—Medications used to treat SLE manifestations include antimalarials (eg, hydroxychloroquine), short-term use of corticosteroids, nonbiologic and biological DMARDs, and NSAIDs.

Physical therapy—Physical therapy interventions are focused on addressing the musculoskeletal manifestations of the disease, as well as concentrating on the decreased level of physical fitness

often found in this population. Each patient is examined and then provided an individualized and effective plan of care to help reduce pain, stiffness, and inflammation, as well as to improve joint ROM and functional mobility. Aerobic exercise has been shown to improve aerobic capacity in patients with mild SLE, while also decreasing overall fatigue.[184]

Differential Diagnosis

The differential diagnosis for SLE is extensive and includes, but is not limited to, scleroderma, rheumatoid arthritis, Lyme disease, Epstein-Barr virus, fibromyalgia, infective endocarditis, acute pericarditis, polymyositis, and Sjögren syndrome.

Psoriatic Arthritis

Psoriatic arthritis is an inflammatory arthritis associated with psoriasis, which affects men and women with equal frequency.[181] Its peak onset is in the fourth decade of life, although it may occur in children and in older adults.

Clinical Significance

Psoriatic arthritis can manifest in one of a number of patterns, including distal joint disease (affecting the DIP joints of the hands and feet), asymmetric oligoarthritis, polyarthritis (which tends to be asymmetric in half the cases), and arthritis mutilans (a severe destructive form of arthritis), and spondyloarthropathy.[181]

Tests and Measures and Response

There are no specific physical therapy tests to diagnose psoriatic arthritis.

Clinical Findings, Secondary Effects, or Complications

- Patients with psoriatic arthritis have less tenderness over both affected joints and tender points than patients with rheumatoid arthritis.[185]
- The spondyloarthropathy of psoriatic arthritis may be distinguished from ankylosing spondylitis (AS) by the pattern of the sacroiliitis.[186] Whereas sacroiliitis in AS tends to be symmetric, affecting both SIJs to the same degree, it tends to be asymmetric in psoriatic arthritis,[181] and patients with psoriatic arthritis do not have as severe a spondyloarthropathy as patients with AS.[175]

    The most telling signs are the skin and nail (occur in more than 80% of patients) changes. The nail changes include discolorations and "pitting"—the formation of depressions in the fingernails or toenails. Another feature of psoriatic arthritis is the presence of dactylitis, tenosynovitis (often digital, in flexor and extensor tendons and in the Achilles tendon), and enthesitis.[186] The presence of erosive disease in the DIP joints is typical.[186]

Diagnostic Tests

The diagnosis is typically made based on the signs and symptoms, the physical examination, the patient's medical and family history, imaging studies, bone density tests, and a series of blood tests (rheumatoid factor [RF] and anti-CCP antibody tests can rule out RA).

Interventions/Treatment

Medical—Psoriatic arthritis is treated in a similar fashion to that of RA. The main goal of treatment is to control joint inflammation through medications.

Pharmacological—The most commonly prescribed medications for psoriatic arthritis include NSAIDs initially and then nonbiologic and/or biological DMARDs as needed.

Physical therapy—The focus of the physical therapy intervention is to use ultraviolet (UV) therapy and thermal modalities to decrease pain. Cryotherapy can be used to reduce joint swelling and tenderness. A recent study indicated that hydrotherapy can improve physical function, sleep and relaxation, energy, work, and cognitive function in patients with psoriatic arthritis.[187]

Differential Diagnosis

The differential diagnosis of psoriatic arthritis includes, but is not limited to, septic arthritis, gout and pseudogout, reactive arthritis, rheumatoid arthritis, and ankylosing spondylitis.

OSTEOMYELITIS

Osteomyelitis is an infectious process of the bone and its marrow. The term can refer to infections caused by pyogenic microorganisms but can also be used to describe other sources of infection such as tuberculosis, or specific fungal infections (mycotic osteomyelitis), parasitic infections (hydatid disease), viral infections, or syphilitic infections (Charcot arthropathy).[188-192]

Clinical Significance

Certain conditions can weaken the immune system, increasing the risk of developing osteomyelitis, including:

- Diabetes (a common cause)
- RA
- HIV or AIDS
- Sickle cell disease
- Intravenous drug use
- Alcoholism
- Long-term use of steroids
- Hemodialysis

Tests and Measures and Response

There are no specific physical therapy clinical tests that can diagnose osteomyelitis.

Clinical Findings, Secondary Effects, or Complications

Findings at physical examination may include the following:

- Fever or no fever
- Edema
- Warmth
- Tenderness to palpation
- Reduction in the use of the extremity

Diagnostic Tests

Diagnosis of osteomyelitis is often based on radiologic results showing a lytic center with a ring of sclerosis, but a culture of material taken from a bone biopsy is needed to identify the specific pathogen.

Interventions/Treatment

Medical—Osteomyelitis may require surgical debridement. Severe cases may lead to the loss of a limb.

Pharmacological—Osteomyelitis often requires prolonged antibiotic therapy, with a course lasting a matter of weeks or months.

Physical therapy—The major physical therapy role in osteomyelitis is one of early detection. In general, rehabilitation is aimed at restoring normal ROM, flexibility, strength, and endurance with the goal of maintaining function and enhancing mobility.

Differential Diagnosis

The differential diagnosis for osteomyelitis is extensive and includes, but is not limited to, sickle cell anemia, septic arthritis, cellulitis, DVT, neoplasm, fracture, and transient synovitis.

OSTEOPOROSIS

Osteoporosis is a systemic skeletal disorder characterized by decreased bone mass and deterioration of bony microarchitecture.[193-203] Osteoporosis results from a combination of genetic and environmental factors that affect both peak bone mass and the rate of bone loss.

Clinical Significance

Skeletal demineralization, caused by an imbalance between bone formation and bone resorption, may be a primary disorder or may be secondary to a variety of other diseases or disorders such as hyperparathyroidism. The term *skeletal demineralization* refers to a loss of mass and calcium content from the bones. Skeletal demineralization can vary in severity:

- Less severe bone loss: osteopenia. Osteopenia may be apparent as radiographic lucency (measured as a T-score—see Tests and Measures and Response) but is not always noticeable until 30% of bone mineral is lost.[204,205]
- More severe bone loss: osteoporosis. Osteoporosis accounts for the largest number of fractures among the elderly.

Risk factors for skeletal demineralization include those that are modifiable and those that are nonmodifiable. The modifiable risk factors include:

- Gender (female > male)
- Race
- Age
- Family history
- Body size
- Early menopause

The nonmodifiable risk factors include:

- Use of specific medications
- Low calcium intake
- Low vitamin D levels
- Estrogen deficiency
- Excessive alcohol intake
- Cigarette smoking
- Physical inactivity
- Prolonged overuse of thyroid hormone

Tests and Measures and Response

The lower a person's T-score, the lower the bone density.

- A T-score of –1.0 or above is normal bone density. Examples are 0.9, 0, and –0.9.
- A T-score between –1.0 and –2.5 indicates low bone density or osteopenia.
- A T-score of –2.5 or below is a diagnosis of osteoporosis.

Clinical Findings, Secondary Effects, or Complications

Osteoporosis may be either primary or secondary.

- Primary. Primary osteoporosis is subdivided into types I and II.
  - Type I, or postmenopausal, osteoporosis is thought to result from gonadal (ie, estrogen, testosterone) deficiency, resulting in accelerated bone loss. An increased recruitment and responsiveness of osteoclast precursors and an increase in bone resorption, which outpaces bone formation, occurs. After menopause, women experience an accelerated bone loss of 1% to 5% per year for the first 5 to 7 years. The end result is a decrease in trabecular bone and an increased risk of Colles and vertebral fractures.
  - Type II, or senile, osteoporosis occurs in women and men because of decreased formation of bone and decreased renal production of 1,25(OH)2 D3 occurring late in life. The consequence is a loss of cortical and trabecular bone and increased risk for fractures of the hip, long bones, and vertebrae.
- Secondary. Secondary osteoporosis, also called type III, occurs secondary to medications, especially glucocorticoids, or other conditions that cause increased bone loss by various mechanisms.

Osteoporosis can occur in either a generalized or a regional form. The cardinal feature is a fracture, and the clinical picture depends on the fracture site. Vertebral fracture often manifests as acute back pain after bending, lifting, or coughing or as asymptomatic progressive kyphosis with loss of height. Most fractures occur in the mid-to-lower thoracic or upper lumbar spine. The pain is described variably as sharp, nagging, or dull; movement may exacerbate pain, and sometimes pain radiates to the abdomen.

Acute pain usually resolves after 4 to 6 weeks. In the setting of multiple fractures with severe kyphosis, or dowager hump, the pain may become chronic. When kyphosis becomes severe, the patient may develop a restrictive pattern of respiratory impairment.

Forearm, hip, and proximal femoral fractures usually occur after falls, with forward falls often resulting in Colles fractures and backward falls resulting in hip fractures. Rib fractures are most often associated with osteoporosis secondary to corticosteroid use or Cushing syndrome, but they can also be observed with other etiologies.

Diagnostic Tests

To definitively diagnose osteoporosis, one must perform some type of quantitative imaging study on the bone in question. Medical and screening tests of bone mineral density are available:

- Screening tests include finger densitometry and heel (calcaneal) ultrasonography.
- Medical tests include single-photon absorptiometry (SPA) and dual energy x-ray absorptiometry (DXA). Radiographs may show fractures or other conditions, such as OA, disk disease, or spondylolisthesis. Osteopenia (low bone density) may be apparent as radiographic lucency but is not always noticeable until 30% of bone mineral is lost.

Bone mineral density (BMD) testing is the best predictor of fracture risk. Although measurement at any site can be used to assess overall fracture risk, measurement at a particular site is the best predictor of fracture risk at that site. BMD is reported as a T-score, which compares the patient's BMD to that of a healthy young adult (see Tests and Measures and Response).

Interventions/Treatment

Medical—Effective medical therapy is available to help prevent and treat osteoporosis, including drug therapy and gonadal hormone replacement.

Pharmacological—A number of pharmaceutical agents are used in the treatment of osteoporosis calcitonin, selective estrogen-receptor modulators, and bisphosphonates.[202] However, these agents reduce bone resorption with little, if any, effect on bone formation.[202]

Physical therapy—The physical therapy intervention for osteoporosis includes:

- Weight-bearing and aerobic exercise, which have been shown to have a positive effect on BMD, although the exact mechanism is not known.[201,206,207] Regular exercise should be encouraged in all patients, including children and adolescents in order to strengthen the skeleton during the maturation process. In addition, exercise improves agility and balance, thereby reducing the risk of falls.
- Postural correction and training—should address walking, standing, and sitting.
- Pain control methods—use of adjunctive interventions including thermal and non-thermal modalities, and transcutaneous electrical nerve stimulation (TENS).

Differential Diagnosis

The differential diagnosis for osteoporosis includes, but is not limited to, osteomalacia, leukemia, lymphoma, pathological fractures secondary to bone metastasis, sickle cell anemia, multiple myeloma, and Paget disease.

GLENOHUMERAL INSTABILITY

Laxity is the physiologic motion and a necessary attribute of the G-H joint that allows normal ROM in an asymptomatic shoulder.[208] Instability is the abnormal symptomatic motion of the G-H joint that affects normal joint kinematics and results in pain, subluxation, or dislocation of the shoulder.[209-212]

Clinical Significance

Characteristic of G-H instability is the complaint of the shoulder "slipping" or "popping out" during overhead activities. Instability of the shoulder can be classified by frequency (acute or chronic), magnitude, direction, and origin.[213] Acute traumatic instability with dislocation of the shoulder is the most dramatic variety, and often requires manipulative reduction. Shoulder instability may also be classified according to the direction of the subluxation as either unidirectional (anterior, posterior, or inferior), bidirectional, or multidirectional. Posterior instability, which results either from avulsion of the posterior glenoid labrum from the posterior glenoid or stretching of the posterior capsuloligamentous structures, is often difficult to diagnose, with no single test having high sensitivity and specificity.

Tests and Measures and Response

A number of physical therapy special tests exist to help confirm a diagnosis of G-H instability (see Special Tests of the Shoulder Complex)

Clinical Findings, Secondary Effects, or Complications

Most patients presenting with hypermobility or instability of the anterior G-H joint are athletic adolescents or young adults with joint laxity.[208,214] Anterior instability occurs when the abducted shoulder is repetitively placed in the anterior apprehension position of external rotation (ER) and horizontal abduction. Such individuals may have pain with overhead movements due to an inability to control the laxity through muscle support. They may develop enough instability directed superiorly that they present with impingement-like symptoms (instability–impingement overlap), especially in positions of abduction and ER.[215] In general, the patients have had normal asymptomatic shoulder function until some event precipitates symptoms. The event usually involves only relatively minor trauma when compared with the traumatic causes of unidirectional instability, or repetitive microtrauma as occurs in patients who participate in swimming and gymnastics.[216] The most common presenting complaint is pain.[217,218]

Diagnostic Tests

Diagnosis of G-H instability is through a thorough history, radiology, and the physical therapy special tests.

Interventions/Treatment

Medical—Two acronyms are commonly used to describe shoulder instability, TUBS (*T*raumatic, *U*nidirectional instability with *B*ankart lesion requiring *S*urgery) and AMBRII (*A*traumatic onset of *M*ultidirectional instability that is accompanied by *B*ilateral laxity or hypermobility. *R*ehabilitation is the primary course of intervention to restore G-H stability. However, if an operation is necessary, a procedure such as a capsulorraphy is performed to tighten the *I*nferior capsule and the rotator *I*nterval).[219]

Pharmacological—The use of medications for G-H instability varies according to severity, but may include NSAIDs and medications for pain relief.

Physical therapy—Intervention goals for G-H instability are to restore dynamic stability and control to the shoulder using the dynamic scapular and G-H stabilizers to contain the humeral head within the glenoid, and to correct any scapular dyskinesis.[215,220-223]

Differential Diagnosis

The differential diagnosis for G-H instability include, but is not limited to, dead arm syndrome, rotator cuff tear, subacromial impingement, internal impingement, and biceps tendinopathy.

SUBACROMIAL IMPINGEMENT SYNDROME

Subacromial impingement syndrome (SIS) is a recurrent and troublesome condition closely related to rotator cuff (RC) disease.[224] The RC problems occur because of trauma, attrition, and the anatomical structure of the subacromial space.

Clinical Significance

In the presence of a normal RC, normal scapular pivoters, and no capsular contractures, the humeral head translates less than 3 mm superiorly during the midranges of active elevation, whereas at the end ranges, A-P and superoinferior translations of 4 to 10 mm do occur, all of which are coupled with specific motions of IR or ER.[221,225-232] An increase in superior translation with active elevation may result in encroachment of the coracoacromial arch.[225,233] This encroachment produces a compression of the suprahumeral structures against the anteroinferior aspect of the acromion and coracoacromial ligament. Repetitive compression of these structures, coupled with other predisposing factors, results in a condition called SIS.

Tests and Measures and Response

A number of physical therapy special tests exist to help confirm a diagnosis of SIS (see Special Tests of the Shoulder Complex)

Clinical Findings, Secondary Effects, or Complications

Both intrinsic and extrinsic factors have been implicated as etiologies of the impingement process, and a number of impingement types have evolved (Table 2–68).

The most common symptoms associated with SIS include:

- Age 40–60
- Painful arc (90°-120° with forward flexion or abduction)

TABLE 2-68 Classification of different shoulder impingement syndromes.

Based on the Stage of Pathology[29]	Based on Direction of Instability	Based on Progressive Microtrauma[30]
Stage I: Edema, hemorrhage (patient usually <25 years of age) Stage II: Tendinitis/bursitis and fibrosis (patient usually 25–40 years of age) Stage III: Bone spurs and tendon rupture (patient usually >40 years of age)	Unidirectional instability (anterior, posterior, or inferior) with or without impingement Multidirectional instability with or without impingement	*Group IA*: This group, typically found in the older population, encompasses those patients with pure and isolated impingement and no instability *Group IB*: This group, typically found in the older population, encompasses those patients with instability secondary to mechanical trauma *Group II*: Patients in this group, who are usually young (<35 year old) overhead athletes, demonstrate instability with impingement secondary to microtrauma that comes from overuse *Group III*: Patients in this group, who are also typically young overhead athletes, demonstrate atraumatic, generalized ligamentous laxity *Group IV*: Patients in this group are young (<35 year old) who have experienced a traumatic event, resulting in instability in the absence of impingement

- Anterior and lateral shoulder pain during arm elevation, but no pain radiating below the elbow
- Increased pain with overhead activities
- Weakness
- Positive impingement tests

Diagnostic Tests

A diagnosis of SIS can usually be made based on the patient history, physical examination, radiographs (A-P view, outlet Y view, and axillary view), and MRI.

Interventions/Treatment

Medical—The extent of the medical intervention depends on the severity and can therefore range between conservative and surgical. The indications for a surgical repair are persistent pain that interferes with ADLs, work, or sports; patients who are unresponsive to a 4- to 6-month period of conservative care; or active young patients (younger than 50 years of age) with an acute full-thickness RC tear.[234]

Pharmacological—NSAIDs.

Physical therapy—Physical therapy typically involves a gradual progression of ROM, and strengthening exercises for the rotator cuff muscles and the scapular stabilizers.[235-238]

Differential Diagnosis

The differential diagnosis for SIS includes, but is not limited to, cervical spondylosis, rotator cuff tendinopathy, subluxing shoulder, A-C joint arthritis, adhesive capsulitis, G-H instability, or nerve compression.

ACROMIOCLAVICULAR JOINT INJURIES

An A-C joint injury, commonly referred to as a shoulder separation, can be caused by direct trauma or overuse.

Clinical Significance

A-C joint injuries typically occur in active or athletic young individuals. The clinical significance of the injury depends on the severity (see Clinical Findings, Secondary Effects, or Complications).

Tests and Measures and Response

The A-C shear test may or may not provide useful information.

Clinical Findings, Secondary Effects, or Complications

Six types of A-C injury have been categorized based on the direction and amount of displacement (Table 2–69).[31,32,239,240]

- Types I, II, III, and V all involve inferior displacement of the acromion with respect to the clavicle. They differ in the severity of injury to the ligaments and the amount of resultant displacement.[242]
- Types I and II usually result from a fall or a blow to the point on the lateral aspect of the shoulder, or a FOOSH, producing a sprain.
- Types III and IV usually involve a dislocation (commonly called A-C separations) and a distal clavicle fracture, both of which commonly disrupt the coracoclavicular ligaments.[30] In addition, damage to the deltoid and trapezius fascia, and rarely the skin, can occur.[30] Type V injuries are characterized by posterior displacement of the clavicle.
- Type VI injuries have a clavicle inferiorly displaced into either a subacromial or subcoracoid position. These types (IV, V, VI) also have complete rupture of all the ligament complexes and are much rarer injuries than types I through III.[30]

Diagnostic Tests

Typically, an A-C joint injury is diagnosed radiographically.

Interventions/Treatment

The intervention for A-C joint injuries has long been the subject of debate.

Medical—Types I and II injuries are typically treated nonoperatively. Types IV, V, and VI generally require surgical repair. However, no real consensus exists regarding the optimal management of acute type III injuries.

Pharmacological—Medications may be prescribed for pain relief.

TABLE 2–69 Classification of A-C injuries and clinical findings.[31,32,241]

Type I	Isolated sprain of A-C ligaments
	Coracoclavicular ligaments intact
	Deltoid and trapezoid muscles intact
	Tenderness and mild pain at A-C joint
	High (160°–180°) painful arc
	Resisted adduction is often painful
	Intervention is with TFM, ice, and pain-free AROM
Type II	A-C ligament is disrupted
	Sprain of coracoclavicular ligament
	A-C joint is wider; may be a slight vertical separation when compared to the normal shoulder
	Coracoclavicular interspace may be slightly increased
	Deltoid and trapezoid muscles intact
	Moderate to severe local pain
	Tenderness in coracoclavicular space
	PROM all painful at end range, with horizontal adduction being the most painful
	Resisted abduction and abduction are often painful
	Intervention initiated with ice and pain-free AROM/PROM; TFM introduced on day 4
Type III	A-C ligament is disrupted
	A-C joint dislocated and the shoulder complex displaced inferiorly
	Coracoclavicular interspace 25%–100% greater than normal shoulder
	Coracoclavicular ligament is disrupted
	Deltoid and trapezoid muscles are usually detached from the distal end of the clavicle
	A fracture of the clavicle is usually present in patients under 13 years of age
	Arm held by patient in adducted position
	Obvious gap visible between acromion and clavicle
	AROM all painful; PROM painless if done carefully
	Piano key phenomenon (clavicle springs back after being pushed caudally) present
Type IV	A-C ligament is disrupted
	A-C joint dislocated and the clavicle anatomically displaced posteriorly into or through the trapezius muscle
	Coracoclavicular ligaments completely disrupted
	Coracoclavicular interspace may be displaced but may appear normal
	Deltoid and trapezoid muscles are detached from the distal end of the clavicle
	Clavicle displaced posteriorly; surgery indicated for types IV–VI
Type V	A-C ligaments disrupted
	Coracoclavicular ligaments completely disrupted
	A-C joint dislocated and gross disparity between the clavicle and the scapula (300%–500% greater than normal)
	Deltoid and trapezoid muscles are detached from the distal end of the clavicle
	Tenderness over entire lateral half of the clavicle
Type VI	A-C ligaments disrupted
	Coracoclavicular ligaments completely disrupted
	A-C joint dislocated and the clavicle anatomically displaced inferiorly to the clavicle or the coracoid process
	Coracoclavicular interspace reversed with the clavicle being inferior to the acromion or the coracoid process
	Deltoid and trapezoid muscles are detached from the distal end of the clavicle
	Cranial aspect of shoulder is flatter than opposite side; often accompanied with clavicle or upper rib fracture and/or brachial plexus injury

A-C, acromioclavicular; AROM, active range of motion; PROM, passive range of motion; TFM, transverse friction massage.

TABLE 2-70 Physical therapy intervention for A-C joint injuries.

Injury Type	Intervention
Type I	Does not require immobilization
	Ice is recommended for pain
	If return to sport involves contact or impact forces, a donut pad placed over the shoulder helps to protect the joint
Type II	Patients are typically prescribed a sling as desired
	ROM exercises are initiated as tolerated, often beginning with PROM to minimize muscle activation of the trapezius and deltoid; however, because the deltoid and trapezius fibers reinforce the AC joint capsule, specific strengthening exercises for these muscles are part of the long-term rehabilitation program
	Return to function usually occurs within 2–3 weeks after injury
Type III	The most appropriate intervention is somewhat controversial and can be either surgical or conservative
	The most commonly used device for reduction is the Kenny–Howard harness

Physical therapy—Physical therapy intervention usually only occurs in types I to III (Table 2–70).

Differential Diagnosis

The differential diagnosis for A-C joint injuries includes clavicle fractures, superior labral lesions, rotator cuff injury, shoulder dislocation, neoplasm, and shoulder impingement.

ADHESIVE CAPSULITIS

Adhesive capsulitis, often termed *frozen shoulder*, is associated with female gender, age older than 40 years, post-trauma, diabetes, prolonged immobilization, thyroid disease, post-stroke or myocardial infarction, certain psychiatric conditions, and the presence of certain autoimmune diseases.[243]

Tests and Measures and Response

The six ROM measurements that should be taken include flexion, external rotation at the side, external rotation in abduction, internal rotation in abduction, horizontal abduction, and functional internal rotation up the back.

Clinical Findings, Secondary Effects, or Complications

The three classic stages of adhesive capsulitis include:[244]

- The early painful stage (freezing). Lasts 2 to 9 months. Patients have diffuse pain, difficulty with sleeping on the affected side, and restricted movement secondary to pain.
- The stiffening stage (freezing). Lasts 4 to 12 months. Characterized by progressive loss of ROM and decreased function.
- Recovery stage (thawing). Lasts 5 to 24 months. Characterized by gradual increases in ROM and decreased pain.

Diagnostic Tests

Adhesive capsulitis is diagnosed primarily by physical examination—patients demonstrate limited active and passive ROM with a capsular pattern of restriction. The capsular pattern of the shoulder is a motion restriction of external rotation > abduction > internal rotation, often noted in frozen shoulders. The reverse capsular pattern of the shoulder is internal rotation > elevation (abduction/flexion), often noted in impingement syndrome.

Interventions/Treatment

Medical—Nash and Hazelman[245] have described the concept of primary and secondary frozen shoulder:

- Primary: Idiopathic in origin and insidious onset.
- Secondary: Either traumatic in origin, or related to a disease process or neurological or cardiac condition.

Surgical intervention (manipulation) is reserved for those patients that do not respond to conservative intervention.

Pharmacological—Most patients with adhesive capsulitis are prescribed NSAIDs, or oral glucocorticoids in cases of severe refractory conditions.

Physical therapy—The primary goal of physical therapy is restoration of ROM, and focuses on the application of controlled tensile stresses using stretching and joint mobilizations to produce elongation of the restricting tissues.

- The patient with capsular restriction and low irritability may require aggressive soft tissue and joint mobilization.
- The patient with high irritability may require pain-easing manual therapy techniques.
- Treatment for the patient with limited ROM due to nonstructural changes is aimed at addressing the cause of the pain.

Differential Diagnosis

The differential diagnosis for adhesive capsulitis includes, but is not limited to, G-H OA, A-C joint dysfunction, rotator cuff tendinopathy or tear (with or without impingement), biceps tendinopathy, autoimmune diseases (eg, SLE, RA), neoplasm, cervical disk degeneration, and subacromial and subdeltoid bursitis.

LATERAL EPICONDYLOSIS (TENNIS ELBOW)

While the terms *epicondylitis* and *tendinopathy* have been commonly used to describe tennis elbow and golfer's elbow, histopathologic studies have demonstrated that these conditions are often not inflammatory conditions; rather, they are degenerative conditions. Therefore, epicondylosis or angioblastic tendinosis, better describe the condition. Lateral epicondylosis represents a pathological condition of the tendons of the muscles that control wrist extension and radial deviation, resulting in pain on the lateral side of the elbow. This pain is aggravated with movements of the wrist, by palpation of the lateral side of the elbow, or by contraction of the extensor muscles of the wrist.

Clinical Significance

Two types of epicondylosis are commonly described: lateral epicondylosis (tennis elbow) and medial epicondylosis (golfer's elbow). Lateral epicondylosis is far more common than medial epicondylosis, with an annual prevalence of 1% to 2% in the general public.[246] Lateral epicondylosis is usually the result of overuse, but can be traumatic in origin. Individuals who perform repetitive wrist extension against resistance are particularly at risk, for example, participants of tennis, baseball, javelin, golf, squash, racquetball, swimming, and weightlifting.

Tests and Measures and Response

A number of physical therapy special tests have been designed to help confirm a diagnosis of lateral epicondylosis (see Special Tests of the Elbow Complex).

Clinical Findings, Secondary Effects, or Complications

A thorough but focused history and physical examination are critical to a timely and accurate diagnosis. Pain is the primary symptom of lateral epicondylosis.[247] The pain is often activity-related. Diffuse achiness and morning stiffness are also common complaints. Occasionally the pain is experienced at night and the patient may report frequent dropping of objects, especially if they are carried with the palm facing down. Tenderness is usually found over the ECRB and ECRL, especially at the lateral epicondyle. The site of maximum tenderness is most commonly over the anterior aspect of the lateral epicondyle.

Diagnostic Tests

In the vast majority of cases, a diagnosis of lateral epicondylosis can be made on the strength of the patient history and physical examination.

Interventions/Treatment

Medical—Lateral epicondylosis is a self-limiting complaint; without intervention, the symptoms will usually resolve within 8 to 12 months.[248] Surgery is indicated if the symptoms do not resolve despite properly performed nonoperative treatments lasting 6 months.

Pharmacological—NSAIDs.

Physical therapy—To date, there is no consensus on the optimal treatment approach for lateral epicondylosis, which is in large part due to its unclear underlying etiology.[249] Poor technique, particularly with racket sports, is the cause of many elbow problems. Emphasis should be placed on recruiting the whole of the shoulder and trunk when hitting the ball so as to dissipate the forces as widely as possible. In addition to correcting poor technique, patient education should address racket size, grip size, and string tension.

An exercise regimen consisting of progressive resistance exercise to the wrist extensors, with the elbow flexed to 90° and also with the elbow straight is recommended.[250] This should be performed as a ten-repetition maximum, morning and night. Gradually the weight must be increased so that the ten-repetition maximum is always maintained. Contrary to popular belief, tennis elbow braces have been shown to have little effect in vibrational dampening.[251]

Differential Diagnosis

The differential diagnosis for lateral epicondylosis includes, but is not limited to, posterior interosseous nerve syndrome (PINS), radial tunnel syndrome, OA of the elbow, cervical radiculopathy, cervical spondylosis, fibromyalgia, and fracture.

MEDIAL EPICONDYLOSIS (GOLFER'S ELBOW)

Medial epicondylosis is only one-third as common as lateral epicondylosis, and primarily involves a tendinopathy of the common flexor origin, specifically the flexor carpi radialis, and the humeral head of the pronator teres.[252] To a lesser extent, the palmaris longus, flexor carpi ulnaris, and FDS may also be involved.[253]

Clinical Significance

The mechanism for medial epicondylosis is not usually related to direct trauma, but rather to overuse. This commonly occurs for three reasons:

- The flexor-pronator tissues fatigue in response to repeated stress.
- There is a sudden change in the level of stress that predisposes the elbow to medial ligamentous injury.[254]
- The ulnar collateral ligament fails to stabilize the valgus forces sufficiently.[255]

Chronic symptoms result from a loss of extensibility of the tissues, leaving the tendon unable to attenuate tensile loads.

Tests and Measures and Response

See Special Tests of the Elbow Complex.

Clinical Findings, Secondary Effects, or Complications

The typical clinical presentation for medial epicondylosis is pain and tenderness over the flexor-pronator origin, slightly distal and anterior to the medial epicondyle, in an aggressive advanced-level athlete. The symptoms are typically exacerbated with either resisted wrist flexion and pronation or passive wrist extension and supination.

Diagnostic Tests

In the vast majority of cases, a diagnosis of lateral epicondylosis can be made on the strength of the patient history and physical examination.

Interventions/Treatment

Medical—A self-limiting complaint; within 8 to 12 months.[248] Surgery is indicated if the symptoms do not resolve despite properly performed nonoperative treatments lasting 6 months.

Pharmacological—NSAIDs.

Physical therapy—The physical therapy intervention for this condition initially involves rest, activity modification, and local modalities. Once the acute phase has passed, the focus is to restore the ROM, and correct imbalances of flexibility and strength. The strengthening program is progressed to include concentric and eccentric exercises of the flexor pronator muscles. Splinting or the use of a counterforce brace may be a useful adjunct.

Differential Diagnosis

The differential diagnosis for medial epicondylosis includes, but is not limited to, cervical radiculopathy, Little League elbow, and an ulnar collateral ligament injury.

LITTLE LEAGUE ELBOW

Little League elbow is a common term for an avulsion lesion to the medial apophysis.

Clinical Significance

Repetitive throwing results in muscular and bony hypertrophic changes about the elbow, and can also result in ligament damage. This has been reflected by an increase in the number of medial ulnar collateral ligament reconstruction ("Tommy John") procedures being performed on injured throwers.[256] The repetitive motions involved in the various phases of throwing place enormous valgus strains on the immature elbow, particularly during the late cocking and acceleration phases, which can result in inflammation, scar formation, loose bodies, ligament sprains or ruptures, and the more serious conditions of osteochondritis, or an avulsion fracture.

Tests and Measures and Response

Complaints of medial elbow pain in an adolescent-aged pitcher (typically aged between 9 to 14), that occurs with throwing and worsens when they throw more innings.

Clinical Findings, Secondary Effects, or Complications

Little League elbow may start insidiously or suddenly. Usually, a sudden onset of pain is secondary to fracture at the site of the lesion. Clinical findings include a history of pain on the medial side of the elbow, with and without throwing. Physical findings relate to the specific lesion, but are commonly a persistent elbow discomfort or stiffness due to aggravation by the injury. A locking or "catching" sensation indicates a loose body.

Diagnostic Tests

Radiographs: An MRI may be required for a closer examination of the growth plates and to evaluate for ligament injury when the radiographic findings are unclear.

Interventions/Treatment

Medical—In the vast majority of cases, a conservative approach is recommended, which typically includes a period of complete rest from throwing for a minimum of 4 to 6 weeks. Surgical intervention is reserved for those patients with symptoms of a loose body, osteochondritis, or who fail to respond to conservative therapy.

Pharmacological—NSAIDs.

Physical therapy—Physical therapy management involves rest and elimination of the offending activity for 3 to 6 weeks. If osteochondritis dissecans is present, the joint needs protection for several months. The patient cannot return to pitching until full and normal motion has returned. To prevent elbow disorders, young athletes should adhere to the rules of Little League, which limit the number of pitches per game, per week, and per season, and the number of days of rest between pitching. The pitch count is the most important of these statistics.

Differential Diagnosis

The differential diagnosis for Little League elbow can include, but is not limited to, ulnar neuritis, C8–T1 radiculopathy (although rare in children), and medial epicondyle fracture.

CARPAL TUNNEL SYNDROME

Carpal tunnel syndrome (CTS) results from entrapment of the median nerve in the relatively unyielding space of the carpal tunnel, which may result in numbness, pain, or paresthesia of the thumb, index, and middle fingers. Compression of the nerve in the carpal tunnel is compounded by an increase in synovial fluid pressure and tendon tension, which decreases the available volume.

Clinical Significance

CTS results from an ischemic compression of the median nerve at the wrist as it passes through the carpal tunnel. CTS more commonly occurs between the fourth and sixth decades. CTS is the most common compression neuropathy, with a prevalence of 9.2% in women and 0.6% of men.[257,258] The compression of the median nerve may result from a wide variety of factors, several of which can easily be remembered using the pneumonic PRAGMATIC:

- **P**regnancy secondary to fluid retention.
- **R**enal dysfunction.
- **A**cromegaly.
- **G**out and pseudogout.
- **M**yxedema or mass.
- **A**myotrophy. Neuralgic amyotrophy is the most likely diagnosis in patients who suddenly develop arm pain followed within a few days by arm paralysis in the distribution of single or multiple nerves or extending over multiple myotomes.
- **T**rauma (repetitive or direct). About half of the cases of CTS are related to repetitive and cumulative trauma in the workplace, making it the occupational epidemic syndrome of our time.

- **I**nfection.
- **C**ollagen disorders. The incidence of carpal tunnel syndrome in patients with polyarthritis is high.

Other causes include rheumatoid arthritis, diabetes, hypothyroidism, and hemodialysis. Less common causes include incursion of the lumbrical muscles within the tunnel during finger movements, and hypertrophy of the lumbricales, lunate laxity or malposition.

Tests and Measures and Response

Physical therapy special tests include Phalen test and Tinel sign; the upper limb tension test (ULTT) for the median nerve,[259-262] which examines the effect of upper extremity position on median nerve tension, has been found to be specific.

Clinical Findings, Secondary Effects, or Complications

The physical assessment focuses on an examination of the motor and sensory functions of the hand as compared to the uninvolved hand.

Diagnostic Tests

The diagnosis of CTS is most reliably made by an experienced clinician after a review of the patient's history and a physical examination.[263] The clinical features of this syndrome include intermittent pain and paresthesias in the median nerve distribution of the hand, which can become persistent as the condition progresses.[259,264-266] The symptoms are typically worse at night, exacerbated by strenuous wrist movements, and can be associated with morning stiffness. The pain may radiate proximally into the forearm and arm.

Muscle weakness and paralysis can occasionally occur, including the thenar muscle group hand branches:

- Recurrent branch: Thenar muscles
- Palmar digital branch:
  - Motor to lateral 2 lumbrical muscles (flex MCP index and middle fingers)
  - Sensory to palmar surface fingertips of lateral 31/2 digits

Interventions/Treatment

Medical—These include the median nerve conduction study (NCS) and electromyography (EMG) study.[267] However, radiculopathy due to disease of the cervical spine, diffuse peripheral neuropathy, or proximal median neuropathy can pose clinical questions that electrodiagnostic testing can settle.[259] A carpal tunnel view radiograph may be the only view that shows abnormalities within the carpal tunnel.[268] Evaluation for surgical management is necessary for patients with atrophy of the thenar muscles, decreased sensation, and persistent symptoms that are intolerable despite conservative therapy.[269]

Pharmacological—NSAIDs and/or diuretics.[270]

Physical therapy—The conservative intervention for mild cases typically includes the use of splints, activity and ergonomic modification, and isolated tendon excursion exercises. Patient education

is also important to avoid sustained pinching or gripping, repetitive wrist motions, and sustained positions of full wrist flexion.

Differential Diagnosis

Cervical dysfunction,[271,272] thoracic outlet syndrome, pronator syndrome,[273] coronary artery ischemia, tendinopathy, fibrositis, and wrist joint arthritis.[274,275]

DEQUERVAIN'S DISEASE

De Quervain's disease is a progressive stenosing tenosynovitis, which affects the tendon sheaths of the first dorsal compartment of the wrist, resulting in a thickening of the extensor retinaculum, a narrowing of the fibroosseous canal, and an eventual entrapment and compression of the tendons, especially during radial deviation.[276]

Clinical Significance

Overuse, repetitive tasks that involve overexertion of the thumb or radial and ulnar deviation of the wrist, and arthritis are the most common predisposing factors, as they cause the greatest stresses on the structures of the first dorsal compartment.[277,278] Such activities include golfing, fly-fishing, typing, sewing, knitting, and cutting.

Tests and Measures and Response

The Finklestein test is commonly used to help confirm the diagnosis (see Special Tests of the Wrist and Hand).

Clinical Findings, Secondary Effects, or Complications

Frequently, patients report a gradual and insidious onset of a dull ache over the radial aspect of the wrist made worse by turning doorknobs or keys. Examination of the wrist may reveal:

- A localized swelling and tenderness in the region of the radial styloid process and wrist pain radiating proximally into the forearm and distally into the thumb.
- Severe pain with wrist ulnar deviation and thumb flexion and adduction. A reproduction of the pain can also be reported with thumb extension and abduction.
- Crepitus of the tendons moving through the extensor sheath.
- Palpable thickening of the extensor sheath and of the tendons distal to the extensor tunnel.
- A loss of abduction of the CMC joint of the thumb.

Diagnostic Tests

De Quervain's tenosynovitis is diagnosed based on the typical appearance, location of pain, and tenderness of the involved wrist.

Interventions/Treatment

Medical—Although the diagnosis is mostly clinical, posterior-anterior and lateral radiographs of the wrist can be obtained to rule out any bony pathology, such as a scaphoid fracture, radioscaphoid, or triscaphoid arthritis, and Kienböck's disease. If a conservative approach does not give relief, surgical tendon sheath release is an option.

Pharmacological—NSAIDs and possibly cortisone injections.

Physical therapy—Physical therapy includes rest, continuous immobilization through splinting with a thumb spica for 3 weeks, and anti-inflammatory medication. Following removal of the splint, ROM exercises are prescribed, with a gradual progression to strengthening.

Differential Diagnosis

The differential diagnosis includes, but is not limited to, OA at the radioscaphoid joint, cervical disk disease/radiculopathy, posterior ganglion at the wrist, Kienböck's disease (osteonecrosis of the lunate), CTS, scaphoid fracture, and OA at the first CMC joint.

DUPUYTREN'S CONTRACTURE

Dupuytren's contracture is a fibrotic condition of the palmar aponeurosis that results in nodule formation in the palmar and digital fascia or scarring of the aponeurosis, and which may ultimately cause finger flexion contractures.

Clinical Significance

The nodules that are associated with this condition occur in specific locations along longitudinal tension lines.[279,280] The appearance of the nodules is followed by the formation of tendon-like cords, which are due to the pathologic change in normal fascia.[281-283] The contractures form at the MCP joint, the PIP joint, and occasionally the DIP joint.[284]

Tests and Measures and Response

The tabletop test can be used to help confirm the diagnosis (see Special Tests of the Wrist and Hand).

Clinical Findings, Secondary Effects, or Complications

The diagnosis of Dupuytren's disease in its early stages may be difficult, and is based on the palpable nodule, characteristic skin changes, changes in the fascia, and progressive joint contracture. The skin changes are caused by a retraction of the skin, resulting in dimples or pits. The disease is usually bilateral, with one hand being more severely involved. However, there appears to be no association with hand dominance. The patient may have one, two, or three rays involved in the more severely affected hand. The most commonly involved digit is the ring finger, which is involved in approximately 70% of patients.

Diagnostic Tests

In most cases, the diagnosis can be made from the physical examination. Other tests are rarely necessary.

Interventions/Treatment

Medical—Needling has been used to break down the tissue cords, although the cords often reappear. Enzyme injections have also been used to help soften the fascia. However, these somewhat conservative interventions have not yet proven to be clinically useful or of any long-term value in the treatment of established contractures. Surgery is the intervention of choice when the MCP joint contracts to 30° and the deformity becomes a functional problem.[285]

Pharmacological—Medications are not typically prescribed for this condition.

Physical therapy—Scar management and splinting are important parts of postoperative management. Active, active-assisted, and passive exercises are usually initiated at the first treatment session.

Differential Diagnosis

The differential diagnosis includes, but is not limited to, fibroma, lipoma, neurofibroma, scarring, diabetic cheiropathy, ganglion cyst, and ulnar nerve palsy.

ACETABULAR LABRAL TEAR

Mechanical impingement and/or instability of the femoroacetabular joint are believed to be common causes of labral chondral pathology. Direct trauma, sporting activities, and certain movements of the hip, including torsional or twisting movements, have been cited to cause labral tears.[286]

Clinical Significance

Labral tears of the hip are more common than previously thought. In patients with mechanical hip pain, the prevalence of labral tears has been reported to be as high as 90%.[287-289] However, a large percentage of labral tears are not associated with any known specific event or cause, and may occur insidiously.[290] Two common types of scenarios have been recognized:

1. A young person with a twisting injury to the hip, usually an external rotation force in a hyperextended position.
2. An older person with a history of hip and/or acetabular dysplasia, or the result of repeated pivoting and twisting.

Tests and Measures and Response

On examination, ROM of the hip may or may not be limited, but in those cases where it is not limited, there may be pain at the extremes.[291] There is little information regarding the sensitivity, specificity, or likelihood ratios associated with a single clinical test or a cluster of tests in diagnosing a labral tear.[292] Generally speaking, the combined movement of flexion and rotation causes pain in the groin.

Diagnostic Tests

Diagnosis can often be made on the basis of the history and physical examination, although the diagnosis is often delayed or the condition is often misdiagnosed due to the fact that labral tears can have a variety of clinical presentations associated with a wide degree of clinical findings.[291,293] Labral tears can be classified according to location, etiology, and type:[294]

- *Location.* Tears can be anterior, posterior, or superior (lateral), although anterior and anterosuperior tears appear to be the most common, with anterior tears being common in patients with a degenerative hip disease or acetabular dysplasia.
- *Etiology.* Tears can be degenerative, dysplastic, traumatic, or idiopathic.
- *Type.* Labral tears have been classified into four types: radial flap (the most common type), radial fibrillated, longitudinal peripheral (least common), and abnormally mobile.[292] All labral tears are associated with increased microvascularity within the substance of the labrum at the base of the tear adjacent to the labrum's attachment to bone. Osteophyte formation is also sometimes seen in labral tears.

Interventions/Treatment

Medical—Conservative intervention has traditionally included bed rest with or without traction, followed by a period of protected weight-bearing. Operative treatment consists of arthrotomy or arthroscopy with resection of the entire labrum or the portion of the labrum that is torn.

Pharmacological—Medications typically include NSAIDs.

Physical therapy—The appropriate physical therapy intervention for a patient with an acetabular labral tear has yet to be established.[286] A common approach, based on clinical findings, typically includes progressive resisted strengthening and closed-chain exercises with emphasis on hip and lumbopelvic stabilization, correction of hip muscular imbalance, and biomechanical control.[295]

Differential Diagnosis

The differential diagnosis of hip/groin pain is broad, including both intra-articular and extra-articular pathology, and varies by age.

ILIOTIBIAL BAND FRICTION SYNDROME

As its name suggests, iliotibial band friction syndrome (ITBFS) is a repetitive stress injury, common in runners and cyclists, caused by friction of the ITB as it slides over the prominent lateral femoral epicondyle at approximately 30° of knee flexion. The friction has been found to occur at the posterior edge of the band, which is felt to be tighter against the lateral femoral condyle than the anterior fibers.

Clinical Significance

ITB syndrome can cause significant morbidity and lead to cessation of exercise. At the hip, an ITB contracture can lead to gluteal tendinopathy by increasing compression and friction of the subgluteus maximus bursa between the ITB and the greater trochanter.[296] Several studies have suggested that pelvic and trunk motion in the coronal plane will be increased in this population, and given the potential for proximal compensations, pelvic and trunk motion should be assessed for abnormal movements during the dynamic examination of this group of patients.[297]

Tests and Measures and Response

The classic test for ITB contracture is the Ober test (see Special Tests of the Hip). Three commonly used physical therapy special tests for ITBFS include Noble's compression and the Renne (creak) test (see Special Tests of the Knee Complex).

Clinical Findings, Secondary Effects, or Complications

Subjectively, the patient reports pain with repetitive motions of the knee. The lateral knee pain is described as diffuse and hard to localize. Although walking on level surfaces does not generally reproduce symptoms, especially if a stiff-legged gait is used, climbing or descending stairs often aggravates the pain. Patients do not complain of pain during sprinting, squatting, or during such stop-and-go activities as tennis or racquetball. The progression of symptoms is often associated with changes in training surfaces, increased mileage, or training on crowned roads.

Objectively, there is localized tenderness to palpation at the lateral femoral condyle and/or Gerdy's tubercle on the anterior-lateral portion of the proximal tibia. The resisted tests are likely to be negative for pain. The special tests for the ITB (Ober's test, prone lying test, and retinacular test) should be positive for pain, crepitus, or both, especially at 30° of weight-bearing knee flexion. In addition to the finding of a tight ITB, a cavus foot (calcaneal varus) structure, leg length difference (with the syndrome developing on the shorter side), fatigue, internal tibial torsion (increased lateral retinaculum tension), an anatomically prominent lateral femoral epicondyle, and genu varum, have all been associated with ITB friction problems, although they have yet to be substantiated.

Diagnostic Tests

The diagnosis for ITBFS is usually based on the history and physical examination. An MRI may be ordered if another joint pathology is suspected or if surgery is being considered. The MRI will show a thickened ITB over the lateral femoral epicondyle in cases of ITBFS, and often detects a fluid collection deep to the ITB in the same region.

Interventions/Treatment

Medical—Surgical intervention, consisting of a resection of the posterior half of the ITB at the level that passes over the lateral femoral condyle, is reserved for the more recalcitrant cases.

Pharmacological—NSAIDs.

Physical therapy—Activity modification to reduce the irritating stress (decreasing mileage, changing the bike seat position, and changing the training surfaces), using new running shoes, heat or ice applications, strengthening of the hip abductors, and stretching of the ITB.

Differential Diagnosis

The differential diagnosis for ITBFS includes, but is not limited to, biceps femoris tendinopathy, LCL sprain, lateral meniscal tear, patellofemoral dysfunction, stress fracture, referred pain from the lumbar spine, or stress fracture.

ANTERIOR CRUCIATE LIGAMENT TEAR

When the outer aspect of the knee receives a direct blow that causes valgus stress, the MCL often is torn first, followed by the ACL, which becomes the second component of a sports-related ACL injury.[298] Approximately 49% of patients with sports-related ACL injuries have meniscal tears.[299]

Clinical Significance

Almost all ACL tears are complete midsubstance tears.[300,301] ACL injury factors have been divided into intrinsic and extrinsic factors:[302]

- Intrinsic factors include a narrow intercondylar notch, a weak ACL, generalized overall joint laxity, and lower extremity malalignment.
- Extrinsic factors include abnormal quadriceps and hamstring interactions, altered neuromuscular control, shoe-to-surface interface, the playing surface, and the athlete's playing style.

ACL injury rates are two to eight times higher in women than in men participating in the same sports.[302,303] Young athletes may sustain growth plate injuries (eg, avulsion fractures) rather than midsubstance tears because the epiphyseal cartilage in their growth plates is structurally weaker than their ligaments, collagen, or bones. Recent studies suggest that young athletes may sustain midsubstance tears similar to adult athletes.[304,305]

Symptomatic ACL deficiencies in young athletes' knee joints are subject to the same long-term detrimental effects that occur in adult athletes.[306] Young athletes also may be more predisposed to more long-term degenerative knee conditions as the result of more years of chronic rotary knee instabilities from ACL deficiencies.[307]

Tests and Measures and Response

Numerous physical therapy special tests exist to aid in the confirmation of an ACL tear (see Special Tests of the Knee Complex).

Clinical Findings, Secondary Effects, or Complications

All ACL tears (ie, sprains) are categorized as grade I, II, or III injuries. Ligament tears are classified according to the degree of injury, which ranges from overstretched ligament fibers (ie, partial or moderate tears) to ligament ruptures (ie, complete tears or disruptions). Patients commonly describe the sensation of their knee "popping" or "giving out" as the tibia subluxes anteriorly. Other signs and symptoms of ACL injuries include pain, immediate dysfunction, instability in the involved knee, and the inability to walk without assistance. In rare instances, when patients have isolated ACL injuries that do not involve related collateral or meniscal tears, local tenderness around the knee joint may be absent.[307] A classic sign of ACL injuries is acute hemarthrosis (ie, extravasation of blood into a joint or synovial cavity).[308] Atrophy of the quadriceps is an almost constant finding with patients who have a torn ACL.[309-313]

Diagnostic Tests

Thorough patient histories and physical examinations are essential for accurate diagnoses of ACL injuries. An arthrometer, such as a KT-1000, is a mechanical testing device for measuring anterior-posterior knee ligament instability. This noninvasive device assesses the amount of displacement between the femur and the tibia at a given force in millimeters. Although most patients who have a complete tear of the ACL have increased tibial translation on instrumented testing,[314] it is not known exactly how many of these patients will have "giving-way" of the knee or how many knees will have overt or latent damage of the cartilage within a few years.[315-317]

MRI scans are useful for diagnosing ACL injuries, although their use in discriminating between complete and partial ACL tears is limited.[304] Diagnostic MRI scans, however, can detect associated meniscal tears that routine radiographs cannot show.[304]

Interventions/Treatment

Medical—The primary healing potential of the ACL has been reported to be extremely poor in both clinical and experimental studies due to its minimal blood supply and the presence of joint fluid, both of which contribute to a reduced healing potential.[318] Patients with either partial (grades I and II) ACL tears (negative pivot shifts) or "isolated" ACL tears, who lead a less active lifestyle and participate in linear, nondeceleration activities, are considered to be candidates for conservative intervention.[319] However, to return to normal preinjury activity levels, patients must be thoroughly rehabilitated, and protective measures (eg, knee bracing and activity restrictions) must be taken to prevent further knee injuries. ACL reconstruction is one of the most commonly performed orthopedic surgeries in the United States. Surgical treatment of the torn ACL includes direct repair, repair with augmentation, and reconstruction with autographs or allografts (single-bundle or double-bundle). The clinical evidence for double-bundle ACL reconstruction is mounting but is still inconclusive.[320] Currently, arthroscopic reconstruction remains the treatment of choice.

Pharmacological—Analgesics both preoperatively and postoperatively.

Physical therapy—Numerous lower extremity rehabilitation protocols following injury or surgery have been reported in the literature.[321-335] Emphasis on regaining extension and closed-chain 0° to 45° strengthening exercises are consistent among most ACL rehab protocols. For the middle-aged and older athlete, physical therapy often is the treatment of choice unless the patient plans to participate in sports activities that expose the knees to vigorous twisting forces. Certain sports activities, however, must be avoided, especially those involving jumping, quick starts and stops, and abrupt lateral movements (eg, soccer, basketball). Identifying the nonoperative patient population who return to an active lifestyle (copers) and those who modify activity level (adapters) from surgical candidates (noncopers) should use an ACL screening examination.[336] The best criteria for this screening examination is an area of ongoing study. Current recommendations include the KOS-Sport, Global Knee Function Rating, hop tests, and Quadriceps Index.

Differential Diagnosis

The differential diagnosis of an ACL tear is dependent on the severity. For example, with a complete tear the differential diagnoses would include meniscal tear, patellar dislocation, MCL tear, PCL tear, or osteochondral fracture.

MENISCAL INJURIES

Meniscal injuries are a common sports-related problem and the most frequent injury to the knee joint. Such injuries are especially prevalent among competitive athletes, particularly those who play soccer, football, and basketball.

Clinical Significance

The outer 25% to 30% of the menisci is known to be vascular.[337] Tears in the vascular region are repairable as well as tears extending into the avascular midsubstance if vascularity is stimulated through abrasion of the perimeniscal synovium and/or implantation of a fibrin clot.[338-341] Next to an adequate blood supply, the most important factor influencing the prognosis of the meniscus repair is ACL stability.

Tests and Measures and Response

Common clinical findings include a twisting mechanism of injury, delayed effusion, and mechanical complaints such as catching or locking.[342] Numerous physical therapy special tests exist to aid in the confirmation of a meniscal injury (see Special Tests of the Knee Complex). The meniscal pathology composite score consisting of mechanical complaints, joint-line tenderness, pain with forced knee hyperextension, pain with maximum passive knee flexion, and pain or audible clinic with McMurray maneuver reports a positive predictive value of 92.3% when all five signs and symptoms are positive.[343]

Clinical Findings, Secondary Effects, or Complications

Meniscal tears can be classified into two types, traumatic and degenerative:

- Traumatic tears: Most commonly found in young, athletically active individuals, not necessarily associated with contact injuries; frequently associated with ACL tears, and less commonly with PCL tears. Vertical longitudinal tears are the most common; transverse or radial tears are also common. Injuries to the healthy meniscus are usually produced by a combination of compressive forces coupled with rotation of the flexed knee as it starts to move into extension. The final type and location of the tear is determined by the direction and magnitude of the force acting on the knee and the position of the knee when injured.
- Degenerative tears: Tend to occur in patients older than 40 years. No history of a traumatic event is present. These tears have minimal or no healing capacity, and horizontal cleavage tears, flap tears, and complex tears are most common.

The most common report following meniscal injury is one of joint-line pain. The patient may also report joint clicking or locking, and the knee giving way. Tests to evaluate the menisci are outlined in the Special Tests of the Knee section.

Severe damage, or loss or removal of the menisci frequently leads to joint instability and later accelerated DJD, resulting in further disability and joint replacement.

Diagnostic Tests

A torn meniscus can often be diagnosed based on the physical examination alone. An MRI is the best imaging study to detect and confirm a torn meniscus.

Interventions/Treatment

Medical—Depending on the type, size, and location of the tear, the initial approach is conservative. If the conservative approach fails, or there is repetitive locking of the knee, a surgical repair of the meniscus is typically recommended.

Pharmacological—Analgesics both preoperatively and postoperatively.

Physical therapy—The process of rehabilitation is based on the healing phases: an initial protection and joint activation phase, followed by a progressive joint loading and functional restoration phase, and finally an activity restoration phase. Patients may progress through the rehabilitation process at different rates, depending on individual characteristics, lesion features, and concomitant pathology.

Differential Diagnosis

The differential diagnosis for a meniscal tear includes, but is not limited to, ACL injury, ITBFS, lumbosacral radiculopathy, medial or lateral collateral ligament injury, medial synovial plica irritation, patellofemoral dysfunction, or pes anserine bursitis.

PATELLAR TENDINOPATHY

Patellar tendinitis (jumper's knee) and quadriceps tendinopathy are overuse conditions that are frequently associated with eccentric overloading during deceleration activities (repeated jumping and landing, downhill running, etc.). The high stresses placed upon these areas during closed kinetic chain functioning place them at high risk for overuse injuries.

Clinical Significance

Chronic tendinopathy.

Tests and Measures and Response

No specific physical therapy special tests exist to confirm a diagnosis.

Clinical Findings, Secondary Effects, or Complications

Patellar tendinopathy is one of many potential diagnoses for a patient presenting with anterior knee pain. Pain upon palpation near the patellar insertion is present in both patellar and quadriceps tendinopathy.

Diagnostic Tests

A comprehensive examination of the complete lower extremity is necessary to identify any relevant deficits at the hip, knee, and ankle/foot regions.

Interventions/Treatment

Medical—These are usually self-limiting conditions. Surgical intervention is only usually required if significant tendinosis develops, and is successful in the majority of patients.

Pharmacological—NSAIDs or analgesics, depending on the severity.

Physical therapy—Patellar tendinopathies typically respond well to rest, stretching, eccentric strengthening, bracing, and other conservative techniques.

A number of protocols have been advocated for the conservative intervention of patellar tendinopathy:

- Grade I lesions. Characterized by no undue functional impairment and pain only after the activity; addressed with adequate warmup before training and ice massage after.
- Grade II-III strains. Activity modification, localized heating of the area, a detailed flexibility assessment, and an evaluation of athletic techniques. In addition, a concentric-eccentric program for the anterior tibialis muscle is prescribed, which progresses into a purely eccentric program as the pain decreases.[344]

Differential Diagnosis

The differential diagnosis for patellar tendinopathy includes, but is not limited to, Osgood-Schlatter syndrome, infrapatellar bursitis, patellofemoral dysfunction, fat pad impingement, and Sinding-Larsen-Johansson syndrome.

PATELLOFEMORAL PAIN SYNDROME

Anterior knee pain, or patellofemoral pain syndrome (PFS), is characterized by pain in the vicinity of the patella, which is worsened by sitting and during activities that require knee flexion and forceful contraction of the quadriceps (eg, during squats, ascending/descending stairs). The pain, which is characteristically located behind the kneecap (ie, retropatellar), and/or along the borders of the patella at the attachment sites of the medial or lateral retinaculum, may worsen in intensity, duration, and rapidity of onset if the aggravating activity is performed repeatedly.

Clinical Significance

Although PFS can occur in anyone—particularly athletes—women who are not athletic appear to be more prone to this problem than men who are not athletic. The impairments resulting from patellofemoral dysfunction have been related to problems that cannot be improved by physical therapy and those that can. The former include anatomical variance (femoral trochlear dysplasia, patellar morphology and the amount of congruence of the patellofemoral joint, the natural positioning of the patella (alta/baja) joint, and gender (females are more predisposed).

Tests and Measures and Response

A number of physical therapy special tests exist to assess the mobility of the patella (see Special Tests of the Knee Complex).

Clinical Findings, Secondary Effects, or Complications

The usual physical findings are localized around the knee.

- Tenderness often is present along the facets of the patella. The facets are most accessible to palpation while the knee is fully extended and the quadriceps muscle is relaxed.
- Tenderness with palpation to medial or lateral retinaculum.
- An apprehension sign may be elicited by manually fixing the position of the patella against the femur and having the patient contract the ipsilateral quadriceps.
- Crepitus may be present, but if present in isolation, crepitus does not allow for definitive diagnosis.
- An alteration in the Q-angle.
- Movement analysis may demonstrate excessive foot pronation, excessive knee valgus, excessive hip internal rotation, an antalgic gait pattern, and excessive hip adduction and internal rotation with squatting, stairs, and landing from a jump.
- Repetitive squatting may reproduce knee pain.
- Genu recurvatum and hamstring weakness.

Diagnostic Tests

PFS is primarily a clinical diagnosis based on a thorough physical examination.

Interventions/Treatment

Medical—PFS is generally treated conservatively. Surgery may be considered for those patients in whom other causes of anterior knee pain have been excluded and whose symptoms persist despite completing at least 6 to 12 months of a thorough program of rehabilitation.

Pharmacological—The physician may prescribe analgesics, depending on the severity.

Physical therapy—The focus of physical therapy intervention is to find the cause of the PFS (eg, muscle imbalance, leg length discrepancy, or other structural problem). Ice, electrical stimulation, and biofeedback may be used. The basic exercise principles for management of PFS are:

- Restoration of muscle balance within the quadriceps group. Quadriceps strengthening traditionally is performed while the knee is flexed 0° to 30°. Controversy remains as to the extent that the individual muscle groups comprising the quadriceps can selectively be strengthened. Stretching of the quadriceps should be of long duration (20–30 seconds) and with low force. In addition, restoration of hip muscle balance should be addressed, with specific attention to the hip abductors and external rotators as well as the gluteus maximus.
- Improving flexibility, including exercises to stretch the ITB, hip, hamstring, and gastrocnemius. Manual stretching of the

lateral retinaculum may be used as a conservative approach, partially mimicking the effect of lateral retinacular release.
- Improving ROM.
- Restricting the offending physical activity.
- Home exercise programs that include both stretching and strengthening exercises.
- Patellar taping techniques (McConnell method) can be used to reduce the friction on the patella. If successful, the clinician can teach the patient self-taping techniques to use at home.
- Proper footwear also is important. The clinician can evaluate the patient's biomechanics and recommend proper shoes and/or orthotics.

Differential Diagnosis

The differential diagnosis for PFS includes, but is not limited to, pes anserine bursitis, prepatellar bursitis, quadriceps tendinopathy, referred pain from the lumbar spinal or hip joint, and saphenous neuritis.

ACHILLES TENDINOPATHY

Achilles tendinopathy is the most common overuse syndrome of the lower leg. Achilles tendinopathy typically occurs as one of two types:[345]

- Insertional: Involving the tendon-bone interface.
- Noninsertional: Occurs just proximal to the tendon insertion on the calcaneus in or around the tendon substance. Can be referred to as peritendinitis, peritendinitis with tendinosis, and tendinosis.[345,346]

Clinical Significance

Clinical symptoms of Achilles tendinitis consist of a gradual onset of pain and swelling in the Achilles tendon 2 to 3 cm proximal to the insertion of the tendon, which is exacerbated by activity. Some patients will present with pain and stiffness along the Achilles tendon when rising in the morning or pain at the start of activity that improves as the activity progresses.

Tests and Measures and Response

A number of tests and measures have been designed specifically to detect Achilles tendinopathy. These can include passive stretching of the tendon to elicit pain, having the patient perform a unilateral heel raise while asking patient to unilaterally hop on the affected side either in place or in a variety of directions. Additional findings include the arc sign and the Royal London Hospital test (see Special Tests of the Ankle and Foot).[143]

A number of factors appear to contribute to the development of Achilles tendinopathy:[347]

- Biomechanical factors: The rapid and repeated transitions from pronation to supination cause the Achilles tendon to undergo a "whipping" or "bowstring" action.[347] Moreover, if the foot remains in a pronated position after knee extension has begun, the external tibial rotation at the knee and the internal tibial rotation at the foot results in a "wringing" or twisting action of the tendon.[348]

- Training variables: A lack of a stretching programs, a faster training pace, and hill training have all been found to correlate with increased incidence.[347]
- Overtraining has been found to correlate to calf muscle fatigue and microtears of the tendon.[348,349]
- Muscular insufficiency has been cited as a significant factor in the inability to eccentrically restrain dorsiflexion during the beginning of the support phase of running.[347,350-352]
- The compensatory overpronation resulting from the inflexibility of the cavus foot is a precursor to Achilles tendinitis.
- Shoe type. Spike shoes lock the feet on the surface during the single support phase in running and increase the athlete's foot grip, but also transfer lateral and torque shear forces directly to the foot and ankle and through to the Achilles tendon.
- Sacroiliac joint dysfunction: Changes in sacroiliac joint mechanics as compared with the contralateral side.[353]

Clinical Findings, Secondary Effects, or Complications

Upon observation, the patient will often be found to have pronated feet, and the presence of swelling is common. Observation during gait may reveal an antalgic gait, with the involved leg held in external rotation during both stance and swing phase.

- Localization of the tenderness with palpation is extremely important.
- Tenderness that is located 2 to 6 cm proximal to the insertion is indicative of noninsertional tendinopathy.
- Pain at the bone-tendon junction is more indicative of insertional tendinopathy.
- If there is an area in the tendon itself that is discrete and painful with side-to-side pressure of the fingers, this often indicates an area of mucoid degeneration or a small partial rupture of the tendon.
- If the tenderness is in the area of the retrocalcaneal bursa, noted by side-to-side pressure in that area, this is the primary area of involvement.

A lack of normal dorsiflexion in knee extension signifies gastrocnemius adaptive shortening, and inability to perform a normal range of dorsiflexion in knee flexion implicates the soleus as well.

There is often pain with resisted testing of the gastrocnemius/soleus complex.

The intervention for Achilles tendonitis varies, with the recommended amount of rest depending on the severity of the symptoms:[354]

- Type I. Characterized by pain that is only experienced after activity. These patients should reduce their exercise by 25%.
- Type II. Characterized by pain that occurs both during and after activity but does not affect performance. These patients should reduce their training by 50%.
- Type III. Characterized by pain after activity but no effect on performance.

Diagnostic Tests

The diagnosis for Achilles tendinopathy is typically made through the description of symptoms and from an examination of the Achilles tendon. An ultrasound scan or MRI is used in cases where the diagnosis is not conclusive.

Interventions/Treatment

Medical—For most individuals, the symptoms of Achilles tendinopathy usually clear with 3 to 6 months of conservative treatment. In cases that do not respond to a conservative approach, surgery may become an option.

Pharmacological—Short-term analgesics are used to help relieve the pain. The use of corticosteroids in the treatment of Achilles tendinopathy has declined due to the adverse effects that these drugs can have on the structure of the tendon.

Physical therapy—The patient should temporarily discontinue any activity that seems to provoke the symptoms.

The intervention strategies for tendon injuries are outlined Intervention Principles for Musculoskeletal Injuries section.

Differential Diagnosis

The differential diagnosis of Achilles tendinopathy includes, but is not limited to, Achilles bursitis, OA, gastrocsoleus muscle strain or rupture, Haglund deformity, syndesmosis, nerve injury, or vascular insufficiency.

LATERAL ANKLE SPRAINS

In the neutral position or dorsiflexion, the ankle is stable because the widest part of the talus is in the mortise. However, in plantarflexion, ankle stability is decreased, as the narrow posterior portion of the talus is in the mortise. Thus, the most common mechanism of an ankle sprain is one of inversion and plantar flexion.

Clinical Significance

Ankle sprains are the most common injuries in sports and recreational activities, and if left untreated can lead to chronic instability and impairment. Most acute ankle injuries occur in people 21 to 30 years old, although injuries in the younger and older age groups tend to be more serious. Sprains of the lateral ligamentous complex represent 85% of ankle ligament sprains.[355,356] Lateral ligament sprains are more common than medial ligament sprains for two major reasons:[357]

- The lateral malleolus projects more distally than the medial malleolus, producing more bony obstruction to eversion than inversion.
- The deltoid ligament is much stronger than the lateral ligaments.

The high ankle sprain, or syndesmotic sprain, which involves disruption of the ligamentous structures between the distal fibula and tibia, just proximal to the ankle joint, occurs less frequently than the lateral ankle sprain.

Tests and Measures and Response

A number of physical therapy special tests exist to help in the diagnosis of a lateral ankle sprain (see Special Tests of the Ankle and Foot).

Clinical Findings, Secondary Effects, or Complications

Lateral ankle sprains can be graded according to severity:

- Grade I sprains are characterized by minimum to no swelling, no laxity, and localized tenderness over the ATFL. These sprains require on the average 11.7 days before full resumption of athletic activities.[358]
- Grade II sprains are characterized by localized swelling and laxity, and more diffuse lateral tenderness. These sprains require approximately 2 to 6 weeks for return to full athletic function.[359,360]
- Grade III sprains are characterized by significant swelling, laxity, pain, and ecchymosis and should be referred to a specialist.[361] Grade III injuries may require greater than 6 weeks to return to full function. For acute grade III ankle sprains, the average duration of disability has been reported anywhere from 4.5 to 26 weeks, and only 25% to 60% of patients are symptom-free 1 to 4 years after injury.[362]

Diagnostic Tests

No single symptom or test can provide a completely accurate diagnosis of a lateral ankle ligament rupture, but the collection of findings can be strongly indicative.[363]

- The absence of swelling at the time of the delayed (after 4 days) physical examination suggests that there is no ligament rupture, whereas extensive swelling at this time is indicative of ligament rupture.[364]
- Pain on palpation of the involved ligament suggests involvement.
- The presence of a hematoma suggests a rupture.
- Positive anterior drawer test suggests a rupture.
- Impairment of walking ability after injury suggests involvement.

According to the Ottawa rules for ankle x-rays (with Buffalo modifications),[365,366] x-rays are indicated to rule out fracture of the ankle when there is bone tenderness in the posterior half of the lower 6 cm of the fibula or tibia and an inability to bear weight immediately after injury.[365-367] Similarly, if there is bone tenderness over the navicular and/or fifth metatarsal and an inability to bear weight immediately after injury, then radiographs of the foot are indicated.

Interventions/Treatment

Medical—Conservative intervention has been found to be consistently effective in treating grades I and II ankle sprains.[368,369] For severe acute ankle sprains, surgical intervention may yield slightly better outcomes for function and instability compared with conservative treatment.[370]

Pharmacological—With the exception of NSAIDs, pharmacological intervention is typically not needed.

Physical therapy—Once pain and inflammation are under control (4–14 days), the patient begins dynamic balance and proprioceptive exercises, with or without an external support. Exercises that promote ankle dorsiflexion past the neutral position, enabling a closer to normal walking pattern, are introduced. Open-chain (non-weightbearing) progressive resistive exercises with rubber tubing resistance are performed (two sets of 30 reps each) for isolated plantarflexion, dorsiflexion, inversion, and eversion. Stationary cycling can also be performed (at a comfortable intensity for up to 30 minutes) to provide cardiovascular endurance training and controlled ankle ROM.[371] Plyometric activities are introduced during the return-to-activity phase.

Differential Diagnosis

The differential diagnosis from lateral ankle sprain includes, but is not limited to, fracture (distal fibula, ankle, and calcaneal) neurovascular compromise, Achilles tendon injuries, ankle impingement syndrome, gout and pseudogout, and stress fracture.

PLANTAR FASCIITIS

Plantar fasciitis is an inflammatory process of the plantar fascia and is reported to be the most common cause of inferior heel pain. The role of the heel spur in plantar fasciitis is controversial.

Clinical Significance

Plantar fasciitis, with or without heel spur, has been experienced by 10% of the population.[372-374] Plantar heel pain is usually unilateral, although in 15% to 30% of people, both feet are affected.[375] Although more common in active individuals, plantar heel pain can also affect the sedentary population, although the reasons for this remain elusive.

NOTE: The clinician should be suspicious of any insidious onset of bilateral plantar fasciitis (or Achilles tendonitis) due to the possibility of a systemic inflammatory condition.

Tests and Measures and Response

A number of special tests are available to help confirm the diagnosis of plantar fasciitis, of which the windlass test (see Special Tests of the Ankle and Foot) is considered the most reliable.

Clinical Findings, Secondary Effects, or Complications

Common findings include a history of pain and tenderness on the plantar medial aspect of the heel and/or plantar surface of foot, especially during initial weight-bearing in the morning. Interference with daily activities is common. Plantar fasciitis is usually unilateral, although both feet can be affected. The heel pain often decreases during the day but worsens with increased activity (such as jogging, climbing stairs, or going up on the toes) or after a period of sitting.

Upon physical examination, there will be localized pain on palpation along the medial edge of the fascia or at its origin on the anterior edge of the calcaneus, although firm finger pressure is often necessary to localize the point of maximum tenderness. The main area of tenderness is typically just over and distal to the medial calcaneal tubercle, and there is usually one small exquisitely painful area. Tenderness in the center of the posterior part of the heel may be due to bruising or atrophy of the heel pad or to subcalcaneal bursitis. Slight swelling in the area is common. To test for plantar fasciitis, the fascia needs to be put on stretch

with a bowstring type test/windlass stretch position. The patient's heel is manually fixed in eversion. The clinician takes hold of the first metatarsal and places it in dorsiflexion before extending the big toe as far as possible. Pain should be elicited at the medial tubercle.

Diagnostic Tests

The clinical diagnosis for plantar fasciitis is normally based on the patient history, evidence of risk factors (eg, pes cavus, excessive foot pronation, obesity, occupations involving prolonged standing/walking), and the physical examination. Imaging, in the form of plain radiography, is only ever used to rule out other heel pathology.

Interventions/Treatment

Medical—In the vast majority of cases, plantar fasciitis responds well to a conservative approach. However, in recalcitrant cases, plantar fascia release surgery may be required.

Pharmacological—NSAIDs.

Physical therapy—A number of physical therapy interventions have been suggested over the years for plantar fasciitis. These include:

- Night splinting
- Orthotics
- Taping
- Heel cups
- Stretching (gastrocnemius) and strengthening of the leg muscles and foot intrinsics
- Progressive loading of the plantar fascia[376]
- Deep frictional massage
- Dexamethasone iontophoresis
- Shoe modifications
- Casting
- Extracorporeal shock wave lithotripsy[377]

Differential Diagnosis

The differential diagnosis for plantar fasciitis includes, but is not limited to, any of the inflammatory spondyloarthropathies, calcaneal stress fracture, nerve entrapment, tumor, peripheral neuropathy, and bone infection.

CERVICOGENIC HEADACHES

A cervicogenic headache (CH) is defined as one that meets the following criteria:[378]

(1) pain localized to the neck and occipital region that may project to the forehead, orbital region, temples, vertex, or ears, (2) pain precipitated or aggravated by specific neck movements or sustained neck posture, and (3) resistance to or limitation of active or passive physiologic and accessory neck movements or abnormal tenderness of neck muscles, or both.

Clinical Significance

CHs are difficult to define and classify because of their variable distribution and character of symptoms.[379]

Tests and Measures and Response

Jull et al.[380] provided a cluster of examination findings to discern CHs from primary headaches. The combination of reduced cervical ROM, painful upper cervical segmental manual palpation, and reduced strength in the cervical cranioflexor muscles delineated people with CHs from those with primary headaches with 100% sensitivity and 90% specificity.[380]

Clinical Findings, Secondary Effects, or Complications

The patient with a CH usually reports a dull, aching pain of moderate intensity, which begins in the neck or occipital region and then spreads to include a greater part of the cranium.[381] CHs can emerge from a number of sources, including:[382]

- Irritation of the posterior (dorsal) root ganglia and nerve root components caused by compression of the C2 posterior (dorsal) root ganglia between the C1 posterior arch and the superior C2 articular process[383]
- Compression of the C2 anterior (ventral) ramus at the articular process of C1–2[384]
- Entrapment of the C2 posterior (dorsal) root ganglia by the C1–2 epistrophic ligament[385]

Diagnostic Tests

According to the International Headache Society (IHS), radiologic examination must reveal at least one of the following: (1) movement abnormalities during flexion–extension, (2) abnormal posture, or (3) fractures, bone tumors, RA, congenital abnormalities, or other distinct pathology other than spondylosis or osteochondrosis.[378]

Interventions/Treatment

Medical—The typical approach for a CH (once other causes have been ruled out) is conservative.

Pharmalogical—Analgesics may be prescribed.

Physical therapy—Several interventions have been recommended for CHs, including posture training, manual therapy, exercise, rest, and minor analgesics.[386] Manual therapy studies have demonstrated positive effects on both the impairment (pain and muscle function) and the disability level, with most studies focusing on short-term outcomes.[387,388] McKenzie[389] recommends a home program of cervical retraction exercises to decrease CH symptoms and maintain correct cervical alignment.

Differential Diagnosis

Neck pain can arise from injuries of the cervical muscles, ligaments, disks, and joints. From lower cervical segments, the pain may be referred to the shoulder and upper limb. From upper segments, neck pain may be referred to the head and manifested as a headache.[390] The clinician must differentiate between:

- Intracranial causes
- Headaches associated with viral or other infective illness
- Drug-induced headache or a headache related to alcohol or substance abuse
- Exercise-related (or exertion-related) headache syndrome
- Vascular, tension, or other causes of a headache

TEMPOROMANDIBULAR JOINT DYSFUNCTION (TMD)

Temporomandibular joint internal derangement is one of the most common forms of TMD and is associated with characteristic clinical findings such as pain, joint sounds, and irregular or deviating jaw function.[391,392] The term *internal derangement* when related to TMD denotes an abnormal positional relationship of the articular disk to the mandibular condyle and the articular eminence.[393] This abnormal positional relationship may result in mechanical interference and restriction of the normal range of mandibular activity.[394-396]

Clinical Significance

Approximately 50% to 75% of the general population has experienced unilateral TMD on a minimum of one occasion, and at least 33% have reported a minimum of one continuing persistent symptom.[397,398]

Tests and Measures and Response

The most common procedure used by physical therapists to detect a TMD is the TMJ screen (see Special Tests of the Cervical Spine and TMJ)

Clinical Findings, Secondary Effects, or Complications

Currently, clinical examination is the gold standard for diagnosing TMDs. Due to the close proximity, the cervical spine must be thoroughly examined in conjunction with the TMJ.

Diagnostic Tests

MRI is currently the most accurate imaging modality for identification of disk positions of the TMJ, and may be regarded as the gold standard for disk position identification purposes.[399]

Interventions/Treatment

Medical—There is lack of a consistent method for identifying and diagnosing TMD. Complicating matters is the fact that the majority of the symptoms associated with TMD are self-limiting and resolve without active intervention.[400]

Pharmacological—Medications may be prescribed for any psychosocial characteristics identified. Analgesics may be prescribed for pain management.

Physical therapy—The physical therapy intervention for this condition depends on the causative factors. Typically, the focus is on:[401]

- Pain management techniques.
- Postural education.
- Elimination of any occlusal disharmony.
- Joint mobilizations to the TMJ and/or subcranial spine.
- Psychological stress reduction. Biofeedback can help the patient recognize periods of stress.
- Habit training to develop a path of mandibular movement that avoids any interference.
- The reduction or elimination of parafunctional habits (cheek biting, nail biting, pencil chewing, teeth clenching or bruxism).
- A reduction in the force of chewing, while encouraging chewing on the affected side to decrease the interarticular pressure.
- Methods to prevent the disk-condyle complex from returning to the closed position. This can be accomplished by applying a permanent stabilization splint for a few months. When symptoms have been reduced, the patient should be weaned off the splint during the day, and eventually, night.

Differential Diagnosis

Differential diagnosis is based on the pain history in combination with the clinical findings of muscle spasm and occlusion in relation to any condylar displacement. Consideration must also be given to a cervical source of the symptoms, dental infections, trigeminal nerve neuralgia, and inner ear infections.

LUMBAR HERNIATED NUCLEUS PULPOSUS

IVD herniation in the lumbar spine may occur from adolescence into old age. Degenerative changes are the body's attempts at self-healing as the body ages. The water-retaining ability of the nucleus pulposus progressively declines with age, resulting in a decrease in the mechanical stiffness of the disk, allowing the annulus to bulge with a corresponding loss of disk and foramina height.

Clinical Significance

The clinical course of low back pain (LBP) can be described as acute, subacute, recurrent, or chronic. Disk deterioration and loss of disk height may shift the balance of weight-bearing to the facet joint. Nuclear material that is displaced into the spinal canal is associated with a significant inflammatory response—macrophages respond to this displaced foreign material and seek to clear the spinal canal. Compression of a motor nerve results in weakness, and compression of a sensory nerve results in numbness. Radicular pain results from inflammation of the nerve. Furthermore, degeneration may result in radial tears and leakage from the nuclear material, which is toxic to the nerves. The resultant inflammatory response causes neural irritation with radiating pain without numbness, weakness, or loss of reflex, as neural compression is absent.

Tests and Measures and Response

One of the best ways to detect lumbar disk pathology is to use the Cyriax scanning examination.

Clinical Findings, Secondary Effects, or Complications

The pertinent historical information begins with an analysis of the chief complaint:

- The provocation of radiating pain down the leg is the most sensitive test for a lumbar disk herniation, while assessing the pattern of pain regarding a dermatomal distribution or in assessing the organicity of the complaints.
- It is important to specifically exclude red flags, such as nonmechanical pain—pain at night unrelated to activity or movement, which may be indicative of a tumor or infection.

The physical examination is essentially a neurological assessment of weakness, dermatomal numbness, reflex change, or, most importantly in the lumbar spine, sciatic or femoral nerve root tension. For a higher lumbar lesion, reverse straight-leg raising or hip extension stretching the femoral nerve is analogous to a straight-leg raising sign.

Diagnostic Tests

Depending on the severity and complexity of the presenting symptoms, any of the following diagnostic test may be used: x-rays, MRI, computed tomography (CT) scan, electrodiagnostics, bone scan, discography.

Interventions/Treatment

Medical—The natural history of radiculopathy and disk herniation is not quite as favorable as for simple LBP, but it is still excellent, with approximately 50% of patients recovering in the first 2 weeks and 70% recovering in 6 weeks.[402] Surgery is often recommended after 4 to 6 weeks if the symptoms persist, following MRI and CT scan findings.[403] However, of those who opt for surgery, 10% to 40% will complain of pain, motor dysfunction, or reduced ADL performance after surgery.[404,405]

Pharmacological—Analgesics, NSAIDs, and cortisone injections.

Physical therapy—In cases of radiculopathy, the goal is to decrease radiating symptoms into the limb and thus centralize the pain by using specific maneuvers or positions, such as the lateral shift correction. Once this centralizing position is identified, the patient is instructed to perform these maneuvers repetitively or sustain certain positions for specific periods throughout the day.[406] In addition, the patient is instructed in a lumbar stabilization program, in which neutral zone mechanics are practiced in various positions to decrease stress to the lumbosacral spine.[404] It is theorized that these types of exercise may strengthen the stabilizer muscles, which control and limit the free movement of one vertebra on the other, thereby accelerating the recovery process of the herniated disk.

Differential Diagnosis

The differential diagnosis for a herniated lumbar disk includes, but is not limited to, acute aortic dissection, nephrolithiasis (kidney stone), osteomyelitis, mechanical back pain, rheumatoid arthritis, pelvic inflammatory disease, and cauda equina syndrome.

SPINAL STENOSIS (DEGENERATIVE)

Degenerative spinal stenosis (DSS) is defined as narrowing of the spinal canal, nerve root canal (lateral recess), or intervertebral foramina of the lumbar spine. It is predominantly a disorder of the elderly and is the most common diagnosis associated with lumbar spine surgery in patients older than 65 years.[407]

Clinical Significance

Spinal stenosis may be classified as central or lateral.[408]

Central stenosis is characterized by a narrowing of the spinal canal around the thecal sac containing the cauda equina in the lumbar spine or the spinal cord in the cervical and thoracic regions. The causes for this type of stenosis include facet joint arthrosis and hypertrophy, thickening and bulging of the ligamentum flavum, bulging of the IVD, osteophytes, instability/spondylolisthesis, or tumor/space-occupying lesion.

Lateral stenosis is characterized by encroachment of the spinal nerve in the lateral recess of the spinal canal or in the intervertebral foramen.[409] The causes for this type include facet joint hypertrophy, loss of IVD height, IVD bulging, or spondylolisthesis.[410] Compression of the nerve within the canal results in a limitation of the arterial supply or claudication due to the compression of the venous return. Compression of the foraminal contents in the canal may occur more with certain movements or changes in posture:[411]

- The length of the canal is shorter in lumbar lordosis than kyphosis.
- Extension and, to a lesser degree, side bending of the lumbar spine toward the involved side produces a narrowing of the canal.
- Flexion of the lumbar spine reverses the process, returning both the venous capacity and blood flow to the nerve.

Tests and Measures and Response

Two commonly used tests in physical therapy to help in the diagnosis of degenerative spinal stenosis are the combination of the bicycle test of van Gelderen and treadmill walking. Both cycling and walking increase symptoms in vascular claudication due to the increased demand for blood supply. However, the symptoms of neurogenic claudication worsen with walking but are unaffected by cycling if the patient leans forward (lumbar spine flexed), due to the differing positions of the lumbar spine adopted in each of these activities. Patients with neurogenic claudication are far more comfortable leaning forward or sitting, which flexes the spine more than walking.[412] The position of forward flexion increases the anteroposterior diameter of the intervertebral canal, which allows a greater volume of the neural elements and improves the microcirculation.

Clinical Findings, Secondary Effects, or Complications

Both the history and the examination findings for DSS are very specific.

Patients with lumbar spinal stenosis who are symptomatic often relate a long history of low back pain. Unilateral or bilateral leg pain is usually a predominant symptom. Approximately 65%

of patients with lumbar spinal stenosis will present with neurogenic claudication (also referred to as pseudoclaudication).[413] Subjectively, the patient reports an increase in symptoms with lumbar extension activities such as walking, prolonged standing, and to a lesser degree, side bending. On observation the patient presents with a flattened lumbar lordosis.

The physical examination usually reveals evidence of reduced flexibility or shortening of the hip flexors (iliopsoas and rectus femoris). The hip extensor muscles (gluteus maximus and hamstrings) are usually lengthened. This lengthening places them at a mechanical disadvantage, which leads to early recruitment of the lumbar extensor muscles and may lead to excessive lumbar extension.[414]

Patients with cervical or thoracic central stenosis can experience UMN signs and symptoms (see Table 2–66) due to compression of the spinal cord. Myelopathy, disease, or compression of the spinal cord, which is the most common in females greater than 45 years old, can be caused by stenosis, tumor, osteophytes, congenital narrowing of central canal, inflammatory process, tumor, encroachment of ligaments/membranes (ligamentum flavum, posterior longitudinal membranes, subcranial membranes), or instability. The signs and symptoms of myelopathy include bilateral or quadrilateral paresthesias in non-dermatomal pattern (glove/stocking distribution), weakness in non-myotomal pattern, ataxic gait, clumsiness, positive pathological reflexes (Babinski, Hoffman, inverted supinator test), hyperreflexia, changes in bowel and bladder, UMN signs and symptoms. A positive in three of the following is considered a high-positive likelihood ratio:[415]

- Gait deviation
- + Hoffman sign
- Inverted supinator sign
- + Babinski test
- Age >45

Diagnostic Tests

Radiographs or MRIs may be ordered to find the site and source of stenosis.

Interventions/Treatment

Medical—An initial conservative approach, including pain medication and physical therapy, is generally recommended for nerve root compression signs and symptoms. Failure to respond to a conservative approach is an indication for nerve root and sinuvertebral nerve infiltration.[416] Permanent relief in lateral recess stenosis has been reported with an injection of local anesthetic around the nerve root.[417] When nerve root infiltration fails, surgical decompression of the nerve root is indicated.

Pharmacological—Analgesics, NSAIDs, and cortisone injections may also be implemented to help control inflammation.

Physical therapy—An MD referral is the first line of treatment in cases of suspected myelopathy. Once evaluated and cleared for therapy, common interventions for cervical spinal stenosis include a therapeutic exercise progression including postural education, stretching of any tight musculature such as the pectorals and suboccipitals, and stabilization exercises targeting the deep neck flexors. For lumbar spine stenosis, the approach includes stretching of the hip flexors and rectus femoris, and stabilization exercises targeting the lumbar paraspinals, transverse abdominals, multifidii, and gluteals, aerobic conditioning, and positioning such as a posterior pelvic tilt.[418-420]

Differential Diagnosis

The differential diagnosis for spinal stenosis includes, but is not limited to, vascular insufficiency, an acute aortic dissection, nephrolithiasis (kidney stone), osteomyelitis, spondylolysis, mechanical back or neck pain, disk herniation, and cauda equina syndrome. Compression of the spinal cord has also been misdiagnosed as amyotrophic lateral sclerosis (ALS), multiple sclerosis (MS), or Parkinson's disease, and therefore also needs to be placed on the differential diagnosis list.

SPONDYLOLYSIS/SPONDYLOLISTHESIS

Spondylolysis is a defect of the pars interarticularis of the spine, which lies between the superior and inferior articular facets of the vertebral arch. The actual defect in the pars covers a broad range of etiologies, from stress fracture to a traumatic bony fracture with separation.

Spondylolisthesis is a diagnostic term that identifies anterior slippage and inability to resist shear forces of a vertebral segment in relation to the vertebral segment immediately below it. Spondylolisthesis usually occurs in the lumbar spine.

Clinical Significance

Newman[421] described five groups represented by this deformity based on etiology:

1. *Congenital* spondylolisthesis. This results from dysplasia of the fifth lumbar and sacral arches and zygapophyseal joints.
2. *Isthmic* spondylolisthesis. This is caused by a defect in the pars interarticularis, which can be an acute fracture, a stress fracture, or an elongation of the pars.
3. *Degenerative* spondylolisthesis. This occurs due to disk and zygapophyseal joint degeneration. Degenerative spondylolisthesis usually affects older people and occurs most commonly at L4-L5. The slip occurs because of arthritis in the zygapophyseal joint with loss of their ligamentous support. The zygapophyseal joints sustain approximately 33% of the static compression load on the lumbar motion segment, and dynamically as much as 33% of the axial load, dependent on spine position.[422]
4. *Traumatic* spondylolisthesis. This fairly rare type occurs with a fracture or acute dislocation of the zygapophyseal joint.
5. *Pathologic* spondylolisthesis. This condition may result from a systemic disease causing a weakening of the pars, pedicle, or zygapophyseal joint, or from a local condition such as a tumor.

Spondylolisthesis aquisita, a sixth etiologic category, was added to represent the slip caused by the surgical disruption of ligaments, bone, and disk.

Tests and Measures and Response

Refer to Tests and Measures and Response in the spinal stenosis section (see Special Tests of the Lumbar Spine and SIJ).

Clinical Findings, Secondary Effects, or Complications

Clinically these patients will complain of low back pain that is mechanical in nature. Mechanical pain is worsened with activity and alleviated with rest. The patients also may complain of leg pain, which can either be of a radicular type pattern, or more commonly will be one of neurogenic claudication. If neurogenic claudication is present, the patient may complain of bilateral thigh and leg tiredness, aches, and fatigue.[423] The questions regarding bicycle use versus walking can be helpful in differentiating neurogenic versus vascular claudication (see earlier). Vascular claudication occurs because not enough blood is flowing to a muscle. While enough blood flows to the muscle to meet the needs of the muscle at rest, when the muscle is involved with exercise the working muscle needs more blood and the narrowed artery may not let enough through. ROM of the lumbar spine flexion frequently is normal with both types of claudication. Some patients will be able to touch their toes without difficulty. Strength is usually intact in the lower extremities. Sensation also is usually intact. A check of distal pulses is important to rule out any coexisting vascular insufficiency. Findings such as hairless lower extremities, coldness of the feet, or absent pulses are signs of peripheral vascular disease. Sensory defects in a stocking glove distribution are more suggestive of diabetic neuropathy. The deep tendon reflexes generally will be normal or diminished. If hyperreflexic symptoms and other upper motor neuron signs such as clonus or a positive Babinski test are found, the cervical, thoracic, and lumbar spine should be investigated to rule out a spinal cord or cauda equina lesion.

Diagnostic Tests
Radiography.

Interventions/Treatment
Medical—The recommended treatment program for an active spondylolysis is bracing to immobilize the spine for a short period (approximately 4 months).

Pharmacological—Analgesics and/or NSAIDs prescribed as needed.

Physical therapy—The therapeutic exercise progression for this population includes postural education, hip flexor, rectus femoris and lumbar paraspinal stretching, lumbar (core) stabilization exercises targeting the abdominals and gluteals, aerobic conditioning, and positioning through a posterior pelvic tilt.[390-392]

Differential Diagnosis

The differential diagnosis for spondylolysis/spondylolisthesis includes, but is not limited to, lumbosacral dysfunctions, facet syndrome, and SIJ dysfunction.

■ SECTION 7: INTERVENTION PRINCIPLES FOR MUSCULOSKELETAL INJURIES

A number of principles should guide the intervention through the various stages of musculoskeletal tissue healing. These include:

- Control pain, inflammation, and swelling (edema)
- Promote and progress healing
- Instructions to the patient on a therapeutic exercise program that:
  - Corrects any imbalances between strength and flexibility
  - Addresses postural and movement dysfunctions
  - Integrates the open and closed kinetic chains
  - Incorporates neuromuscular re-education
  - Maintains or improves overall strength and fitness
  - Improves the functional outcome of the patient

CONTROL OF PAIN AND INFLAMMATION

The clinician has a number of tools at his or her disposal to help to control pain, inflammation and swelling (edema). These include the application of electrotherapeutic and physical modalities, gentle ROM exercises, and graded manual techniques. During the acute stage of healing the principles of POLICE (Protection, Optimal Loading, Ice, Compression, Elevation) are recommended. The modalities used during the acute phase involve the application of cryotherapy, electrical stimulation, pulsed ultrasound, and iontophoresis. Modalities used during the later stages of healing include thermotherapy, phonophoresis, electrical stimulation, ultrasound (US), iontophoresis, and diathermy. The applications of cold and heat are taught to the patient at the earliest opportunity.

Gentle manual techniques (grade I or II joint mobilizations) may also be used to help with pain. As the patient progresses, gentle passive muscle stretching may be introduced. Self-stretching and self-mobilization techniques are taught to the patient at the earliest and appropriate opportunity.

The goals of the acute phase should include:

- Maximizing patient comfort by decreasing pain and inflammation
- Protection of the injury site
- Restoration of pain-free ROM throughout the entire kinetic chain
- Retardation of muscle atrophy
- Minimizing the detrimental effects of immobilization and activity restriction[424–429]
- Attainment of early neuromuscular control
- Improving soft tissue extensibility
- Increasing functional tolerance
- Maintaining general fitness
- Appropriate management of scar tissue
- Encouraging the patient toward independence with the home exercise program
- Progression of the patient to the functional stage

PROMOTE AND PROGRESS HEALING

The promotion and progression of tissue repair involves a delicate balance between protection and the application of controlled functional stresses to the damaged structure. Tissue repair can be viewed as an adaptive life process in response to both intrinsic and extrinsic stimuli.[430] These stimuli can be in the form of manual techniques and/or therapeutic exercises. Although physical therapy cannot accelerate the healing process, it can ensure that the healing process is not delayed or disrupted, and that it occurs in an optimal environment.[431] In addition to excess stress, detrimental environments include prolonged immobilization,

High-Yield Terms to Learn

Primary joint replacement or arthroplasty	The first replacement surgery.
Revision surgery	A second or succeeding surgery performed usually for an unstable, loose, or painful joint replacement.
Total hip replacement (THR) or total hip arthroplasty (THA)	Replacement of the femoral head and the acetabular articular surface.
Hemiarthroplasty	Replacement of the femoral head only.
Bipolar hemiarthroplasty	A specific form of hemiarthroplasty using a femoral prosthesis with an articulating acetabular component. The acetabular cartilage is not replaced. The principle of this procedure is to decrease the frictional wear between the femoral head prosthesis and the cartilage of the acetabulum.
POLICE	Acronym for the treatment of acute injuries that has replaced the former acronym PRICE (protection, rest, ice, compression, elevation) with protection, optimal loading, ice, compression, elevation.

which must be avoided. The rehabilitation procedures chosen to progress the patient will depend on the type of tissue involved, the extent of the damage, and the stage of healing. The intervention must be related to the signs and symptoms present rather than the actual diagnosis.

The functional phase addresses any tissue overload problems and functional biomechanical deficits. The goals of the functional phase should address:

- Attainment of full range of pain-free motion
- Restoration of normal joint kinematics
- Improvement of muscle strength to within normal limits
- Improvement of neuromuscular control
- Restoration of normal muscle force couples
- Correction of any deficits in the whole kinetic chain that are involved in an activity to which the patient is planning to return
- Performance of activity-specific progressions before full return to function

The selection of intervention procedures, and the intervention progression, must be guided by continuous reexamination of the patient's response to a given procedure, making the reexamination of patient dysfunction before, during, and after each intervention essential.[57] There are three possible scenarios following a reexamination:

1. The patient's function has improved. In this scenario, the intensity of the intervention may be incrementally increased.
2. The patient's function has diminished. In this scenario, the intensity and the focus of the intervention must be changed. Further review of the home exercise program may be needed. The patient may require further education on activity modification and the use of heat and ice at home. The working hypothesis must be reviewed. Further investigation is needed.
3. There is no change in the patient's function. Depending on the elapse of time since the last visit, there may be a reason for the lack of change. This finding may indicate the need for a change in the intensity of the intervention. If the patient is in the acute or subacute stage of healing, a decrease in the intensity may be warranted to allow the tissues more of an opportunity to heal. In the chronic stage, an increase in intensity may be warranted.

Tendon Injury

For the treatment of a tendon injury, the following five-step plan is recommended:

1. The principles of POLICE to aid healing.
2. A gradual progression of therapeutic exercise, focusing on progression toward eccentric exercises and the removal of intrinsic deficits: increasing flexibility, and muscle imbalances.
3. Removal of any extrinsic factors (damaging stimuli). This often involves absence from abuse rather than absolute rest.
4. Identification of any faulty mechanics/technique. When treating overuse injuries, it is essential that the clinician limits both the chronic inflammation and degeneration by working on both sides of the problem—tissue strength should be maximized through proper training, and adequate healing time must be allowed before returning to full participation.
5. Application of cross-section massage to the tendon as tolerated.

Ligament Injury

Intervention in the acute stage centers around aggressive attempts to:

- Minimize effusion so as to speed healing (cryotherapy, compression, and elevation).
- Promote early protected motion and early supported/protected weight-bearing as tolerated/appropriate using low load cyclic loading. For example, with an ankle sprain, protected weight-bearing with an orthosis is permitted, with weight-bearing to tolerance as soon as possible following injury.
- Protected return to activity. As the healing progresses and the patient is able to bear more weight through the joint, there is a corresponding increase in the use of weight-bearing (closed chain) exercises.
- Prevention of reinjury.

Bursitis

Most forms of bursitis are treated conservatively to reduce inflammation. Conservative treatment includes rest, cold and heat treatments, elevation, and NSAIDs. Patients with suspected septic bursitis are treated with antibiotics while awaiting culture results.

ORTHOPEDIC SURGICAL REPAIRS

Lumbar Diskectomy

Lumbar diskectomy involves removing a small window of bone in the spine, moving the nerve to one side, and removing either some or the entire herniated disk. Percutaneous diskectomy uses x-ray and a video screen to guide small instruments toward the disk. Postoperative recovery is relatively fast, with relief from nerve root compression often immediate.

Laminectomy

Laminectomy is the most commonly performed surgery on the lower spine, and involves removing part or all of the lamina to remove pressure on one or more nerve roots. Because the procedure requires an incision of 2 more inches, a hospital stay is required.

Vertebroplasty

This procedure, usually performed on an outpatient basis, is used to repair a fractured vertebra. A small incision is made in the skin over the affected area and a cement-like mixture is injected into the vertebra. The cement hardens to stabilize the bones of the spine.

Kyphoplasty

Kyphoplasty is similar to vertebroplasty, and involves making a small incision in the back and injecting a cement-like material to repair a fractured vertebra(e). However, in kyphoplasty, prior to injecting the cement, the surgeon inserts a balloon device to help restore the height and shape of the spine.

Foraminotomy

This procedure, used to enlarge the foramen, involves removing any bone or tissue that is obstructing the foramen and compressing the nerve root. This procedure is often combined with other procedures such as a laminectomy.

Total Joint Replacement

Total joint replacement (arthroplasty) represents a significant advance in the treatment of painful and disabling joint pathologies. Total joint replacement can be performed on any joint of the body including the hip, knee, ankle, foot, shoulder, elbow, wrist, and fingers. Cemented joint replacement or arthroplasty is a procedure in which bone cement or polymethylmethacrylate (PMMA) is used to fix the prosthesis in place in the joint. Ingrowth or cementless joint replacement or arthroplasty does not involve bone cement to fix the prosthesis in place. An anatomic or press fit with bone ingrowth into the surface of the prosthesis leads to a stable fixation. This procedure is based on a fracture-healing model.

Of the total joint replacement procedures, hip and knee total joint replacements are by far the most common.

Standard precautions given to patients to prevent posterior hip dislocation include the following for 3 months postsurgery:

- Maintain appropriate weight-bearing status
- Do not cross legs (avoid hip adduction) when sitting or lying
- Put a pillow between legs if lying on side
- Do not turn leg inward (avoid internal rotation of the hip)
- Do not pivot toward the surgical side
- Sit only on elevated chairs or toilet seats
- Do not lean forward to get up from a chair
- Do not bend over from the hips toward the ground to reach objects or tie shoes

With an anterior approach, the surgery is performed without violating any of the hip's posterior structures, and thus hip precautions are not required.

Flexor Tendon Repair

One of the main purposes of the hand is to grasp; therefore, the loss of flexor tendons imposes a catastrophic functional loss.[432] The purpose of a flexor tendon repair is to restore maximum active flexor tendon gliding to ensure effective finger joint motion.

Most flexor tendon ruptures occur silently after prolonged inflammatory tenosynovitis, although the causes also can be traumatic. Researchers have shown that early mobilization can prevent the formation of scar tissue without jeopardizing tendon healing, and they have developed many different forms of early mobilization programs.[433] Several postsurgical protocols and modifications exist, based on individual characteristics, the zone involved, the suture strength, and physician preferences.

QUESTIONS

1. Your patient dove into the pool and hit his head. You perform the Sharp-Purser test and get a "clunk." Which upper cervical structure are you most concerned with based on this examination finding?
   A. Alar ligament
   B. Transverse ligament
   C. Tectorial membrane
   D. Posterior occipital membrane

2. Your patient has a positive Wartenberg sign, paresthesias along the medial hand and finger, and weakness with gripping objects. Which peripheral nerve is most likely involved?
   A. Ulnar nerve
   B. Median nerve
   C. Radial nerve
   D. Anterior interosseous nerve

3. Your patient fell on an outstretched arm and complains of clicking and pain when he raises his arm overhead or lifts something heavy. You find a (+) O'Brien test. Which of the following structures is most likely involved?
   A. Rotator cuff
   B. Hypomobile capsule
   C. Glenoid labrum
   D. Superior G-H ligament

4. In reference to the patient described in Question 3 above, which of the following descriptions best fits the patient's examination findings?
   A. SLAP tear
   B. Bankhart lesion
   C. Hill-Sachs lesion
   D. Supraspinatus tear

5. Your patient was struck on the outside knee while playing soccer. You perform an examination to assess for tissue damage. If your patient has a (+) Lachman test, (+) valgus stress test, and a (−) McMurray test, which structure(s) are most likely damaged?
   A. ACL, MCL
   B. ACL, MM
   C. MCL, MM
   D. MCL, LCL

6. You are rehabilitating a patient who is status-post ACL reconstructive surgery 2 weeks ago. Which of the following exercises would put the most stress through the new ACL graft?
   A. Quad sets pressing into towel roll
   B. Closed-chain knee extension 0° to 30°
   C. Open-chain knee extension 0° to 40°
   D. Long-arc quad sets 90° to 45°

7. The Benediction sign is a result of damage to which nerve?
   A. Median or anterior interosseous nerves
   B. Ulnar or posterior interosseous nerves
   C. Radial or recurrent branch nerves
   D. Palmar cutaneous or sinuvertebral nerves

8. Which structure provides the most stability to the distal radioulnar joint complex?
   A. Flexor and extensor tendons crossing the wrist
   B. Wrist joint capsule
   C. TFCC
   D. Flexor and extensor retinacula

9. Your patient is 78 years old with a complaint of stiffness and pain in her hands. She was diagnosed with osteoarthritis and wants you to tell her what the new tender bumps she is feeling on her DIP joints are. Which of the following best names these bumps?
   A. Bouchard's nodes
   B. Heberden's nodes
   C. Swan-neck deformity
   D. Boutonniere deformity

10. A 30-year-old man with complaint of LBP and radiating pain into his right lower extremity is seen for an examination after lifting a heavy truck tire into the back of his truck 2 weeks ago. He has a (+) SLR at 45°, a right lateral shift with left lower extremity pain, and weakness with testing left ankle dorsiflexion (DF). Which of the following best describes this patient's problem?
   A. Discogenic with left L4 nerve root compression
   B. Discogenic with left L5 nerve root compression
   C. Central stenosis with left L4 nerve root compression
   D. Lateral foraminal stenosis with left L5 nerve root compression

11. Your 75-year-old patient presents with gradual onset of right hip pain over the past 6 months, worse with walking, better with lying down. Radiographs show osteophytes, sclerosing, and decreased joint space of the right hip. Which of the following motions would you expect to find the most limited during your AROM and PROM testing?
   A. External rotation and flexion
   B. Internal rotation and extension
   C. External rotation and extension
   D. Internal rotation and flexion

12. A 56-year-old man presents with insidious onset of right shoulder pain 3 months ago he describes as constant, but states he notices it worsens after he eats. He states he can find no position of his shoulder that either worsens or relieves his pain. What is the most likely cause of this patient's pain?
   A. Prostate referral
   B. Spleen referral
   C. Heart attack referral
   D. Gallbladder referral

ANSWERS

1. The answer is **B**. The Sharp-Puser test is used to check the integrity of the transverse ligament.

2. The answer is **A**. Wartenberg's sign, the involuntary abduction of the fifth finger, is indicative of an injury to the ulnar nerve.

3. The answer is **C**. O'Brien's test is designed to help detect glenohumeral joint labral tears.

4. The answer is **A**. O'Brien's test is designed to specifically test for SLAP (superior labral tear from anterior to posterior) lesions.

5. The answer is **A**. The Lachman test detects ACL lesions, the valgus stress test detects MCL lesions, and the McMurray test detect MM lesions.

6. The answer is **C**. Open-chain knee extension between 0 and 40 degrees has been demonstrated to put the most stress through the ACL.

7. The answer is **A**. The hand of benediction, also known as benediction sign, occurs as a result of prolonged compression or injury of the median/anterior interosseous nerve.

8. The answer is **C**. The TFCC provides load transmission across the ulnocarpal joint and allows forearm rotation by providing stabilization between the distal radius and ulna, and the ulnar portion of the carpus.

9. The answer is **B**. Heberden's nodes, a sign of osteoarthritis, are hard or bony swellings that can develop in the distal interphalangeal (DIP) joints.

10. The answer is **A**. These are the classic signs of a L4 nerve root compression.

11. The answer is **D**. The capsular pattern of the hip includes limited motion with internal rotation and flexion.

12. The answer is **D**. Given the fact that motion does not appear to influence the pain and the distribution of the symptoms, the gall bladder is the best choice.

SKILL KEEPER QUESTIONS

1. *Compare and contrast the examination findings you would get with a bicep tendonitis and a bicep muscle strain. What would be the best test to differentiate the two?*

2. *Your patient presents with bilateral lower extremity paresthesia in a stocking distribution when he walks his dog, so you perform the treadmill test to differentiate the cause. He is able to walk on an incline longer than on flat surface. Does this suggest vascular or neurogenic claudication?*

3. *Compare and contrast the neurovascular assessment findings you would get with an entrapment of the median nerve versus spinal cord compression at the C5–6 level*

SKILL KEEPER ANSWERS

1. *Both are contractile tissues so would likely have pain with contraction (MMT), pain with lengthening the tissues (in the case of a bicep tendon or muscle involvement, lengthening with elbow extension, pronation, and shoulder extension), and pain with palpation over the involved area. The best way to differentiate which is the culprit is to palpate the location; the tendon will be painful with tendinitis and the bicep muscle belly will be tender with a muscle strain.*

2. *Neurogenic claudication, because the incline would cause a positional change in the spine to a more flexed posture, which would decrease the venous congestion due to the stenosis. A person's symptoms with vascular claudication would worsen, as the incline requires more intensity, which increases the oxygen demand to the muscles and therefore the paresthesia would worsen.*

3. *This is comparing an LMN and a UMN presentation. (See Table 2–66 for details on LMN versus UMN signs, symptoms, and findings.)*

REFERENCES

1. Prentice WE. Understanding and managing the healing process. In: Prentice WE, Voight ML, eds. *Techniques in Musculoskeletal Rehabilitation*. New York, NY: McGraw-Hill; 2001:17-41.

2. Engles M. Tissue response. In: Donatelli R, Wooden MJ, eds. *Orthopaedic Physical Therapy*. 3rd ed. Philadelphia, PA: Churchill Livingstone; 2001:1-24.

3. Garrett WE. Muscle strain injuries. *Am J Sports Med*. 1996;24:S2-S8.

4. Safran MR, Seaber AV, Garrett WE. Warm-up and muscular injury prevention: an update. *Sports Med*. 1989;8: 239-249.

5. Huijbregts PA. Muscle injury, regeneration, and repair. *J Man Manip Ther*. 2001;9:9-16.

6. Armstrong RB, Warren GL, Warren JA. Mechanisms of exercise-induced muscle fibre injury. *Med Sci Sports Exerc*. 1990;24:436-443.

7. Hall SJ. The biomechanics of human skeletal muscle. In: Hall SJ, ed. *Basic Biomechanics*. New York, NY: McGraw-Hill; 1999:146-185.

8. Boeckmann RR, Ellenbecker TS. Biomechanics. In: Ellenbecker TS, ed. *Knee Ligament Rehabilitation*. Philadelphia, PA: Churchill Livingstone; 2000:16-23.

9. Brownstein B, Noyes FR, Mangine RE, Kryger S. Anatomy and biomechanics. In: Mangine RE, ed. *Physical Therapy of the Knee*. New York, NY: Churchill Livingstone; 1988: 1-30.

10. Deudsinger RH. Biomechanics in clinical practice. *Phys Ther*. 1984;64:1860-1868.

11. Hall SJ. Kinematic concepts for analyzing human motion. In: Hall SJ, ed. *Basic Biomechanics*. New York, NY: McGraw-Hill; 1999:28-89.

12. Luttgens K, Hamilton N. The center of gravity and stability. In: Luttgens K, Hamilton N, eds. *Kinesiology: Scientific Basis of Human Motion*. 9th ed. Dubuque, IA: McGraw-Hill; 1997:415-442.

13. Cyriax J. *Textbook of Orthopaedic Medicine, Diagnosis of Soft Tissue Lesions*. 8th ed. London: Bailliere Tindall; 1982.

14. Hayes KW. An examination of Cyriax's passive motion tests with patients having osteoarthritis of the knee. *Phys Ther*. 1994;74:697.

15. Rothstein JM. Cyriax reexamined. *Phys Ther*. 1994;74:1073.

16. Oakes BW. Acute soft tissue injuries: nature and management. *Austr Family Physician*. 1982;10:3-16.

17. Garrick JG. The sports medicine patient. *Nurs Clin N Am*. 1981;16:759-766.

18. Muckle DS. Injuries in sport. *Royal S Health J*. 1982;102:93-94.

19. Kellett J. Acute soft tissue injuries: a review of the literature. *Med Sci Sports Exerc*. 1986;18:5.

20. Prentice WE. Understanding and managing the healing process through rehabilitation. In: Voight ML, Hoogenboom BJ, Prentice WE, eds. *Musculoskeletal Interventions: Techniques for Therapeutic Exercise*. New York, NY: McGraw-Hill; 2007:19-46.

21. Orgill D, Demling RH. Current concepts and approaches to wound healing. *Crit Care Med*. 1988;16:899.

22. Cook JL, Rio E, Purdam CR, Docking SI. Revisiting the continuum model of tendon pathology: what is its merit in clinical practice and research? *Br J Sports Med*. 2016;50:1187-1191.

23. Coombes BK, Bisset L, Vicenzino B. A new integrative model of lateral epicondylalgia. *Br J Sports Med*. 2009;43:252-258.

24. Rio E, Kidgell D, Purdam C, et al. Isometric exercise induces analgesia and reduces inhibition in patellar tendinopathy. *Br J Sports Med*. 2015;49:1277-1283.

25. Loghmani MT, Warden SJ. Instrument-assisted cross-fiber massage accelerates knee ligament healing. *J Orthop Sports Phys Ther*. 2009;39:506-514.

26. Loghmani MT, Warden SJ. Instrument-assisted cross fiber massage increases tissue perfusion and alters microvascular morphology in the vicinity of healing knee ligaments. *BMC Complement Altern Med*. 2013;13:240.

27. American College of Sports Medicine. *ACSM's Guidelines for Exercise Testing and Prescription*. 8th ed. Philadelphia, PA: Lippincott Williams & Wilkins; 2010.

28. Kiser DM. Physiological and biomechanical factors for understanding repetitive motion injuries. *Semin Occup Med*. 1987;2:11-7.

29. Wiater JM. Functional anatomy of the shoulder. In: Placzek JD, Boyce DA, eds. *Orthopaedic Physical Therapy Secrets*. Philadelphia, PA: Hanley & Belfus; 2001:243-248.

30. Turnbull JR. Acromioclavicular joint disorders. *Med Sci Sports Exerc*. 1998;30:S26-32.

31. Rockwood CA Jr. Injuries to the acromioclavicular joint. In: Rockwood CA Jr, Green DP, eds. *Fractures in Adults*. 2nd ed. Philadelphia, PA: JB Lippincott; 1984:860-910.

32. Rockwood CA Jr, Young DC. Disorders of the acromioclavicular joint. In: Rockwood CA, Jr, Matsen FA III, eds. *The Shoulder*. Philadelphia, PA: WB Saunders; 1990: 413-468.

33. Keele CA, Neil E. *Samson Wright's Applied Physiology*. 12th ed. London: Oxford University Press; 1971.

34. de Seze MP, Rezzouk J, de Seze M, et al. Does the motor branch of the long head of the triceps brachii arise from the radial nerve? An anatomic and electromyographic study. *Surg Radiol Anat*. 2004;26:459-461.

35. Cummings GS. Comparison of muscle to other soft tissue in limiting elbow extension. *J Orthop Sports Phys Ther*. 1984;5:170.

36. Kapandji IA. *The Physiology of the Joints, Upper Limb*. New York, NY: Churchill Livingstone; 1991.

37. Hammer WI. *Functional Soft Tissue Examination and Treatment By Manual Methods*. Gaithersburg, MD: Aspen; 1991.

38. Hume MC, Gellman H, McKellop H, Brumfield RH. Functional range of motion of the joints of the hand. *J Hand Surg*. 1990; 15A:240-243.

39. Tubiana R, Thomine J-M, Mackin E. *Examination of the Hand and Wrist*. London: Mosby; 1996.

40. Patterson RM, Nicodemus CL, Viegas SF, Elder KW, Rosenblatt J. High-speed, three-dimensional kinematic analysis of the normal wrist. *J Hand Surg* [Am]. 1998;23:446-453.

41. Sun JS, Shih TT, Ko CM, Chang CH, Hang YS, Hou SM. In vivo kinematic study of normal wrist motion: an ultrafast computed tomographic study. *Clin Biomech (Bristol, Avon)*. 2000;15:212-216.

42. Moore JS. De Quervain's tenosynovitis: stenosing tenosynovits of the first dorsal compartment. *J Occup Environ Med.* 1997;39:990-1002.

43. Verdan CE. Primary repair of flexor tendons. *J Bone Joint Surg Am.* 1960;42-A:647-657.

44. Cibulka MT, Sinacore DR, Cromer GS, Delitto A. Unilateral hip rotation range of motion asymmetry in patients with sacroiliac joint regional pain. *Spine.* 1998;23: 1009-1015.

45. Afoke NYP, Byers PD, Hutton WC. Contact pressures in the human hip joint. *J Bone Joint Surg Br.* 1987;69B:536.

46. Oatis CA. Biomechanics of the hip. In: Echternach J, ed. *Clinics in Physical Therapy: Physical Therapy of the Hip.* New York, NY: Churchill Livingstone, 1990:37-50.

47. Kapandji IA. *The Physiology of the Joints, Lower Limb.* New York, NY: Churchill Livingstone; 1991.

48. Pauwels F. *Biomechanics of the Normal and Diseased Hip.* Berlin: Springer-Verlag; 1976.

49. Maquet PGJ. *Biomechanics of the Hip as Applied to Osteoarthritis and Related Conditions.* Berlin: Springer-Verlag; 1985.

50. Menke W, Schmitz B, Schild H, Köper C. Transversale Skelettachsen der unteren extremitat bei coxarthrose. *Zeitschr Orthop.* 1991;129:255-259.

51. Pizzutillo PT, MacEwen GD, Shands AR. Anteversion of the femur. In: Tonzo RG, ed. *Surgery of the Hip Joint.* New York, NY: Springer-Verlag; 1984.

52. Lausten GS, Jorgensen F, Boesen J. Measurement of anteversion of the femoral neck, ultrasound and CT compared. *J Bone Joint Surg Br.* 1989;71B:237.

53. Gross MT. Lower quarter screening for skeletal malalignment — suggestions for orthotics and shoewear. *J Orthop Sports Phys Ther.* 1995;21:389-405.

54. Deusinger R. Validity of pelvic tilt measurements in anatomical neutral position. *J Biomech.* 1992;25:764.

55. Kaltenborn FM. *Manual Mobilization of the Extremity Joints: Basic Examination and Treatment Techniques.* 4th ed. Oslo, Norway: Olaf Norlis Bokhandel, Universitetsgaten; 1989.

56. Williams PL, Warwick R, Dyson M, Bannister LH. *Gray's Anatomy.* 37th ed. London: Churchill Livingstone; 1989.

57. Yoder E. Physical therapy management of nonsurgical hip problems in adults. In: Echternach JL, ed. *Physical Therapy of the Hip.* New York, NY: Churchill Livingstone; 1990:103-137.

58. Dye SF. An evolutionary perspective of the knee. *J Bone Joint Surg Am.* 1987;69A:976-983.

59. Davids JR. Pediatric knee. Clinical assessment and common disorders. *Pediatr Clin North Am.* 1996;43:1067-1090.

60. McGinty G, Irrgang JJ, Pezzullo D. Biomechanical considerations for rehabilitation of the knee. *Clin Biomech.* 2000;15:160-166.

61. Kendall FP, McCreary EK, Provance PG. *Muscles: Testing and Function.* Baltimore: Williams & Wilkins; 1993.

62. Brownstein B, Noyes FR, Mangine RE, Kryger S. Anatomy and biomechanics. In: Mangine RE, ed. *Physical Therapy of the Knee.* New York, NY: Churchill Livingstone; 1988:1-30.

63. Desio SM, Burks RT, Bachus KN. Soft tissue restraints to lateral patellar translation in the human knee. *Am J Sports Med* 1998;26:59-65.

64. Fulkerson JP. *Disorders of the Patellofemoral Joint.* Baltimore: Williams & Wilkins; 1997.

65. Grelsamer RP, McConnell J. *The Patella: A Team Approach.* Gaithersburg, MD: Aspen; 1998.

66. Woodland LH, Francis RS. Parameters and comparisons of the quadriceps angle of college aged men and women in the supine and standing positions. *Am J Sports Med.* 1992;20:208-11.

67. Olerud C, Berg P. The variation of the quadriceps angle with different positions of the foot. *Clin Orthop.* 1984; 191:162-165.

68. Rand JA. The patellofemoral joint in total knee arthroplasty. *J Bone Joint Surg Am.* 1994;76:612-620.

69. Aglietti P, Insall JN, Walker PS, Trent P. A new patella prosthesis. *Clin Orthop.* 1975;107:175-187.

70. McConnell J, Fulkerson JP. The knee: patellofemoral and soft tissue injuries. In: Zachazewski JE, Magee DJ, Quillen WS, eds. *Athletic Injuries and Rehabilitation.* Philadelphia, PA: WB Saunders; 1996:693-728.

71. Fujikawa K, Seedholm BB, Wright V. Biomechanics of the patellofemoral joint. Parts 1 and 2. Study of the patellofemoral compartment and movement of the patella. *Eng Med.* 1983;12:3-21.

72. Goodfellow JW, Hungerford DS, Woods C. Patellofemoral joint mechanics and pathology: I and II. *J Bone Joint Surg.* 1976;58B:287-299.

73. Hehne H-J. Biomechanics of the patellofemoral joint and its clinical relevance. *Clin Orthop.* 1990;258:73-85.

74. Huberti HH, Hayes WC. Patellofemoral contact pressures. The influence of Q-angle and tendofemoral contact. *J Bone Joint Surg Am.* 1984;66-A:715-724.

75. Carson WG, James SL, Larson RL, et al. Patellofemoral disorders - physical and radiographic examination. Part I. Physical examination. *Clin Orthop.* 1984;185:178-186.

76. Hungerford DS, Barry M. Biomechanics of the patellofemoral joint. *Clin Orthop.* 1979;144:9-15.

77. Steinkamp LA, Dilligham MF, Markel MD, Hill JA, Kaufman KR. Biomechanical considerations in patellofemoral joint rehabilitation. *Am J Sports Med.* 1993;21: 438-444.

78. Grelsamer RP, McConnell J. Applied mechanics of the patellofemoral joint. *The Patella: A Team Approach.* Maryland: Aspen; 1998:25-41.

79. Beynnon BD, Fleming BC, Johnson RJ, Nichols CE, Renstrom PA, Pope MH. Anterior cruciate ligament strain behavior during rehabilitation exercises in vivo. *Am J Sports Med.* 1995;23:24-34.

80. Lutz GE, Palmitier RA, An KN, Chao EY. Comparison of tibiofemoral joint forces during open-kinetic-chain and closed-kinetic-chain exercises. *J Bone Joint Surg Am.* 1993;75:732-739.

81. Reilly DT, Martens M. Experimental analysis of the quadriceps muscle force and patello-femoral joint reaction force for various activities. *Acta Orthop Scand.* 1972;43: 126-137.

82. Powers CM. The influence of abnormal hip mechanics on knee injury: a biomechanical perspective. *J Orthop Sports Phys Ther.* 2010;40:42-51.

83. Lundberg A, Goldie I, Kalin B, et al. Kinematics of the ankle/foot complex: plantar flexion and dorsiflexion. *Foot Ankle.* 1989;9:194-200.

84. Levens AS, Inman VT, Blosser JA. Transverse rotations of the lower extremity in locomotion. *J Bone Joint Surg Am.* 1948;30A:859-872.

85. Oatis CA. Biomechanics of the foot and ankle under static conditions. *Phys Ther.* 1988;68:1815-1821.

86. Subotnick SI. Biomechanics of the subtalar and midtarsal joints. *J Am Podiatry Assoc.* 1975;65:756-764.

87. Elftman H. The transverse tarsal joint and its control. *Clin Orth Rel Res.* 1960;16:41-45.

88. White AA, Johnson RM, Panjabi MM, et al. Biomechanical analysis of clinical stability in the cervical spine. *Clin Orthop.* 1975;109:85-96.

89. Panjabi M, Dvorak J, Crisco J, et al. Flexion, extension, and lateral bending of the upper cervical spine in response to alar ligament transections. *J Spinal Disord.* 1991;4:157-167.

90. Vangilder JC, Menezes AH, Dolan KD. *The Craniovertebral Junction and its Abnormalities.* Mount Kisco, NY: Futura; 1987.

91. Buckworth J. Anatomy of the suboccipital region. In: Vernon H, ed. *Upper Cervical Syndrome.* Baltimore: Williams & Wilkins; 1988.

92. Bogduk N. Innervation and pain patterns of the cervical spine. In: Grant R, ed. *Physical Therapy of the Cervical and Thoracic Spine.* New York, NY: Churchill Livingstone; 1988.

93. Swash M, Fox K. Muscle spindle innervation in man. *J Anat.* 1972;112:61-80.

94. Lazorthes G. Pathology, classification and clinical aspects of vascular diseases of the spinal cord. In: Vinken PJ, Bruyn GW, eds. *Handbook of Clinical Neurology.* Oxford: Elsevier; 1972:494-506.

95. Janda V. Muscles and motor control in cervicogenic disorders: assessment and management. In: Grant R, ed. *Physical Therapy of the Cervical and Thoracic Spine.* New York, NY: Churchill Livingstone; 1994:195-216.

96. Jull GA, Janda V. Muscle and Motor control in low back pain. In: Twomey LT, Taylor JR, eds. *Physical Therapy of the Low Back: Clinics in Physical Therapy.* New York, NY: Churchill Livingstone; 1987:258-278.

97. Bergmark A. Stability of the lumbar spine. *Acta Orthop Scand Suppl.* 1989;230:1-54.

98. Mayoux-Benhamou MA, Revel M, Valle C, et al. Longus colli has a postural function on cervical curvature. *Surg Radiol Anat.* 1994;16:367-371.

99. Conley MS, Meyer RA, Bloomberg JJ, et al. Noninvasive analysis of human neck muscle function. *Spine.* 1995;20:2505-2512.

100. Viener AE. Oral surgery. In: Garliner D, ed. *Myofunctional Therapy.* Philadelphia, PA: WB Saunders; 1976.

101. Castaneda R. Occlusion. In: Kaplan AS, Assael LA, eds. *Temporomandibular Disorders Diagnosis and Treatment.* Philadelphia, PA: WB Saunders; 1991:40-49.

102. Andriacchi T, Schultz A, Belytschko T, Galante J. A model for studies of mechanical interactions between the human spine and rib cage. *J Biomech.* 1974;7:497-505.

103. Shea KG, Schlegel JD, Bachus KN, et al, eds. *The Contribution of the Rib Cage to Thoracic Spine Stability.* Vermont: International Society for the Study of the Lumbar Spine; 1996.

104. Jette AM. Toward a common language for function, disability, and health. *Phys Ther.* 2006;86:726-734.

105. Goodman CC, Snyder TK. Introduction to the interviewing process. In: Goodman CC, Snyder TK, eds. *Differential Diagnosis in Physical Therapy.* Philadelphia, PA: WB Saunders; 1990:7-42.

106. Maitland G. *Vertebral manipulation.* Sydney: Butterworth; 1986.

107. American Physical Therapy Association. Guide to physical therapist practice. *Phys Ther.* 2001;81:S13-S95.

108. Meadows J. *Orthopedic Differential Diagnosis in Physical Therapy.* New York, NY: McGraw-Hill; 1999.

109. White DJ. Musculoskeletal examination. In: O'Sullivan SB, Schmitz TJ, eds. *Physical Rehabilitation.* 5th ed. Philadelphia, PA: FA Davis; 2007:159-192.

110. Farfan HF. The scientific basis of manipulative procedures. *Clin Rheum Dis.* 1980;6:159-177.

111. McKenzie R, May S. Physical Examination. In: McKenzie R, May S, eds. *The Human Extremities: Mechanical Diagnosis and Therapy.* Waikanae, NZ: Spinal Publications New Zealand; 2000:105-121.

112. Cyriax J. *Textbook of Orthopaedic Medicine, Diagnosis of Soft Tissue Lesions.* 8th ed. London: Bailliere Tindall; 1982.

113. Petersen CM, Hayes KW. Construct validity of Cyriax's selective tension examination: association of end-feels with pain ath the knee and shoulder. *J Orthop Sports Phys Ther.* 2000;30:512-527.

114. Wintz MN. Variations in current manual muscle testing. *Phys Ther Rev.* 1959;39:466-475.

115. Sapega AA. Muscle performance evaluation in orthopedic practice. *J Bone Joint Surg.* 1990;72A:1562-1574.

116. Iddings DM, Smith LK, Spencer WA. Muscle testing. Part 2. Reliability in clinical use. *Phys Ther Rev.* 1961;41:249-256.

117. Silver M, McElroy A, Morrow L, Heafner BK. Further standardization of manual muscle test for clinical study: applied in chronic renal disease. *Phys Ther.* 1970;50:1456-1465.

118. Marx RG, Bombardier C, Wright JG. What we know about the reliability and validity of physical examination tests used to examine the upper extremity. *J Hand Surg.* 1999;24A:185-193.

119. Palmer ML, Epler M. Principles of examination techniques. In: Palmer ML, Epler M, eds. *Clinical Assessment Procedures in Physical Therapy.* Philadelphia, PA: JB Lippincott; 1990:8-36.

120. Frese E, Brown M, Norton B. Clinical reliability of manual muscle testing: middle trapezius and gluteus medius muscles. *Phys Ther.* 1987;67:1072-1076.

121. Daniels K, Worthingham C. *Muscle Testing Techniques of Manual Examination.* 5th ed. Philadelphia, PA: WB Saunders; 1986.

122. Tovin BJ, Greenfield BH. *Impairment-Based Diagnosis for the Shoulder Girdle. Evaluation and Treatment of the Shoulder: An Integration of the Guide to Physical Therapist Practice.* Philadelphia, PA: FA Davis; 2001:55-74.

123. Riddle DL. Measurement of accessory motion: critical issues and related concepts. *Phys Ther.* 1992;72:865-874.

124. Calis M, Akgun K, Birtane M, Karacan I, Calis H, Tuzun F. Diagnostic values of clinical diagnostic tests in subacromial impingement syndrome. *Ann Rheum Dis.* 2000;59:44-47.

125. Post M, Cohen J. Impingement syndrome: a review of late stage II and early stage III lesions. *Clin Orth Rel Res.* 1986;207:127-132.

126. Ure BM, Tiling T, Kirchner R, Rixen D. Zuverlassigkeit der klinischen untersuchung der schulter im vergleich zur arthroskopie. *Unfallchirurg.* 1993;96:382-386.

127. Leroux JL, Thomas E, Bonnel F, et al. Diagnostic value of clinical tests for shoulder impingement. *Rev Rheum.* 1995;62:423-428.

128. Clarnette RG, Miniaci A. Clinical exam of the shoulder. *Med Sci Sports Exerc.* 1998;30:1-6.

129. Yergason RM. Rupture of biceps. *J Bone Joint Surg.* 1931;13:160.

130. Kibler WB. Specificity and sensitivity of the anterior slide test in throwing athletes with superior glenoid labral tears. *Arthroscopy.* 1995;11:296-300.

131. Neer CSI, Foster CR. Inferior capsular shift for involuntary inferior and multidirectional instability of the shoulder. *J Bone Joint Surg.* 1980;62A:897-908.

132. Rockwood CA. Subluxations and dislocations about the shoulder. In: Rockwood CA, Green DP, eds. *Fractures in Adults - I.* Philadelphia, PA: JB Lippincott; 1984.

133. Zimney NJ. Clinical reasoning in the evaluation and management of undiagnosed chronic hip pain in young adult. *Phys Ther.* 1998;78:62-73.

134. Davis DS, Quinn RO, Whiteman CT, Williams JD, Young CR. Concurrent validity of four clinical tests used to measure hamstring flexibility. *J Strength Cond Res.* 2008;22:583-538.

135. Hanten WP, Pace MB. Reliability of measuring anterior laxity of the knee joint using a knee ligament arthrometer. *Phys Ther.* 1987;67:357-359.

136. Hughston JC, Andrews JR, Cross MJ, Moschi A. Classification of knee ligament instabilities. Part 2. *J Bone Joint Surg.* 1976;58A:173-179.

137. Hughston JC, Andrews JR, Cross MJ, Moschi A. Classification of knee ligament instabilities. Part 1. *J Bone Joint Surg.* 1976;58A:159-172.

138. Shino K, Horibe S, Ono K. The voluntary evoked posterolateral drawer sign in the knee with posterolateral instability. *Clin Orthop.* 1987;215:179-186.

139. Winkel D, Matthijs O, Phelps V. *Examination of the Knee.* Frederick, MD: Aspen; 1997.

140. Apley AG. The diagnosis of meniscus injuries: some new clinical methods. *J Bone Joint Surg Am.* 1947;29B:78-84.

141. Renne JW. The iliotibial band friction syndrome. *J Bone Joint Surg Am.* 1975;57:1110-1111.

142. Noble HB, Hajek MR, Porter M. Diagnosis and treatment of iliotibial band tightness in runners. *Phys Sports Med.* 1982;10:67-74.

143. Carcia CR, Martin RL, Houck J, Wukich DK. Orthopaedic Section of the American Physical Therapy Association. Achilles pain, stiffness, and muscle power deficits: achilles tendinitis. *J Orthop Sports Phys Ther.* 2010;40:A1-26.

144. Patla CE, Abbott JH. Tibialis posterior myofascial tightness as a source of heel pain: diagnosis and treatment. *J Orthop Sports Phys Ther.* 2000;30:624-632.

145. Australian Physiotherapy Association. Protocol for premanipulative testing of the cervical spine. *Aust J Physiother.* 1988;34:97-100.

146. Fast A, Zincola DF, Marin EL. Vertebral artery damage complicating cervical manipulation. *Spine.* 1987;12:840.

147. Golueke P, Sclafani S, Phillips T. Vertebral artery injury—diagnosis and management. *J Trauma.* 1987;27:856-865.

148. Aspinall W. Clinical testing for cervical mechanical disorders which produce ischemic vertigo. *J Orthop Sports Phys Ther.* 1989;11:176-182.

149. Evans RC. *Illustrated Essentials in Orthopedic Physical Assessment.* St. Louis: Mosby-Year Book; 1994.

150. Kanchandani R, Howe JG. Lhermitte's sign in multiple sclerosis: a clinical survey and review of the literature. *J Neurol Neurosurg Psychiatry.* 1982;45:308-312.

151. Smith KJ, McDonald WI. Spontaneous and mechanically evoked activity due to central demyelinating lesion. *Nature.* 1980;286:154-155.

152. Uchihara T, Furukawa T, Tsukagoshi H. Compression of brachial plexus as a diagnostic test of a cervical cord lesion. *Spine.* 1994;19:2170-2173.

153. Landi A, Copeland S. Value of the Tinel sign in brachial plexus lesions. *Ann R Coll Surg Engl.* 1979;61:470-471.

154. Selke FW, Kelly TR. Thoracic outlet syndrome. *Am J Surg.* 1988;156:54-57.

155. Nichols AW. The thoracic outlet syndrome in athletes. *J Am Board Fam Pract.* 1996;9:346-355.

156. Roos DB. Congenital anomalies associated with thoracic outlet syndrome. *J Surg.* 1976;132:771-778.

157. Wright IS. The neurovascular syndrome produced by hyperabduction of the arms. *Am Heart J.* 1945;29:1-19.

158. Thompson JF, Jannsen F. Thoracic outlet syndromes. *Br J Surg.* 1996;83:435-436.

159. Roos DB. The place for scalenectomy and first-rib resection in thoracic outlet syndrome. *Surgery.* 1982;92:1077-1085.

160. Deyo RA, Weinstein JN. Low back pain. *N Engl J Med.* 2001;344:363-370.

161. Fahrni WH. Observations on straight leg raising with special reference to nerve root adhesions. *Can J Surg.* 1966;9:44-48.

162. Kirkaldy-Willis WH. *Managing Low Back Pain.* 2nd ed. New York, NY: Churchill Livingstone; 1988.

163. Lee DG. *The Pelvic Girdle: An Approach to the Examination and Treatment of the Lumbo-Pelvic-Hip Region.* 2nd ed. Edinburgh: Churchill Livingstone; 1999.

164. Potter NA, Rothstein JM. Intertester reliability for selected clinical tests of the sacroiliac joint. *Phys Ther.* 1985;65:1671.

165. Meadows J, Pettman E, Fowler C. Manual therapy. NAIOMT Level II & III course notes. Denver: North American Institute of Manual Therapy; 1995.

166. Pearle AD, Warren RF, Rodeo SA. Basic science of articular cartilage and osteoarthritis. *Clin Sports Med.* 2005;24:1-12.

167. Vereeke West R, Fu F. Soft tissue physiology and repair. *Orthopaedic Knowledge Update 8: Home Study Syllabus.* Rosemont, IL: American Academy of Orthopaedic Surgeons; 2005:15-27.

168. Woolf AD, Pfleger B. Burden of major musculoskeletal conditions. *Bull World Health Organ.* 2003;81:646-656.

169. Jinks C, Jordan K, Ong BN, Croft P. A brief screening tool for knee pain in primary care (KNEST). 2. Results from a survey in the general population aged 50 and over. *Rheumatology.* 2004;43:55-61.

170. Roberts WN, Williams RB. Hip pain. *Primary Care.* 1988;15:783-793.

171. Hammer WI. The use of transverse friction massage in the management of chronic bursitis of the hip or shoulder. *J Man Physiol Ther*. 1993;16:107-111.

172. Guccione AA, Minor MA. Arthritis. In: O'Sullivan SB, Schmitz TJ, eds. *Physical Rehabilitation*. 5th ed. Philadelphia, PA: FA Davis; 2007:1057-1085.

173. Roubenoff R. Gout and hyperuricaemia. *Rheum Dis Clin North Am*. 1990;16:539-550.

174. Isomaki H, von Essen R, Ruutsalo H-M. Gout, particularly diuretics-induced, is on the increase in Finland. *Scand J Rheumatol*. 1977;6:213-216.

175. Gladman DD, Brubacher B, Buskila D, et al. Differences in the expression of spondyloarthropathy: a comparison between ankylosing spondylitis and psoriatic arthritis: genetic and gender effects. *Clin Invest Med*. 1993;16:1-7.

176. Haslock I. Ankylosing spondylitis. *Baillieres Clin Rheumatol*. 1993;7:99.

177. Deyo RA, Rainville J, Kent DL. What can the history and physical examination tell us about low back pain? *JAMA*. 1992;268:760-765.

178. Turek SL. *Orthopaedics–Principles and Their Application*. 4th ed. Philadelphia, PA: JB Lippincott; 1984.

179. Gran JT. An epidemiologic survey of the signs and symptoms of ankylosing spondylitis. *Clin Rheumatol*. 1985;4:161-169.

180. Cohen MD, Ginsurg WW. Late onset peripheral joint disease in ankylosing spondylitis. *Arthritis Rheum*. 1983;26:186-190.

181. Gladman DD. Clinical aspects of the spondyloarthropathies. *Am J Med Sci*. 1998;316:234-238.

182. Calin A, Porta J, Fries JF, Schurman DJ. Clinical history as a screening test for ankylosing spondylitis. *JAMA*. 1977;237:2613-2614.

183. Kraag G, Stokes B, Groh J, et al. The effects of comprehensive home physiotherapy and supervision on patients with ankylosing spondylitis: an 8-month follow-up. *J Rheumatol*. 1994;21:261-263.

184. Tench CM, McCarthy J, McCurdie I, White PD, D'Cruz DP. Fatigue in systemic lupus erythematosus: a randomized controlled trial of exercise. *Rheumatology*. 2003;42:1050-1054.

185. Buskila D, Langevitz P, Gladman DD, et al. Patients with rheumatoid arthritis are more tender than those with psoriatic arthritis. *J Rheumatol*. 1992;19:1115-1119.

186. Gladman DD. Psoriatic arthritis. In: Kelley WN, Harris ED, Ruddy S, Sledge CB, eds. *Textbook of Rheumatology*. 5th ed. Philadelphia, PA: WB Saunders; 1997:999-1005.

187. Lindqvist MH, Gard GE. Hydrotherapy treatment for patients with psoriatic arthritis--a qualitative study. *Open J Ther Rehab*. 2013;1:22-30.

188. Kankate RK, Selvan TP. Primary haematogenous osteomyelitis of the patella: a rare cause for anterior knee pain in an adult. *Postgrad Med J*. 2000;76:707-709.

189. Dich VQ, Nelson JD, Haltalin KC. Osteomyelitis in infants and children: a review of 163 cases. *Am J Dis Child*. 1975;129:1273-1278.

190. Roy DR. Osteomyelitis of the patella. *Clin Orthop Relat Res*. 2001;389:30-34.

191. Lew DP, Waldvogel FA. Osteomyelitis. *Lancet*. 2004; 364:369-379.

192. Lew DP, Waldvogel FA. Osteomyelitis. *N Engl J Med*. 1997;336:999-1007.

193. Bukata SV, Rosier RN. Diagnosis and treatment of osteoporosis. *Curr Opin Orthop*. 2000;11:336-340.

194. Lane JM, Russell L, Khan SN. Osteoporosis. *Clin Orthop*. 2000;372:139-150.

195. Eisman JA. Genetics of osteoporosis. *Endocrine Rev*. 1999;20:788-804.

196. Scheiber LB, Torregrosa L. Early intervention for postmenopausal osteoporosis. *J Musculoskel Med*. 1999;16: 146-157.

197. Lane JM, Riley EH, Wirganowicz PZ. Osteoporosis: diagnosis and treatment. *J Bone Joint Surg*. 1996;78A:618-632.

198. Block J, Smith R, Black D, Genant H. Does exercise prevent osteoporosis. *JAMA*. 1987;257:345.

199. NIH Consensus Development Panel on Osteoporosis Prevention D, and Therapy. Osteoporosis prevention, diagnosis, and therapy. *JAMA*. 2001;285:785-795.

200. Sran MM, Khan KM. Is spinal mobilization safe in severe secondary osteoporosis? A case report. *Man Ther*. 2005;29:29.

201. Shea B, Bonaiuti D, Iovine R, Negrini S, Robinson V, Kemper HC, et al. Cochrane Review on exercise for preventing and treating osteoporosis in postmenopausal women. *Eura Medicophys*. 2004;40:199-209.

202. O'Connell MB. Prescription drug therapies for prevention and treatment of postmenopausal osteoporosis. *J Manag Care Pharm*. 2006;12:S10-19; quiz S26-8.

203. Compston J. Does parathyroid hormone treatment affect fracture risk or bone mineral density in patients with osteoporosis? *Nat Clin Pract Rheumatol*. 2007;1:1.

204. Cummings SR. A 55-year-old woman with osteopenia. *JAMA*. 2006;296:2601-2610.

205. Dupree K, Dobs A. Osteopenia and male hypogonadism. *Rev Urol*. 2004;6:S30-34.

206. Bonaiuti D, Shea B, Iovine R, et al. Exercise for preventing and treating osteoporosis in postmenopausal women. *Cochrane Database Syst Rev*. 2002;3.

207. Marcus R. Role of exercise in preventing and treating osteoporosis. *Rheum Dis Clin North Am*. 2001;27: 131-141, vi.

208. Brown GA, Tan JL, Kirkley A. The lax shoulder in females. Issues, answers, but many more questions. *Clin Orthop Relat Res*. 2000;372:110-122.

209. Flatow EL, Warner JJP. Instability of the shoulder: complex problems and failed repairs: Part I. Relevant biomechanics, multidirectional instability, and severe glenoid loss. *Instr Course Lect*. 1998;47:97-112.

210. Kennedy JC, Alexander IJ, Hayes KC. Nerve supply of the human knee and its functional importance. *Am J Sports Med*. 1982;10:329-335.

211. Rowe CR, Sakellarides HT. Factors related to recurrences of anterior dislocations of the shoulder. *Clin Orthop*. 1961;20:40.

212. Rowe CR, Zarins B. Recurrent transient subluxation of the shoulder. *J Bone Joint Surg Am*. 1981;63:863-872.

213. Brody LT. Shoulder. In: Wadsworth C, ed. *Current Concepts of Orthopedic Physical Therapy—Home Study Course*. La Crosse, WI: Orthopaedic Section, APTA; 2001.

214. Garth WP, Allman FL, Armstrong WS. Occult anterior subluxations of the shoulder in noncontact sports. *Am J Sports Med.* 1987;15:579-585.

215. Jobe FW, Tibone JE, Jobe CM, et al. The shoulder in sports. In: Rockwood CA Jr, Matsen FA III, eds. *The Shoulder.* Philadelphia, PA: WB Saunders; 1990:963-967.

216. Pagnani MJ, Warren RF. Stabilizers of the glenohumeral joint. *J Shoulder Elbow Surg.* 1994;3:173-190.

217. Schenk TJ, Brems JJ. Multidirectional instability of the shoulder: pathophysiology, diagnosis, and management. *J Am Acad Orthop Surgeons.* 1998;6:65-72.

218. Hawkins RJ, Abrams JS, Schutte J. Multidirectional instability of the shoulder--an approach to diagnosis. *Orthop Trans.* 1987;11:246.

219. Lippitt SB, et al. Diagnosis and management of AMBRII syndrome. *Tech Orthop.* 1991;6:61.

220. Perry J. Muscle control of the shoulder. In: Rowe CR, ed. *The Shoulder.* New York, NY: Churchill Livingstone; 1988:17-34.

221. Poppen NK, Walker PS. Normal and abnormal motion of the shoulder. *J Bone Joint Surg Am.* 1976;58A:195-201.

222. Burkhead WZ Jr, Rockwood CA Jr. Treatment of instability of the shoulder with an exercise program. *J Bone Joint Surg Am.* 1992;74A:890-896.

223. Matsen FA, Harryman DT, Sidles JA. Mechanics of glenohumeral instability. *Clin Sports Med.* 1991;10:783-788.

224. Chard M, Sattele L, Hazleman B. The long-term outcome of rotator cuff tendinitis--a review study. *Br J Rheum.* 1988;27:385-389.

225. Deutsch A, Altchek DW, Schwartz E, Otis JC, Warren RF. Radiologic measurement of superior displacement of the humeral head in the impingement syndrome. *J Shoulder Elbow Surg.* 1996;5:186-193.

226. Karduna AR, Williams GR, Williams JL, Iannotti JP. Kinematics of the glenohumeral joint: Influences of muscle forces, ligamentous constraints, and articular geometry. *J Orthop Res.* 1996;14:986-993.

227. Kelkar R, Flatow EL, Bigliani LU, Mow VC. The effects of articular congruence and humeral head rotation on glenohumeral kinematics. *Adv Bioeng.* 1994;28:19-20.

228. Kelkar R, Newton PM, Armengol J, et al. Glenohumeral kinematics. *J Shoulder Elbow Surg.* 1993;2(Suppl):S28.

229. Poppen NK, Walker PS. Forces at the glenohumeral joint in abduction. *Clin Orthop.* 1978;135:165-170.

230. Howell SM. Normal and abnormal mechanics of the glenohumeral joint in the horizontal plane. *J Bone Joint Surg.* 1988;70:227-235.

231. Kibler WB. Shoulder rehabilitation: principles and practice. *Med Sci Sports Exerc.* 1998;30:40-50.

232. Kibler BW. Normal shoulder mechanics and function. *Instr Course Lect.* 1997;46:39-42.

233. Neer CS II. Anterior acromioplasty for the chronic impingement syndrome in the shoulder: a preliminary report. *J Bone Joint Surg Am.* 1972;54:41-50.

234. Gartsman GM. Arthroscopic rotator cuff repair. *Clin Orthop Relat Res.* 2001;390:95-106.

235. Gordon EJ. Diagnosis and treatment of common shoulder disorders. *Med Trial Tech Q.* 1981;28:25-73.

236. Nixon JE, DiStefano V. Ruptures of the rotator cuff. *Orthop Clin North Am.* 1975;6:423-445.

237. Ellman H. Diagnosis and treatment of incomplete rotator cuff tears. *Clin Orthop.* 1990;254:64-74.

238. Goldberg BA, Nowinski RJ, Matsen FA III. Outcome of nonoperative management of full-thickness rotator cuff tears. *Clin Orthop Relat Res.* 2001;1:99-107.

239. Williams GR, Nguyen VD, Rockwood CA Jr. Classification and radiographic analysis of acromioclavicular dislocations. *Appl Radiol.* 1989;29-34.

240. Wirth MA, Rockwood CA Jr. Chronic conditions of the acromioclavicular and sternoclavicular joints. In: Chapman MW, ed. *Operative Orthopaedics.* 2nd ed. Philadelphia, PA: JB Lippincott; 1993:1673-1683.

241. Allman FL Jr. Fractures and ligamentous injuries of the clavicle and its articulation. *J Bone Joint Surg.* 1967;49A:774-784.

242. Rockwood CA. *Rockwood and Green's Fractures in Adults.* Philadelphia, PA: Lippincott; 1991:1181-1239.

243. Brue S, Valentin A, Forssblad M, Werner S, Mikkelsen C, Cerulli G. Idiopathic adhesive capsulitis of the shoulder: a review. *Knee Surg Sports Traumatol Arthrosc.* 2007;15(8): 1048-1054.

244. Reeves B. The natural history of the frozen shoulder syndrome. *Scand J Rheumatol.* 1975;4:193-196.

245. Nash P, Hazelman BD. Frozen shoulder. *Baillieres Clin Rheumatol.* 1989;3.

246. Shiri R, Viikari-Juntura E, Varonen H, Heliovaara M. Prevalence and determinants of lateral and medial epicondylitis: a population study. *Am J Epidemiol.* 2006;164:1065-1074.

247. Hong QN, Durand MJ, Loisel P. Treatment of lateral epicondylitis: where is the evidence? *Joint Bone Spine.* 2004;71:369-373.

248. Bailey RA, Brock BH. Hydrocortisone in tennis-elbow: a controlled series. *Proc R Soc Med.* 1957;50:389-390.

249. Bhatt JB, Glaser R, Chavez A, Yung E. Middle and lower trapezius strengthening for the management of lateral epicondylalgia: a case report. *J Orthop Sports Phys Ther.* 2013;43:841-847.

250. Johnson EW. Tennis elbow. Misconceptions and widespread mythology. *Am J Phys Med Rehabil.* 2000;79:113.

251. Chiumento AB, Bauer JA, Fiolkowski P. A comparison of the dampening properties of tennis elbow braces. *Med Sci Sports Exerc.* 1997;29:123.

252. Jobe FW, Ciccotti MG. Lateral and medial epicondylitis of the elbow. *J Am Acad Orthop Surgeons.* 1994;2:1-8.

253. Nirschl RP. Prevention and treatment of elbow and shoulder injuries in the tennis player. *Clin Sports Med.* 1988;7:289-308.

254. Krischek O, Hopf C, Nafe B, Rompe JD. Shock-wave therapy for tennis and golfer's elbow–1 year follow-up. *Arch Orthop Trauma Surg.* 1999;119:62-66.

255. Glousman RE, Barron J, Jobe FW, Perry J, Pink M. An electromyographic analysis of the elbow in normal and injured pitchers with medial collateral ligament insufficiency. *Am J Sports Med.* 1992;20:311-317.

256. Dun S, Loftice J, Fleisig GS, Kingsley D, Andrews JR. A biomechanical comparison of youth baseball pitches: is the curveball potentially harmful? *Am J Sports Med.* 2008;36:686-692.

257. DeKrom MC, Knipschild PG, Kester AD, et al. Carpal tunnel syndrome: prevalence in the general population. *J Clin Epidemiol.* 1992;45:373-376.

258. Stevens JC, Sun S, Beard CM, et al. Carpal tunnel syndrome in Rochester, Minnesota, 1961-1980. *Neurology.* 1988;38:134-138.

259. D'Arcy CA, McGee S. Does this patient have carpal tunnel syndrome? *JAMA.* 2000;283:3110-3117.

260. Heller L, Ring H, Costeff H, Solzi P. Evaluation of Tinel's and Phalen's signs in diagnosis of the carpal tunnel syndrome. *Eur Neurol.* 1986;25:40-42.

261. Kenneally M, Rubenach H, Elvey R. The upper limb tension test: the SLR of the arm. In: Grant R, ed. *Physical Therapy of the Cervical and Thoracic Spine.* New York, NY: Churchill Livingstone; 1988.

262. Kleinrensink GJ, Stoeckart R, Vleeming A, et al. Mechanical tension in the median nerve. The effects of joint positions. *Clin Biomech.* 1995;10:240-244.

263. Katz JN, Larson MG, Sabra A, et al. The carpal tunnel syndrome: diagnostic utility of the history and physical examination findings. *Ann Intern Med.* 1990;112:321-327.

264. Barnes CG, Currey HL. Carpal tunnel syndrome in rheumatoid arthritis: a clinical and electrodiagnostic survey. *Ann Rheum Dis.* 1970;26:226-233.

265. Feuerstein M, Burrell LM, Miller VI, Lincoln A, Huang GD, Berger R. Clinical management of carpal tunnel syndrome: a 12 year review of outcomes. *Am J Ind Med.* 1999;35: 232-245.

266. Szabo RM. Carpal tunnel syndrome-general. In: Gelberman RH, ed. *Operative Nerve Repair and Reconstruction.* Philadelphia, PA: JB Lippincott; 1991:882-883.

267. Onieal M-E. *Essentials of Musculoskeletal Care.* Rosemont, IL: American Academy of Orthopaedic Surgeons; 1997.

268. Taleisnik J. Classification of carpal instability. In: Taleisnik J, ed. The wrist. New York, NY: Churchill Livingstone; 1985: 229-238.

269. Von Schroeder HP, Botte MJ. Carpal tunnel syndrome. *Hand Clin.* 1996;12:643-655.

270. Chang MH, Chiang HT, Lee SSJ, et al. Oral drug of choice in carpal tunnel syndrome. *Neurology.* 1998;51:390-393.

271. De-la-Llave-Rincon AI, Fernandez-de-las-Penas C, Palacios-Cena D, Cleland JA. Increased forward head posture and restricted cervical range of motion in patients with carpal tunnel syndrome. *J Orthop Sports Phys Ther.* 2009;39: 658-664.

272. Bowles AP Jr, Asher SW, Pickett JB. Use of Tinel's sign in carpal tunnel syndrome [letter]. *Ann Neurol.* 1983;13:689-690.

273. Hartz CR, Linscheid RL, Gramse RR, et al. The pronator teres syndrome: compressive neuropathy of the median nerve. *J Bone Joint Surg.* 1981;1981:885-890.

274. Anto C, Aradhya P. Clinical diagnosis of peripheral nerve compression in the upper extremities. *Orthop Clin North Am.* 1996;27:227-245.

275. Cambell WW. diagnosis and management of common compression and entrapment neuropathies. *Neurol Clin.* 1997;15:549-567.

276. Lapidus PW, Fenton R. Stenosing tenovaginitis at the wrist and fingers: report of 423 cases in 269 patients. *Arch Surg.* 1952;64:475-487.

277. Muckart RD. Stenosing tendovaginitis of abductor pollicis brevis at the radial styloid (de Quervain's disease). *Clin Orthop.* 1964;33:201-208.

278. Finkelstein H. Stenosing tenovaginitis at the radial styloid process. *J Bone Joint Surg.* 1930;12A:509.

279. McFarlane RM, Albion U. Dupuytren's disease. In: Hunter JM, Schneider LH, Mackin EJ, Callahan AD, eds. *Rehabilitation of the Hand.* 3rd ed. St. Louis: CV Mosby; 1990:867.

280. Saar JD, Grothaus PC. Dupuytren's disease: an overview. *Plast Reconstr Surg.* 2000;106:125-136.

281. Hill NA, Hurst LC. Dupuytren's contracture. In: Doyle JR, ed. *Landmark Advances in Hand Surgery.* Philadelphia, PA: WB Saunders; 1989:349.

282. Luck JV. Dupuytren's contracture: a new concept of the pathogenesis correlated with surgical management. *J Bone Joint Surg Am.* 1959;41:635.

283. Rayan GM. Clinical presentation and types of Dupuytren's disease. *Hand Clin.* 1999;15:87.

284. Strickland JW, Leibovic SJ. Anatomy and pathogenesis of the digital cords and nodules. *Hand Clin.* 1991;7:645.

285. Eckhaus D. Dupuytren's disease. In: Clark GL, Aiello B, Eckhaus D, Shaw Wilgis EF, Valdata Eddington L, eds. *Hand Rehabilitation.* Edinburgh: Churchill Livingstone; 1993:37-42.

286. Lewis CL, Sahrmann SA. Acetabular labral tears. *Phys Ther.* 2006;86:110-121.

287. Byrd JW, Jones KS. Hip arthroscopy for labral pathology: prospective analysis with 10-year follow-up. *Arthroscopy.* 2009;25:365-368.

288. Fagerson TL. Hip. In: Wadsworth C, ed. *Current Concepts of Orthopedic Physical Therapy—Home Study Course.* La Crosse, WI: Orthopaedic Section, APTA; 2001.

289. Byrd JW. Labral lesions: an elusive source of hip pain case reports and literature review. *Arthroscopy.* 1996;12:603-612.

290. Groh MM, Herrera J. A comprehensive review of hip labral tears. *Curr Rev Musculoskelet Med.* 2009;2:105-117.

291. Narvani AA, Tsiridis E, Tai CC, Thomas P. Acetabular labrum and its tears. *Br J Sports Med.* 2003;37:207-211.

292. Martin RL, Enseki KR, Draovitch P, Trapuzzano T, Philippon MJ. Acetabular labral tears of the hip: examination and diagnostic challenges. *J Orthop Sports Phys Ther.* 2006;36:503-515.

293. Byrd JW, Jones KS. Diagnostic accuracy of clinical assessment, magnetic resonance imaging, magnetic resonance arthrography, and intra-articular injection in hip arthroscopy patients. *Am J Sports Med* 2004;32:1668-1674.

294. McCarthy J, Noble P, Aluisio F, Schuck M, Wright J, Lee J. Anatomy, pathologic features, and treatment of acetabular labral tears. *Clin Orthop Relat Res.* 2003;406:38-47.

295. Yazbek PM, Ovanessian V, Martin RL, Fukuda TY. Nonsurgical treatment of acetabular labrum tears: a case series. *J Orthop Sports Phys Ther.* 2011;41:346-353.

296. Fagerson TL. Hip pathologies: diagnosis and intervention. In: Magee DJ, Zachazewski JE, Quillen WS, eds. *Pathology and Intervention in Musculoskeletal Rehabilitation.* St. Louis, MO: Saunders; 2009:497-527.

297. Reddy A, Bage J, Levine D. The hip. *Independent Home Study Course.* LaCrosse, WI: Orthopedic Section, APTA; 2014.

298. Stanish WD, Lai A. New concepts of rehabilitation following anterior cruciate reconstruction. *Clin Sports Med.* 1993;12:25-58.

299. Daniel DM, et al. Fate of the ACL-injured patient. *Am J Sports Med.* 1994;22:642.

300. Arnoczky SP. Anatomy of the anterior cruciate ligament. In: Urist MR, ed. *Clinical Orthopedics and Related Research.* Philadelphia, PA: JB Lippincott; 1983:19-20.

301. Cabaud HE. Biomechanics of the anterior cruciate ligament. In: Urist MR, ed. *Clinical Orthopedics and Related Research.* Philadelphia, PA: JB Lippincott; 1983:26-30.

302. Arendt E, Dick R. Knee injury patterns among men and women in collegiate basketball and soccer. NCAA data and review of literature. *Am J Sports Med.* 1995;23:694-701.

303. Bjordal JM, Arnly F, Hannestad B, Strand T. Epidemiology of anterior cruciate ligament injuries in soccer. *Am J Sports Med.* 1997;25:341-345.

304. Clasby L, Young MA. Management of sports-related anterior cruciate ligament injuries. *AORN J.* 1997;66:609-625, 28, 30; quiz 32-36.

305. Mizuta H, et al. The conservative treatment of complete tears of the anterior cruciate ligament in skeletally immature patients. *J Bone Joint Surg Br.* 1995;77:890.

306. Parker AW, Drez D, Cooper JL. Anterior cruciate injuries in patients with open physes. *Am J Sports Med.* 1994;22:47.

307. Micheli LJ, Jenkins M. Knee injuries. In: Micheli LJ, ed. *The Sports Medicine Bible.* Scranton, PA: Harper Row; 1995:118-51.

308. Liu SH, et al. The diagnosis of acute complete tears of the anterior cruciate ligament. *J Bone Joint Surg Br.* 1995;77:586.

309. Gerber C, Hoppeler H, Claassen H, Robotti G, Zehnder R, Jakob RP. The lower-extremity musculature in chronic symptomatic instability of the anterior cruciate ligament. *J Bone Joint Surg Am.* 1985;67-A:1034-1043.

310. Kariya Y, Itoh M, Nakamura T, Yagi K, Kurosawa H. Magnetic resonance imaging and spectroscopy of thigh muscles in cruciate ligament insufficiency. *Acta Orthop Scand.* 1989;60:322-325.

311. Lorentzon R, Elmqvist LG, Sjostrom M, Fagerlund M, Fuglmeyer AR. Thigh musculature in relation to chronic anterior cruciate ligament tear: muscle size, morphology, and mechanical output before reconstruction. *Am J Sports Med.* 1989;17:423-429.

312. Noyes FR, Mangine RE, Barber S. Early knee motion after open and arthroscopic anterior cruciate ligament reconstruction. *Am J Sports Med.* 1987;15:149-160.

313. Yasuda K, Ohkoshi Y, Tanabe Y, Kaneda K. Quantitative evaluation of knee instability and muscle strength after anterior cruciate ligament reconstruction using patellar and quadriceps tendon. *Am J Sports Med.* 1992;20:471-475.

314. Daniel DM, Malcom LL, Losse G, Stone ML, Sachs R, Burks R. Instrumented measurement of anterior laxity of the knee. *J Bone Joint Surg.* 1985;67-A:720-725.

315. Indelicato PA, Bittar ES. A perspective of lesions associated with ACL insufficiency of the knee. A review of 100 cases. *Clin Orthop.* 1985;198:77-80.

316. Irvine GB, Glasgow MMS. The natural history of the meniscus in anterior cruciate insufficiency. Arthroscopic analysis. *J Bone Joint Surg.* 1992;74-B:403-405.

317. Frank CB, Jackson DW. The science of reconstruction of the anterior cruciate ligament. *J Bone Joint Surg.* 1997;79:1556-1576.

318. Kurosaka M, Yoshiya S, Mizuno T, Mizuno K. Spontaneous healing of a tear of the anterior cruciate ligament. A report of two cases. *J Bone Joint Surg Am.* 1998;80:1200-1203.

319. Williams JS, Bernard RB. Operative and nonoperative rehabilitation of the ACL-injured knee. *Sports Med Arth Rev.* 1996;4:69-82.

320. Hensler D, Van Eck CF, Fu FH, Irrgang JJ. Anatomic anterior cruciate ligament reconstruction utilizing the double-bundle technique. *J Orthop Sports Phys Ther.* 2012;42:184-195.

321. Antich TJ, Brewster CE. Rehabilitation of the nonreconstructed anterior cruciate ligament-deficient knee. *Clin Sports Med.* 1988;7:813-826.

322. Bynum WF. An experiment that failed: malaria control at Mian Mir. *Parassitologia.* 1994;36:107-120.

323. Frndak PA, Berasi CC. Rehabilitation concerns following anterior cruciate ligament reconstruction. *Sports Med.* 1991;12:338-346.

324. Mangine RE, Noyes FR, DeMaio M. Minimal protection program: advanced weight bearing and range of motion after ACL reconstruction-Weeks 1 to 5. *Orthopedics.* 1992;15:504-515.

325. Paulos LE, Noyes FR, Grood ES. Knee rehabilitation after anterior cruciate ligament reconstruction and repair. *Am J Sports Med.* 1981;9:140-149.

326. Pevsner DN, Johnson JRG, Blazina ME. The patellofemoral joint and its implications in the rehabilitation of the knee. *Phys Ther.* 1979; 59:869-874.

327. Seto JL, Brewster CE, Lombardo SJ. Rehabilitation of the knee after anterior cruciate ligament reconstruction. *J Orthop Sports Phys Ther.* 1989;11:8-18.

328. Shelbourne KD, Nitz P. Accelerated rehabilitation after anterior cruciate ligament reconstruction. *Am J Sports Med.* 1990;18:292-299.

329. Shelbourne KD, Wilckens JH. Current concepts in anterior cruciate ligament rehabilitation. *Orthop Rev.* 1990;19:957-964.

330. Silfverskold JP, Steadman JR, Higgins RW. Rehabilitation of the anterior cruciate ligament in the athlete. *Sports Med.* 1988;6:308-319.

331. Steadman JR. Rehabilitation of acute injuries of the anterior cruciate ligament. *Clin Orthop.* 1983;172:129-132.

332. Steadman JR, Forster RS, Silfverskold JP. Rehabilitation of the knee. *Clin Sports Med.* 1989;8:605-627.

333. Steadman JR, Sterett WI. The surgical treatment of knee injuries in skiers. *Med Sci Sports Exerc.* 1995;27:328-333.

334. Timm KE. Postsurgical knee rehabilitation. A five-year study of four methods and 5,381 patients. *Am J Sports Med.* 1988;16:463-468.

335. Zappala FG, Taffel CB, Scuderi GR. Rehabilitation of patellofemoral joint disorders. *Orthop Clin North Am.* 1992;23:555-565.

336. Kaplan Y. Identifying individuals with an anterior cruciate ligament-deficient knee as copers and noncopers: a narrative literature review. *J Orthop Sports Phys Ther.* 2011;41:758-766.

337. Arnoczky SP, Warren RF. Microvasculature of the human meniscus. *Am J Sports Med.* 1982;10:90-95.

338. Arnoczky SP, McDevitt CA, Schmidt MB, Mow VC, Warren RF. The effect of cryopreservation on canine menisci: a biochemical, morphologic, biomechanical evaluation. *J Orthop Res.* 1988;6:1-12.

339. Henning CE, Lynch MA, Yearout KM. Arthroscopic meniscal repair using an exogenous fibrin clot. *Clin Orthop.* 1990;252:64-72.

340. Henning CE, Lynch MA, Glick C. An in vivo strain gauge study of elongation of the anterior cruciate ligament. *Am J Sports Med.* 1985;13:22-26.

341. Henning CE. Current status of meniscal salvage. *Clin Sports Med.* 1990;9:567-576.

342. Logerstedt DS, Snyder-Mackler L, Ritter RC, Axe MJ, Orthopedic Section of the American Physical Therapy A. Knee pain and mobility impairments: meniscal and articular cartilage lesions. *J Orthop Sports Phys Ther.* 2010;40:A1-A35.

343. Lowery DJ, Farley TD, Wing DW, Sterett WI, Steadman JR. A clinical composite score accurately detects meniscal pathology. *Arthroscopy.* 2006;22:1174-1179.

344. Black JE, Alten SR. How I manage infrapatellar tendinitis. *Physician Sports Med.* 1984;12:86-90.

345. Clain MR, Baxter DE. Achilles tendinitis. *Foot Ankle.* 1992;13:482-487.

346. Puddu G, Ippolito E, Postacchini F. A classification of Achilles tendon disease. *Am J Sports Med.* 1976;4:145-150.

347. McCrory JL, Martin DF, Lowery RB, Cannon DW, Curl WW, Read HM Jr, et al. Etiologic factors associated with Achilles tendinitis in runners. *Med Sci Sports Exerc.* 1999;31:1374-1381.

348. Clement DB, Taunton JE, Smart GW. Achilles tendinitis and peritendinitis: etiology and treatment. *Am J Sports Med.* 1984;12:179-183.

349. James SL, Bates BT, Osternig LR. Injuries to runners. *Am J Sports Med.* 1978;6:40-49.

350. Clement DB, Taunton JE, Smart GW, McNicol KL. A survey of overuse running injuries. *Physician Sportsmed.* 1981;9:47-58.

351. Renstrom P, Johnson RJ. Overuse injuries in sports: a review. *Sports Med.* 1985;2:316-333.

352. Hess GP, Cappiello WL, Poole RM, Hunter SC. Prevention and treatment of overuse tendon injuries. *Sports Med.* 1989;8:371-384.

353. Voorn R. Case report: can sacroiliac joint dysfunction cause chronic Achilles tendinitis? *J Orthop Sports Phys Ther.* 1998;27:436-443.

354. Nichols AW. Achilles tendinitis in running athletes. *J Am Bd Fam Pract.* 1989;2:196-203.

355. Garrick JG. The frequency of injury, mechanism of injury, and epidemiology of ankle sprains. *Am J Sports Med.* 1977;5:241-242.

356. O'Donoghue DH. Treatment of ankle injuries. *Northwest Med.* 1958;57:1277-1286.

357. Attarian DE, McCracken HJ, Devito DP, McElhaney JH, W.E. Garrett J. Biomechanical characteristics of human ankle ligaments. *Foot Ankle.* 1985;6:54-58.

358. Thorndike A. *Athletic Injuries: Prevention, Diagnosis and Treatment.* Philadelphia, PA: Lea and Febiger; 1962.

359. Inman VT. Sprains of the ankle. In: Chapman MW, ed. *AAOS Instructional Course Lectures.* 1975;294-308.

360. O'Donoghue DH. *Treatment of Injuries to Athletes.* Philadelphia, PA: WB Saunders; 1976:698-746.

361. Gronmark T, Johnson O, Kogstad O. Rupture of the lateral ligaments of the ankle. *Foot Ankle.* 1980;1:84-89.

362. Iversen LD, Clawson DK. *Manual of Acute Orthopaedics.* Boston: Little, Brown and Company; 1982.

363. van Dijk CN, Lim LSL, Bossuyt PMM, Marti RK. Physical examination is sufficient for the diagnosis of sprained ankles. *J Bone Joint Surg Br.* 1996;78-B:958-962.

364. Prins JG. Diagnosis and treatment of injury to the lateral ligament lesion of the ankle: a comparative clinical study. *Acta Chir Scand.* 1978;(Suppl)486:3-149.

365. Stiell IG, McKnight RD, Greenberg GH, et al. Implementation of the Ottawa Ankle Rules. *JAMA.* 1994;271:827-832.

366. Leddy JJ, Smolinski RJ, Lawrence J, Snyder JL, Priore RL. Prospective evaluation of the Ottawa Ankle Rules in a University Sports Medicine Center. With a modification to increase specificity for identifying malleolar fractures. *Am J Sports Med.* 1998;26:158-165.

367. Stiell IG, Greenberg GH, McKnight RD, et al. Decision rules for the use of radiography in acute ankle injuries: refinement and prospective validation. *JAMA.* 1994;269:1127-1132.

368. van Rijn RM, van Os AG, Bernsen RM, Luijsterburg PA, Koes BW, Bierma-Zeinstra SM. What is the clinical course of acute ankle sprains? A systematic literature review. *Am J Med.* 2008;121:324-331, e6.

369. Balduini FC, Tetzelaff J. Historical perspectives on injuries of the ligaments of the ankle. *Clin Sports Med.* 1982;1:3-12.

370. Kerkhoffs GM, Handoll HH, de Bie R, Rowe BH, Struijs PA. Surgical versus conservative treatment for acute injuries of the lateral ligament complex of the ankle in adults. *Cochrane Database Syst Rev.* 2007:CD000380.

371. Roy S, Irvin R. *Sports Medicine—Prevention, Evaluation, Management, and Rehabilitation.* Englewood Cliffs, NJ: Prentice-Hall; 1983.

372. Crawford F. Plantar heel pain and fasciitis. *Clin Evid.* 2004;1589-1602.

373. Crawford F, Thomson C. Interventions for treating plantar heel pain. *Cochrane Database Syst Rev.* 2003;3.

374. Crawford F, Atkins D, Edwards J. Interventions for treating plantar heel pain. *Cochrane Database Syst Rev.* 2000;3.

375. Charles LM. Why does my foot hurt? Plantar fasciitis. *Lippincotts Prim Care Pract.* 1999;3:408-409.

376. Rathleff MS, Molgaard CM, Fredberg U, et al. High-load strength training improves outcome in patients with plantar fasciitis: a randomized controlled trial with 12-month follow-up. *Scand J Med Sci Sports.* 2015;25:e292-300.

377. Rompe JD, Schoellner C, Nafe B. Evaluation of low-energy extracorporeal shock-wave application for treatment of chronic plantar fasciitis. *J Bone Joint Surg Am.* 2002;84-A:335-341.

378. International Headache Society. The International Classification of Headache Disorders. 2nd ed. *Cephalalgia.* 2004;24:9-160.

379. Bogduk N. The anatomical basis for cervicogenic headache. *J Manip Physiol Ther.* 1992;15:67-70.

380. Jull G, Amiri M, Bullock-Saxton J, Darnell R, Lander C. Cervical musculoskeletal impairment in frequent intermittent headache. Part 1: Subjects with single headaches. *Cephalalgia.* 2007;27:793-802.

381. Nicholson GG, Gaston J. Cervical headache. *J Orthop Sports Phys Ther.* 2001;31:184-193.

382. Sizer PS, Jr., Phelps V, Brismee J-M. Diagnosis and management of cervicogenic headache and local cervical syndrome with multiple pain generators. *J Man Manip Ther.* 2002;10:136-152.

383. Lu J, Ebraheim NA. Anatomical consideration of C2 nerve root ganglion. *Spine.* 1998;23:649-652.

384. Bogduk N. An anatomical basis for the neck-tongue syndrome. *J Neurol Neurosurg Psychiatry.* 1981;44:202-208.

385. Polletti CE, Sweet WH. Entrapment of the C2 root and ganglion by the atlanto-epitrophic ligament: clinical syndrome and surgical anatomy. *Neurosurgery.* 1990;27:288-290.

386. Welch KM. A 47-year-old woman with tension-type headaches. *JAMA.* 2001;286:960-966.

387. McDonnell MK, Sahrmann SA, Van Dillen L. A specific exercise program and modification of postural alignment for treatment of cervicogenic headache: a case report. *J Orthop Sports Phys Ther.* 2005;35:3-15.

388. Hurwitz EL, Aker PD, Adams AH, Meeker WC, Shekelle PG. Manipulation and mobilization of the cervical spine. A systematic review of the literature. *Spine.* 1996;21: 1746-1759; discussion 59-60.

389. McKenzie RA. *The Cervical and Thoracic Spine: Mechanical Diagnosis and Therapy.* Waikanae, NZ: Spinal Publications; 1990.

390. Sjaastad O, Fredriksen TA, Pfaffenrath V. Cervicogenic headache: diagnostic criteria. The Cervicogenic Headache International Study Group. *Headache.* 1998;38:442-445.

391. Isacsson G, Linde C, Isberg A. Subjective symptoms in patients with temporomandibular disk displacement versus patients with myogenic craniomandibular disorders. *J Prosthet Dent.* 1989;61:70-77.

392. Paesani D, Westesson P-L, Hatala M, et al. Prevalence of temporomandibular joint internal derangement in patients with craniomandibular disorders. *Am J Orthod Dentofacial Orthop.* 1992;101:41-47.

393. Dolwick MF. Clinical diagnosis of temporomandibular joint internal derangement and myofascial pain and dysfunction. *Oral Maxillofac Surg Clin North Am.* 1989; 1:1-6.

394. Juniper RP. Temporomandibular joint dysfunction: a theory based upon electromyographic studies of the lateral pterygoid muscle. *Br J Oral Maxillofac Surg.* 1984; 22:1-8.

395. Porter MR. The attachment of the lateral pterygoid muscle to the meniscus. *J Prosthet Dent.* 1970;24:555-562.

396. Wongwatana S, Kronman JH, Clark RE, et al. Anatomic basis for disk displacement in temporomandibular joint (TMJ) dysfunction. *Am J Orthod Dentofacial Orthop.* 1994;105: 257-264.

397. Nassif NJ, Al-Salleeh F, Al-Admawi M. The prevalence and treatment needs of symptoms and signs of temporomandibular disorders among young adult males. *J Oral Rehabil.* 2003;30:944-950.

398. Reneker J, Paz J, Petrosino C, Cook C. Diagnostic accuracy of clinical tests and signs of temporomandibular joint disorders: a systematic review of the literature. *J Orthop Sports Phys Ther.* 2011;41:408-416.

399. Tasaki MM, Westesson PL. Temporomandibular joint: diagnostic accuracy with sagittal and coronal MR imaging. *Radiology.* 1993;186:723-729.

400. Carlsson GE, LeResche L. Epidemiology of temporomandibular disorders. In: Sessle BJ, Bryant PS, Dionne RA, eds. *Temporomandibular Disorders and Related Pain Conditions, Progress in Pain Research and Management.* Seattle: IASP Press; 1995:211-226.

401. Bell WE. *Orofacial Pains: Classification, Diagnosis, Management.* 3rd ed. Chicago: New Year Medical Publishers; 1985.

402. Weinstein JN. A 45-year-old man with low back pain and a numb left foot. *JAMA.* 1998;280:730-736.

403. Ito T, Takano Y, Yuasa N. Types of lumbar herniated disc and clinical course. *Spine.* 2001;26:648-651.

404. Bakhtiary AH, Safavi-Farokhi Z, Rezasoltani A. Lumbar stabilizing exercises improve activities of daily living in patients with lumbar disc herniation. *J Back Musculoskel Rehabil.* 2005;18:55-60.

405. Manniche C, Asmussen KH, Vinterberg H, Rose-Hansen EB, Kramhoft J, Jordan A. Back pain, sciatica and disability following first-time conventional haemilaminectomy for lumbar disc herniation. Use of "Low Back Pain Rating Scale" as a postal questionnaire. *Dan Med Bull.* 1994;41:103-106.

406. Saal JS, Franson R, Dobrow RC, et al. High levels of phopholipase A2 activity in lumbar disc herniation. *Spine.* 1990;15:674-678.

407. Turner JA, Ersek M, Herron L, Deyo R. Surgery for lumbar spinal stenosis: attempted meta-analysis of the literature. *Spine.* 1992;17:1-8.

408. Arnoldi CC, Brodsky AE, Cauchoix J. Lumbar spinal stenosis and nerve root encroachment syndromes: definition and classification. *Clin Orthop.* 1976;115:4-5.

409. Verbiest H. A radicular syndrome from developmental narrowing of the lumbar vertebral canal. *J Bone Joint Surg.* 1954;26B:230.

410. Huijbregts PA. Lumbopelvic region: aging, disease, examination, diagnosis, and treatment. In: Wadsworth C, ed. *Current Concepts of Orthopaedic Physical Therapy—Home Study Course.* La Crosse, WI: Orthopaedic Section, APTA; 2001.

411. Cailliet R. *Low Back Pain Syndrome.* 4th ed. Philadelphia, PA: FA Davis; 1991:263-268.

412. Postacchinia F, Perugia D. Degenerative lumbar spondylolisthesis. Part I: Etology, pathogenesis, pathomorphology, and clinical features. *Ital J Orthop Traumatol.* 1991;17:165-173.

413. Katz JN, Dalgas M, Stucki G, et al. Degenerative lumbar spinal stenosis: diagnostic value of the history and physical examination. *Arthritis Rheum.* 1995;38:1236-1241.

414. Weinstein SM, Herring SA. Rehabilitation of the patient with low back pain. In: DeLisa JA, Gans BM, eds. *Rehabilitation Medicine: Principles and Practice.* 2nd ed. Philadelphia, PA: JB Lippincott; 1993:996-1017.

415. Cook C, Brown C, Isaacs R, Roman M, Davis S, Richardson W. Clustered clinical findings for diagnosis of cervical spine myelopathy. *J Man Manip Ther.* 2010;18:175-180.

416. Dooley JF, McBroom RJ, Taguchi T, Macnab I. Nerve root infiltration in the diagnosis of radicular pain. *Spine.* 1988;13:79-83.

417. Tajima T, Furakawa K, Kuramochi E. Selective lumbosacral radiculography and block. *Spine.* 1980;5:68-77.

418. Fast A. Low back disorders: conservative management. *Arch Phys Med Rehabil.* 1988;69:880-891.

419. Fritz JM, Erhard RE, Vignovic M. A nonsurgical treatment approach to patients with lumbar spinal stenosis. *Phys Ther.* 1997;77:962-973.

420. Bodack MP, Monteiro M. Therapeutic exercise in the treatment of patients with lumbar spinal stenosis. *Clin Orthop Relat Res.* 2001;384:144-152.

421. Newman PH. The etiology of spondylolisthesis. *J Bone Joint Surg.* 1963;45B:39-59.

422. Yang K, King A. Mechanism of facet load transmission as a hypothesis for low back pain. *Spine.* 1984;9:557-565.

423. Laus M, Tigani D, Alfonso C, et al. Degenerative spondylolisthesis: lumbar stenosis and instability. *Chir Organi Mov.* 1992;77:39-49.

424. Booth FW. Physiologic and biochemical effects of immobilization on muscle. *Clin Orthop Relat Res.* 1987;219:15-21.

425. Eiff MP, Smith AT, Smith GE. Early mobilization versus immobilization in the treatment of lateral ankle sprains. *Am J Sports Med.* 1994;22:83-88.

426. Akeson WH, Amiel D, Mechanic GL, Woo SL, Harwood FL, Hamer ML. Collagen cross-linking alterations in the joint contractures: changes in the reducible cross-links in periarticular connective tissue after 9 weeks immobilization. *Connect Tissue Res.* 1977;5:15-19.

427. Akeson WH, Amiel D, Abel MF, et al. Effects of immobilization on joints. *Clin Orthop.* 1987;219:28-37.

428. Akeson WH, Amiel D, Woo SL-Y. Immobility effects on synovial joints: the pathomechanics of joint contracture. *Biorheology.* 1980;17:95-110.

429. Woo SL-Y, Matthews J, Akeson WH, Amiel D, Convery R. Connective tissue response to immobility: a correlative study of biochemical and biomechanical measurements of normal and immobilized rabbit knee. *Arthritis Rheum.* 1975;18:257-264.

430. Dehne E, Tory R. Treatment of joint injuries by immediate mobilization based upon the spiral adaption concept. *Clin Orthop.* 1971;77:218-232.

431. McKenzie R, May S. Introduction. In: McKenzie R, May S, eds. *The Human Extremities: Mechanical Diagnosis and Therapy.* Waikanae, NZ: Spinal Publications New Zealand Ltd; 2000:1-5.

432. Ertel AN, Millender LH, Nalebuff E. Flexor tendon ruptures in patients with rheumatoid arthritis. *J Hand Surg Am.* 1988;13A:860-866.

433. Stewart KM. Review and comparison of current trends in the postoperative management of tendon repair. *Hand Clin.* 1991;7:447-460.

CHECKLIST

When you complete this chapter you should be able to:

❑ Describe the various structures of the musculoskeletal system.

❑ Describe the axes and planes of motion about which body movements occur.

❑ Differentiate between osteokinematic and arthrokinematic motion.

❑ Explain the importance of the concave-convex rule as it pertains to joint mobilizations.

❑ Describe how the various musculoskeletal tissues respond to injury.

❑ Describe the various clinical signs and symptoms seen during the healing process of each of the musculoskeletal tissues.

❑ Describe how each of the various energy systems produce energy.

❑ Describe how each of the various energy systems work together during various levels of exercise intensity.

❑ Describe the functional anatomy and biomechanics of all of the major joints in the body.

❑ List the various components of a musculoskeletal physical therapy examination.

❑ Be able to describe and perform the various special tests designed for each of the major regions.

❑ Have a working knowledge of the more common orthopedic conditions in terms of their clinical significance, the tests and measures used to diagnose them, the interventions for each, and the differential diagnoses for each.

❑ Describe the various intervention principles used to treat orthopedic conditions.

❑ Outline the different kinds of orthopedic surgical repairs.

Neuromuscular Physical Therapy

Kristen Johnson and Heather David

■ ANATOMY AND PHYSIOLOGY OF THE NERVOUS SYSTEM

OVERVIEW

The nervous system is divided into the central nervous system (CNS) and the peripheral nervous system (PNS). The CNS contains the brain and spinal cord, while the PNS involves the spinal and cranial nerves and ganglia, the autonomic nervous system. Understanding neuroanatomy is critical to understanding brain functioning. Figure 3–1 illustrates the gross anatomical divisions of the CNS.

In the nervous system, it is important to understand the directional locations and planes of motion. Because the CNS bends around the closed system within the skull, planes are ventral-dorsal rather than anterior-posterior as noted in musculoskeletal anatomy. See Figure 3–2 for the directional planes in the nervous system.

High-Yield Terms to Learn

Neuroplasticity	An emerging body of research evidence to support the hypothesis that brain remodeling throughout life is possible and is enhanced by the type and amount of practice related to skill acquisition.
Neurologic examination	An essential component of a comprehensive physical examination, and includes the systems review and a comprehensive and systematic examination of both the central and peripheral nervous system in conjunction with other body systems. The examination should determine impairments in body function and structure, limitations in functional activities, and participation restrictions.
Cerebrovascular accident/ stroke	Occurs when there is interruption of blood flow within brain blood vessels, which can be a narrowing or blockage of the vessel (ischemia) or can be a rupture of a vessel (hemorrhage).
Traumatic brain injury (TBI)	Can result from a blow to the head and/or sudden acceleration–deceleration of the head, such as in motor vehicle accidents. TBIs can be closed or open, in terms of whether or not the skull is fractured.
Mild TBI (mTBI)	A brain injury that causes microscopic damage that may not be detectable on neuroimaging and may or may not involve a loss of consciousness.
Brain tumor	A mass or growth of abnormal cells in the brain.
Spinal cord injury (SCI)	An injury most commonly when there is fracture, dislocation, and/or subluxation of the vertebrae into the spinal cord.
Multiple sclerosis (MS)	A chronic, progressive, inflammatory disease that affects neurons in the central nervous system.
Parkinson's disease (PD)	The second most common, progressive neurodegenerative disorder with deficits in the basal ganglia and its connections to motor, cognitive, and psychiatric functions.
Huntington's disease (HD)	A progressive neurodegenerative disorder caused by an autosomal dominant mutation where there is a severe loss of neurons in the caudate and putamen of the basal ganglia.
Amyotrophic lateral sclerosis (ALS)	A slow, progressive, asymmetric atrophy with muscular weakness and hyperreflexia.

High-Yield Terms to Learn (continued)

Guillain–Barre syndrome (GBS)	A group of neuropathic conditions that affect the peripheral nervous system, causing progressive weakness due to motor neuropathy and diminished or absent reflexes.
Post-polio syndrome (PPS)	A condition that affects people who have a history of polio, followed by a period of neurological stability, and then develop new or exacerbated symptoms several years after the acute poliomyelitis infection.
Peripheral neuropathy	Damage to nerves which leads to impaired sensation, movement, gland, or organ function.
Vestibular disorders	Categorized by their location as peripheral, central, or both. Peripheral vestibular disorders involve the peripheral sensory apparatus and/or inner ear structures and/or the vestibular nerve. Central vestibular disorders result from damage to the vestibular nuclei, the cerebellum, and the brainstem, including vestibular pathways within the brainstem that mediate vestibular reflexes.
Outcome measure	A type of test and measure that can be used in the patient management process to assist in the diagnosis and prognosis of patient care in addition to tracking changes in human performance and health status.
Clinical practice guideline (CPG)	Recommendations based on the systematic review and evaluation of research evidence used to guide best practice for a specific condition.

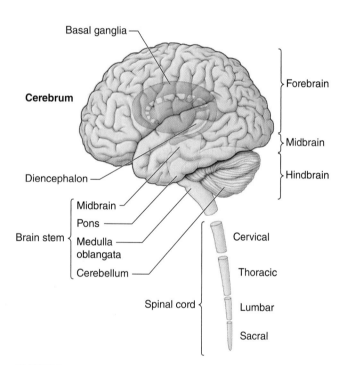

FIGURE 3–1 Gross anatomical divisions of the CNS. The cerebral hemispheres are found at the rostral end of the nervous system. The basal ganglia are contained within the cerebrum. The midbrain, pons, and medulla oblongata together are called the brainstem, and caudal to that is the spinal cord. Rostral to the midbrain is the diencephalon, the thalamus, and hypothalamus, which together with the cerebrum is called the forebrain. In this scheme (forebrain, midbrain, and hindbrain), the midbrain is itself, and the hindbrain is the pons, medulla, and cerebellum. (Adapted with permission, from Kandel ER, Schwartz JH, Jessell TM, Siegelbaum SA, Hudspeth AJ. Principles of Neural Science, 5th ed. New York, NY: McGraw-Hill; 2013, Box 1-1, Pg 9.)

Important distinctions in the nervous system are differences between gray and white matter. Gray matter includes neurons, glial cells, axons, and their synapses into and out of tissues. White matter is made up of myelin, axons, and glial cells. See Figure 3–3 for a visual depiction of gray and white matter in the nervous system.

Neuroanatomy can be clinically relevant when structure identification is paired with function. Understanding basic terms is critical in how nervous system structures work together, and they are often repeated and used interchangeably. See Table 3–1 for common neuroscience terms.

Central Nervous System

The CNS is composed of the brain and spinal cord. It is critical to understand how structures are connected to each other for functional clinical significance. It is important to understand the types of neurons, physiology, and mode of communication that is involved regarding how structures communicate with one another to command the PNS. Components of the CNS are identified in the following sections.

Cerebral Hemispheres

These involve a left and right hemisphere and collectively are referred to as the cerebrum. The cerebral hemispheres support functions of consciousness, memory, movement, sensation, emotion, and voluntary movement. The outermost layer is gray matter and is referred to as the cerebral cortex. Underneath this gray matter lie many additional gray matter structures, referred to as deep nuclei, such as the basal ganglia, which are interspersed with white matter structures that work to connect the cerebral hemispheres with other structures in the brain.

Meninges

The meninges are a set of membranes that encase the CNS. From outermost to innermost layer they are:

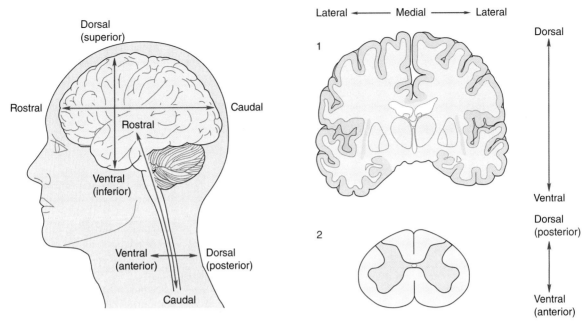

FIGURE 3-2 The directions used in the nervous system. The rostral direction is toward the nose and caudal is toward the tail. In the head of a person standing, rostral and anterior are roughly the same direction, and caudal and posterior are the same for the cerebral cortex. However, as the brainstem forms and descends into the spinal cord, the meanings of rostral and caudal shift. In the brainstem, rostral would be closer to the cerebrum and caudal would be closer to the spinal cord. Within the spinal cord, rostral would be toward the brainstem and caudal would be toward the coccygeal segments. In the person standing, for the spinal cord, rostral and superior are the same, and caudal and inferior are the same. The other directions used in the nervous system are dorsal, toward the back, and ventral, toward the front. The ventral side of the nervous system is the anterior part of the brainstem and spinal cord and the inferior part of the cerebrum. The dorsal part is the superior part of the cerebrum and the posterior part of the brainstem and spinal cord. Medial and lateral directions in the nervous system have the same meaning as in the regular cardinal planes. (Adapted with permission from Kandel ER, Schwartz JH, Jessell TM, et al. *Principles of Neural Science.* 5th ed. New York, NY: McGraw-Hill; 2013.)

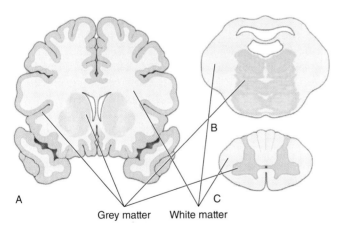

1. Dura matter, with its specialized infoldings of the falx cerebri and cerebellar tentorium, protects the brain and does not permit fluid to pass, with the exception of exchange through blood vessels.
2. Arachnoid matter is the middle layer and does not cover all surfaces of the brain as does the dura matter; directly under the arachnoid matter is the cerebrospinal fluid (SCF) and dural sinuses.
3. Pia mater is the innermost layer of meninges, which also seals and protects the brain as a component of the blood–brain barrier; it is very thin and is adherent to the nervous system within the deep crevices of the nervous tissue.

See Figure 3–4 for more details about the meninges.

FIGURE 3-3 Brain, brainstem, and spinal cord sections showing gray and white matter. All levels of the central nervous system have a combination of gray matter and white matter. Gray matter is composed of the neurons and the supporting cells, along with the connections between neurons. The gray matter is where the information processing of the brain occurs. White matter is composed of axons carrying information between parts of the nervous system. In the cerebral hemispheres, there is white matter in the middle forming connections, and gray matter at the surface and in nuclei within the brain. In the brainstem and spinal cord, there is white matter on the outside, and gray matter within. (Part B: Used with permission of John A. Buford, PT, PhD. Part C: Adapted with permission from Kandel ER, Schwartz JH, Jessell TM, Siegelbaum SA, Hudspeth AJ. *Principles of Neural Science.* 5th ed. New York, NY: McGraw-Hill; 2013, Fig 16–1, p 357.)

Lobes of the Brain

The cerebral hemispheres can be divided into four major lobes: frontal, parietal, occipital, and temporal. Two additional regions, once considered lobes, are the limbic and insular regions. See Figure 3–5 for details regarding lobes of the brain.

Frontal lobe—Begins at the central sulcus, and everything rostral is the frontal lobe. This lobe is responsible for thoughts, planning, decision-making, and actions. It is large in humans, and typically size is related to intelligence.

TABLE 3–1 Common terms in neuroscience.

Term	General Usage
Nucleus	A group of neurons in a gray matter structure that is anatomically relatively distinct from the surrounding tissue. A subnucleus would be a small nucleus that is a relatively distinct part of a larger nucleus.
Ganglion	Typically a nucleus located around the origin of a nerve; occasionally used instead of nucleus.
Cortex	The outer layer of the brain of both the cerebrum and the cerebellum, composed of gray matter.
Peduncle	A large bundle of axons that physically connects one structure to another.
Commissure	A group of axons travelling together to cross the midline.
Tract	A bundle of axons having a common origin, destination, and function.
Pathway	A route through which information travels, usually involving connections among multiple neurons. For example, there is a pathway from the cerebral cortex to the cerebellum that involves a connection with neurons in the brainstem. If the axons traveled directly from the cortex to the cerebellum, it would be called a tract, but because there is a connection to a neuron in the brainstem along the way, it is a pathway.
Lamina	A thin layer of white matter separating nuclei or subnuclei in gray matter.
Mesial	An inner surface formed by the apposition of two structures; in the nervous system, most commonly used along the midline where left and right parts of the brain are touching each other.

From Nichols-Larsen DS et al. *Neurologic Rehabilitation: Neuroscience and Neuroplasticity in Physical Therapy Practice.* New York, NY: McGraw Hill Professional; 2015. Table 1–1.

Parietal lobe—The rostral boundary is the central sulcus and the caudal boundary is the parietal-occipital sulcus. The parietal lobe is responsible for sensation and perceptions from the somatosensory systems of the skin, muscles, and joints but not special senses such as vision and hearing. The parietal lobe does integrate information from the special senses as related to our sense of overall perception.

Occipital lobe—Is bounded by the parietal lobe medially and the temporal lobe laterally. The occipital lobe's main function is for the special sense of vision. There are two specialized pathways for vision: the dorsal visual stream and the ventral visual stream. The dorsal visual stream is responsible for locating objected and integration vision into perception, along with the support of the parietal lobe. The ventral visual stream travels to the temporal lobe for object recognition and naming of objects.

Temporal lobe—Has no clear boundary between the temporal and occipital lobes; however, it is separated from the parietal and frontal lobes by the lateral sulcus. The temporal lobe is responsible for auditory processing as well as identification of objects, and memory.

Insular region/cortex—Is located deep in the lateral sulcus between the temporal and parietal lobes. This region can be identified in Figure 3–6. The insular region is responsible for digestive and eating functions, autonomic functions, and sensations of pain or pleasure.

Limbic region/cortex—Specifically the cingulate cortex, can be located superior to the corpus collasum and is responsible for basic functions and motivation for hunger, emotions, and initiation.

Subcortical Structures

These include important white and gray matter structures, as listed below.

Thalamus—A major gray matter nucleus comprised of multiple nuclei that serves as a major relay station for motor and sensory projections to and from the cerebral cortex. See Figure 3–6.

Basal ganglia—A collection of nuclei within the cerebral hemispheres that process information and send information by way of the thalamus back to the cortex. See Figures 3–1 and 3–6. Specific basal ganglia nuclei include the caudate and putamen (together called the striatum), the globus pallidus, the subthalamic nucleus, and the substantia nigra. The latter is located in the dorsal midbrain rather than within the cerebral hemispheres, and the subthalamic nucleus sits just below the thalamus within the portion of the brain known as the diencephalon (eg, thalamus, hypothalamus, epithalamus, and subthalamus). The caudate nucleus borders and follows the lateral ventricles. The globus pallidus and putamen appear as a single nucleus, referred to as the lenticular nucleus, just medial to the insular region.

Hypothalamus—Located inferior to the thalamus (see Figure 3–6) and is where hormones are regulated by the brain for thirst and hunger and are detected based on physiologic signals, sleep–wake cycles are determined, and many other basic physiological functions for homeostasis are regulated.

Hippocampal formation—Located in the medial aspect of the temporal lobe on the inferior surface of the brain. It is responsible for declarative memory, the ability to memorize information and experiences.

Amygdala—A nucleus located in the temporal lobe that can be found at the most rostral end of the hippocampal formation. It is responsible for the creation of memories, especially those related to intense emotions such as anger and fear.

Corpus callosum—Made up of axons that connect the right and left hemispheres primarily in the frontal and parietal lobes. See Figure 3–6.

Anterior commissure—A white matter structure that links the left and right hemispheres.

Internal capsule—Another white matter pathway that sends and receives information to/from the cerebral cortex, connecting information from the spinal cord and brainstem.

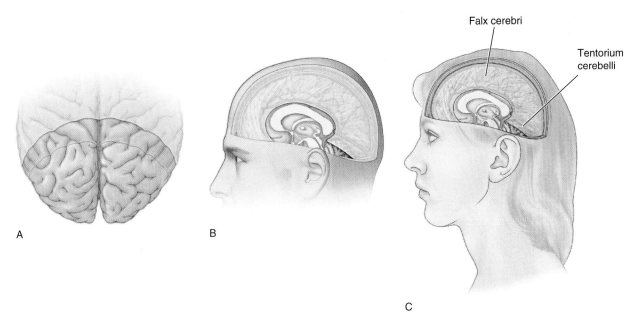

FIGURE 3–4 The meninges. A and B. This image of a brain shows layers of meninges removed, revealing the tough dura matter and the thinner arachnoid. The pia is continuous with the brain surface and cannot be distinguished without a microscope. C. The falx cerebri is a dura mater structure that separates the two cerebral hemispheres. (Part C: Reproduced with permission from Martin JH. *Neuroanatomy Text and Atlas*. 4th ed. New York, NY: McGraw-Hill; 2012, Figure 1–16B, p 25.)

Corona radiate—A significant amount of white matter which comprises the majority of the subcortical white matter, and due to its spanning bulk is not typically pictured on images. Most axons communicate from one portion of the cortex to another without passing through the thalamus.

Ventricular System

The ventricular system consists of the "spaces," or cavities, inside the brain and includes the ventricles, passageways between the ventricles, and structures called the choroid plexus that secrete and reabsorb CSF. The choroid plexus can be located within the lateral and fourth ventricles. The ventricular system consists of two lateral ventricles, one in each of the cerebral hemispheres, and a third and fourth ventricle. The third ventricle is a midline cavity located around the level of the midbrain, and the fourth ventricle is located between the brainstem and the cerebellum. CSF passes between the lateral and third ventricle through the interventricular foramen and between the third and fourth ventricles by the cerebral aqueduct.

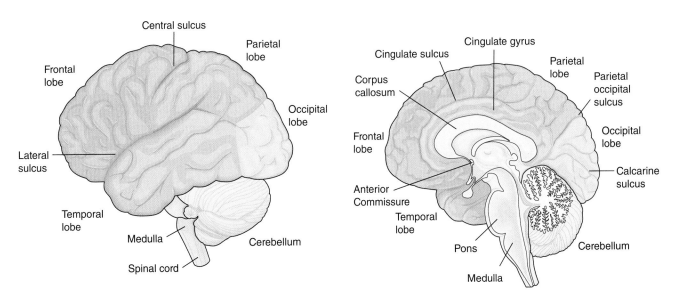

FIGURE 3–5 Lobes of the cerebral cortex and the landmarks structures that form their boundaries. On the left, a lateral view of the brain shows the four major lobes. The central sulcus and the lateral sulcus are visible here. On the right, the medial view of the brain is shown, with the brain split in the sagittal plane, along the midline. The parietal–occipital sulcus is visible here, along with the cingulate gyrus. (Adapted with permission from Martin JH. *Neuroanatomy Text and Atlas*. 3rd ed. New York, NY: McGraw-Hill; 2003. Figure 1–9, p 14.)

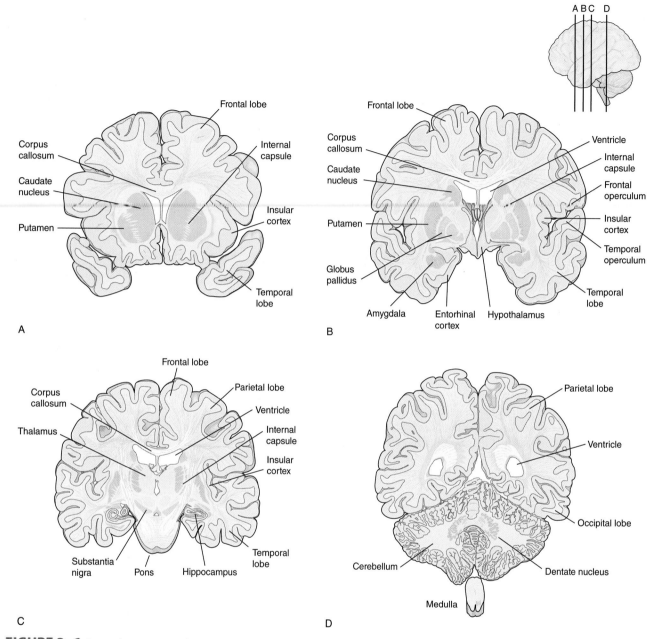

FIGURE 3–6 Internal structures in the cerebral cortex. The lateral view at the top right shows where each section was made. (Reproduced with permission from Nieuwenhuys R, Voogd J, and van Huijzen C. *The Human Central Nervous System: A Synopsis and Atlas.* 4th ed. Berlin: Springer-Verlag; 2008.)

- CSF travels the path as described above and exits through one of three major openings: the foramen of Magendie, which is a midline opening from the fourth ventricle to the posterior aspect of the medulla in the brainstem, and two lateral apertures, a left and right, called the foramina of Luschka, coming out from each side of the fourth ventricle in the space between the cerebellum and pons. The central canal of the spinal cord, forming in the caudal medulla, is also a place for CSF to leave the fourth ventricle; however, this space is small compared to the three major openings described above.
- Outside the ventricular system, CSF is in the subarachnoid space between the arachnoid and pia mater. Additionally,

venous sinuses are located in the dura mater, called arachnoid villi, and they permit slow leaking of the CSF into the venous blood to allow the fluid to return to its circulatory path.

Cerebellum

Cerebellum means "little brain" and has a major role in motor learning and coordination of voluntary movement. The cerebellum, like the cerebral hemispheres, has an outer layer of gray matter and an inner layer of white matter that works to connect the nervous system through the pathways connecting the brainstem, spinal cord, and cerebrum. See Figure 3–7. Cerebellar anatomy is described below.

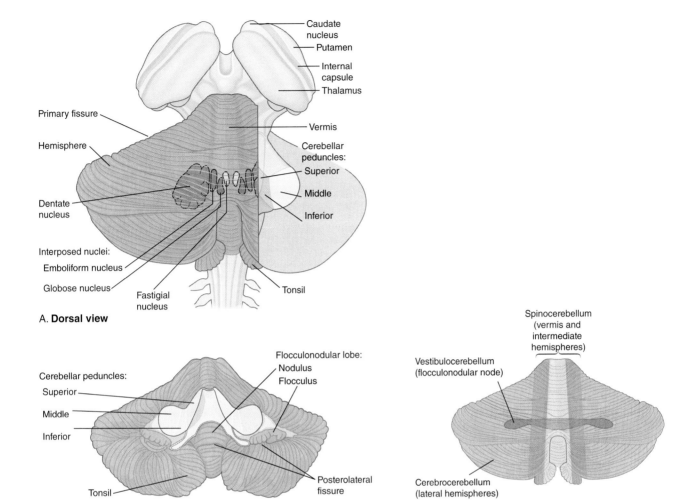

FIGURE 3–7 The cerebellum. **A.** The deep cerebellar nuclei within the cerebellum are illustrated. On the right, the cerebellum has been removed to show how the cerebellar peduncles come from the brainstem. **B.** This is the view of the cerebellum that would be seen from the front if it was removed from the brainstem. **C.** The functional regions of the cerebellum are shown. (Reproduced with permission from Nieuwenhuys R. *Chemoarchitecture of the Brain*. New York, NY: Springer-Verlag, 1985.)

Cerebellar cortex—Has three layers, each named by its structural features: a parallel fiber layer, a Purkinje layer, and a granular layer.

Deep cerebellar nuclei (DCN)—Deep gray matter structures that connect with specific areas of the cerebellar cortex. There are four specific DCN: the fastigial nucleus, the globose and emboliform nuclei, and the dentate nucleus.

Lobes of the cerebellum—The cerebellum can be divided into three lobes. The anterior lobe is the part underneath the occipital lobe, rostral to a cerebellar cortex structure called the primary fissure. The posterior cerebellum is everything else, with the exception of a small structure called the flocculonodular lobe, which is at the opposite end of the cerebellum from the anterior lobe and can be found on the anterior surface, opposed to the fourth ventricle. See Figure 3–7.

Functional divisions—The cerebellum can also be divided into functional divisions from a rehabilitation perspective. They are the vestibulocerebellum, the spinocerebellum, and the cerebrocerebellum. See Figure 3–7.

Connections—Each of the DCN is connected mainly with a certain functional division of the cerebellum.

- Vestibulocerebellum is connected to the fastigial nucleus, and its function relates to vestibular control of eye movement, posture, and balance.
- Spinocerebellum is connected to the fastigial, globose, and emboliform nuclei, receiving postural sensory information via the spinocerebellar tracts and projecting to the medial descending system (rubrospinal, vestibulospinal, and reticulospinal tracts) to control postural stability.
- Cerebrocerebellum is connected to the dentate nucleus, sending efferents via the thalamus to the motor cortex and other cortical areas to participate in motor planning and motor control.

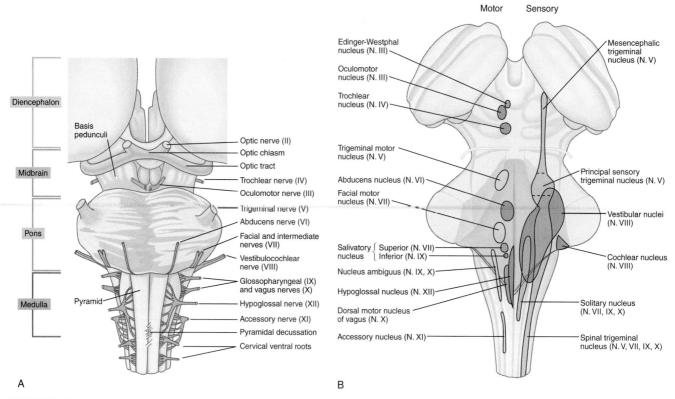

FIGURE 3–8 The cranial nerves. On the left (A), a ventral view of the brainstem and diencephalon shows where each of the cranial nerves exits the brainstem. On the right (B), a dorsal view shows where the cranial nerve nuclei are located for motor outputs and sensory inputs. (Modified with permission from Kandel ER, Schwartz JH, Jessell TM, Siegelbaum SA, Hudspeth AJ. *Principles of Neural Science*. 5th ed. New York, NY: McGraw-Hill; 2013, Figures 45–1 and 45–5, p 1020 and 1025.)

Cerebellar peduncles—There are three white matter connections located on each side of the cerebellum and brainstem. They are the inferior, middle, and superior cerebellar peduncles. See Figure 3–8.

Brainstem

The brainstem involves the midbrain, pons, and medulla, and all white matter communication between the brain and spinal cord passes through the brainstem. This major relay station is critical for many vital functions such as sensory, motor, and autonomic, and includes a role in more basic functions such as taste, eating, hearing, balance, and vision. In addition, the brainstem assists with the modulation of pain and supports functions such as posture, locomotion, and perception along with arousal and cardio-respiratory function. See Figure 3–8.

Brainstem structures—Some structures are isolated to a particular region of the brainstem, while others span the length of the brainstem in a rostro-caudal fashion.

- Trigeminal nucleus runs from the midbrain to the medulla to support both the sensory and motor functions of the trigeminal nerve.
- Reticular formation, which is a long column of gray matter found ventrolateral to the cerebral aqueduct and fourth ventricle extending from the midbrain to the medulla and supports the reticulospinal tracts, which are key regulators for posture, locomotion, and gross limb movements.

- Raphe nuclei have a variety of functions that regulate the state of other parts of the nervous system, including arousal, the spinal cord circuits for control of walking, and the transmission and modulation of pain.

Midbrain—This is the most rostral level of the brainstem and contains the most visible white matter structures, called the cerebral peduncles, which contain the axons from the cerebrum to the brainstem and spinal cord. Also within the midbrain are several important structures: substantia nigra, periaqueductal gray, red nucleus, superior colliculus, and the inferior colliculus.

Pons—The pons and medulla are distinguished from each other by the middle cerebellar peduncle. Within the pons, the ventral aspect contains the pontine nuclei in which synapses occur as information enters the cerebellum. In the dorsal aspect of the pons, the trigeminal nuclei for the fifth cranial nerve (CN V), the nucleus for the sixth cranial nerve, abducens (CN VI), and the nucleus for the seventh cranial nerve, the facial nerve (CN VII) can be located. The vestibular nuclei are in the pons slightly lateral to midline and just ventral to the fourth ventricle.

Medulla—The medulla is the caudal-most aspect of the brainstem, and its most prominent surface features anteriorly are the medullary pyramids and the inferior olives. In addition, there are other important nuclei, including the cranial nerve nuclei for nerves IX–XII (glossopharyngeal, vagus, spinal accessory, and hypoglossal) and the cardiorespiratory regulation centers.

Cranial nerves—See Table 3–2.

Major fiber tracts—There are major tracts on the surface of the brainstem including the cerebral and cerebellar peduncles, the medullary pyramids, and the dorsal columns. There are also certain internal white matter tracts of importance in rehabilitation. (See Figure 3–9.)

Spinal Cord

The spinal cord is the direct source of connection between the brain and the body. There are spinal nerves that exit at both the left and right sides of each vertebral body that receive afferent sensory information and transmit efferent motor information. Like the CNS, the spinal cord is surrounded by meninges to include the dura, arachnoid, and pia mater. Two special meningeal extensions of the spinal cord include the denticulate ligaments, which attach the spinal cord to the dura mater to assist with stability, and the filum terminale, which is an extension of the pia mater at the most caudal end of the cord. See Figure 3–10 for details.

When viewing the spinal cord, note the dorsal aspect containing the dorsal columns, which contain sensory fibers ascending toward the medulla. The ventral roots are formed by efferent axons of motor and autonomic projections from the spinal cord to the body. Two specialized regions of the spinal cord involve the cervical and lumbosacral regions; there is a lateral expansion of the ventral horns where limb muscle motoneurons are located.

Segmental organization of the spinal cord is organized for the vertebral bone that is formed alongside that particular segment during embryological development. Each segment contains a combination of the dorsal and ventral roots; the first spinal nerve exits the intervertebral foramen above the first cervical vertebra, and the eighth spinal nerve exits below the seventh cervical vertebra (above T1). These segments are referred to as the eight cervical segments. From here, each spinal segment is named by the vertebra above the exit of its spinal nerve, so the first thoracic segment has a spinal nerve that exits below the first thoracic vertebra. In summary, there are 8 cervical spinal segments, 12 thoracic, 5 lumbar, 5 sacral, and 1 coccygeal segmental levels in the human spinal cord, and an equal number of spinal nerves on each side.

In addition, the spinal cord supports complex communication within its own gray matter circuits for functions of flexor withdrawal, reflexive control of bowel and bladder function, and neural control of ambulation.

Sensory Pathways

Our sensation is comprised of complex networks, allowing humans to sense the perception of touch, muscle stretch and tension, joint pressure and motion, pain, pressure, temperature, vibration, and itch. The two essential sensory pathways, the dorsal column medial leminiscal system and the anterior lateral system should be reviewed relative to Figure 3–11.

Motor Pathways

Each of the four major descending motor systems has specific functions to support motor control. These systems are the corticospinal system, the rubrospinal tract, the reticulospinal system, and the vestibulospinal system. They should be reviewed with regard to origin, decussation as appropriate, and termination relative to Figure 3–11.

Peripheral Nervous System

The PNS is composed of the sensory and motor axons traveling into and out of the CNS. In the PNS, Schwann cells create the myelin. These cells cover only one segment of an axon. In most parts of the PNS, the spinal nerves exit the spinal cord and travel individually to innervate specific locations in the body; however, in both the lower cervical to include T1 and in the lumbosacral regions, spinal nerves are combined together to form a bundle of plexus of spinal nerves which innervate the arms, legs, and skin.

Autonomic Nervous System

The ANS is composed of two divisions: the sympathetic and parasympathetic divisions, which function to regulate vasculature, glands, and visceral organs. The sympathetic division is often known as the fight-or-flight response system because it is engaged when we are aroused, for example, in response to fear. The sympathetic division also contains the sympathetic chain ganglia, which are positioned along the length of the spinal cord to send efferent information to target organs. The parasympathetic division is often known as the rest-and-digest response system because it is engaged when we are relaxing; for example, when we are sleeping. In addition, the parasympathetic division also involves the cranial nerves, cranial nerve nuclei, and specialized structures in the sacral spinal cord. In the parasympathetic division, there are preganglionic neurons that project to target ganglia in the periphery, and postganglionic neurons that project to the target organs. These two powerful PNS divisions work together in conjunction with the CNS.

Summary

Table 3–3 provides an overview of the important structures and functions of the CNS.

Embryological Development of the Nervous System and Neuroplasticity

The nervous system arises from neural crest cells within the ectodermal layer of the developing embryo. The neural plate is altered by cell proliferation which then translates the neural plate into the neural tube. Further cell proliferation takes place and fosters the development of three vesicles into a five-vesicle structure identified by the telencephalon (cerebral hemispheres), diencephalon (retina, hypothalamus, thalamus, epithalamus, and

TABLE 3–2 Cranial nerves.

	Nerve	Name	Cranial Foramina	Functional component	Nucleus	Target	Function
Forebrain	I	Olfactory	Cribriform plate	SVA	Connects directly with forebrain	Nose: Olfactory mucosa	Smell
	II	Optic	Optic	SSA	Thalamus, lateral geniculate nucleus	Eye: Retina	Vision
Midbrain	III	Oculomotor	Superior orbital fissure	GSE	Oculomotor nucleus	Eyelid: Levator palpebrae superioris	Lid movements
						Eye muscles: Superior rectus, inferior rectus, medial rectus, inferior oblique	Eye movements
				GVE (Parasympathetic)	Edinger-Westphal nucleus	Pupil: Sphincter pupillae / Intraocular lens: Ciliary muscles	Pupillary constriction / Accommodation (focus of the eye)
	IV	Trochlear	Superior orbital fissure	GSE	Trochlear nucleus	Superior oblique muscle	Eye movement
	V	Trigeminal	V3, foramen ovale	GSA	Mesencephalic nucleus	Muscles of mastication	Proprioception
Pons	V	Trigeminal		GSA	Principal sensory nucleus	Face	Discriminative touch and vibration sense
				SVE	Motor nucleus	Muscles of mastication	Movement of mandible
	VI	Abducens	Superior orbital fissure	GSE	Abducens nucleus	Eye: Lateral rectus	Abduction of the eye
	VII	Facial	Internal auditory meatus	SVE	Facial nucleus	Face	Movement of muscles of facial expression; stylohyoid and posterior belly of digastric; stapedius
				GSA	Spinal nucleus of CN V	Ear	Sensation from external acoustic meatus and skin posterior to ear
				GVE (Parasympathetic)	Superior salivatory nucleus	Lacrimal, sublingual, and sub-mandibular glands	Lacrimation and salivation
				SVA	Nucleus solitarius	Anterior 2/3 of tongue	Taste
Medulla	VIII	Vestibulocochlear	Internal auditory meatus	SSA	Vestibular nuclear complex	Vestibulospinal tracts, vestibular nuclei, and cerebellum	Balance and reflex eye movements
				SSA	Cochlear nuclei	Inner ear: Organ of Corti	Hearing
	IX	Glossopharyngeal	Jugular	GSA	Spinal nucleus of V	Posterior 1/3 of tongue, tonsil, external ear, internal tympanic membrane, pharynx	Somatic sensation

Region	CN	Nerve	Foramen	Fiber type	Nucleus	Structure	Function
				GVA	Nucleus solitarius	Tongue and pharynx; Carotid body	Gag reflex; Chemoreceptors and baroreceptors
				SVA	Nucleus solitarius	Posterior 1/3 of tongue	Taste
				SVE	Nucleus ambiguus	Stylopharyngeus	Motor
				GVE (Parasympathetic)	Inferior salivatory nucleus	Parotid gland	Salivation
Medulla	V	Trigeminal		GSA	Spinal nucleus of V	Face	Pain and temperature
	X	Vagus	Jugular	GSA	Spinal nucleus of CN V	Posterior meninges, external acoustic meatus, skin posterior to ear	Somatic sensation
				GVA	Nucleus solitarius	Larynx, trachea, esophagus, thoracic viscera, abdominal viscera	Somatic sensation
						Aortic arch	Stretch and chemoreceptors for cardio-pulmonary system reflexes
				SVA	Nucleus solitarius	Taste buds in epiglottis	Taste
				SVE	Nucleus ambiguus	Pharyngeal muscles and intrinsic muscles of the larynx	Muscles of phonation and deglutition
				GVE (Parasympathetic)	Dorsal motor nucleus of vagus	Cervical, thoracic, and abdominal viscera; ganglion neurons located in/near target organ	Smooth muscle and glands of pharynx, larynx, thoracic viscera, abdominal viscera
				GVE	Nucleus ambiguus	Cardiac muscle	Decrease heart rate and blood pressure
	XI	Accessory	Jugular	SVE	Spinal accessory nucleus; nucleus ambiguus	Sternocleidomastoid and trapezius	Shoulder and neck movement
	XII	Hypoglossal	Hypoglossal canal	GSE	Hypoglossal nucleus	Hyoglossus, genioglossus, styloglossus, intrinsic muscles of tongue	Movement of the tongue

From Mosconi T, Graham V. *Neuroscience for Rehabilitation.* New York, NY: McGraw Hill Professional; 2018. Table 6–2.

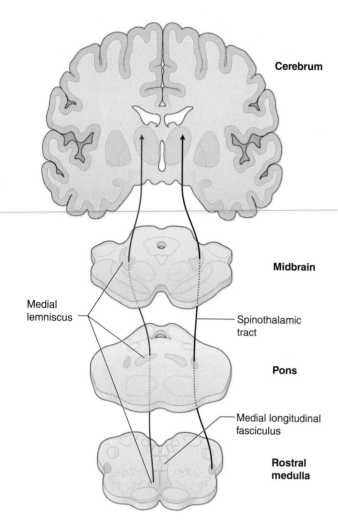

Cerebrum

Midbrain

Medial lemniscus

Spinothalamic tract

Pons

Medial longitudinal fasciculus

Rostral medulla

FIGURE 3–9 Selected fiber tracts in the brainstem. The medial lemniscus and spinothalamic tracts carry sensory information upward toward the brain. The medial longitudinal fasciculus carries oculomotor control signals as well as commands for head and neck movements. (From Nichols-Larsen DS, Kegelmeyer DA, Buford JA, Kloos AD, Heathcock JC, Basso D. *Neurologic Rehabilitation: Neuroscience and Neuroplasticity in Physical Therapy Practice*; 2016 Available at: http://accessphysiotherapy.mhmedical.com/content.aspx?bookid =1760&sectionid=120047286. Accessed January 04, 2018.)

subthalamus), mesencephalon (midbrain), metencephalon (pons, cerebellum), and myelencephalon (medulla), which is contiguous with the remainder of the neural tube that forms the spinal cord. The space or lumen of the neural tube eventually develops into the entire ventricular system and central spinal canal. See Figure 3–12 for identification of further developing cellular layers. Additional terms related to developmental neuroplasticity are listed below. Figure 3–12 provides an image and further explanation.

- **Neurogenesis** refers to the development of neurons, and **gliogenesis** is the development of glial cells; these are inter-related processes.
- **Pruning** is the elimination of unnecessary axon collaterals.
- **Programmed cell death** is the destruction of neurons.

- **Long-term potentiation (LTP)** is associated with well-established connections in developing synapses and relates to axon survival and the entire strengthening of the neuronal network.

Adult Neurogenesis

Gliogenesis continues throughout the brain and spinal cord into adult life, while neurogenesis is mainly related to embryological and early postnatal development. The one noted exception is that neurogenesis does occur in adults in locations near the hippocampus and olfactory bulb. Synaptogenesis in damaged pathways due to disease is unlikely.

Learning-Associated Neuroplasticity

There is an emerging body of research evidence to support the hypothesis that brain remodeling throughout life is possible and is enhanced by the type and amount of practice related to skill acquisition. LTP is mediated by several neurotransmitters and endogenous factors, along with brain-derived neurotrophic factor (BDNF) appearing to assist with synaptogenesis and supporting the formation of the synapse as related to the motor map reorganization. This then leads to angiogenesis, expansion of the capillary beds, and permits an increased vascular density that supports the new synaptic communication.

Neuronal Response to Injury

Below are several important definitions related to the CNS's response to injury:

- **Focal degeneration**—disruption of cellular function within the cell body of the neuron and leads to cell death.
- **Remote neurodegeneration**—commonly occurs after neural injury and leads to the loss of neurons in the area surrounding the focal injury and at sites distal to but functionally related to the injured area.
- **Inflammation**—occurs at the site of injury as well as in areas distant from the initial injury over approximately a 2- to 3-week period.
- **Excitotoxicity**—the excessive release of glutamate, dopamine, and norepinephrine that occurs as a result of CNS trauma or ischemia.
- **Apoptosis**—programmed cell death that occurs in neural development but also in response to neural injury.
- **Autophagy**—a natural process to eliminate damaged proteins or organelles within the cell body to promote optimal cell functioning.

Neuroplasticity after CNS Injury

Plasticity Promoters

Post injury, there are neural changes that work to support and strengthen the surviving neurons and their synapses to facilitate new axon and dendrite connections. The several known endogenous promotors of plasticity include neurotrophins such as BDNF and neurotrophin-3 (NT-3) that assist post CNS injury. These endogenous neurotrophins can be enhanced by exercise both in the spinal cord and in the muscles.

Spontaneous Recovery

Spontaneous recovery is dependent on the integrity of the surrounding CNS tissue. After neural shock, research has shown

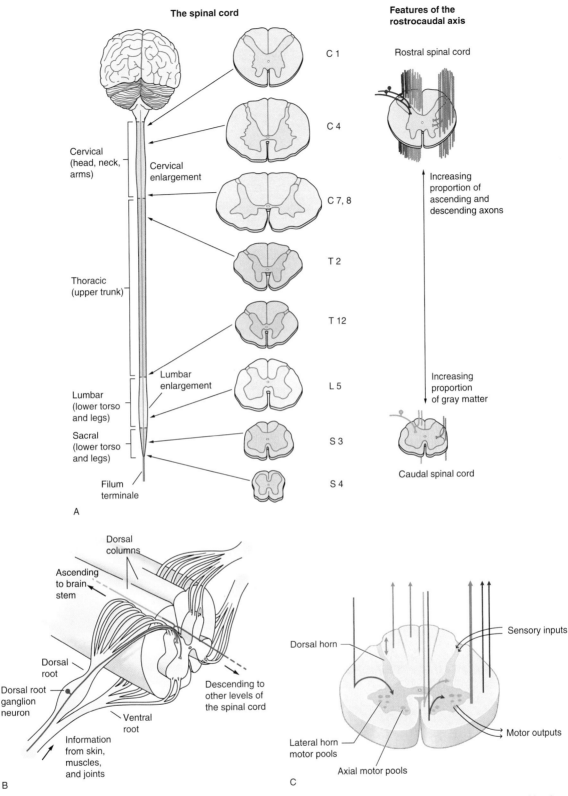

The spinal cord

C 1

C 4

C 7, 8

T 2

T 12

L 5

S 3

S 4

Cervical (head, neck, arms)

Cervical enlargement

Thoracic (upper trunk)

Lumbar enlargement

Lumbar (lower torso and legs)

Sacral (lower torso and legs)

Filum terminale

A

Features of the rostrocaudal axis

Rostral spinal cord

Increasing proportion of ascending and descending axons

Increasing proportion of gray matter

Caudal spinal cord

Dorsal columns

Ascending to brain stem

Dorsal root

Dorsal root ganglion neuron

Ventral root

Information from skin, muscles, and joints

Descending to other levels of the spinal cord

B

Dorsal horn

Lateral horn motor pools

Axial motor pools

Sensory inputs

Motor outputs

C

FIGURE 3–10 The spinal cord. A. The spinal cord carries all information between the brain and the body except that carried by the cranial nerves. There are enlargements at the cervical and lumbosacral levels to contain the extra gray and white matter for the arms and legs. Cross-sections representative of each segmental level are illustrated. Note how the relative proportion of white matter decreases at lower levels; few sensory axons have accumulated from below, and most motor axons have already terminated at levels above. B. The organization of a typical spinal segment is shown, including the dorsal roots, ventral roots, dorsal root ganglion, and spinal nerve. C. The general organization of information moving up and down the spinal cord is shown. Descending fibers (red) can travel in the lateral or ventral funiculus. Ascending fibers travel in the lateral and dorsal funiculus, some bound for the brain (green) and some for the cerebellum (purple). Special systems also descend to release neuromodulators that regulate spinal cord circuits (orange). (A: Reproduced with permission from Kandel ER, Schwartz JH, Jessell TM, Siegelbaum SA, Hudspeth AJ. *Principles of Neural Science.* 5th ed. New York, NY: McGraw-Hill; 2013, Figure 16–2, p 359. B: Reproduced with permission from Kandel ER, Schwartz JH, Jessell TM, Siegelbaum SA, Hudspeth AJ. *Principles of Neural Science.* 5th ed. New York, NY: McGraw-Hill; 2013, Figure 16–3 p 360.)

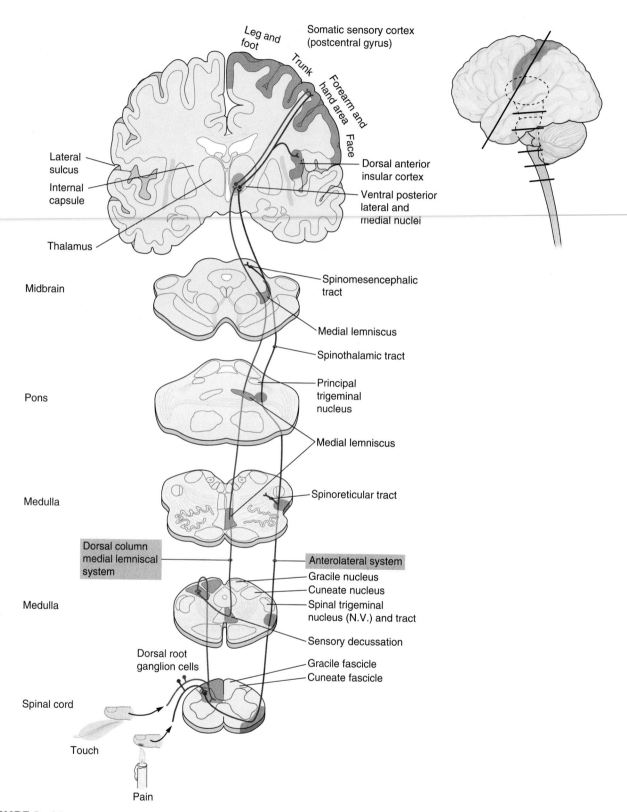

FIGURE 3–11 Ascending somatosensory pathways. (Reproduced with permission from Kandel ER, Schwartz JH, Jessell TM, Siegelbaum SA, Hudspeth AJ. *Principles of Neural Science.* 5th ed. New York, NY: McGraw-Hill; 2013, Figure 22–11, p 493.)

TABLE 3–3 Major structures and landmarks in the nervous system, with emphasis on function in sensory and motor systems.

Structure	Functions
Meninges	Protect the brain and spinal cord
Lobes of the Cerebrum	
Frontal	Motor planning and initiation, language output, personality, problem solving, insight, and foresight
Parietal	Sensory perception and integration, visual location, auditory location, music appreciation
Occipital	Vision (primary visual cortex and visual association cortex)
Temporal	Auditory processing, especially language, identification of objects, learning, and memory
Insular	Gustatory (taste) perception
Limbic	Emotional responses, drive-related behavior, and emotional memory
Major Cortical Landmarks	
Central sulcus	Divides frontal and parietal lobes
Parieto–occipital sulcus	Divides parietal and occipital lobes
Lateral sulcus	Superior border of temporal lobe
Cingulate sulcus	Superior border of limbic lobe
Precentral gyrus	Primary motor cortex
Postcentral gyrus	Primary sensory cortex
Posterior parietal association area	Integration of body awareness with visual perception
Subcortical Structures	
Lateral ventricle	C-shaped chambers in each cerebral hemisphere where most of the cerebrospinal fluid (CSF) is made; communicate with the third ventricle via the two interventricular foramen
Third ventricle	Midline cavity in diencephalon that connects with the fourth ventricle via the cerebral aqueduct
Fourth ventricle	Tent-like cavity between the cerebellum posteriorly and the pons and rostral medulla anteriorly that communicates with subarachnoid space
Choroid plexus	Vascularized tissue that secretes CSF
Cerebral aqueduct	Narrow channel through the midbrain that connects the third and fourth ventricles
Foramen of Magendie	Median aperture (opening) of fourth ventricle through which CSF flows into the subarachnoid space
Foramina of Luschka	Two lateral apertures of fourth ventricle through which CSF flows into the subarachnoid space
Basal Ganglia	Initiation and selection of thoughts and especially actions
Caudate nucleus	Receives information primarily from association areas of the cerebral cortex; important for cognitive functions of the basal ganglia
Head	Rostral—main target for prefrontal cortex
Body	Superior—parietal areas
Tail	Wraps around into the temporal lobe—temporal areas
Putamen	Functionally and cellularly just like the caudate, but anatomically separated from caudate by fibers of the internal capsule. Receives information primarily from motor and somatosensory areas of the cerebral cortex; important for motor functions of the basal ganglia
Striatum	A name used to refer to the caudate and putamen in combination
Globus pallidus—external segment (GPe)	One target of output from striatum. Involved in intermediate stage of basal ganglia processing
Globus pallidus—internal segment (GPi)	Final output nucleus targeted by GPe and STN—has neurons with axons leaving basal ganglia to go to the thalamus and thereby influence cortex and the control of movement
Subthalamic nucleus	Works with GPe for intermediate steps in basal ganglia processing
Substantia nigra	The largest nucleus in the midbrain
Pars compacta (SNpc)	Location of dopamine-producing cells that project into the striatum (caudate and putamen) to control movement
Pars reticulata (SNpr)	Just like cells in GPi but SNpr cells control eye movements, while GPi cells are for the rest of the body
Internal capsule	Funnel-shaped region separating the thalamus from the basal ganglia; contains fiber tracts that relay almost all of the information going to and from the cerebral cortex and other (noncortical) parts of the brain
Hippocampus	Memory formation (declarative)

(Continued)

TABLE 3–3 Major structures and landmarks in the nervous system, with emphasis on function in sensory and motor systems. (*Continued*)

Structure	Functions
Amygdala	Emotions, learning whether something is "good" or "bad," aggression
Thalamus	Receives, filters, and distributes information bound for the cerebral cortex
Hypothalamus	Autonomic functions, drives, hormones
Cerebellum	Receives information from sensory systems, the cerebral cortex and other sites, and participates in the planning and coordination of movement
Cerebellar cortex	Three-layered structure that receives cerebellar inputs and projects them to the deep cerebellar nuclei
Folia	Repeated horizontal folds or gyri of the cerebellum
Vermis	Midline lobe of the cerebellum important for cerebellar control of body and posture
Flocculonodular lobe	Cerebellar control for vestibular responses and eye movements
Spinocerebellum	Consists of the vermis and medial parts of the lateral cerebellar hemispheres that receive spinal inputs; involved with regulation of posture and coordination of limb movements
Lateral cerebellar hemispheres	Main lobes of the cerebellum on each side of the vermis; medial part is part of spinocerebellum as stated above; lateral parts are part of the cerebrocerebellum, a functional division that communicates with the cerebral cortex for the coordination of motor planning and to some extent the coordination of higher order thought processes
Deep cerebellar nuclei	Location for cells send axons projecting out of the cerebellum to affect other parts of the nervous systems, especially the brainstem and (via the thalamus) the cortex
Brainstem	Consists of the midbrain, pons, and medulla
Midbrain	The most rostral of the three subdivisions of the brainstem
Cerebral peduncles	Two large cylindrical masses on ventral surface of midbrain containing descending motor fibers from the cortex
Red nucleus	Involved in cerebellar circuitry and in control of limb movements, especially shaping the hand during reaching
Cerebral aqueduct—PAG	Site of origin of a descending pain-control pathway
Superior colliculi	Involved in directing visual attention and controlling eye movements
Inferior colliculi	Major link in the auditory system
Pons	The second of the three parts of the brainstem, continuous rostrally with the midbrain and caudally with the medulla
Pontine nuclei	Nuclei in the basal pons that receive inputs from the cerebral cortex and project to contralateral cerebellum
Cerebellar peduncles	Three paired fiber bundles connecting the cerebellum and brainstem via cerebellar afferents and efferents
Vestibular nuclei	Involved in regulating posture and coordinating eye and head movements
Reticular formation	Complex network of nuclei involved in integrative functions such as control of complex movements, transmission of pain information, vital functions, and arousal and consciousness
Medulla	The most caudal of the three subdivisions of the brainstem
Pyramids	Two rounded masses on the ventral surface of the medulla containing motor fibers
Inferior olivary complex	Origin of "climbing fibers" to cerebellum that are involved in motor learning
Dorsal column nuclei	Nuclei for relay of proprioceptive and discriminative touch for dorsal column-medial lemniscus system
Vestibular nuclei	Involved in regulating posture and coordinating eye and head movements
Reticular formation	Complex network of nuclei involved in integrative functions such as control of complex movements, transmission of pain information, vital functions, and arousal and consciousness
Spinal cord	Conducts sensory/motor information to/from the brain; contains central pattern generators for control of walking
White matter	Fiber tracts (ie, myelinated axons) that carry information up and down
Gray matter	Contains neuronal cell bodies and reflex circuits
Cervical enlargement (C5–T1)	Expanded gray matter to control the arms, and expanded white matter for incoming and outgoing information
Lumbar enlargement (L2–S3)	Expanded gray area to control the legs, and expanded white matter for incoming and outgoing information
Dorsal roots	Incoming (sensory) information
Ventral roots	Outgoing (motor) commands
Spinal nerves	Where dorsal and ventral roots fuse before exiting the intervertebral foramina
Cauda equina	Spinal nerves in lower vertebral column on their way to their original foramina (vertebral column longer than spinal cord in adults)
Sympathetic chain	Series of interconnected ganglia that lie ventral and lateral to the vertebral column that contain cell bodies of post-ganglionic neurons in the sympathetic nervous system
Corpus callosum	White matter fiber tracts connecting left and right cerebral hemispheres

From Nichols-Larsen DS et al. *Neurologic Rehabilitation: Neuroscience and Neuroplasticity in Physical Therapy Practice*. New York, NY: McGraw Hill Professional; 2015. Unnumbered table, Chapter 1.

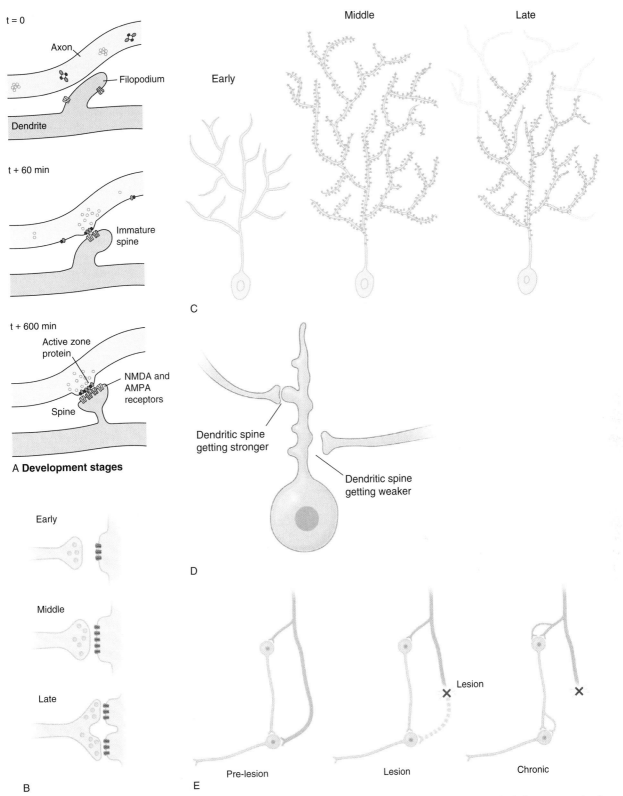

FIGURE 3–12 Synaptogenesis, pruning, and sprouting—mechanisms of neural development and injury repair. A. An axon passing by a cell can develop a new branch called a filopodium, which begins to form a synapse, and eventually becomes functional. The postsynaptic member begins to develop a synaptic spine. B. When a synapse strengthens over time, the presynaptic and postsynaptic elements can enlarge, and eventually, a second synapse can develop. C. As neurons develop, they initially lack synaptic spines. In the middle phase of development, they have an overabundance. As the connections mature, there is pruning, and some spines are eliminated. D. A dendritic spine can become stronger or weaker over time as the plasticity develops. E. In a circuit with alternative pathways, if one route is lesioned, the other can become stronger and replace the lost function. (A: Reproduced with permission from Kandel ER, Schwartz JH, Jessell TM, Siegelbaum SA, Hudspeth AJ. *Principles of Neural Science.* 5th ed. New York, NY: McGraw-Hill; 2013. Figure 55–14A, p 1250. C: From Kandel ER, Schwartz JH, Jessell TM, Siegelbaum SA, Hudspeth AJ. *Principles of Neural Science.* 5th ed. New York, NY: McGraw-Hill; 2013. Figure 54–3, p 1213. Reproduced, with permission, from Prof. Dr. Stefan W. Hell. Parts B, D, and E: Used with permission of John A. Buford, PT, PhD.)

neuronal outgrowth, local sprouting, synaptogenesis, and angiogenesis. Sprouting is a mechanism by which axons grow additional distal projections to fill empty receptor sites.

Experience-Dependent Plasticity

This depends on the activities of the patient post injury, and can be influenced by physical therapy interventions. The physical therapist must be aware that plasticity can be both adaptive and maladaptive.

Maladaptive plasticity—Can be best described as learned nonuse. Nonuse is a process in which patients experience negative feedback—for example, when attempting to use their paretic arm after a stroke—and this experience discourages use of the extremity even though spontaneous recovery is occurring. In addition, the patient will then use the less-involved extremity and is thus rewarded to complete compensatory strategies which result in less and less use of the more involved extremity.

Adaptive plasticity—Is best described through the research of constraint-induced movement therapy (CIMT). See Figure 3–13.

One of the seminal articles by Kleim and colleagues outline the key principles related to adaptive plasticity. See outline in Box 3–1.

Physical therapists, along with other members of the rehabilitation team, play a critical role in neural recovery when, using research and theories of neuroplasticity, they direct targeted intervention programs. The potentially critical period post injury is when the nervous system has the greatest opportunity for remodeling. Physical therapists should emphasize task-specific training for new skill acquisition in addition to translating the research regarding the importance of aerobic activity to raise BDNF, protein, and microRNA levels that support neuroplasticity mechanisms.

Special Senses that Interact with CNS

The special senses of vision, smell, taste, vestibular, hearing, and proprioception and their interactions with the central nervous system are reviewed in the following sections.

Vision

The eye—Figure 3–14 represents the anatomy of the eye and Box 3–2 outlines the major functions.

Visual field(s)—Is the view of the environment without eye movement. See Figure 3–15 for the schematic of visual fields.

Visual receptors—Are the rod and cone cells, which are both photosensitive.

Visual processing—This is complex pathway, as visual projection is supported on the cornea and the pathway eventually ends up at the visual cortex. Figure 3–16 represents this pathway.

Eye movement and visual pursuit—The eye has six muscles, which are innervated by cranial nerves (CN) III, IV, and VI.

CN III innervates the superior rectus, inferior rectus, medial rectus, and inferior oblique. CN IV innervates the superior oblique, and CN VI innervates the lateral rectus. The medial and lateral recti produce medial (adduction) and lateral (abduction) horizontal movements. Similarly, the superior and inferior recti pull the eye upward (elevation) and downward (depression), respectively, but because of their oblique insertions on the eye, also pull the eyes inward, so with superior rectus contraction the eye moves up and in, and conversely, the inferior rectus contraction pulls the eye down and in to look at the tip of the nose. Both oblique muscles attach to the eye on the posterolateral surface, the superior oblique attaches on the superior aspect of the eye and orients the eye downward and laterally, while the inferior oblique attaches on the inferior aspect and orients the eye upward and laterally.

Smell

Olfaction—This is phylogenetically the oldest sensory system, and in nonhumans plays a critical role in survival to locate food.

Olfactory receptors—These are in the bipolar cells of the nasal epithelium and project multiple cilia into the mucosa that covers the epithelial layer. Only airborne chemicals that are soluble in the mucosa can activate the olfactory neurons, and these axons pass through the bony cribriform plate at the top of the nasal passage and make up CN I—olfactory nerve. A synapse occurs in the olfactory bulb and magnifies the olfactory communication. From here the olfactory tract projects to the higher cortical centers for processing. See Figure 3–17 for more details.

Cortical processing of olfaction—This can be viewed in Figure 3–18.

Taste

Gustation—Like taste, relies on the transduction of chemicals to perceive the sense of taste.

Taste receptors—The five tastes that have been identified are salty, sweet, sour, bitter, and savory. Taste receptors die after about 10 days and are replaced with new cells. Taste is functionally important so that people can identify potentially dangerous poisons or impurities in food.

Central processing of taste—This is supported by three cranial nerves: VII (anterior 2/3 of the tongue), IX (posterior 1/3 of tongue, pharynx), and X (epiglottis, larynx). Figure 3–19 illustrates the central processing of taste.

Vestibular and Hearing

Ear anatomy—The ear has two functions: hearing and vestibular. See Figure 3–20 for the components of the ear and Figure 3–21 for understanding central auditory processing.

Vestibular system—Detects motion and position of the head through several receptors. The labyrinths are made up of three semicircular canals and two otolithic organs called the utricle and the saccule. The outermost labyrinth is called the bony labyrinth

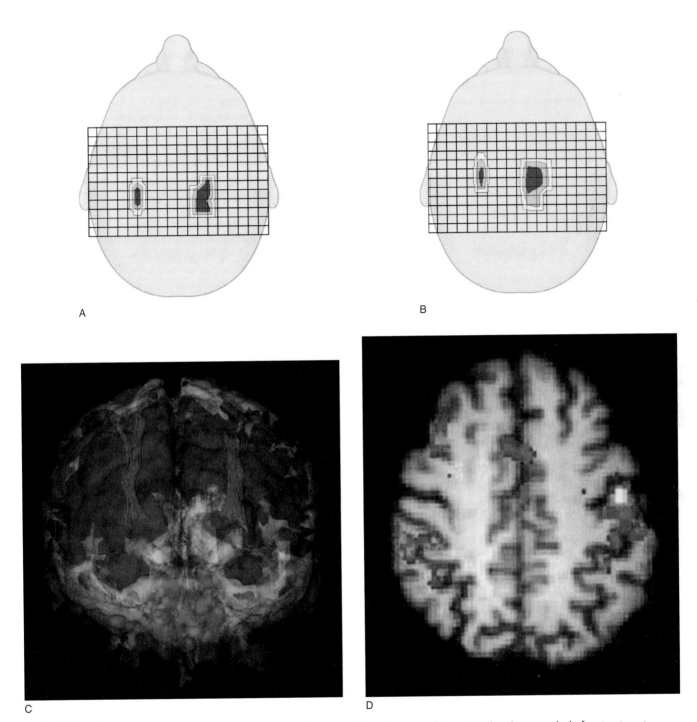

FIGURE 3–13 Imaging documentation of neural remodeling. **A.** Initial motor map of the paretic hand post-stroke before treatment; **B.** Post-training motor map illustrating expansion of the ipsilesional (right) motor cortex; **C.** Diffusion tensor imaging illustrates integrity of fibers within the internal capsule, associated with improved function, which could be the product of greater neuronal survival, enhanced sprouting, or a combination of the two; and **D.** Demonstrates localized activity in the sensory discrimination network (ipsilesional primary sensory cortex, contralesional secondary sensory cortex, and right superior frontal cortex) of a left stroke survivor with full recovery of sensory ability (imaging view—right is anatomical left). (C and D: Used with permission of Deborah S. Nichols Larsen, PT, PhD. The Ohio State University.)

BOX 3-1 Critical Factors for Adaptive Neural Plasticity

- Activity must target neural networks, in which plasticity is desired.
- Activity can prevent secondary damage.
- Activity must target specific movements and skills that are salient to the patient to induce change in desired neural networks; saliency may activate critical emotional networks to facilitate plasticity.
- Neural plasticity requires repetition at an intensity that challenges the nervous system.
- The timing of activity is critical: (1) too much too early can exacerbate the lesion; (2) some early level of activity may be neuroprotective; (3) there may be a critical period or periods when plasticity is more likely; and (4) the window for plasticity is restricted and does not continue indefinitely.
- Older brains do not have the same capacity for remodeling that is available to younger brains.
- Plasticity in one neural network may facilitate (transference) or inhibit (interference) plasticity in other networks.

From Nichols-Larsen DS et al. *Neurologic Rehabilitation: Neuroscience and Neuroplasticity in Physical Therapy Practice.* New York, NY: McGraw Hill Professional; 2015.

and is filled with perilymphatic fluid, and the innermost labyrinth, called the membranous labyrinth, is filled with endolymphatic fluid. Figure 3–22 illustrates the cochlea and vestibular labyrinth.

Receptors—The sensory cells in each of the above-named organs contain hair cells, which translate signals into neural fining.

Semicircular canals—These sense angular acceleration; for example, with rotations, tilting, or turning of the head. There are three semicircular canals: horizontal, anterior, and posterior. The semicircular canals are oriented with the extraocular eye muscles.

Utricle and saccule—These detect linear acceleration and static head position; for example when leaning one side or riding in an elevator.

Vestibular pathways—The primary afferents have cell bodies in Scarpa's ganglion, and from here information travels along CN VIII and enters the brainstem at the pons–medulla junction. The target areas for this information are the vestibular nuclei and the cerebellum. From here projections are sent to the oculomotor nuclei, which are CN III, IV, and VI, which regulate the vestibular-ocular reflex (VOR). The VOR allows humans to maintain an image stable on the fovea of the retina during the presence of head movement. In addition, efferent projections are communicated to the spinal cord in the form of the medial and lateral vestibulospinal tracts to support the activation of muscles

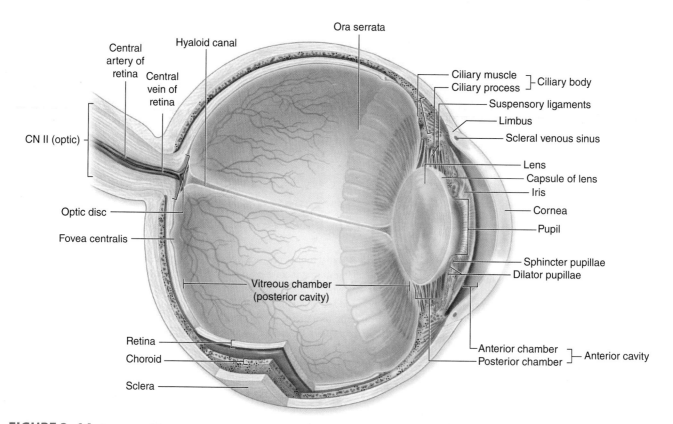

FIGURE 3–14 Anatomy of the eye. (Reproduced with permission from McKinley M, O'Laughlin VD. *Human Anatomy.* 3rd ed. New York, NY: McGraw-Hill; 2012, Figure 19–12B, p 576.)

BOX 3–2 Pupil and Lens Control

Pupillary Reflexes

Constriction: When a strong light hits the retina, it induces constriction of the pupil through a reflexive response. This reflex is mediated by sequential projections from the retina to the midbrain's pretectal nucleus, to the Edinger–Westphal nuclei (also in the midbrain), to the ciliary ganglion and ultimately to the ciliary muscles that constrict the pupil via parasympathetic fibers in CN III. Each Edinger–Westphal muscle connects to its counterpart on the opposite side such that pupillary constriction occurs bilaterally and symmetrically.

Dilation: Dilation can be achieved by inhibition of the reflexive loop that produces constriction or activation of the iris dilator muscle via the sympathetic nervous system component of the ciliary ganglion.

Accommodation

Changing of the shape of the lens within the eye allows us to orient to objects near to us as well as those far away. To allow us to focus on objects in the distance, the lens becomes elongated, associated with ciliary muscle relaxation, while focus on near objects is achieved by a thickening of the lens via ciliary muscle contraction; both of these changes serve to focus the image on the retina. The ciliary muscles of the lens create this change in lens shape through the same series of projections that control the pupillary reflexes; in fact, accommodation for near vision is also associated with pupil constriction and eye convergence (slight adduction), requiring integration via these brainstem nuclei.

Myopia (nearsightedness): Light is focused short of the retina, making distance vision poor, associated with poor elongation of the lens or an eye that is too long.

Hyperopia (farsightedness): Poor near vision caused by poor accommodation (inability of the lens to achieve a sufficiently round shape) or an eye that is too short.

Presbyopia: Age-induced change in the ability to accommodate, resulting in poorer near vision.

From Nichols-Larsen DS et al. *Neurologic Rehabilitation: Neuroscience and Neuroplasticity in Physical Therapy Practice*. New York, NY: McGraw Hill Professional; 2015.

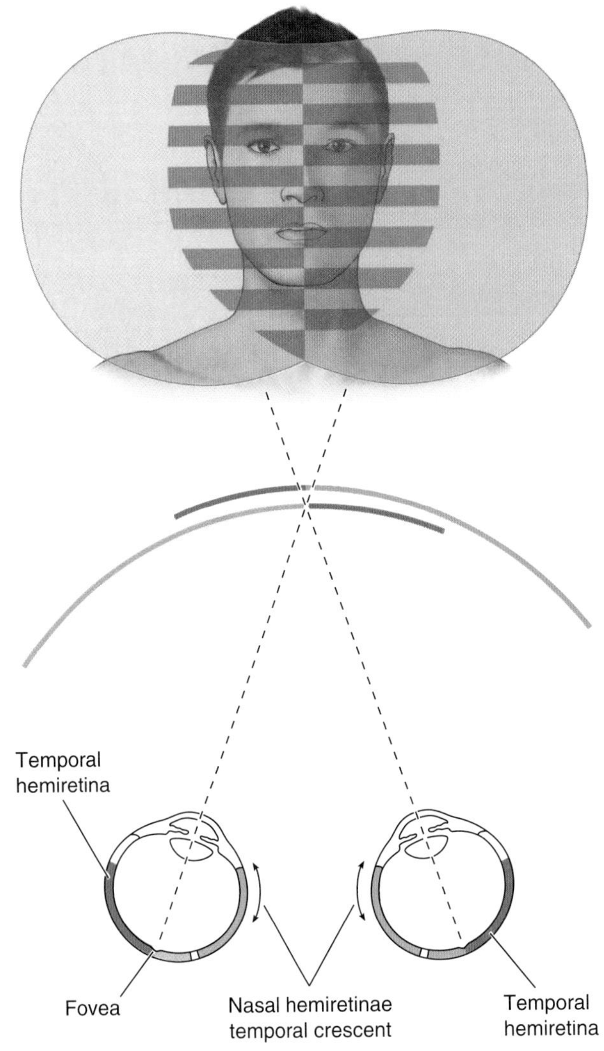

FIGURE 3–15 Schematic of visual field projections. Projections to the retina: The central striped area illustrates the overlapping binocular visual field, conveyed to the temporal retina of each eye. The solid colored fields are unique to each eye. The right monocular visual field (green) is transmitted to the right nasal retina while the left (blue) is transmitted to the left nasal retina. This allows the projections from the right field to come together as the nasal fibers cross at the optic chiasm. (Reproduced with permission from Martin JH. *Neuroanatomy Text and Atlas*. 4th ed. New York, NY: McGraw-Hill; 2012, Figure 7–5, p 161.)

for postural responses. See Figure 3–23 for a schematic of the vestibular pathway.

Balance/postural control—The ability of the body to maintain an upright position requires adequate balance and use of perception. Perception is the integration of sensory information to assess the position and motion of the body in space, involving sensory and higher-level cognitive processes. The three main specialized sensory systems used for balance are the visual, somatosensory, and vestibular systems.

Specialized Functions of the CNS— Cognition, Commutation, and Language

Cognition is an expansive term used to describe our ability to perceive the world around us, interact with it, remember our past experiences in it, and imagine potential experiences with it; the concepts of thinking, memory, imagery, problem-solving, and decision-making are all included within the term cognition. These complex skills involve multiple neural pathways.

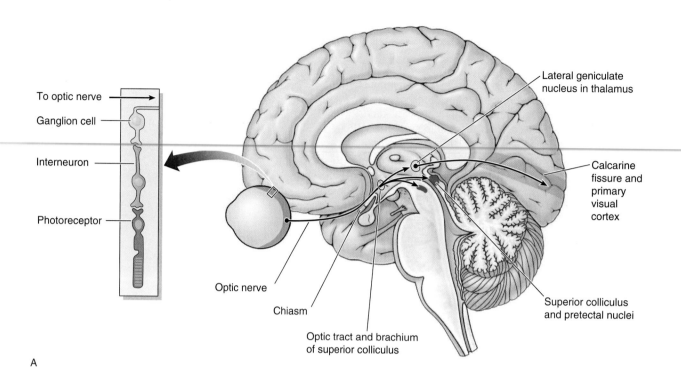

A

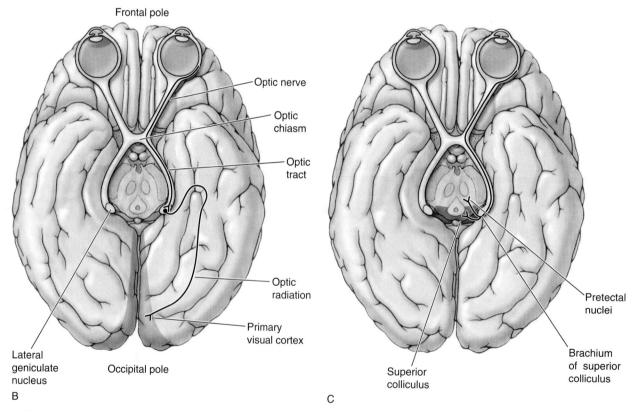

B   C

FIGURE 3–16 Visual projections from the retina to the visual cortex. (Reproduced with permission from Martin JH. *Neuroanatomy Text and Atlas*. 4th ed. New York, NY: McGraw-Hill; 2012, Figure 7–2, p 158.)

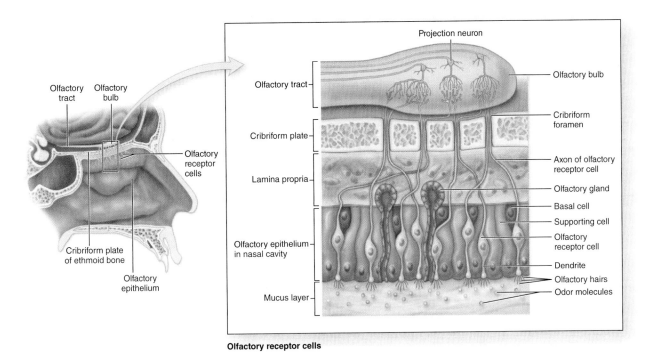

Olfactory receptor cells

FIGURE 3–17 Olfactory receptors and projections. Bipolar cells within the nasal epithelium project through the cribriform plate to the olfactory tubercle, activating mitral cells that project as the olfactory tract to the olfactory cortex in structures on the dorsum of the brain. (Reproduced with permission from McKinley M, O'Laughlin VD. *Human Anatomy*. 3rd ed. New York, NY: McGraw-Hill; 2012, Figure 19–9A, p 572.)

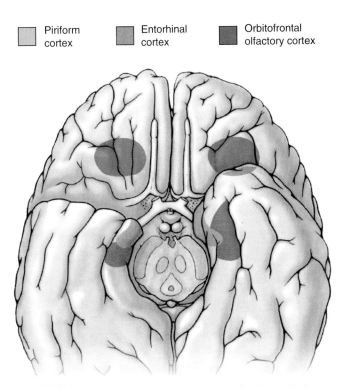

FIGURE 3–18 Olfactory cortex. (Reproduced with permission from Martin JH. *Neuroanatomy Text and Atlas*. 4th ed. New York, NY: McGraw-Hill; 2012, Figure 9–11, p 215.)

Executive Function

Executive function refers to a spectrum of abilities, including attention, working memory, inhibition, task switching, abstract thought, and behavioral regulation as well as decision-making, sequence planning, and initiation.

Attention—The ability to focus awareness on visual, auditory, tactile, or other sensory stimuli, but also involves the ability to prioritize attention on one among competing stimuli as well as to switch attention from one stimulus to another.

Task switching—The ability to focus on one task, and then immediately switch to another task.

Perseveration—Failure to switch attention to attend to a new appropriate cue, and instead continue the current task.

Working memory—The ability to retain or manipulate information cognitively for immediate use.

Memory

The concepts of learning and memory coexist. There are different types of learning and memory, defined below. Implicit and explicit memory systems are organized in Figure 3–24.

Emotions—These are complex learned responses elicited by sensory stimuli that produce a motor response, physiologic changes, and/or motivate us to some type of action. Emotions, along with memory, are controlled and regulated by the limbic system.

Language—Is a higher-level skill that differentiates humans from other animals. Our language abilities are usually divided into receptive and expressive language skills. The anatomical language centers are identified as Broca's area and Wernicke's area. These locations are depicted in Figure 3–25.

NEUROLOGICAL EXAMINATION

The examination of the neurologic system is an essential component of a comprehensive physical examination. It includes the systems review or screening and a comprehensive and systematic examination of both the central and peripheral nervous system in conjunction with other body systems. The examination should determine impairments in our body function and structure, limitations in our functional activities, and participation restrictions consistent with the World Health Organization's

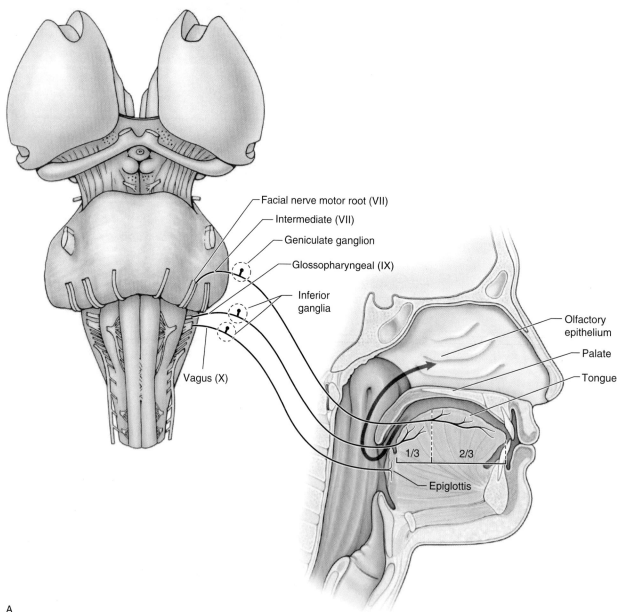

A

FIGURE 3–19 Cranial nerve projections of taste. A. The three cranial nerves (VII, IX, and X) innervate the oral cavity through long dendritic projections from the cells within the peripheral ganglia (inferior, geniculate) with axonal projections to the solitary nucleus. B. Gustatory projections from the solitary nucleus project to the ventral posterior medial nucleus of the thalamus. (Reproduced with permission from Martin JH. *Neuroanatomy Text and Atlas*. 4th ed. New York, NY: McGraw-Hill; 2012, Figures 9–4 and 9–5, p 206 and 207.)

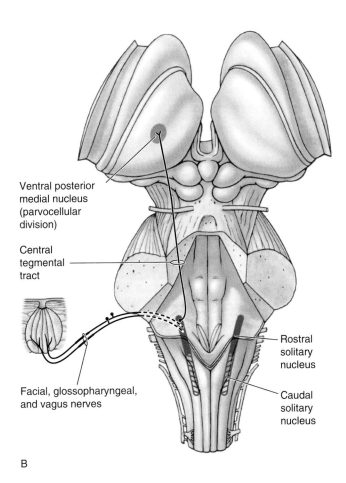

Ventral posterior
medial nucleus
(parvocellular
division)

Central
tegmental
tract

Facial, glossopharyngeal,
and vagus nerves

Rostral
solitary
nucleus

Caudal
solitary
nucleus

B

FIGURE 3–19 (*Continued*)

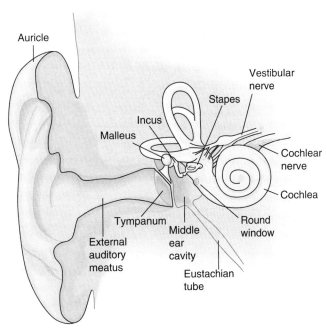

Auricle

Vestibular
nerve

Stapes

Incus

Malleus

Cochlear
nerve

Cochlea

Tympanum

Round
window

External
auditory
meatus

Middle
ear
cavity

Eustachian
tube

FIGURE 3–20 The three components of the ear. The ear has three functional components: (1) the external ear (auricle, external acoustic meatus, and tympanic membrane) that funnels sound to the interior of the ear; (2) the middle ear (auditory ossicles—malleus, incus, and stapes) that transmits vibration to the ear drum; and (3) the inner ear (cochlea) that allows the transduction of sound to neural signals. (Reproduced with permission from Kandel ER, Schwartz JH, Jessell TM, Siegelbaum SA, Hudspeth AJ. *Principles of Neural Science*. 5th ed. New York, NY: McGraw-Hill; 2013, Figure 30–1, p 655.)

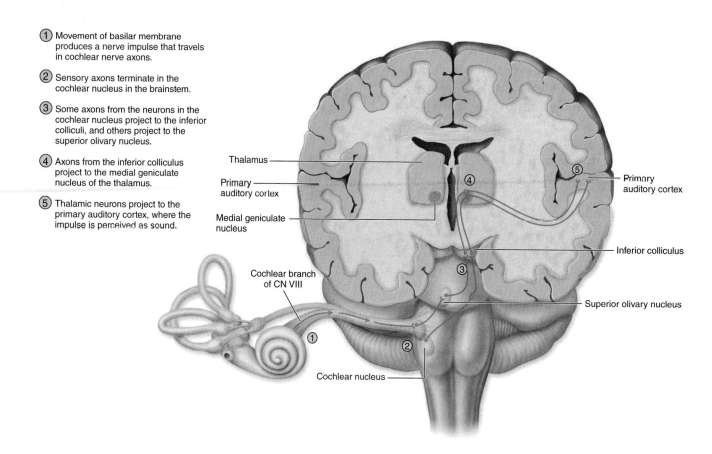

1. Movement of basilar membrane produces a nerve impulse that travels in cochlear nerve axons.

2. Sensory axons terminate in the cochlear nucleus in the brainstem.

3. Some axons from the neurons in the cochlear nucleus project to the inferior colliculi, and others project to the superior olivary nucleus.

4. Axons from the inferior colliculus project to the medial geniculate nucleus of the thalamus.

5. Thalamic neurons project to the primary auditory cortex, where the impulse is perceived as sound.

FIGURE 3–21 Auditory projections. (Reproduced with permission from McKinley M, O'Laughlin VD. *Human Anatomy*. 3rd ed. New York, NY: McGraw-Hill; 2012, Figure 19–30, p 598.)

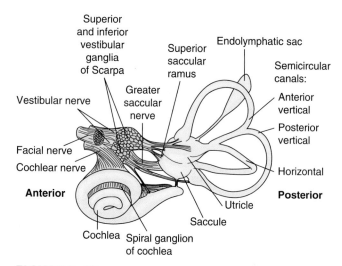

FIGURE 3–22 Vestibular labyrinths: This schematic illustrates the relationship of the cochlea and the components of the vestibular labyrinth: the vestibule with its saccule and utricle and the three semicircular canals. (Reproduced with permission from Kandel ER, Schwartz JH, Jessell TM, Siegelbaum SA, Hudspeth AJ. *Principles of Neural Science*. 4th ed. New York, NY: McGraw-Hill; 2000; Figure 40–1, p 918.)

International Classification of Functioning, Disability, and Health (ICF).

The examination begins with a thorough history and interview to attempt to localize patient- and therapist-identified problems. Movement analysis is an important part of the examination process and can assist in the development of hypotheses related to the movement deficits. Tests and measures, including standardized outcome measures, are performed to measure specific impairments in body function and body structure, activity limitations, and participation restrictions and test-identified hypotheses. The information gained during this process is organized and informs the decision-making of the therapist to identify a physical therapy diagnosis and prognosis, set anticipated goals and outcomes, and design interventions to meet the identified goals and outcomes. During and after interventions, responses are measured and observed and the original hypotheses are modified as necessary. This should be thought of as a cyclical process whereby the examination informs the intervention, which in turn informs the examination. See Figure 3–26.

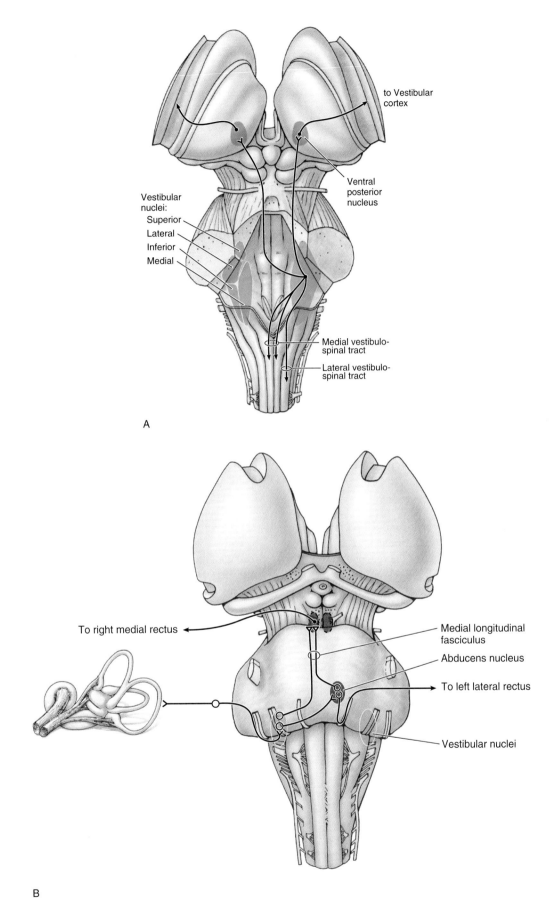

A

B

FIGURE 3–23 A and B. The vestibular nuclei. The four vestibular nuclei can be visualized in this diagram along with their projections to the thalamus and spinal cord. (Reproduced with permission from Martin JH. *Neuroanatomy Text and Atlas*. 4th ed. New York, NY: McGraw-Hill; 2012. Figure 12–2 (A) and 12–6 (B) p 280 and 285, respectively.)

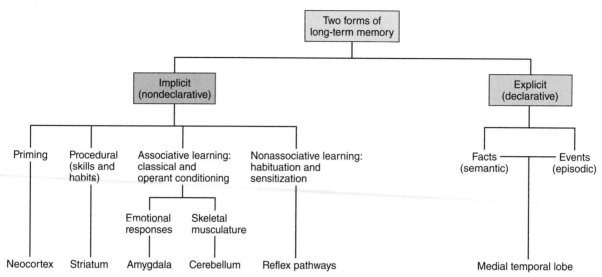

FIGURE 3–24 Schematic of implicit and explicit memory systems. Long-term memory can be divided into explicit (semantic—facts; episodic—events) and implicit (procedural) memories. Explicit memories are encoded by the medial temporal lobe structures and their connections to the anterior cingulate and prefrontal cortices. Implicit memories are generated within an array of networks, including the sensory cortices (priming), striatum of the basal ganglia and cerebellum (motor skills, habits), the cerebellum and amygdala (classical and operant conditioning), and reflex networks of the brainstem. (Reproduced with permission from Kandel ER, Schwartz JH, Jessell TM, Siegelbaum SA, Hudspeth AJ. *Principles of Neural Science*. 5th ed. New York, NY: McGraw-Hill; 2013. Figure 66–1 top section, p 1462.)

Components of the Neurologic Examination

History

The history should be concise and comprehensive to generate several hypotheses as to why the patient is experiencing the signs, symptoms, and limitations with the function. The history includes pertinent information such as name, age, and current and past medical history. In addition, the physical therapist should identify medications and supplements that have been prescribed. Lastly, the physical therapist needs to find out the patient's goals for therapy.

Systems Review

Systems review is a screening and general review of each body system, and guides which systems then require further examination and referral to another medical professional. At the minimum, the systems review should include assessment of the following:

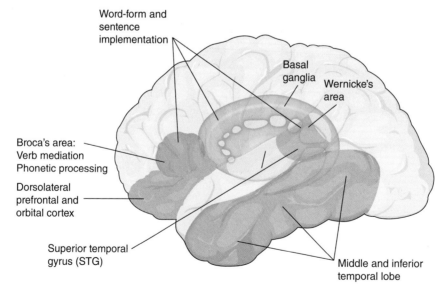

FIGURE 3–25 Language centers. The historic Broca's and Wernicke's areas are depicted in association with the surrounding areas that contribute to language skills (dorsolateral and orbitofrontal cortex, middle and inferior temporal lobes, basal ganglia). (Reproduced with permission from Kandel ER, Schwartz JH, Jessell TM, Siegelbaum SA, Hudspeth AJ. *Principles of Neural Science*. 5th ed. New York, NY: McGraw-Hill; 2013. Figure 60–5, p 1364.)

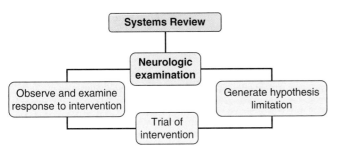

FIGURE 3–26 Diagram of the relationship between evaluation and treatment. (From Nichols-Larsen DS, Kegelmeyer DA, Buford JA, Kloos AD, Heathcock JC, Basso D. *Neurologic Rehabilitation: Neuroscience and Neuroplasticity in Physical Therapy Practice*; 2016 Available at: http://accessphysiotherapy.mhmedical.com/content.aspx?bookid =1760&sectionid=120047974. Accessed March 04, 2018.)

- Communication/cognition: Mental status, alertness, orientation, memory, communication abilities.
- Integumentary: Examine for the presence of incisions, wounds, burns, inflammation.
- Cardiovascular/pulmonary: Vitals—heart rate, blood pressure, respiration rate.
- Musculoskeletal: Rule out contraindications for further evaluation and treatment. Is the patient capable of doing examination activities? This should include a gross screen of strength and range of motion (ROM).
- Neuromuscular: Screen for muscle tone, strength, and functional movement/coordination by observing mobility as the patient enters the evaluation area and performs gross movements. When individuals have a known neurologic disorder or are found to have deficits in the systems review of the neuromuscular system, the physical therapist should progress to the neurologic examination, targeting those areas of concern from the screening.

Neurologic Examination

This should be performed on any individual suspected of having any neurologic disorder or psychological disease. The examination should be performed in a systematic and comprehensive order and consists of several thorough and in-depth assessments: mental status, cranial nerves, motor examination, reflexes, sensory examination, and posture and mobility analysis.

Mental status examination—This is the first item to be examined. It is not possible to conduct the rest of the examination without first determining how the individual follows directions and interacts with the environment and if he/she is able to follow directions. If an individual is suspected of having a neurologic disorder, mental status should be examined in more detail. Further detail regarding the mental status examination can be found in Table 3–4. Standardized outcome measures for mental status should be reviewed in the appendices of this chapter in alignment with the Academy of Neurologic Physical Therapy (ANPT) recommendations for entry-level Doctor of Physical Therapy (DPT) education. The basic mental status examination should include:

- **Immediate recall**—can assessed by determining the number of digits that can be repeated in sequence from a string recited by the examiner.

- **Recent memory**—typically examined by testing recall of a series of three to five objects immediately, then after 5 and 15 minutes with intervening activities.
- **Remote memory**—assessed by asking the patient to review in a chronological fashion his or her illness or personal life events that the patient feels comfortable disclosing.
- **Higher-order functioning**—assessed by spontaneous speech and repetition, reading, naming, writing, and comprehension of written and oral information.

Communication—It is important for the physical therapist to understand the patient's ability to communicate. First, it is essential to understand the patient's ability to hear and accurately report the patient's level of comprehension and ability to express himself verbally or nonverbally. Standardized outcome measures that include communication should be reviewed in the appendices of this chapter in alignment with the ANPT recommendations for entry-level DPT education. The examination should answer the following questions:

- Can the client communicate? Does the patient have word finding problems consistent with expressive aphasia or trouble enunciating consistent with dysarthria?
- Note voice quality; is volume adequate?
- Does the individual understand language or show signs of receptive aphasia?

Motor examination—Assess muscle strength and tone, and compare active to passive range of motion. These findings, along with use of observation skills, should indicate whether the patient has a muscular, neural, or perceptual disorder that impairs their motor function. Abnormal and involuntary movements should also be noted. See below for an additional description of motor components of the neurologic examination.

Strength (force production)—Assessment can be challenging for a patient with neurologic diagnoses as they often lack the isolated, active range of motion and often have impaired trunk control, which often limits their abilities to stabilize their trunk while being engaged in manual muscle testing. Manual muscle testing should only be utilized when voluntary, isolated active range of motion is present. The physical therapist should document the available range the patient was able to move through, if gravity eliminated or not, and if there was presence of an abnormal synergy involved with the movement. If the active range of motion is limited, a functional strength test is suggested.

- Functional **muscle testing**—is assessing the patient's performance during activities under normal daily conditions. The physical therapist should document a detailed description of the motion. For example, the therapist might comment on the base of support, use of one or both of the upper extremities, and whether or not the patient can manipulate objects in the environment.
- **Tone**—is assessed by performing passive range of motion in a pain-free range, both in a slow and fast manner. The physical therapist will note any resistance during the motion. An increase in tone, **hypertonicity**, is present when the examiner notes an increased resistance to passive movement. There are two types of hypertonicity: spasticity and rigidity. **Spasticity** is characterized by increased resistance to passive movement, as the velocity

TABLE 3–4 Mental function assessment for the physical therapist.

Area to be Examined	What to Look For	Insight
Appearance	Clothes, posture, grooming, alertness	Ability to take care of themselves; mood/affect
Behavior	Impulse control, fidgeting, overall movements	
Speech	Volume/Rate	Mood (eg, loud and fast speech—related to mania; soft and slow—related to depression)
	Coherence	Indication of higher level processing
Mood/Affect	Flat—minimal or absent affective response to situation	Signs of mental illness or cortical disease
	Labile—shifting emotional outbursts (eg, crying/laughing)	
	Blunted—some emotional response but less than would be expected for the situation	
	Constructed/Inappropriate—responses that are inconsistent with the situation (eg, laughing at a sad situation)	
Thought processing	Word usage	Language issues (agnosia, expressive aphasia)
	Thought stream	Slow versus overabundant gives an indication of mood and cognition
	Continuity—coherence of thought and idea association	Ability to follow the discussion and respond accordingly—higher-level cognition or receptive language problems
	Content—complete/incomplete responses	Higher-level cognition/language issues, delusions suggest mental disorders
Perception	Screening of vision, hearing, touch, taste, and smell	General system integrity/dysfunction; potential medication side effects
Attention/Concentration	Ability to stay focused on a task	Frontal lobe dysfunction; anxiety
Memory	Long-term and current episodic memory (client's history and current events); immediate memory (naming 3 objects immediately and then in 5 and 15 minutes)	Temporal and frontal lobe function/dysfunction
Judgment	Decision-making in complex situations (safe versus unsafe)	Executive function (frontal lobe function)
Intelligence	Requires specific testing but a general sense can be obtained by responses to questions, general language used, etc.	Overall ability to participate in treatment/cortical deficits
Insight	Understanding of the current illness and potential limitations	Executive function

From Nichols-Larsen DS et al. *Neurologic Rehabilitation: Neuroscience and Neuroplasticity in Physical Therapy Practice.* New York, NY: McGraw Hill Professional; 2015. Table 9–1.

of the movement is increased (velocity dependent), and by hyperreflexia (exaggerated monosynaptic reflexes). **Rigidity** is increased resistance throughout the ROM that is independent of the velocity of the movement; reflexes are typically normal with rigidity. The causes of spasticity and rigidity are different and will be discussed in later sections specific to neurologic diagnoses. A limb that feels heavy or "floppy" is **hypotonic**, demonstrating limited resistance to passive movement and poor ability to sustain power or maintain a given posture. Hypotonia can be caused by both central and peripheral nervous system disorders. Reflexes can be decreased (hyporeflexia), normal, or exaggerated (hyperreflexia), depending on the cause of the hypotonia. It is important to note that tone can fluctuate depending on time of day and other environmental and personal stimuli; therefore testing should be performed at the same time each day and with the same examiner. Standardized outcome measures for tone and spasticity should be reviewed in the appendices of this chapter in alignment with the ANPT recommendations for entry-level DPT education.

- **Reflexes**—are tested by using a reflex hammer. The physical therapist will tap over key tendon insertions in the arms (biceps, triceps, brachioradialis), knees (quadriceps, hamstrings), and heels (Achilles). A comparison should always be made between the left and right sides, and a difference between the arms and legs usually indicates a spinal cord lesion. If only one extremity is involved, this is usually indicative of a peripheral nerve lesion. Hyperactive reflexes indicate a lesion in the upper motor neuron or central nervous system. Deep tendon reflexes are typically documented using a numerical scale, which can be viewed in Table 3–5. In addition, the reflex exam should include the Hoffman and Babinski reflex testing when a CNS deficit is suspected.

Cranial nerves—Cranial nerves (CN) originate in the brainstem and support the muscles of the face and eyes, the sensory receptors, and support specialized senses such as hearing, vision, smell, taste, and vestibular function. See Table 3–6 for further detail regarding cranial nerve function and screening.

TABLE 3-5 Deep tendon reflex grades.

Reflex Grade	Evaluation	Response Characteristics
0	Absent	No visible or palpable muscle contraction
1+	Hyporeflexia	Slight or sluggish muscle contraction with little or no joint movement Reinforcement may be required to elicit a reflex response
2+	Normal	Slight muscle contraction with slight joint movement
3+	Hyperreflexia	Clearly visible, brisk muscle contraction with moderate joint movement
4+	Abnormal	Strong muscle contraction with one to three beats of clonus Reflex spread to contralateral side may be noted
5+	Abnormal	Strong muscle contraction with sustained clonus Reflex spread to contralateral side may be noted

From Nichols-Larsen DS et al. *Neurologic Rehabilitation: Neuroscience and Neuroplasticity in Physical Therapy Practice.* New York, NY: McGraw Hill Professional; 2015. Table 9–2.

Sensory examination—Requires the patient to have concentration and cooperation during the examination of the five primary senses: vibration, joint position and awareness, light touch, pinprick, and temperature. Patients with sensory deficits may have a lesion at any place along the sensory pathways as described in the sensory pathways content. Ideally, the sensory examination starts out with basic testing procedures and becomes more detailed to include all the other sensory modalities as limitations are identified.

- **Tests of Proprioception**
  - *Movement sense (kinesthesia)*—The physical therapist has the patient close their eyes and then moves the extremity through a small ROM. The patient is asked to verbally indicate the direction of movement while the extremity is in motion. Prior to performing the test, the physical therapist should demonstrate the examination to the patient with their eyes open to establish understanding. Communication should be simple, for example, "up," "down," or "in" and "out." The physical therapist should hold the patient's extremities using bony prominences to minimize additional sensory input.
  - *Position sense*—The physical therapist places the patient's extremity in a position, and the patient is then asked to verbally communicate the position.
  - *Vibration testing*—Is the most reliable and valid way to test dorsal column–medial lemniscal system. A 250-mHz tuning fork is suggested, and the physical therapist should strike the fork against the palm of their hand and then place it on a bony prominence while asking the patient what they feel.

- **Cutaneous Sensation** is commonly tested by: (1) monofilament testing for sensory threshold; (2) pinprick for pain; and (3) water vials for hot and cold modalities. First, the physical therapist should screen for the ability to sense and localize touch. This can be achieved by applying a light touch across the surface of both upper/lower limbs, and the individual is asked if she "can feel it" and "does it feel the same." Then the same examination should be completed with the patient's eyes closed and asked to identify the location of the randomly applied stimulus. If deficits are found, a more thorough sensory exam should be completed, including pinprick and temperature. Additional tests include identifying common objects, shapes of varying weight, etc. See Table 3–7 for common sensory deficits and options for testing and documenting each.

Coordination and balance—Is the ability to execute smooth, accurate, controlled movements. It is characterized by appropriate speed, distance, direction, rhythm, muscle tension, and synergistic movements accomplished via orchestrated reversals of opposing muscle group activations. Proximal stabilization is critical in order to achieve distal movement when performing many of these tests. Coordination involves nonequilibrium, which involves assessment of the extremities, and equilibrium, which involves upright postural control. Typically, nonequilibrium tests are completed first, followed by the equilibrium tests. The physical therapist should observe the quality of movement, note time to complete the test, monitor the patient's speed, and whether adjustments are needed to be successful with the task at hand. In addition, nonequilibrium tests should include unilateral and bimanual tasks with eyes open and closed and with altering speeds. Nonequilibrium tests are outlined in Box 3–3. Equilibrium testing then begins with observing the patient's standing posture, and progresses as described in Box 3–4. Table 3–8 outlines common movement and coordination abnormalities and their assessment methods.

Balance—Is a composite impairment and involves a systematic aspect of the examination due to the complexity. Physical therapists should examine static and dynamic balance in a seated and standing position. Balance is best assessed using standardized outcome measures that capture a variety of aspects of the feedforward and feedback postural control systems under a variety of functional and environmental conditions. Standardized outcome measures for balance should be reviewed in the appendices of this chapter in alignment with the ANPT recommendations for entry-level DPT education. Further resources in the appendices should be used to assist in the decision-making process for both balance and gait standardized outcome measures with respect to the patient diagnosis and clinical practice setting.

Transfers—Includes an examination of the patient's ability to change positions in bed, and to transition from sitting to standing and standing to sitting from a variety of support surfaces. The physical therapist should note and document the level of assistance, movement strategies that are unsafe or inefficient, the environment in which the activity is taking place, and use of any assistive devices or adaptive equipment. Refer to Table 3–9 for descriptions of assistance levels. Standardized outcome measures for transfers and functional mobility should be reviewed in the

TABLE 3–6 Cranial nerve function and screening methods.

Cranial Nerve	Name	Function	Screening
I	Olfactory	Smell	Have patient identify familiar smells (vanilla); there are vials that can be purchased or therapists can make their own.
II	Optic	Vision	Reading close and distant items.
III	Oculomotor	Eye movement, pupillary reflexes	Eye tracking in all directions, pupillary response to light; at rest, eye will be slightly depressed and rotated toward the nose when damaged.
IV	Trochlear	Superior oblique eye muscle innervation	Observe eye position at rest; will be elevated if there is a problem.
V	Trigeminal	Muscles of mastication and sensation of the face	Observe jaw motion (resistance to motion, opening, side-to-side mobility), temporalis muscles can be palpated.
VI	Abducens	Lateral rectus of the eye innervation	Look at eye movement; if damaged, there will be an inability to look outward (abduct the eye).
VII	Facial	Muscles of facial expression, taste for the anterior 2/3 of tongue	Look for facial asymmetries, observe motions (raising eyebrows, wrinkling forehead, closing eyes, frowning/smiling, lip pursing, etc.). Taste with common liquids (lemon juice, honey) can also be tested.
VIII	Vestibulocochlear	Hearing and vestibular	Can use the "rub test"—rub thumb and forefinger together next to the ear. Ask the patient to point to which ear they hear it in. Check both. Look for differences. You can use a tuning fork, which tests for air conduction and structural problems that can occur inside the ear—strike tuning fork on your hand and place behind the ear on the bony surface. Observe balance.
IX	Glossopharyngeal	Sensation and taste for posterior tongue and pharynx	Ask about swallowing, which may be impaired; have patient say "ahh" and watch for palatal-uvula movement; unilateral nerve damage can yield asymmetric motion; absent gag reflex is also a sign of damage (stimulate with tongue depressor).
X	Vagus	Innervates epiglottis and larynx, parasympathetic innervation of internal organs	Voice hoarseness with increased heart and respiration rate are signs of CN X damage.
XI	Accessory	Trapezius and sternocleidomastoid muscle innervation	Observe ability to shrug shoulders and turn head to both sides.
XII	Hypoglossal	Tongue muscles	Observe tongue protrusion and mobility; unilateral lesions will result in lateral movement when protruding tongue.

From Nichols-Larsen DS et al. Neurologic *Rehabilitation: Neuroscience and Neuroplasticity in Physical Therapy Practice*. New York, NY: McGraw Hill Professional; 2015. Table 9–3.

appendices of this chapter in alignment with the ANPT recommendations for entry-level DPT education.

Gait/locomotion—Consists of many components such as power, coordination, sensation, and balance working together in a coordinated fashion to achieve this complex process. Observational gait analysis can assist in detecting a variety of diagnoses. For example, ataxic gait with a wide base of support indicates involvement of the cerebellum. The patient's gait should be carefully analyzed using each of the subphases: initial contact, stance (early, mid, and late), push-off, and swing. Some considerations during the gait analysis should include:

- Assistance, assistive device, use of an orthotic device
- Description of the gait pattern on a variety of support surfaces, directions, and incorporating turns and velocity at a comfortable, self-selected speed

- Loss of balance and direction if appropriate
- Stair climbing
- Use of a wheelchair on a variety of support surfaces

Research on gait speed correlates with aspects of health, and should be determined to understand overall activity status. Standardized outcome measures for gait should be reviewed in the appendices of this chapter in alignment with the ANPT recommendations for entry-level DPT education. Further resources in the appendices of this chapter should be used to assist in the decision-making process for both balance and gait standardized outcome measures with respect to the patient diagnosis and clinical practice setting.

- **Evaluation**—is the physical therapist's thought process and should discuss how they either accepted or rejected hypotheses regarding the cause of the movement disorders. Here examination data are synthesized and a problem list is documented.

TABLE 3-7 Common sensory impairments and assessment methods.

Name of Sensory Impairment	Definition of Sensory Impairment	Assessment
Abarognosis	Inability to recognize weight	Hold objects of varying weights in each hand and have patient state which is heavier (or the same)
Allodynia	Pain is caused by nonpainful stimuli such as light touch	Uncovered in the sensory exam when light touch or other nonpainful stimuli elicit pain
Analgesia	Complete loss of pain sensitivity	Lack of pinprick sensation along with findings from the history
Astereognosis	Inability to use touch to recognize the shape or form of an object	Have patient identify shapes of objects while eyes are closed; use common shapes like square and ball
Atopognosia	Inability to localize a sensation	During light touch testing, ask patient to localize the touch with eyes closed
Dysesthesia	Abnormal touch sensation that may be experienced as unpleasant or painful	Typically determined during cutaneous testing (touch localization)
Hyperalgesia	Increased sensitivity to pain	Senses pinprick as being more painful than is typical and discovered through the history
Hyperesthesia	Increased sensitivity to sensory stimuli	Noted throughout the exam as an increased sensitivity to stimuli as compared to normal
Hypoalgesia	Decreased response to pain	Identified with the pinprick testing
Paresthesia	Abnormal sensation such as prickly or burning feeling that has no apparent cause	Noted during the history or when asked if they have any burning or prickling sensations

From Nichols-Larsen DS et al. *Neurologic Rehabilitation: Neuroscience and Neuroplasticity in Physical Therapy Practice*. New York, NY: McGraw Hill Professional; 2015. Table 9–4.

- **Diagnosis**—should describe how physical therapy intervention can impact the impairments in body structure/function and activity limitations that prevent the patient from their desired participation roles. The diagnosis should include the relevant International Classification for Disease 10 Code (ICD 10) and involve the use of clinical practice guidelines where available.
- **Prognosis**—goals and outcomes—Long-term functional prognosis, as well as identifying the short-and long-term goal, are essential to establish a plan of care for this episode of care (level of care). With an emphasis on long-term functional prognosis, the physical therapist should consider and prioritize the impact on neuroplasticity and negative consequences of compensation techniques. The prognosis statement should identify a time frame for care and address the potential for participation, specific motor functions, as well as positive influences and identification of any potential barriers that could prevent achievement of goals.
- **Short-term and long-term goals**—All goals need to be measurable and functional. Impairments related to body structure/function are acceptable as short-term goals. Long-term goals should incorporate activities from the problem list and/or the reported participation restrictions as identified from the patient during the history and interview.

NEUROLOGICAL DEFICITS/DIAGNOSES

Stroke

Pathophysiology

Stroke, or cerebrovascular accident, is the leading cause of adult disability and represents the greatest rehabilitation diagnosis. An estimated 15 million people around the world experience a stroke each year, and it affects more than 7 million people in the United States. A stroke occurs when there is interruption of blood flow within brain blood vessels, which can be a narrowing or blockage of the vessel, called ischemia, or can be a rupture of a vessel, called a hemorrhage. Hemorrhagic strokes often result in increased disability and death as compared to ischemic strokes. Ischemic strokes are seven times more common than hemorrhagic strokes.

Ischemic strokes—Result from either an embolism, which is a moving thrombus, or a thrombus, which is the blockage of an artery.

Transient ischemic attacks (TIAs)—Are the result of brief blockages with associated stroke symptoms that resolve quickly (<24 hours) and are not associated with permanent consequences, however indicate negative changes in circulation and should be further evaluated by the medial team.

Hemorrhagic strokes—Are more typical with poorly controlled and long-term hypertension, which cause weakening of the vascular wall. Hemorrhage within the cerebral vessels is referred to as an **intracerebral hemorrhage** and hemorrhage in the subarachnoid space is referred to as **subarachnoid hemorrhage**.

Stroke Risk Factors

Stroke risk factors and their cardiovascular consequences are listed in Table 3–10.

BOX 3–3 Nonequilibrium Coordination Tests

Most of these tests should be performed first with eyes open and then with eyes closed to examine the influence of vision on the individual's coordination. After doing each test at a comfortable pace, instruct the client to move faster and examine the influence of speed on coordination:

1. *Finger to nose:* With shoulder in a flexed position, bring the finger to the tip of the nose and back out to the examiner's hand or just straight out in front, repeating several times.

2. *Finger to therapist's finger:* Therapist sits in front of the client and has them alternately touch the therapist's fingertip. The therapist places their fingertip at nose height, arm's length away from the client. The movement is alternated. The therapist can also try moving their own finger so that the client has to make contact with the finger in different locations and can also move their finger, while the client is reaching, to observe how easily and smoothly he can change the trajectory of this movement in response to a moving target.

3. *Opposition of fingers:* The thumb is touched to the tip of each finger on the same hand, moving in order from the index finger to the pinky and back down to the index finger. Be sure that the client is instructed to fully abduct the thumb after each digit is touched.

4. *Grasp:* The hand is opened and closed with gradually increasing speed. Encourage the client to fully open the hand with each repetition. Failure to fully open the hand or progressive shrinking of movement may be indicative of basal ganglia disorder.

5. *Alternating pronation and supination:* The client is asked to alternately pronate and supinate with the arms held at the sides and elbows flexed (hands can be placed

on legs while seated so that palms and back of hands alternately touch the thighs).

6. *Tapping (hand and/or foot):* The arm is placed on a table or on the client's leg and they are instructed to tap the hand on the table or on his knee. For the foot, the client is seated with the knee flexed and foot flat on the floor; then, ask him to tap his toe on the ground.

7. *Rebound test:* The client is positioned with the elbow in 90° of flexion and the therapist applies resistance to elbow flexion. The client is instructed to maintain the flexed posture. The therapist then suddenly releases their resistance and observes the response; since the elbow flexors are active, the arm will begin to flex when the resistance is released. A normal response involves the opposing muscle group (triceps) rapidly checking the flexion movement with little motion occurring. Abnormal tests involve a large flexion of the elbow or a loss of trunk control in response to the sudden change in resistance.

8. *Heel on shin:* In supine or sitting, the client is asked to slide the heel up the shin from the ankle to the knee and back down again. Any movement off of the shin is considered a coordination deficit.

9. *Toe to examiner's finger:* Examiner holds their finger out and the client is asked to point to it with their great toe. This motion can be alternated.

10. *Drawing a circle:* The client is asked to draw a circle on the floor with the big toe. A figure of eight can also be used. In supine, they can be asked to draw the figure in the air. This test can also be done with the upper extremity, using the finger to draw an imaginary circle in the air.

From Nichols-Larsen DS et al. *Neurologic Rehabilitation: Neuroscience and Neuroplasticity in Physical Therapy Practice.* New York, NY: McGraw Hill Professional; 2015.

Cerebral Circulation and Why Results of Stroke are Variable

The brain is supported by a complex arterial system which involves two components: anterior and posterior circulation. The complex nature of perfusion can be viewed in Figure 3–27. In this figure, it is important to identify the carotid artery system consisting of the internal carotid arteries, the anterior, middle, and the posterior arteries. This anterior circulation is further supported by the anterior and the posterior communicating arteries. The second component of the perfusion system, referred to as posterior circulation, begins with identifying the vertebral arteries, the basilar artery, the anterior inferior cerebellar artery, the **superior cerebellar artery**, and finally the **posterior cerebral artery**.

Stroke Syndromes

Specific stroke symptoms are associated with the vasculature distribution that is damaged. This is outlined in Table 3–11, and Figure 3–28 demonstrates deficits and corresponding impairments at the level of the brainstem. Patients present with a varying number and degree of these symptoms based on the amount of damage in the circulation.

Acute Management

Ischemic stroke—A comprehensive history should be taken to attempt to discover the time of onset of stroke symptoms. If medically appropriate, the patient will receive tissue-type plasminogen activator (rTPA or TPA) to assist in breaking down the clot and

BOX 3-4 Equilibrium Coordination Tests

Tests are listed from least to most difficult

1. Standing in normal, comfortable posture
2. Standing, feet together (narrow base of support)
3. Standing, with one foot directly in front of the other in tandem position (toe of one foot touching heel of other foot)
4. Standing on one foot
5. Arm position may be altered in each of the above postures (ie, arms at side, overhead, hands on waist, and so forth)
6. Displacing balance unexpectedly (while carefully guarding the patient, wearing gait belt)
7. Standing, alternate between forward trunk flexion and return to neutral
8. Standing, laterally flex trunk to each side
9. Standing; eyes open to eyes closed; ability to maintain an upright posture without visual input is referred to as a **positive Romberg sign**
10. Standing in tandem position eyes open to eyes closed—**Sharpened Romberg**
11. Walking, placing the heel of one foot directly in front of the toe of the opposite foot (tandem walking)
12. Walking along a straight line drawn or taped to the floor, or placing feet on floor markers while walking
13. Walking sideways, backward, or cross-stepping
14. Marching in place
15. Altering speed of ambulatory activities; observe patient walking at normal speed, as fast as possible, and as slow as possible
16. Stopping and starting abruptly while walking
17. Walking and pivoting (turn 90°, 180°, or 360°)
18. Walking in a circle, alternate directions
19. Walking on heels and then on toes
20. Walking with horizontal and vertical head turns
21. Stepping over or around obstacles
22. Stair climbing with and without using handrail; one step at a time versus step over step
23. Performing agility activities (coordinated movement with upright balance)—jumping jacks; alternate flexing and extending the knees while sitting on a Swiss ball

From Nichols-Larsen DS et al. *Neurologic Rehabilitation: Neuroscience and Neuroplasticity in Physical Therapy Practice.* New York, NY: McGraw Hill Professional; 2015.

TABLE 3-8 Movement and coordination impairments with assessment methods.

Impairment	Definition	Sample Test
Dysdiadochokinesia	Impaired alternating movements	Finger to nose Alternate nose to finger Pronation/supination Knee flexion/extension Walking, alter speed or direction
Dysmetria	Uncoordinated movement, characterized by over- or undershooting intended position	Pointing to a target Drawing a circle or figure eight Heel on shin Placing feet on floor markers while walking
Dyssynergia	Movement decomposition and loss of coordination	Finger to nose Finger to therapist's finger Alternate heel to knee Toe to examiner's finger
Hypotonia	Diminished muscle tone	Passive movement Deep tendon reflexes
Tremor (resting)	Oscillating movements at rest	Observation of patient at rest Observation during functional activities (tremor will diminish or disappear with movement)

(Continued)

TABLE 3–8 Movement and coordination impairments with assessment methods. (*Continued*)

Impairment	Definition	Sample Test
Tremor (intentional)	Oscillating movements with movement	Observation during functional activities Alternate nose to finger Finger to finger Finger to therapist's finger Toe to examiner's finger
Tremor (postural)	Oscillating trunk movements	Observation of steadiness of normal standing posture
Asthenia	Diminished strength	Fixation or position holding (UE and LE) Application of manual resistance to assess muscle strength
Rigidity	Hypertonia with normal reflexes	Passive movement Observation during functional activities Observation of resting posture(s)
Bradykinesia	Slowness of movement and loss of associated movements (eg, arm swing)	Walking, observation of arm swing and trunk motions Walking, alter speed and direction Request that a movement or gait activity be stopped abruptly Observation of functional activities; timed tests
Disturbances of posture	Inability to maintain a given position, react to displacement, or adjust one's posture to changing expectations	Fixation or position holding (UE and LE) Displace balance unexpectedly in sitting or standing Standing—alter base of support (eg, one foot directly in front of the other; standing on one foot)
Disturbance of gait	Any change in the ability to walk under varying conditions	Walk along a straight line Walk sideways, backward March in place Alter speed and direction of ambulatory activities Walk in a circle

UE, upper extremity; LE, lower extremity.

From Nichols-Larsen DS et al. *Neurologic Rehabilitation: Neuroscience and Neuroplasticity in Physical Therapy Practice*. New York, NY: McGraw Hill Professional; 2015. Table 9–5.

TABLE 3–9 Terminology for levels of assistance.

Independence	Completes the activity with no assistance and is safe while doing it.
Modified independence	Completes the activity with no assistance and is safe but requires the use of an assistive device or orthosis.
Supervision	Completes the activity with no assistance but is not safe <50% of the time. The level of safety risk is minimal. Assistance provided is that of the therapist being in close proximity in order to assist if needed, but not touching the client.
Contact guard assist (CGA)	Completes the activity with no assistance but there are consistent safety concerns or periodic losses of balance requiring light assistance to regain balance.
Minimal assistance (Min)	Assistance is required but no more than 25% of the work is done by the person helping, during times of assistance.
Moderate assistance (Mod)	Assistance is required but no more than 75% of the work is done by the person helping, during times of assistance.
Maximal assistance (Max)	The majority of the work is done by the person helping (>75%).
Total assist	The patient does not do anything and all work is done by the person(s) helping.

Additional items to document: Number of helpers should be included. Typically this is documented as +1 Min assist, meaning only one person helped. +2 Mod assist would mean that two people helped. Any assistive device that is used should also be documented; ie, +1 Min assist with walker.

From Nichols-Larsen DS et al. *Neurologic Rehabilitation: Neuroscience and Neuroplasticity in Physical Therapy Practice*. New York, NY: McGraw Hill Professional; 2015. Table 9–6.

TABLE 3–10 Stroke risk factors and their cardiovascular consequences.

Risk Factor	Explanation of Relationship with Stroke[*][**][***][****]
Age	With increasing age, the frequency and severity of many other risk factors increases and multiple comorbidities are common, thus increasing the risk for stroke.
Gender	Men are more likely to have strokes at younger ages, but more women than men have strokes annually, perhaps due to the greater number of women living longer.
Race	Stroke is more common in African, Asian, and Hispanic Americans than in Caucasians. This partially reflects disparities in health care and the delay in diagnosis and treatment of risk factors in these racial groups. It may also relate to differences in diet or access to health literature.
Hypertension	Uncontrolled hypertension stresses blood vessels, decreasing their pliability and causing thickening of the arterial walls, which in turn makes them susceptible to clot formation and hemorrhage.
High cholesterol	Cholesterol is an essential lipid for cell maintenance; cholesterol, specifically low density lipoproteins (LDL), contributes to plaque formation in vessel walls.
Obesity	Stresses the cardiovascular system and is often associated with hypertension, high cholesterol, and diabetes (metabolic syndrome).
Atrial fibrillation	AF is associated with a high incidence of embolism formation and subsequent embolic stroke.
Congenital heart anomaly	A high incidence of stroke has been associated with a patent foramen ovale (PFO), which is the persistence of the fetal connection between the right and left atria that typically closes at birth. PFO is associated with embolitic stroke.
Atherosclerosis	Plaque buildup in blood vessels (atherosclerosis) throughout the body is associated with both embolitic and thrombotic stroke.
Diabetes	Vascular changes are common in type II diabetes, increasing the stiffness of the vascular wall and resulting in decreased capacity for vasodilation.
Alcohol abuse	Excessive alcohol consumption is associated with increased clotting and thereby stroke.
Smoking	Smoking increases the likelihood of blood clots and contributes to the development of atherosclerosis.
Drug abuse	Many drugs (cocaine, LSD, amphetamines, heroin, opiates, Ecstasy, PCP) are associated with risk of stroke, often associated with induced hypertension, vasospasm with/without tachycardia. Heroin/opiates/LSD are more likely to induce stroke by cardioembolism.

[*]Ihle-Hansen H, Thommassen B, Wyllar TB, Engedal K, Fure B. Risk factors for and incidence of subtypes of ischemic stroke. *Funct Neurol.* 2012;27(1):35-40.

[**]Roda L, McCrindle BW, Manlhiot C, et al. Stroke recurrence in children with congenital heart disease. *Ann Neurol.* 2012;72:103-111.

[***]Esse K, Fossati-Bellani M, Traylor A, Martin-Schild S. Epidemic of illicit drug use, mechanisms of action/addition and stroke as a health hazard. *Brain Behav.* 2011;1(1):44-54.

[****]Parry CD, Patra J, Rehm J. Alcohol consumption and non-communicable diseases: epidemiology and policy implications. *Addiction.* 2011;106:1718-1724.

From Nichols-Larsen DS et al. *Neurologic Rehabilitation: Neuroscience and Neuroplasticity in Physical Therapy Practice.* New York, NY: McGraw Hill Professional; 2015. Table 10–1.

opening the narrowed vessel. There are important inclusion and exclusion criteria as to if the patient should receive this drug, and the medical team synthesizes the current and past medical history to make this determination. TPA is most effective if given within the first 4.5 hours of the onset of stroke symptoms. Imaging is used to rule out a hemorrhage prior to administering TPA.

Hemorrhagic stroke—A pooling of blood, which results in cerebral edema and potentially hydrocephalus. Hemorrhagic stroke is more likely to cause the patient to lose consciousness, and often intracranial pressures are increased. These patients require careful monitoring and support to minimize demise.

Measuring stroke severity—This can be achieved using a variety of standardized outcome measures; however, in the acute setting, it is most common for the medical team to use the NIH Stroke Scale (NIHSS) or its **modified version**, the mNIHSS, the modified Rankin, and the Glascow Coma Scale (GCS). These measures can be located using the resources outlined in the appendices of this chapter.

Initial Stroke Outcomes

About 20% of individuals admitted into an acute care hospital will die because of a stroke, and another 20% will return home. It is estimated that 60% of individuals who survive their stroke often require rehabilitation support at varying levels of care; this may be a skilled nursing facility (SNF), or an inpatient rehabilitation hospital, depending on the ability of the individual to participate in 3 hours of therapy each day.

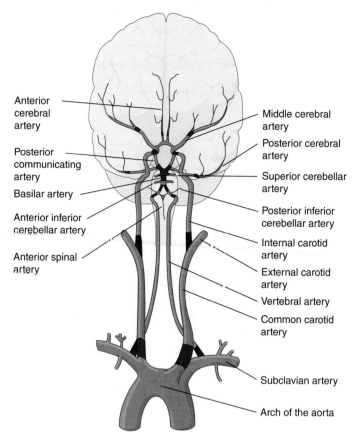

A

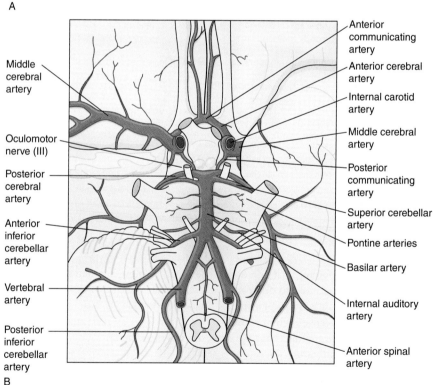

B

FIGURE 3–27 Schematic of the major blood vessels of the brain and the Circle of Willis. A. The brain is supplied by two networks, arising from the aorta: the internal carotid network, branching into the anterior and middle cerebral arteries that supply the anterior 2/3 of the cerebral hemispheres and the vertebral artery system that supplies the posterior 1/3 and the brainstem and cerebellum. B. The Circle of Willis is comprised of the anterior cerebral arteries, the anterior communicating arteries, and the internal carotid arteries (components of the carotid artery system), as well as the posterior communicating arteries and the posterior cerebral arteries (components of the vertebral artery system). The vertebral artery distribution illustrated on the dorsal surface of the brainstem, supplies the brainstem and cerebellum as well as the posterior cerebrum. (Reproduced with permission from Kandel ER, Schwartz JH, Jessell TM, Siegelbaum SA, Hudspeth AJ. *Principles of Neural Science.* 5th ed. New York, NY: McGraw-Hill; 2013. Figure C–1, p 1551.)

TABLE 3–11 Stroke syndromes and associated symptoms.

Artery	Areas of Damage	Common Symptoms
Anterior cerebral **A**[*]	Frontal lobe	
	Medial surface	Apathy/lack of spontaneity
	Anterior and superior aspect of primary motor area	Contralateral motor dysfunction of the lower leg and foot
		Bladder incontinence
		Gait apraxia
	Anterior and superior aspect of premotor cortex	
	Parietal lobe	
	Medial surface	Contralateral sensory dysfunction of leg and foot
	Superior aspect of lateral surface	
Middle cerebral **B**[****]	Lateral surface of frontal lobe	Contralateral hemiparesis (UE > LE)
	Primary motor area	Apraxia
	Premotor area	Expressive aphasia (left)[**]
	Broca's area	Contralateral hemisensory loss
	Lateral surface of parietal lobe	Contralateral neglect syndrome (right)
	Parietal lobe projections to frontal lobe and contralesional parietal lobe	
		Bilateral sensory discrimination loss
	Internal capsule (posterior limb)	Contralateral hemiparesis and hemisensory loss
	Optic radiations	
	Superior (parietal lobe)	Inferior quadrantanopia
	Inferior (temporal lobe, "Meyer's loop")	Superior quadrantanopia
	Both	Homonymous hemianopia
	Temporal lobe (Wernicke's area)	Receptive aphasia (left)[**]

Anterior cerebral artery infarct

Superior frontal gyrus

Cingulate gyrus

Thalamus

Third ventricle

Corpus callosum

Insular cortex

Putamen

Globus pallidus

Middle cerebral artery infarct

Cingulate gyrus

Caudate nucleus, head

Internal capsule, anterior limb

External capsule

Putamen

Insular cortex

Claustrum

Globus pallidus

Anterior commissure

Optic tract

(Continued)

TABLE 3–11 Stroke syndromes and associated symptoms. *(Continued)*

Artery	Areas of Damage	Common Symptoms
Carotid artery	Distribution of both anterior and middle cerebral arteries	Combination of anterior and middle cerebral artery symptoms
Posterior cerebral	Occipital lobe	Contralateral hemianopia or quadrantanopia
		Cortical blindness (bilateral)
		Visual agnosia, agraphia (dominant)
		Prosopagnosia—loss of facial recognition
	Thalamus	Contralateral hemisensory loss
	Hippocampus (temporal lobe)	Memory loss (dominant hemisphere)
	Cerebral peduncle/midbrain	
	Lateral geniculate	Hemianopia/quadrantanopia
	Cranial nerve III	Ophthalmoplegia:
		Ipsilateral gaze deviation—down and out (unopposed pull of superior oblique and lateral rectus)
		Double vision lack of accommodation
Basilar	Medulla	Death is common due to loss of medullary centers associated with respiration control
	Reticular activating system	Loss of consciousness, coma
	Cranial nerve disruption	
	Cr N IX and XII	Tongue paresis, loss of taste, swallowing deficits (dysphagia) Vocal loss (dysphonia)
		Ipsilateral/bilateral
	Pons	
	Cr N III	Dilated pupil(s)—ipsilateral/bilateral
	Cr N V and VII	Facial muscle paresis and sensory loss (dysarthria)—ipsilateral/bilateral
	Cr N VI	Horizontal gaze paresis: bilateral eye turns in—ipsilateral
	Descending motor fibers	Contralateral hemiparesis or quadreparesis (pure motor stroke)
	Ascending sensory fibers	Contralateral hemisensory loss
	Cerebellum	Ipsilateral/bilateral ataxia, vertigo, nystagmus (ipsilateral/bilateral)
	Distribution of posterior cerebral artery	Same symptoms as above

Artery	Structure affected	Signs and symptoms
Anterior inferior cerebellar	Lateral Pontine syndrome	
	Vestibular nuclei	Vertigo, nystagmus, nausea, ipsilesional falling
	Cochlear nucleus	Ipsilateral tinnitus and deafness
	Trigeminal nucleus	Ipsilateral sensory loss to face; ipsilateral paresis of muscles of mastication (dysarthria, dysphagia)
Posterior inferior cerebellar	Wallenberg syndrome (lateral medulla)	
	Cerebellum/peduncles	Ipsilateral limb and gait ataxia
	Vestibular nuclei	Vertigo, nystagmus, nausea
	Cr N IX	Dysphagia
	Cr N X	Dysphonia
	Horner's syndrome	
	Postganglionic sympathetic neuron damage	Ipsilateral ptosis, miosis, and anhidrosis
	Cr N V—sensory portion	Ipsilateral facial sensory loss
	Second-order spinothalamic neurons	Contralateral loss of pain and temperature in extremities
Superior cerebellar	Cerebellum/peduncles	Ipsilateral ataxia (mild trunk, severe limb and gait), vertigo/dizziness, nausea, vomiting, dysarthria, dysmetria, optokinetic nystagmus
	Medial lemniscus/spinal lemniscus (midbrain)	Contralateral sensory loss (touch, pain and temperature)
	Corticospinal fibers (pons)	Contralateral paresis

*Strokes of the anterior cerebral artery are uncommon, most likely due to the redundancy of circulation from the right and left systems.

**Damage to both areas results in global aphasia (both expressive and receptive).

***A. Reproduced, with permission, from Afifi AK, Bergman RA. *Functional Neuroanatomy*. 2nd ed. New York, NY: McGraw-Hill; 2005, Fig 28–2, pg. 361.

****B. Reproduced, with permission, from Afifi AK, Bergman RA. *Functional Neuroanatomy*. 2nd ed. New York, NY: McGraw-Hill; 2005, Fig 28–1, pg. 360.

From Nichols-Larsen DS et al. *Neurologic Rehabilitation: Neuroscience and Neuroplasticity in Physical Therapy Practice*. New York, NY: McGraw Hill Professional; 2015. Table 10–2.

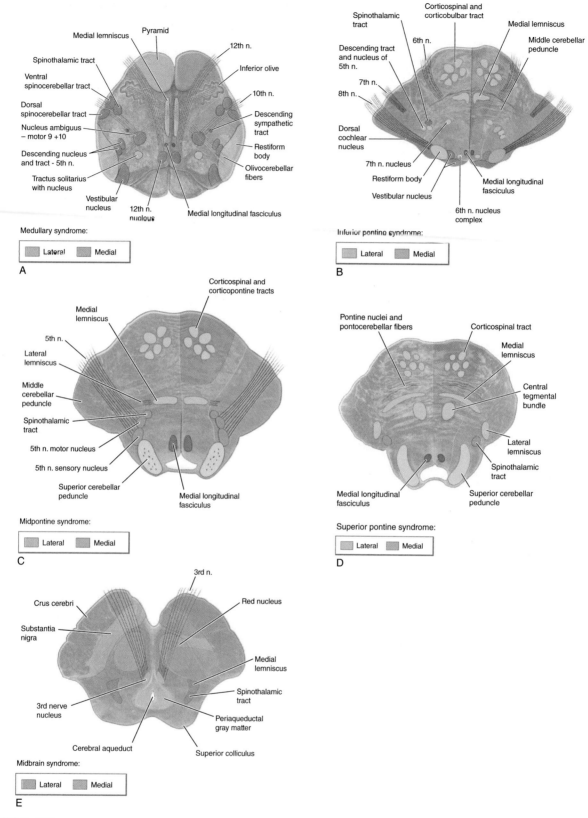

FIGURE 3–28 A–E. Brainstem circulation and stroke syndromes. Ascending syndromes A–E, from the medulla (A) to the midbrain (E), illustrate the complexity of structures damaged with lateral and medial stroke syndromes at each level. Damage to the corticospinal tracts, medial lemniscus, and spinothalamic tract result in loss of function contralateral to the lesion; damage at the level of the lower medulla often results in bilateral loss of corticospinal and medial lemniscal function because of the decussation of these fibers at this level. Typically cranial nerve, spinocerebellar or cerebellar peduncle or medial longitudinal fasciculus symptoms are ipsilateral to the lesion. Thus, brainstem syndromes often present with contralateral or bilateral changes in the limbs, ipsilateral or bilateral changes in balance/proprioception, and ipsilateral or bilateral changes in cranial nerve function. (Reproduced with permission from Jameson JL, Fauci AS, Kasper DL, et al, eds. *Harrison's Principles of Internal Medicine.* 20th ed. New York, NY: McGraw-Hill; 2018, Figures 419–7 through 419–11, pp 3073–3077.)

Acute Neuroplasticity Post-Stroke

The brain attempts to heal itself to return to a state of homeostasis. This neuroplasticity term is referred to as **spontaneous reorganization**. The stroke itself causes neuronal cell death and the area surrounding the cell death, called the ischemic penumbra, is further susceptible to cause an increase in cell death. Early medical interventions attempt to minimize the penumbra and support **angiogenesis** for increased healing and work toward homeostasis. Minimizing the cascade of inflammatory processes is dependent on the activity of surviving neurons and a balance of excitatory and inhibitory connections.

Traumatic Brain Injury

Traumatic brain injury (TBI) is estimated to affect up to 10 million people worldwide and is a leading cause of long-term disability, with 500,000 new cases and an estimated annual cost of $17 billion dollars in the United States. This cost does not reflect the growing number of mild TBIs or concussions. This is more common in men between 17 and 24 years of age, but is becoming more gender-neutral in the current population.

TBI can result from a blow to the head and/or sudden acceleration–deceleration of the head, such as in a motor vehicle accident. TBIs can be closed or open, in terms of whether or not the skull is fracture. Closed TBIs are more common due to car accidents, falls, and blows to the head from falls or assaults. Injuries penetrating the skull can occur from anything that will penetrate the skull; for example, a bullet. TBIs are classified as mild, moderate, or severe, depending on the initial clinical presentation and length of time the person is unconsciousness. The GCS, seen in Box 3–5, is most often used to capture this initial clinical presentation.

Pathophysiology of TBI

TBIs are either focal or diffuse. **Focal injury** occurs at the area of contact between the brain and the skull. Focal damage is characterized by (1) **contusions**—bruising of the brain surface, (2) **lacerations**—tearing of the pia or arachnoid matter or the brain tissue, and/or (3) **hematomas**—bleeding within the subdural or epidural spaces or within the brain tissue, referred to as **intraparenchymal**. These hemorrhages occur due to rupture of the blood vessels within these areas: (1) subdural—tearing of cerebral arteries or veins that bleed into the space between the dura and arachnoid matters, (2) epidural—tearing of meningeal arteries of the dura with bleeding into the space between the dura and the skull, and (3) intraparenchymal—tearing of the penetrating intracerebral arteries with bleeding into the brain tissue.

Diffuse axonal injury (DAI) results from the tearing of axons that comprise the white matter due to rotational forces as the brain moves within the cranium. Most often DAI occurs with motor vehicle accidents; however, is also becoming more common with minor TBI, or concussions. DAI is most common in white matter structures of the brainstem, corpus callosum, and some white matter projections in lateral hemispheres.

The degree of severity and consequences of TBI are dependent upon the areas of focal damage and the amount of white matter damage.

BOX 3–5   Glasgow Coma Scale

The Glasgow Coma Scale (GCS) was developed in the 1970s and assesses eye movements, verbal responses, and motor behavior, looking for spontaneous versus responsive activity, with each scale recorded numerically as indicated here.

Score	Eye Opening	Verbal Responsiveness	Motor Behavior
1	None	None	None
2	Opens in response	Makes sounds	Limbs in extension to deep pressure
3	Opens to verbal stimulation	Saying words	Limbs in flexion
4	Spontaneously opens	Confused but talking	Flexor withdrawal of limb to stimulus
5	N/A	Oriented	Localized response to stimulus
6	N/A	N/A	Moves to commands

Adapted from Teasdale G, Maas A, Lecky F, et al. The Glasgow Coma Scale at 40 years: standing the test of time. *Lancet Neurol.* 2014;13(8):844-854.

TBI Consequences

Coma, post-traumatic amnesia, and executive dysfunction—

As noted with the GCS, initially after TBI there is a loss of consciousness, which can be seconds to weeks. When the loss of consciousness exceeds 6 hours, it is defined as a coma, which is characterized by a lack of responsiveness, volitional movement, and a sleep–wake cycle. Some people after sustaining a severe TBI will enter what is known as a **vegetative state**, which is characterized by an emergence of a sleep–wake cycle and a generalized response to stimuli. Many move through this state to one of minimal consciousness, indicated by specific responses to stimulation but no ability to speak.

Patients who recover from coma after a moderate to severe TBI progress through the vegetative state to a gradual state of responsiveness and severe confusion, abnormal behavior, and memory deficits, defined as **post-traumatic amnesia** (PTA). As the patient moves through the recovery process and the PTA decreases, the patient often has impairment of multiple systems. A tool frequently used to characterize and document changes in behavior, memory, and awareness is the Rancho Los Amigos (RLA) Cognitive Recovery Scale. Additional outcome measures are available in the appendices at the end of this chapter.

Secondary Impairments Following TBI

Respiratory distress syndrome—A common secondary complication of TBI is acute respiratory distress syndrome (ARDS), which occurs in up to 31% of TBI admissions and ultimately is the leading cause of death after TBI. ARDS is defined as inflammation of the lung lining, disruption of gas exchange, and hypoxia.

Interventions involve respiratory support for those with a GCS of ≤8. Those patients who can breathe on their own may require continuous positive airway pressure (CPAP), provided through a mask, or positive pressure support, provided through a nasal cannula.

Intracranial hypertension—Post-traumatic intracranial hypertension (ICH) occurs from hematomas that may create increased pressure, or the shifting of the brain tissue across the midline. Also, if there is compromised blood perfusion, this will exacerbate ICH and cause increased in the intracranial pressure.

It is critical to monitor the patient's intracranial pressure (ICP) when a hematoma has been diagnosed, and this is typically performed with an ICP monitor. If the hematoma is large, it may require immediate surgical removal to decrease the secondary effects.

Epilepsy—Approximately 25% of patients with severe TBI will develop post-traumatic epilepsy. This can occur within the first week of the injury and up to a year or more post-injury. The cause of PTE is unknown, and many theories exist to support these clinical findings.

Many patients who experience PTE are supported with antiepileptic medications. Use and weaning of these medications is dependent on seizure activity and accomplished with the support of the MD.

Dysautonomia/paroxysmal sympathetic hyperactivation—Dysautonomia, more recently renamed paroxysmal sympathetic hyperactivation (PSH), is a dysregulation of autonomic function that presents in 10% to 12% of TBI hospital admissions. It is noted to occur more frequently with severe TBI and those who have fractures, infections, or prolonged ventilation. The theory is that PSH occurs as a result of damage between the hypothalamus and cortex. This causes a loss of inhibition and hypersensitivity to stimuli, and the patient has periods from minutes to hours of tachycardia, hyperpyrexia (fever), elevated blood pressure, extensor posturing (decorticate or decerebrate), and excessive sweating.

Medications are the most common intervention and may include baclofen, beta blockers, benzodiazepine, and morphine.

Neuropsychiatric changes—Some of the most debilitating secondary affects after TBI are the neuropsychiatric changes. Two common behavioral syndromes are emotional and behavioral dyscontrol. **Emotional dyscontrol** manifests itself in up to 62% of TBI survivors as agitation, irritability, restlessness, pathologic laughing/crying, and/or emotional lability. **Behavioral dyscontrol** is characterized by disinhibition and sometimes aggression;

this can result in the pulling out of IV lines and feeding tubes, fighting and swearing early in recovery, as well as hypersexual behavior and excessive risk-taking in later recovery. Many TBI survivors will experience additional psychiatric conditions, especially depression.

The most effective intervention for the common neuropsychiatric diagnoses is behavior modification and management. In some cases, pharmacologic management should be considered or is required.

Mild TBI and concussion—Mild TBI (mTBI) and concussion are discussed as one category, as a concussion is defined as a mild form of a TBI. In both conditions, there is microscopic damage that may not be detectable on neuroimaging, and the injury may or may not involve a loss of consciousness.

It is more common to see mTBI and concussions in the younger population, of which many are still developing brain function and capacity. It is critical that the public is educated on how to prevent mTBI and concussions as related to athletic events. Screening instruments can be found using the resources outlined in the appendices of this chapter. Table 3–12 details the symptoms of concussion.

Brain Tumor

Types of Primary Brain Tumors

Primary brain tumors are somewhat uncommon, with only 200,000 diagnoses each year worldwide. These types of tumors are most common in children, second to the childhood diagnosis of leukemia, that cause death in children. Primary brain tumors are defined as abnormal cell proliferation of neurons or glia within the brain, meninges, vasculature, or pituitary or pineal glands.

Glioma—This is the most common type of tumor in adults and children, and can be further subdivided into astrocytomas, oligodendrogliomas, ependymomas, and mixed gliomas, which typically involve both astrocytes and oligodendrocytes. Gliomas are staged from I (least benign) to stage IV (malignant) based on their

TABLE 3–12 Symptoms of concussion or mTBI.

Cognitive	Physical	Emotional	Sleep
Poorer concentration	Blurred vision	Irritability	Drowsiness/lethargy
Memory disturbance	Headache	Depression	Increased sleepiness
Slower processing	Nausea/vomiting	Hyper-emotionality	Insomnia
	Noise and/or light sensitivity	Anxiety	
	Poor balance/coordination		

From Nichols-Larsen DS et al. *Neurologic Rehabilitation: Neuroscience and Neuroplasticity in Physical Therapy Practice.* New York, NY: McGraw Hill Professional; 2015. Table 11–7.

TABLE 3–13 Tumor locations and characteristics.

Tumor Type	Common Locations	Characteristics
Ependymoma	Usually infratentorial but can be supratentorial (parietal or temporal lobe)	Arise from ventricular ependymal cells (lining of the ventricles); infratentorial tumors are typically Stage III, while supratentorial tumors are typically Stage II.
Gliomas	Anywhere	Arise from glial cells—astrocytes (astrocytoma), oligodendrocytes (oligodendrocytoma); can range from grade I to IV glioblastomas. Stage IV astrocytoma stimulates abnormal angiogenesis, creating highly vascularized tumors. Prognosis is poor.
Glioneuronal	Temporal or frontal lobes; cerebellum	Tumor comprised of both glial cells and neuronal components, arising from neuroepithelial tissues; most common in temporal lobe. Associated with epilepsy that is pharmacologically resistant.
Medulloblastoma	Cerebellum and vermus	Fast-growing malignant posterior fossa tumor in children <7; associated with hydrocephalus.
Meningioma	Arachnoid matter	Stages I–III (most are stage I); multiple genetic contributions. Stages I and II are effectively treated with surgery and radiation.
Pituitary adenoma	Pituitary gland	Benign tumors of one of the six cell types of the pituitary, leading to abnormal secretion of the respective secretory hormones (adenocorticotropic, growth, prolactin, thyroid-stimulating, follicle-stimulating, and luteinizing) with associated symptomology. Tumor growth may disrupt pituitary function. Commonly treatable with gamma knife surgery.
Primitive neuroectodermal tumors (PNETs)	Supratentorial—often within pineal gland	Metastasize easily, so staged according to: 0 = no metastases; 1 = cells in CSF; 2 = supratentorial metastases; 3 = spinal metastases. Fatal in almost 50% (only 20% if in pineal gland), especially once metastasized. Treated with surgery and radiation, sometimes with chemotherapy.

From Nichols-Larsen DS et al. *Neurologic Rehabilitation: Neuroscience and Neuroplasticity in Physical Therapy Practice.* New York, NY: McGraw Hill Professional; 2015. Table 11–10.

rate of growth and whether they have penetrated the surrounding tissue. Table 3–13 describes tumor locations and characteristics.

Tumor Symptoms

Symptoms are often specific to the neuroanatomical location of the tumor itself; however, an increase in ICP is often the first indication of a tumor. Like TBI, tumors may cause nausea, headaches, blurred vision, and fatigue. Many tumors may cause seizures and ultimately epilepsy due to the irritation and eventual death of adjacent cells. Memory or executive function changes occur when the temporal or frontal lobe are involved. Tumors of the posterior frontal/parietal lobe can present with contralateral sensorimotor disturbances such as a stroke. It is common for these symptoms to be initially mild and progress as the tumor increased in size. Tumors located in the posterior fossa disrupt the cerebellum and brainstem, leading to clinical presentations similar to brainstem strokes, that include lack of coordination, dizziness, ataxia, and deficits in the cranial nerves.

Tumor Diagnosis

Imaging is the best diagnostic tool to identify the presence of a tumor. Tumors on a CT scan appear as areas of hypointensity (lighter than the normal surrounding tissue) and therefore an MRI is used for tumor identification.

Medical Treatment of Brain Tumors

Medical treatment needs to be aggressive to minimize secondary neuronal damage. Medical interventions could include surgical resection, radiation, and chemotherapy, depending on tumor type and location.

Spinal Cord Injury

Pathophysiology

Spinal cord injury (SCI) occurs most commonly when there is fracture, dislocation, and/or subluxation of the vertebrae into the spinal cord. Neurological damage from a SCI may occur as a result of primary (or direct) injury and secondary injury. The primary injury is at the site of dysfunction occurring initially, and the **secondary injury** occurs because of inflammation and an increased level of toxicity from the primary injury.

Epidemiology

Each year approximately 12,000 people have a traumatic SCI from car accidents (36%), falls (28%), violence (14%), or sports (9%). About half of all SCIs occur in people under the age of 30, and more SCIs occur in men than women. Additional causes of SCI include transverse myelitis, spinal stenosis, spinal abscess, or tumor.

Classifications of Spinal Cord Injury

SCI is classified by the level and severity of the primary pathology using the **ASIA Impairment Scale** (AIS) and the **International Standards for Neurological Classification of SCI** (ISNCSCI). These resources can be located in the appendices at the end of this chapter.

The severity of SCI is classified into four categories: ASIA A, B, C, and D. Please see Table 3–14 for details.

TABLE 3–14 Classification of SCI.

AIS A	Complete; no sensory or motor function below the level of the injury
AIS B	Incomplete; no motor function but some sensation below the injury, including in the anal sphincter region (S4–5)
AIS C	Incomplete; some sensory and motor function below the injury but most of these muscles score below 3 on MMT
AIS D	Incomplete; sensory and motor function with at least half of the muscle groups scoring 3 or higher on MMT
AIS E	Normal motor and sensory function

SCI, spinal cord injury; ASIA, American Spinal Injury Association; AIS, ASIA Impairment Scale; MMT, manual muscle test.

From Nichols-Larsen DS et al. *Neurologic Rehabilitation: Neuroscience and Neuroplasticity in Physical Therapy Practice.* New York, NY: McGraw Hill Professional; 2015. Table 12–1.

Clinical Syndromes of SCI

Brown-Sequard injury—Is an injury to primarily one side of the cord, leaving the other side relatively intact. See Figure 3–29 for details.

Central cord syndrome—Is caused by a lesion of the center core of the gray matter and occurs with trauma, tumors, or syrinxes, and presents with lower motor neuron (LMN) signs of the upper extremities, with less severe impairments of the lower extremities. See Figure 3–30 for details.

Anterior spinal cord syndrome—Is a lesion of the anterior two-third of the spinal cord and is caused by damage or infarction of the anterior spinal artery. See Figure 3–31 for details.

Posterior spinal cord syndrome—Is a lesion in the posterior part of the spinal cord and can be caused by a penetrating wound to the back or hyperextension that fractures the vertebral arch. See Figure 3–32 for details.

Conus medullaris—Is an injury to the conus medullaris occurs at the L1 vertebral level, which is where the spinal cord tapers to an end. See Figure 3–33 for details.

Cauda equina syndrome—Similar to a conus medullaris injury, and is named as such because of damage to the nerves below the L2 vertebral level. See Figure 3–33 for details.

Medical Management

Acute medical management begins in the community when the injury is traumatic, or in the emergency room for nontraumatic SCIs.

The medical team will make an early decision regarding spinal stabilization and whether surgery is indicated. Once the patient

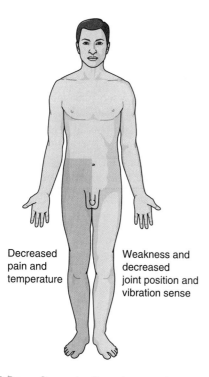

A Brown-Sequard pattern of sensory loss

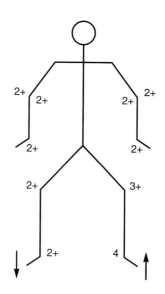

B Hyperreflexia in the weak leg

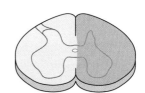

C Extradural compression at T8

FIGURE 3–29 Brown-Sequard pattern of injury. The primary symptoms of a BS pattern are ipsilesional motor and somatosensory dysfunction with contralesional loss of pain and temperature (A); hyperreflexia in the ipsilesional leg (B); and a lesion confined to one side of the spinal cord (C). (Reproduced with permission from Kandel ER, Schwartz JH, Jessell TM, Siegelbaum SA, Hudspeth AJ. *Principles of Neural Science.* 5th ed. New York, NY: McGraw-Hill; 2013. Figure B–5, p 1545.)

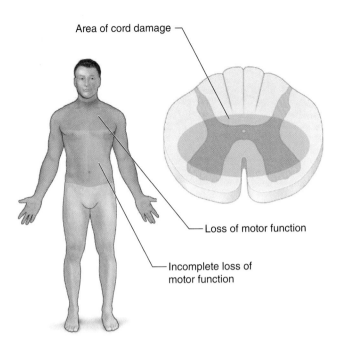

FIGURE 3–30 Central cord syndrome. This shows a lesion in the central gray matter, sparing a peripheral rim of white matter (right). The shaded areas (left) show the regions with complete loss of motor function (dark) and incomplete, mild loss of motor function (light). (From Nichols-Larsen DS, Kegelmeyer DA, Buford JA, Kloos AD, Heathcock JC, Basso D. *Neurologic Rehabilitation: Neuroscience and Neuroplasticity in Physical Therapy Practice*. 2016. Available at: http://accessphysiotherapy.mhmedical.com/content.aspx?bookid=1760&sectionid=120048525. Accessed March 12, 2018.)

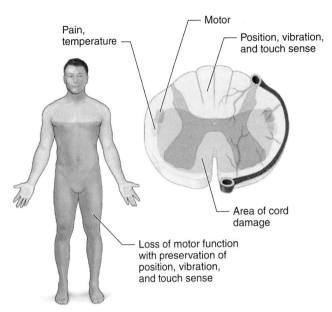

FIGURE 3–31 Anterior spinal cord injury. The lesion location in the ventral gray and white matter is shown on the right image of the cord. The shaded regions on the left show loss of motor function and pain and temperature sensation. Vibration and position sense remain. (From Nichols-Larsen DS, Kegelmeyer DA, Buford JA, Kloos AD, Heathcock JC, Basso D. *Neurologic Rehabilitation: Neuroscience and Neuroplasticity in Physical Therapy Practice*. 2016. Available at: http://accessphysiotherapy.mhmedical.com/content.aspx?bookid=1760&sectionid=120048525. Accessed March 12, 2018.)

has been stabilized and medically cleared, the interprofessional rehabilitation process begins. It is important that the physical therapist be mindful of several body systems that if not managed can pose life-threatening conditions. These systems include: (1) cardiovascular and pulmonary system, (2) bladder and bowel functioning, (4) respiratory system, and (5) integumentary system. Significant attention should be paid to these systems and the possible deficits that can occur with persons after sustaining a SCI. Below is a list of possible medical complications common for individuals with SCI that should be considered and reviewed in further detail.

- Autonomic dysfunction and autonomic dysreflexia
- Cardiac and vasomotor changes—hypotension, bradycardia, arrhythmia
- Deep vein thrombosis
- Bladder and bowl dysfunction
- Pressure ulcer and skin integrity

Multiple Sclerosis

Multiple sclerosis (MS) is a chronic, progressive, inflammatory disease that affects neurons in the CNS.

The incidence of MS is 30 to 80 per 100,000 population; about 400,000 people are affected with the disease in the

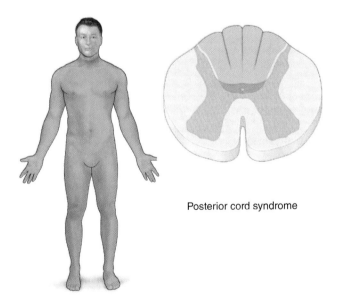

Posterior cord syndrome

FIGURE 3–32 Posterior cord syndrome. The shaded region depicted in the right image of the cord shows the lesion located in the dorsal columns. The affected body regions are shown on the left which have loss of vibration and position sense. (From Nichols-Larsen DS, Kegelmeyer DA, Buford JA, Kloos AD, Heathcock JC, Basso D. *Neurologic Rehabilitation: Neuroscience and Neuroplasticity in Physical Therapy Practice*. 2016. Available at: http://accessphysiotherapy.mhmedical.com/content.aspx?bookid=1760&sectionid=120048525. Accessed March 12, 2018.)

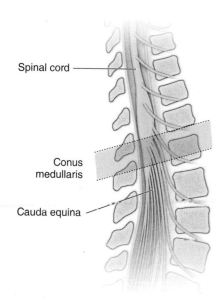

FIGURE 3–33 Conus medullaris and cauda equina injuries. The conus medullaris injury damages the distal portion of the spinal cord at L1; the cauda equina injury damages the spinal nerves, located in the spinal segments below the end of the cord. (From Nichols-Larsen DS, Kegelmeyer DA, Buford JA, Kloos AD, Heathcock JC, Basso D. *Neurologic Rehabilitation: Neuroscience and Neuroplasticity in Physical Therapy Practice.* 2016. Available at: http://accessphysiotherapy .mhmedical.com/content.aspx?bookid=1760&sectionid=120048525. Accessed March 12, 2018.)

United States. It typically affects people between the ages of 20 and 50 and is one of the most common causes of neurologic disability in young adults. MS is two to three times more common in women than in men, and whites of European descent have a higher incidence of MS than any other ethnicity. An increased risk of MS is also associated with smoking and low blood levels of vitamin D.

Pathophysiology

Environmental agents specific to certain viruses are believed to be possible triggers for MS; however, the exact cause is unknown. Although specific genes have not been directly linked to MS, there is one gene, human leukocyte antigen (HLA), located on chromosome 6, that is strongly associated with development of the disease.

MS is an autoimmune disease and involves its own attack on the CNS, which is mediated in part by activated T-cells that travel through the blood–brain barrier. This immune response results in inflammatory damage to the myelin covering as well as the axons themselves. See Figure 3–34 for details.

Various types of MS exist. Box 3–6 describes the clinical presentation of each MS subgroup.

MS has a variety of symptoms and lacks a definitive diagnostic test. An MS diagnosis remains a clinical diagnosis whereby the practitioner considers the patient's history after clinical neurologic examination. Neurologic symptoms related to the demyelinated anatomical locations in the CNS are separated in time and space.

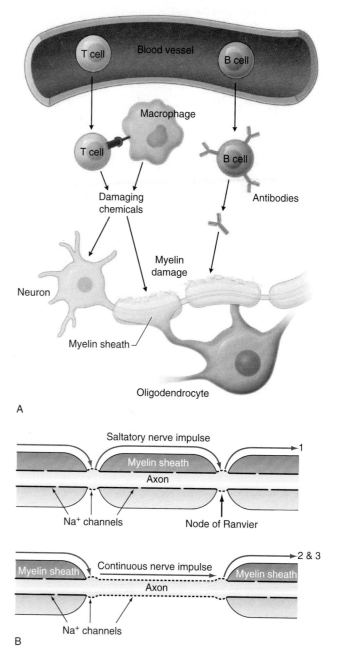

FIGURE 3–34 A. Autoimmune process of myelin damage: activated T cells and potentially B cells, followed by macrophage activity, induce myelin inflammation that can damage the myelin. During the inflammatory phase, conduction is impaired, producing symptoms associated with the involved axons; as inflammation recedes, recovery of symptoms occurs if remyelination is achieved. B. Schematic representation of demyelination and axonal degeneration in MS. 1) schematic of normal neural function in a myelinated axon; 2) in acute demyelination, action potentials can't cross the open space due to low numbers of voltage-gated sodium channels in the internodal axonal regions and stop; 3) in a demyelinated axon, conduction can take place if voltage gated sodium channels are added to the axon membrane through neuroplasticity. but is much slower; 4) with further loss of myelin, axon degeneration occurs (not shown). (B: Reproduced with permission from Hauser SL (ed). *Harrison's Neurology in Clinical Medicine.* 3rd ed. New York, NY: McGraw-Hill; 2013, Figure 39–1, p 475.)

BOX 3–6 Types of Multiple Sclerosis

The clinical disease course varies widely and is unpredictable from person to person and within a particular person over time. However, there are four main subtypes that describe the most frequent clinical course for multiple sclerosis (MS).

Relapsing-Remitting MS

Most individuals (about 85%) diagnosed with MS are initially diagnosed with relapsing-remitting MS (RRMS). People with RRMS have clearly defined relapses, also called attacks, flare-ups, or exacerbations, during which neurologic function worsens. These relapses are followed by remissions, defined as periods during which the disease does not progress and individuals experience complete or incomplete recovery of neurologic function. Incomplete recovery leads to incremental worsening of disability over time. Relapse rates for untreated RRMS are about one to two relapses a year and are correlated with disability.

Secondary Progressive MS

Following an initial period of RRMS, many people develop a secondary-progressive (SPMS) disease course, in which the disease steadily worsens, with or without notable relapses and remissions or plateaus. Approximately 50% of people with RRMS developed SPMS within 10 years of diagnosis before the advent of disease-modifying medications. Long-term data are not yet available to determine if this transition is delayed in treated individuals.

Primary Progressive MS

Primary progressive MS (PPMS) affects approximately 10% of people and is characterized by slowly worsening neurologic function from the time of diagnosis with no distinct relapses or remissions. The rate of progression may vary over time, with occasional plateaus and temporary minor improvements. Individuals with PPMS tend to be older (ie, around 40 years old) at the time of onset.

Progressive-Relapsing MS

Progressive-relapsing MS (PRMS) includes about 5% of people with MS who experience steadily worsening disease from the beginning, with superimposed relapses followed by no or little recovery along the way. In contrast to RRMS, the disease continues to progress and disability increases even during the time between relapses.

In rare cases, individuals with MS experience a very mild disease course called benign MS, in which full neurologic function is preserved 15 years after disease onset. On the other extreme, some individuals experience a very rapid disease course called malignant MS (Marburg disease), leading to death within a short time of onset.

From Nichols-Larsen DS et al. *Neurologic Rehabilitation: Neuroscience and Neuroplasticity in Physical Therapy Practice.* New York, NY: McGraw Hill Professional; 2015.

Imaging and other diagnostic tests help confirm an MS diagnosis. Box 3–7 provides a list of common symptoms associated with MS. These symptoms should be explored in further detail.

Medical Management

Medical management is best achieved with an interprofessional team. Long-term management should be supported with disease-modifying immunomodulatory pharmacological drugs. Acute symptoms and relapses are most notably treated with high-dose intravenous corticosteroids for a period of 3 to 5 days. Drug side effects of both types of intervention should be considered. Pain management is usually managed with anticonvulsant medications, including gabapentin, pregabalin, and carbamazepine. Medications and many rehabilitation interventions are often used to support varying levels of spasticity, fatigue, ataxia and tremor, cognition, emotion, and bowel, bladder, and sexual issues.

Life expectancy is near normal for most people with MS, and the majority of persons with MS do not become severely disabled. The prognostic indicators for MS are variable from person to person; however, the guidelines below are suggested for the most accurate prognosis.

- Gender
- Age
- Symptom
- Progression of disease
- Neurological findings at 5 years
- MRI findings

Parkinson's Disease

Parkinson's disease (PD) is the second most common progressive neurodegenerative disorder, with deficits in the basal ganglia and its connections to motor, cognitive, and psychiatric functions.

PD is estimated to affect 1 million Americans and 7 to 10 million people worldwide. There are approximately 60,000 new cases of PD annually in the United States, with an average age of onset of 60 years old. PD affects men 1.5 times more than women, with the highest incidence among Hispanics.

Etiology and Risk Factors

Parkinsonism is a group of disorders which including slowing movement, tremor, rigidity or stiffness, and balance problems. Parkinsonism includes idiopathic PD and secondary parkinsonism. **Parkinson-plus syndromes** mimic PD in some ways, but are caused by other neurodegenerative disorders.

Idiopathic Parkinson's disease—Idiopathic PD is the most common form of parkinsonism, affecting 78% of individuals with

BOX 3–7 Common Symptoms of Multiple Sclerosis

Sensory Symptoms
  Hypoesthesia, numbness
  Paresthesias
Pain
  Dysesthesias
  Optic or trigeminal neuritis
  Lhermitte's sign
  Chronic pain
Visual Symptoms
  Blurred or double vision
  Diminished acuity/loss of vision
  Scotoma
  Internuclear ophthalmoplegia
  Nystagmus
Motor Symptoms
  Weakness or paralysis
  Fatigue
  Spasticity
  Impaired balance
  Ataxia and intention tremor
  Impaired gait and mobility
  Impaired speech and swallowing
Cognitive Symptoms
  Decreased information processing speed
  Short-term memory problems

  Decreased attention and concentration
  Executive function problems
  Impaired visual spatial processing
  Impaired verbal fluency
Emotional/Behavioral Symptoms
  Depression
  Pseudobulbar affect
  Euphoria
  Lack of insight
  Adjustment disorders
  Obsessive–compulsive disorders
Cardiovascular dysautonomia
Bladder and Bowel Symptoms
  Urinary urgency, frequency
  Nocturia
  Urinary hesitancy, dribbling
  Constipation
  Diarrhea
  Incontinence
Sexual Symptoms
  Erectile and ejaculatory dysfunction
  Decreased vaginal lubrication
  Decreased libido
  Decreased ability to achieve orgasm

From Nichols-Larsen DS et al. *Neurologic Rehabilitation: Neuroscience and Neuroplasticity in Physical Therapy Practice.* New York, NY: McGraw Hill Professional; 2015.

parkinsonism. Most scientists believe PD is caused by an interaction between genetic and environmental factors, although the exact cause remains unknown.

Secondary parkinsonism—Toxins, trauma, multiple strokes, infections, metabolic disorders, and drugs are the known causes of secondary parkinsonism. **Toxic parkinsonism can be caused by such toxins as carbon monoxide, mercury, and cyanide poisoning.** Post-traumatic parkinsonism can be caused by severe or frequent head injuries and is also associated with dementia. Vascular parkinsonism is caused by one or more small, sudden strokes to the basal ganglia (BG).

Pathophysiology

PD is caused by degeneration of nigrostriatal dopamine-containing neurons whose cell bodies are in the **substantia nigra pars compacta** (SNpc) of the midbrain and project primarily to the putamen. The loss of dopamine causes numerous motor deficits; however, by the time the patient experiences any clinical

symptoms, approximately 60% of the SNpc neurons have already been lost. The effects produce increased activity in the indirect motor pathway and decreased activity in the direct pathway. The patient will experience a state of stiffness, or muscle rigidity, and an inability to activate and relax muscles needed for functional activities. In addition, a patient with PD experiences symptoms of slow movement (bradykinesia) and a reduction in the amplitude of movement (hypokinesia).

Clinical Presentation
Primary motor symptoms

- **Tremor** is the initial symptom for patients with PD in approximately 70% of individuals, and typically presents as an involuntary slow oscillation in the hand or fingers on one side of the body. This is defined as resting tremor, and is often referred to as a pill-rolling tremor.
- **Bradykinesia** is defined as slowness of voluntary movement, and typically poses challenges when individuals attempt initiation of movements. A reduction of movement amplitude

(hypokinesia) affects all movements and is a primary cause of reduced gait speed and step length.

- **Rigidity**, which can be cogwheel rigidity or lead pipe rigidity, affects proximal musculature of the shoulders and neck, and later progresses to the muscles of the face and extremities.
- **Postural instability** typically occurs in the later stages of PD and will worsen over time. Declining balance poses an increase in fall risks and loss of overall independence and function. Postural instability in patients with PD causes (1) reduced limits of stability, (2) reduced magnitude of postural responses, (3) impaired postural adaptations, and (4) altered anticipatory postural adjustments. Many of these deficits cause postural deformities as the disease progresses. This posture is characterized by rounded shoulders and a forward head with increased trunk, hip, and knee flexion.

Secondary motor symptoms—Muscle performance and strength of both the upper and lower extremities have been noted to decline over time in persons with PD.

Gait deficits are more common in the middle to late stages of PD and contribute to falls, loss of independence, and hospitalization. PD will cause slower gait velocity, shorter step length, an increased step variability and an increased time in double limb support. In addition, trunk rotation is decreased, which then causes a reduction in arm swing. **Dystonia**, involuntary sustained muscular contractions that cause abnormal movements and/or postures, often interfere with gait, with involvement of the foot and ankle. Additional characteristics of a parkinsonian gait include **festination** and freezing, which may contribute to the increased number of falls.

Freezing of gait is a manifestation of akinesia, and a person with PD will have the appearance that their feet are glued to the floor.

Dual-tasking during gait is also impaired in persons with PD because of the decreased gait speed and increased gait variability.

Other motor symptoms—Patients with PD often have speech disorders and dysphagia due to bulbar dysfunction. These occur because of the rigidity and bradykinesia of the orofacial and laryngeal muscles.

- **Motor learning**—Because the striatum is involved in all stages of motor learning, most importantly when learning new skills that consist of a sequence of movements, research has shown that learning of new motor skills or fine-tuning of skills is preserved in early stages of PD for those without dementia, but individuals with PD generally take longer to learn motor tasks than healthy controls. In patients with PD, motor learning has also been shown to benefit from the use of external auditory or visual cueing, particularly with respect to gait.

Non-motor symptoms—Non-motor symptoms are common for individuals with PD. These include autonomic dysfunction, cognitive/behavioral disorders, and sensory and sleep abnormalities.

Medical Diagnosis and Progression

PD is generally based on the patient's clinical presentation; however, differentiation of PD from other forms of parkinsonism is essential. PD usually progresses slowly in the first 5 years, followed by a gradual increase in symptoms for approximately 13 years. The average rate of progression can be seen in Table 3–15.

Two outcome measures that are widely used to measure disease progression and severity of symptoms are the Unified Parkinson's Disease Rating Scale (UPDRS) and the Hoehn–Yahr Classification of Disability Scale. Please view the appendices at the end of this chapter for additional resources.

Medical Management

Pharmacological management—There is no cure for PD. Medical management aims to slow down the progression of the disease through neuroprotective strategies as well as treatment

TABLE 3–15 Progression of symptoms across disease stages in Parkinson's disease (PD) and Huntington's disease (HD).

Disease	Premanifest	Early	Middle	Late
PD	• Hyposmia • Constipation • Depression/anxiety • Rapid eye movement (REM) sleep behavior disorder • Reduced arm swing • Mild motor function changes	• Unilateral tremor • Rigidity • Mild gait hypokinesia • Micrographia • Reduced speech volume	• Bilateral bradykinesia, axial and limb rigidity • Balance and gait deficits/falls • Speech impairments • May need assistance toward end of stage	• Severe voluntary movement impairments • Pulmonary function and swallowing compromised • Dependence in mobility, self-care, and activities of daily living
HD	• Mild motor symptoms (rapid alternating movements, fine coordination, gait) • Difficulty with complex thinking tasks • Depression, aggression, irritability	• Mild chorea (mainly hands) • Mild balance problems (turns) • Abnormal extraocular movements • Mild visuospatial and cognitive deficits • Depression, irritability	• Chorea, dystonia • Voluntary movement abnormalities • Balance and gait deficits/falls • Cognitive/behavioral problems • Weight loss • Difficulties with self-care	• Bradykinesia, rigidity • Severe dysarthria, dysphagia • Chorea (may be less) • Global dementia • Psychosis • Dependence in mobility, self-care, and activities of daily living

From Nichols-Larsen DS et al. *Neurologic Rehabilitation: Neuroscience and Neuroplasticity in Physical Therapy Practice.* New York, NY: McGraw Hill Professional; 2015. Table 14–5.

TABLE 3–16 Medications for PD.

Drug	Action	Side Effects	Brand Names
Levodopa/Carbidopa	L-dopa converted to dopamine in brain to restore DA levels	Orthostatic hypotension, dyskinesias, hallucinations, sleepiness	Sinemet, immediate and sustained release; Parcopa
Dopamine agonists	Directly stimulate postsynaptic dopamine receptors	Nausea, sedation, dizziness, constipation, hallucinations Linked to impulse control disorders (eg, pathological gambling, compulsive shopping, hypersexuality)	Pramipexole (Mirapex), ropinirole (Requip), piribedil (Trivastal), rotigotine transdermal patch (Neupro), apomorphine (Uprima)
Anticholinergics	Block acetylcholine receptors and may inhibit dopamine reuptake in striatum	Blurred vision, dry mouth, dizziness, and urinary retention; toxicity causes impaired memory, confusion, hallucinations, and delusions	Trihexyphenidyl HCl (Artane), benztropine mesylate (Cogentin), procyclidine hydrochloride (Kemadrin)
Catechol-o-methyl transferase (COMT) inhibitors	Inhibits enzyme COMT to prevent degradation of dopamine	Dyskinesia, nausea, vomiting, orthostatic hypotension, sleep disorders, hallucinations, diarrhea, liver damage with tolcapone	Entacapone (Comtan), entacapone and levodopa (Stalevo), tolcapone (Tasmar)
Monoamine oxidase B (MAO-B) inhibitors	Inhibits enzyme MAO-B to prevent degradation of dopamine	Mild nausea, dry mouth, dizziness, orthostatic hypotension, confusion, hallucinations, insomnia	Selegiline hydrochloride (Eldepryl), rasagiline (Azilect)
Amantadine	Increases release of dopamine presynaptically; blocks acetylcholine receptors	Dizziness, nausea, and anorexia; livedo reticularis (ie, purplish red blotchy spots on skin), leg edema, confusion, hallucinations	Amantadine hydrochloride (Symmetrel), Symadine

From Nichols-Larsen DS et al. *Neurologic Rehabilitation: Neuroscience and Neuroplasticity in Physical Therapy Practice.* New York, NY: McGraw Hill Professional; 2015. Table 14–7.

of motor and non-motor symptoms. A wide range of first-line medications support the neuroprotective aspects and assist with symptom management. See Table 3–16 for details.

Deep brain stimulation—Deep brain stimulation (DBS) can be used to change the firing of the brain circuits; however, it does not slow down the progression of the disease. DBS is reserved for patients who do not have success with pharmacological management.

Huntington's Disease

Epidemiology

Huntington's disease (HD) occurs in the United States in about 1 in every 10,000 people—about 30,000 people in all. There are another 250,000 Americans at risk of having HD. The onset is typically between the ages of 30 and 50. HD affects females slightly more than men and is more common in white people of Western European descent than in those of Asian or African ancestry.

Etiology and Risk Factors

HD is caused by an autosomal dominant mutation, which was mapped to chromosome 4 in 193, in either of an individual's two copies of a gene called *Huntingtin*. Any child from a person having HD has a 50% chance of inheriting the disease.

Pathophysiology

There is severe loss of neurons in the caudate and putamen nuclei of the BG with the diagnosis of HD. These areas have a decreased size, and as such an increase in the ventricular space.

Clinical Presentation

Symptoms typically evolve slowly over time and will vary from person to person, even within the same family. There are motor, cognitive, and behavioral deficits.

Motor symptoms—Patients with HD typically have involuntary movements such as **chorea** and **dystonia**. Choreic movements start out as general restlessness and progress to involve the face, head, lips, tongue, and trunk, and cause flailing movements, called **ballismus**.

Voluntary motor impairments may present in the form of apraxia and persistence of nonfunctional movements. In addition, there are musculoskeletal impairments related to muscle performance, posture, and tone that can negatively impact activity and participation for the patient.

Speech and swallowing impairments develop over time for persons with HD, and patients have difficulty with articulation, alternations in pitch, and a reduction in the rate of speech. In addition, dysphagia will appear as the disease progresses.

Changes in motor learning are similar to those persons with PD.

Cognitive symptoms—In early stages of HD, cognitive problems arise. These may include impaired perception of time, decreased speed of processing, impaired visuospatial perception, short-term memory decline, and executive function deficit; however in later stages patients with HD often have global dementia.

Behavioral symptoms—With HD, emotional and behavioral changes often present prior to the onset of motor symptoms; these include depression, anxiety, and apathy.

Other symptoms—Sleep disturbances are common with HD and often sleep studies are warranted.

Sensory disturbances typically present in the form of pain from dystonias and the alterations in muscle imbalances.

Cardiovascular and respiratory function are compromised due to declines in abnormal changes in both metabolic and physiologic responses to aerobic exercise. In addition, inactivity causes long-term deconditioning and negative changes in overall endurance.

Falls are very common due to the degree of involuntary movements and changes in the muscle performance and musculoskeletal system.

Weight loss is often common with HD and although the causes are not clearly understood, referrals should be made for further support.

Diagnosis

An HD diagnosis is typically made with genetic testing to determine whether a person carries the HD gene. In addition, if there is the presence of motor signs and a positive family history, a clinical diagnosis can be made.

Clinical Course

The clinical course of HD can be divided into five approximate stages: premanifest, prediagnostic, early, middle, and late. Typical progression of HD across the disease stages can be viewed in Table 3–17.

The Unified Huntington's Disease Rating Scale (UHDRS) is the standardized outcome measure used to quantify disease

TABLE 3-17 Total functional capacity staging of HD.

Stage	TFC Scores	Description
Stage I (early)	11–13	No limitations in any area
Stage II (middle)	7–10	Some problems with work and financial capacity but still able to meet responsibilities at home and complete all ADLs
Stage III (middle)	3–6	Limited work ability, needs assistance with finances and home responsibilities; some difficulty with ADLs but still living at home
Stage IV (late)	1–2	No longer working or able to take care of finances or home chores; increased difficulty with ADLs and may no longer be living at home
Stage V (late)	0	Requires a total care facility and is unable to care for self

From Nichols-Larsen DS et al. *Neurologic Rehabilitation: Neuroscience and Neuroplasticity in Physical Therapy Practice.* New York, NY: McGraw Hill Professional; 2015. Table 14–9.

TABLE 3-18 Medications used to treat HD.

Subclass of Drug	Example Medications	Potential Side Effects
Antichoreic Drugs		
Dopamine-depleting medication	Tetrabenazine (Xenazine)	Depression, extrapyramidal symptoms, drowsiness, akathisia
Atypical antipsychotics	Olanzapine (Zyprexa), risperidone (Risperdal)	Extrapyramidal symptoms, drowsiness, akathisia
Neuroleptics (dopamine-blocking agents)	Haloperidol (Haldol), fluphenazine (Prolixin)	Extrapyramidal symptoms, sedation, akathisia
Antidepressants (used for depression and sometimes for irritability and anxiety)		
Selective serotonin reuptake inhibitors (SSRIs)	Fluoxetine (Prozac), citalopram (Celexa), sertraline (Zoloft), paroxetine (Paxil)	Insomnia, gastrointestinal upset, restlessness, weight loss, dry mouth, anxiety, headache
Tricyclic antidepressant	Amytriptyline (Elavil), nortriptyline (Pamelor)	Same as SSRIs
Other medications	Bupropion (Wellbutrin), venlafaxine (Effexor)	Insomnia, headache
Antipsychotics (used for psychosis and sometimes for irritability or for chorea suppression)		
Atypical antipsychotics	Olanzapine (Zyprexa), quetiapine (Seroquel), ziprasidone (Geodon), aripiprazole (Abilify)	Extrapyramidal symptoms, drowsiness, akathisia
Neuroleptics (dopamine-blocking agents)	Haloperidol (Haldol), fluphenazine (Prolixin)	Extrapyramidal symptoms, sedation, akathisia

From Nichols-Larsen DS et al. *Neurologic Rehabilitation: Neuroscience and Neuroplasticity in Physical Therapy Practice.* New York, NY: McGraw Hill Professional; 2015. Table 14–10.

severity and to track symptom changes over time. Please see the appendices at the end of this chapter for further details.

Medical Management

Pharmacological management assists in supporting the motor, cognitive, and emotional/behavioral symptom management. Typical medications and their side effects used for symptom management are summarized in Table 3–18.

MOTOR NEURON DISEASE AND NEUROPATHY

Motor neuron disease and neuropathies involve diseases that affect the neurons and affect how the nerves and muscles are activated. Initial examination is typically with electrophysiologic studies. These may be a variety of tests, including nerve conduction studies to detect demyelination and a reduced conduction velocity and clinical electromyography, which determines if the axons themselves are injured, using needle electrodes.

Amyotrophic Lateral Sclerosis

Epidemiology and Risk Factors

Amyotrophic lateral sclerosis (ALS) is classified as a rare disease; however it is the most common type of motor neuron disease. There are approximately two new cases per year per 100,000 population, with an increased the incidence until age 80, where there are few cases reported. In the United States, non-Hispanic Caucasians are twice as likely as African American and Hispanic populations to develop ALS.

Known risk factors for ALS include age, gender, family history, disease-causing mutations, and living in geographic areas where clusters of patients with ALS have been reported. ALS primarily affects adults between the ages of 40 and 70 and is more frequent in men than women. There is some research to suggest links to lifestyle behaviors. However, there is currently insufficient evidence to determine if any lifestyle influences increase the risk of ALS.

Pathophysiology

ALS is named for atrophy of the muscle fibers and the hardening of the corticospinal neurons in the spinal cord. See Figure 3–35. The etiology of ALS remains unknown. Several suspected neurodegenerative processes, such as genetic mutations, glutamate excitotoxicity, mitochondrial dysfunction, neurofilament aggregation, neurotrophic factor deficits, ribonucleic acid (RNA) metabolism disorders, autoimmune reaction, and programmed cell death (apoptosis) may play a role. By the time most patients report motor deficits, they have already lost as much as 50% of the motor neurons.

Clinical Presentation and Progression

ALS is slow, progressive asymmetric atrophy with muscular weakness and hyperreflexia. For a majority of patients, symptoms begin in the extremities with 20% to 30% of patients presenting with bulbar symptoms (ie, bulbar-onset ALS). See Table 3–19 for details.

Diagnosis and Variants of ALS

The diagnosis of ALS is made on clinical presentation, as there are no biological markers or definitive diagnostic tests. Often

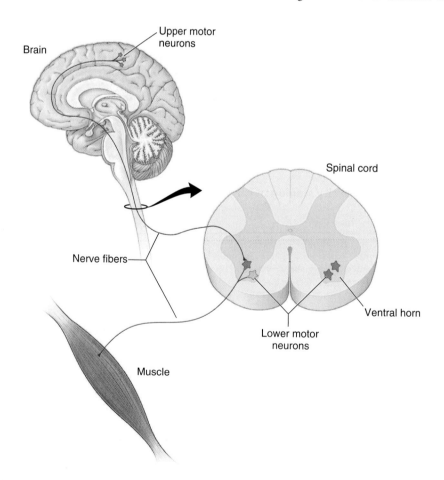

FIGURE 3–35 Pathophysiology of ALS. ALS affects upper motor neurons that arise from the cortex and brainstem as well as cranial and spinal lower motor neurons that arise from the brainstem and spinal cord. (From Nichols-Larsen DS, Kegelmeyer DA, Buford JA, Kloos AD, Heathcock JC, Basso D. *Neurologic Rehabilitation: Neuroscience and Neuroplasticity in Physical Therapy Practice.* 2016 Available at: http://accessphysiotherapy.mhmedical.com/content.aspx?bookid=1760&sectionid=120049201. Accessed March 14, 2018.)

TABLE 3-19 Motor neuron pathology and associated signs and symptoms in ALS.

Motor Neuron Type	Affected Neurons	Associated Signs and Symptoms
Upper motor neurons (UMNs)	Pyramidal Betz motor neurons in the cerebral cortex, corticospinal, and corticobulbar tracts	Loss of dexterity or the ability to coordinate movements; muscle paresis; spasticity; Hoffmann and Babinski reflexes; hyperreflexia; spastic dysarthria
Brainstem motor neurons (bulbar)	Cranial nerve nuclei: V (trigeminal), VII (facial), IX (glossopharyngeal), X (vagus), and XII (hypoglossal)	Difficulty with chewing; dysphagia; flaccid dysarthria/anarthria
Lower motor neurons (LMNs)	Ventral horn cells in the spinal cord	Muscle paralysis and atrophy; fasciculations; flaccid tone; hyporeflexia; respiratory problems

From Nichols-Larsen DS et al. *Neurologic Rehabilitation: Neuroscience and Neuroplasticity in Physical Therapy Practice.* New York, NY: McGraw Hill Professional; 2015. Table 15–3.

neuroimaging and electrophysiological studies are used to support the clinical diagnosis and rule out other disorders.

Medical Prognosis

The medical prognosis is harsh, as death occurs due to respiratory failure within 3 to 5 years of diagnosis, due to the progressive nature of the disease.

Medical Management

Medical management should involve an interprofessional team of healthcare practitioners. There is no cure for ALS; however, research trials using various medications to slow down the progression of the disease and assist with managing symptoms are currently underway.

Guillain–Barré Syndrome

Guillain–Barré syndrome (GBS) is a group of neuropathic conditions that affect the PNS, causing progressive weakness due to motor neuropathy and diminished or absent reflexes. Autonomic and sensory deficits are also possible.

Incidence and Risk Factors

The incidence of GBS is about 2 per 100,000 persons, and an estimated 3000 to 6000 people develop GBS each year in the United States. The incidence of GBS increases with age, and people over age 50 are at greatest risk for developing GBS, with males being more likely than females to develop GBS.

Etiology and Pathophysiology

Many patients with GBS have respiratory and gastrointestinal types of infections that precede the onset of the disease by 1 to 3 weeks. A clinical diagnosis of GBS is related to the following two pathologies: acute inflammatory demyelinating polyradiculoneuropathy (AIDP)—more common—and acute motor axonal neuropathy (AMAN). See Table 3–20 for details.

Clinical Presentation

GBS is characterized by weakness, numbness, tingling, pain in the limbs, or some combination of these symptoms. With AIDP, symptoms progress rapidly and are fairly symmetric. Respiratory failure is common in patients with rapid progression of the disease. This weakness can continue and progress for up to 1 to 3 weeks after the onset of GBS, followed by a plateau of symptoms. It is estimated that 20% of patients remain unable to walk after 6 months from the onset of symptoms. Additional symptoms include cranial neuropathies, sensory disturbances, pain, and autonomic disturbances.

Diagnosis

Diagnosis of GBS is based on clinical presentation of progressive, relatively symmetrical weakness with decreased or absent deep tendon reflexes. In addition, electrodiagnostic and hemodynamic studies and CSF analysis assist in supporting a definitive diagnosis.

Prognosis

Overall mortality is estimated to be 5% related to conditions of sepsis, pulmonary emboli, or unexplained cardiac arrest, possibly related to dysautonomia. The degree of recovery will depend on the degree of remyelination and axonal regrowth.

Medical Management

Patients with GBS should be hospitalized for observation and support of cardiac, respiratory, bowel, and bladder functions until there is evidence of clinical disease progression. Medical treatments to assist recovery and/or eliminate symptoms of GBS include plasma exchange and intravenous immunoglobulin (IVIg).

Acute Poliomyelitis and Postpolio Syndrome

Acute anterior poliomyelitis is a viral disease in which the *poliovirus* enters the body by oral ingestion and multiplies in the intestine. The majority of infected individuals (95%–99%) remain asymptomatic; but 1% to 5% of persons develop fever, fatigue, headache, vomiting, stiffness in the neck, and pain in the limbs, similar to viral meningitis. It can strike at any age but affects mainly children under 3 (over 50% of all cases). It has largely been eradicated through vaccination programs, but 416 cases were reported in 2013. Polio leads to asymmetric, flaccid paralysis, with the legs more commonly involved than the arms. In 10% to 15% of all paralytic cases, severe bulbar weakness occurs. After the initial infection, the virus is shed in feces for several weeks and can spread rapidly through a community.

TABLE 3–20 GBS subtypes.

Type	Pathologic Features	Clinical Features	Nerve Conduction Studies
Acute inflammatory demyelinating polyradiculoneuropathy (AIDP)	• Multifocal peripheral demyelination • Slow remyelination • Probably both humeral and cellular immune mechanisms	• Progressive, symmetrical weakness; hyporeflexia or areflexia • Often accompanied by sensory symptoms, CN* weakness, and autonomic involvement	Demyelinating polyneuropathy
Acute motor axonal neuropathy (AMAN)	• Antibodies against gangliosides GM1, GD1a/b, GalNAc-GD1a in peripheral motor nerve axons; no demyelination	• Strongly associated with *Campylobacter jejuni* infection; more common in the summer, in younger patients, and in eastern Asia • Only motor symptoms; CN involvement uncommon • Deep tendon reflexes may be preserved	Axonal polyneuropathy, normal sensory action potential
Acute motor and sensory axonal neuropathy (AMSAN)	• Mechanism similar to AMAN, but with sensory axonal degeneration	• Similar to those of AMAN, but with predominantly sensory involvement	Axonal polyneuropathy, reduced or absent sensory action potential
Miller Fisher syndrome	• Antibodies against gangliosides GQ1b, GD3, and GT1a • Demyelination	• Bilateral ophthalmoplegia • Ataxia • Areflexia • Facial, bulbar weakness occurs in 50% of cases • Trunk, extremity weakness occurs in 50% of cases	Generally normal, sometimes discrete changes in sensory conduction or H-reflex detected
Pharyngeo-cervico-brachial variant	• Antibodies against mostly gangliosides GT1a, occasionally GQ1b, rarely GD1a; no demyelination	• Weakness particularly of the throat muscles, face, neck, and shoulder muscles	Generally normal, sometimes axonal neuropathy in arms

*CN, cranial nerve.

From Nichols-Larsen DS et al. *Neurologic Rehabilitation: Neuroscience and Neuroplasticity in Physical Therapy Practice.* New York, NY: McGraw Hill Professional; 2015. Table 15–11.

Pathology of the Polio Virus

The pathological findings consist of inflammation of meninges and anterior horn cells, with loss of spinal and bulbar motor neurons. Less common findings include abnormalities in the cerebellar nuclei, basal ganglia, reticular formation, hypothalamus, thalamus, cortical neurons, and dorsal horn. Recovery begins in weeks and reaches a plateau in 6 to 8 months. The extent of neurological and functional recovery is determined by three major factors:

1. The number of motor neurons that recover and resume their normal function
2. The number of motor neurons that sprout axons to reinnervate muscle fibers left denervated by the death of motor neurons (ie, collateral sprouting)
3. The degree of muscle hypertrophy wherein muscle fibers may increase in size from 2 to 3 times normal size

Due to collateral sprouting, a single motor neuron that normally innervates 100 muscle fibers might eventually innervate 700 to 2000 fibers. As a result, survivors of acute polio have a few significantly enlarged motor units doing the work previously performed by many units. Fiber type grouping occurs in the reinnervated muscle, and the normal mosaic interspersion of Type I and Type II fibers will be diminished or absent. Compensation by collateral sprouting and muscle hypertrophy may result in normal manual muscle tests even though more than half the original anterior horn cells are destroyed in some patients.

Postpolio Syndrome Presentation

Postpolio syndrome (PPS) is a condition that affects people who have a history of polio, followed by a period of neurological stability, and then develop new or exacerbated symptoms several years after the acute poliomyelitis infection. The exact incidence of PPS is unknown. Evidence suggests that PPS affects 25% to 40% of polio survivors.

Patients with PPS identify fatigue as their most debilitating symptom. In addition, PPS causes weakness in the muscles that were involved in the initial infection of polio. Often muscle weakness is asymmetrical, and pain is a common complaint with PPS.

Diagnosis

The diagnosis of PPS first rules out other diagnoses, and the physician will order a blood test to determine if the creatine kinase level is elevated. The cause of PPS remains unknown.

Medical Management and Prognosis

Management is directed at treating the symptoms, as there is no specific pharmaceutical treatment for the diagnosis. PPS has periods of stability or a plateau, and is a very slowly progressing condition. In addition, EMG studies are typically ordered and will display chronic denervations.

Peripheral Neuropathies

Peripheral neuropathy is defined as damage to nerves which leads to impaired sensation, movement, gland, or organ function. If the damage involves one nerve it is defined as **mononeuropathy**. If it involves multiple nerves it is defined as **polyneuropathy**. Neuropathies occur in 3% to 4% of persons over the age of 55 due to the common nature of diabetes. Neuropathies also occur due to trauma, infection, autoimmune disorders, and inherited disorders. See Table 3–21 for causes of peripheral neuropathies.

Effects of Muscle Denervation

If muscles become denervated, they undergo several changes in structure, including the proliferation of extrajunctional acetylcholine receptors, which are normally found only at the neuromuscular junction, and atrophy of both Type I and II fibers. Surgical repair may be indicated and may involve a nerve graft.

Peripheral and Central Vestibular Disorders

It is estimated that as many as 35% of adults aged 40 years or older in the United States have experienced some form of vestibular dysfunction. In addition, up to 65% of individuals older than 60 years of age experience dizziness or loss of balance, often on a daily basis.

Vestibular disorders can be categorized by their location as peripheral, central, or both. Peripheral vestibular disorders involve the peripheral sensory apparatus and/or inner ear structures and/or the vestibular nerve. Central vestibular disorders result from damage to the vestibular nuclei, the cerebellum, and the brainstem, including vestibular pathways within the brainstem that mediate vestibular reflexes.

TABLE 3–21 Causes of peripheral neuropathies.

Category	Mechanism of Nerve Damage	Examples
Trauma		
Stretch injury	Severance or tearing of the nerve due to a traction force	• Brachial plexus damage at birth (Erb's palsy) • Radial nerve injury secondary to a humeral fracture
Lacerations, stab wounds, and penetrating trauma	Partial or complete severing of the nerve	• May be a cleancut (surgical incision, glass) or • Irregular (blunt instruments, knife stabbings)
Compression	Mechanical deformation and ischemia	• "Saturday night palsy" in which the radial nerve is compressed while sleeping either from a partner laying on the arm or from placement of the arm under the body; known as "Saturday night palsy" because it is thought to be more common when the person is impaired by alcohol • Bone displacement from fracture • Hematoma • Compartment syndrome—swelling within the facial sheath following severe trauma
Repetitive stress injury	Repetitive flexing of a joint leads to irritation and swelling When swelling is in a constricted area through which a nerve passes, the nerve becomes compressed	• Carpal tunnel is a well-known condition thought to be caused by repetitive stress such as typing or working with a jackhammer
Systemic Disease		
Diabetes I and II	Most common form in the United States; mechanism is usually loss of peripheral blood flow leading to ischemia of the distal nerve endings	• Usually a symmetrical distal polyneuropathy • Sensorimotor neuropathy found in up to 50% of patients involves paresthesia, hyperesthesia, sensory loss of vibration, pressure, pain and temperature; presence of a foot ulcer may clue physician into diagnosis • Acute diabetic mononeuropathy (carpal tunnel, cranial nerves): common nerves compressed are the median at the wrist (carpal tunnel), ulnar at the elbow, peroneal at the fibular head, and lateral cutaneous nerve of the thigh at the inguinal ligament • Diabetic autonomic neuropathy is a widespread disorder of the cholinergic, adrenergic, and peptidergic autonomic fibers that leads to dysregulation of one or more of the following systems: cardiac, sexual, gastrointestinal, sudomotor (sweating), pupillomotor (blurred vision), and bladder dysfunction
Kidney disorders	Leads to high levels of ammonia in the blood	• Caused by uremic toxicity

(Continued)

TABLE 3–21 Causes of peripheral neuropathies. (*Continued*)

Category	Mechanism of Nerve Damage	Examples
Autoimmune diseases	• Sjogren syndrome • Lupus • Rheumatoid arthritis and other connective tissue disorders • Acute inflammatory demyelinating neuropathy (Guillain–Barré syndrome) • Chronic inflammatory demyelinating polyradiculopathy (CIDP) • Multifocal motor neuropathy	• Immune system attacks the body's own tissues, leading to nerve damage • Inflammation in tissues around nerves can spread directly into nerve fibers • Over time, these chronic autoimmune conditions can destroy joints, organs, and connective tissues, making nerve fibers more vulnerable to compression injuries and entrapment • Guillain-Barré can damage motor, sensory, and autonomic nerve fibers • CIDP usually damages sensory and motor nerves, leaving autonomic nerves intact • Multifocal motor neuropathy affects motor nerves exclusively; it may be chronic or acute
Vitamin deficiencies and alcoholism	• Deficiencies of vitamins E, B1, B6, B12, niacin, thiamine • Alcohol abuse	• Damage to the nerves associated with long-term alcohol abuse may not be reversible when a person stops drinking alcohol • Chronic alcohol abuse also frequently leads to nutritional deficiencies (including B_{12}, thiamine, and folate) that contribute to the development of peripheral neuropathy
Vascular disease	Lack of blood to the nerves, most commonly the terminal nerve endings leads to ischemia	• Vasculitis leads to loss of distal blood supply and anoxic damage to distal nerve fibers
Cancers	Neuroblastomas, tumors, paraneoplastic syndromes	• Cancer can infiltrate nerve fibers or exert damaging compression forces on nerve fibers • Tumors also can arise directly from nerve tissue cells • Paraneoplastic syndromes can indirectly cause widespread nerve damage • Toxicity from the chemotherapeutic agents and radiation used to treat cancer also can cause peripheral neuropathy
Infections	• Herpes varicella zoster (shingles), Epstein-Barr virus, West Nile virus, cytomegalovirus, and herpes simplex members of the large family of human herpes viruses • Lyme disease, diphtheria, and leprosy are bacterial diseases • Human immunodeficiency virus (HIV) leading to AIDs • Lyme disease, diphtheria, and leprosy	• The viruses can severely damage sensory nerves, causing attacks of sharp, lightning-like pain; post-herpetic neuralgia is long-lasting, particularly intense pain that often occurs after an attack of shingles • The bacterial infections are characterized by extensive peripheral nerve damage • A rapidly progressive, painful polyneuropathy affecting the feet and hands is often the first clinically apparent sign of HIV infection • Bacterial diseases characterized by extensive peripheral nerve damage

Inherited neuropathies	• Charcot-Marie-Tooth disease
	• Mutations in genes that produce proteins involved in the structure/function of the peripheral nerve axon or the myelin sheath
		• Symptoms include:
		  • Extreme weakening and wasting of muscles in the lower legs and feet
		  • Foot deformities, such as high arches and hammertoes
		  • Gait abnormalities: foot drop and a high-stepped gait
		  • Loss of tendon reflexes and numbness in the lower limbs
		  • Decreased or increased sensation
		  • Dutonomic changes: decreased sweating; edema; uncontrolled BP, HR; bowel and bladder problems
		  • Motor changes: weakness or paralysis; muscle atrophy
		  • Trophic changes: shiny skin, brittle nails, neurogenic joint damage

Toxins		
Heavy metals and environmental toxins	Lead, mercury, arsenic, insecticides, and solvents	
Drugs	• Anticonvulsants • Antiviral agents • Antibiotics • Some heart and blood pressure medications • Chemotherapy drugs	• In most cases, the neuropathy resolves when these medications are discontinued or dosages are adjusted. • About 30%–40% of people who undergo chemotherapy develop peripheral neuropathy, and it is a leading reason why people with cancer stop chemotherapy early • The severity of chemotherapy-induced peripheral neuropathy (CIPN) varies from person to person

From Nichols-Larsen DS et al. *Neurologic Rehabilitation: Neuroscience and Neuroplasticity in Physical Therapy Practice.* New York, NY: McGraw Hill Professional; 2015. Table 15–16.

Peripheral Vestibular Disorders

Peripheral vestibular disorders, based on the anatomy involved, can be further divided into the following three types: (1) acute unilateral vestibular hypofunction, (2) bilateral vestibular hypofunction, and (3) recurrent pathological excitation or inhibition of the peripheral vestibular system.

Unilateral vestibular hypofunction—Unilateral vestibular hypofunction (UVH) is a decrease in peripheral vestibular function that can be caused by viral or bacterial infections, head trauma, vascular occlusion, and unilateral vestibulopathy. It can also occur following some surgical procedures. Individuals with UVH experience symptoms of acute vertigo, nystagmus, oscillopsia, postural instability, nausea and vomiting, and impaired vestibular ocular reflex (VOR).

Vestibular neuritis—Is the second most common cause of peripheral vestibular pathologies. It typically affects people between 30 and 60 years of age, with a higher incidence in women in their fourth and men in their sixth decade of life. Vestibular neuritis can be unilateral or bilateral, and often occurs after a viral infection. Patients will have severe symptoms of rotational vertigo for 48 to 72 hours and note gradual improvement over a 6-week period, while hearing remains intact. Medications are only indicated initially, and physical therapy interventions are recommended for those who remain with impairments in their postural control and gaze abilities.

Vestibular labyrinthitis—Is an inflammatory disorder where the deficit occurs in the membranous labyrinth, typically caused by viral and bacterial infections. This condition affects individuals of all ages, but more often in adults in their fourth to seventh decades of life. The patient experiences vertigo, nystagmus, postural instability, nausea, tinnitus, and hearing loss. Medical intervention attempts to decrease the infection, and if residual symptoms persist, physical therapy is indicated.

Vestibular Schwannoma of an acoustic neuroma—Is the slowest growing tumor in the human body. Vestibular Schwannomas are usually benign. They originate from the Schwann cells and are located along the vestibular portion of CN VIII. When the tumor grows, it causes additional impairments involving other cranial nerves and causes compression of the brainstem or cerebellum.

Bilateral vestibular hypofunction—Is typically caused by persons taking ototoxic medications but can also occur after an infection, with autoimmune disorders, and with normal aging. Patients typically report disequilibrium, severe postural instability that results in gait ataxia, and oscillopsia with head movement.

Recurrent Vestibular Disorders

These include benign paroxysmal positional vertigo, Ménière's disease (endolymphatic hydrops), and perilymphatic fistula. These disorders are characterized by periods of normal functioning with intermittent periods of vestibular symptoms.

Benign paroxysmal positional vertigo—Benign paroxysmal positional vertigo (BPPV) is the most common peripheral vestibular disorder. It typically affects women more than men, in their fourth and fifth decades of life, and is the cause of approximately 50% of complaints of dizziness in older people. BPPV occurs because of otoconia detaching from the otolithic membrane in the utricle and moving into one of the semicircular canals (SCCs). BPPV has two forms: **canalithiasis**, where otoconia are free-floating in the SCC, or **cupulolithiasis**, where the otoconia are attached to the cupula. Posterior SCC canalthiasis accounts for 81% to 90% of all cases. Physical therapy for assessment and intervention consists of head maneuvers and vestibular rehabilitation exercises as the first choice of treatment.

Ménière's disease—Ménière's disease is a disorder of the inner ear, also known as **idiopathic endolymphatic hydrops**, and involves increased pressure caused by malabsorption of the endolymph in the duct and sac which inappropriately excites the nerve. It more commonly affects women than men, in their fourth and fifth decades of life. An attack involves symptoms such as aural fullness, a reduction in hearing, and tinnitus, followed by rotational vertigo, postural imbalance, nystagmus, and nausea and vomiting after a few minutes. Typically, an attack lasts 24 to 72 hours with improvement of symptoms. Medical treatment supports fluid buildup along with dietary restrictions of salt, caffeine, and alcohol. Pharmacologic treatments include treatment of symptoms with use of vestibular suppressants, antiemetics, and antinausea medications during acute episodes. Long-term, many patients with Ménière's disease benefit from psychological support to manage the lifestyle changes.

Perilymphatic fistula—A perilymphatic fistula (PLF) is commonly caused by a tear or defect in the oval and/or round windows that separate the air-filled middle ear and the fluid-filled perilymphatic space of the inner ear. Because of this small opening, perilymph leaks into the middle ear. A PLF is usually caused by head trauma (often minor), excessive intracranial or atmospheric pressure changes as in rapid airplane descent or scuba diving, extremely loud noises, objects perforating the tympanic membrane, ear surgery (stapedectomy), or vigorous straining as in lifting a heavy object, and physical therapy is contraindicated. Medical treatment involves bed rest with the head elevated for 5 to 10 days and if symptoms persist, surgery is indicated. Table 3–22 outlines and compares peripheral vestibular symptoms and conditions.

Central Vestibular Disorders

Central vestibular disorders occur because of vertebrobasilar ischemic disease, traumatic head injury, migraine-associated dizziness, and conditions that affect the brainstem and cerebellum. Vertebrobasilar ischemic stroke and insufficiency relate to insufficient blood supply to the brainstem, cerebellum, and inner ear. Symptoms could include vertigo, Wallenberg's syndrome, blurred vision or diplopia, drop attacks, syncope (fainting) or weakness, ataxia, and headaches depending on the vasculature involved.

TABLE 3–22 Symptomatology of peripheral vestibular disorders.

	UVH	BVH	BPPV	Ménière's Disease	Perilymphatic Fistula
Vertigo	+	−	+	+	+
Nystagmus	+	−	+	+	−/+
Duration of vertigo	Days to weeks	N/A	30 seconds–2 minutes	30 minutes–24 hours	Seconds to minutes
Nausea	+	−	−/+	+	−/+
Postural imbalance	+	++	+	+	+
Specific symptoms	Acute onset, tinnitus, hearing loss with labyrinthitis	Gait ataxia	Onset latency, adaptation	Fullness of ear, tinnitus, hearing loss	Loud tinnitus, Tullio's phenomenon
Precipitating event	Upper respiratory or gastrointestinal infection	Treatment with antibiotics (gentamicin, streptomycin)	Looking up, turning in bed		Head trauma, ear surgery, coughing, sneezing, straining
Outcome	Resolution of most symptoms by 1 year; dark vertigo may be permanent	Symptoms are typically permanent	Resolved with PT or surgery in most people	Vertigo severity diminishes but hearing loss is often permanent	Usually resolves in 4 weeks

−, Absent; +, present; ++, very strong.

From Nichols-Larsen DS et al. *Neurologic Rehabilitation: Neuroscience and Neuroplasticity in Physical Therapy Practice.* New York, NY: McGraw Hill Professional; 2015. Table 16–1.

Traumatic brain injury—This was discussed previously as a neurologic diagnosis. The incidence of central vestibular pathology occurs in about 50% to 70% of all individuals sustaining an mTBI, and almost all moderate TBIs report varying levels of vertigo.

Migraine-associated dizziness (vestibular migraine)—Involves 10% of all Americans and affects women more than men between the ages of 25 and 55. These individuals could experience episodic symptoms of vertigo, dizziness, imbalance, and motion sickness that can last minutes to hours and which may or may not involve a headache.

Conditions affecting the brainstem and cerebellum—Including diagnoses such as Friedreich's ataxia, cerebellar atrophy, brain tumor, and multiple sclerosis.

Central versus peripheral vestibular pathology—Differentiating peripheral from central vestibular pathology is critical for assessment and intervention. Table 3–23 provides key features to differentiate peripheral from central vestibular pathologies.

TABLE 3–23 Common symptoms differentiating central versus peripheral vestibular pathology.

Central Vestibular Pathology	Peripheral Vestibular Pathology
Uncommon to have hearing loss	Symptoms may include hearing loss, fullness in ears, tinnitus
Nystagmus direction is purely vertical or torsional	Nystagmus is horizontal and torsional
Pendular nystagmus (eyes oscillate at equal speeds)	Jerk nystagmus (nystagmus has slow and fast phases)
Nystagmus either does not change or reverses direction with gaze	Nystagmus increases with gaze toward the direction of the fast phase (ie, away from the side of the lesion)
Nystagmus either does not change or it increases with visual fixation	Nystagmus is decreased with visual fixation
Symptoms of acute vertigo not usually suppressed by visual fixation	Symptoms of acute vertigo usually suppressed by visual fixation
Nausea/vomiting more mild	Nausea/vomiting usually severe
Oscillopsia is severe	Oscillopsia is mild unless lesion is bilateral
Abnormal performance on smooth pursuit and/or saccades	Smooth pursuit tracking and saccade performance normal
If sudden onset, patient likely not able to stand and walk even with assistance (severe ataxia)	If sudden onset, patient can stand and walk with assistance (mild ataxia)
Other neurologic symptoms are present	Other neurologic symptoms are rare
Symptoms may recover slowly or never resolve	Symptoms usually resolve within 7 days in people with UVH

UVH, unilateral vestibular hypofunction.

From Nichols-Larsen DS et al. *Neurologic Rehabilitation: Neuroscience and Neuroplasticity in Physical Therapy Practice.* New York, NY: McGraw Hill Professional; 2015. Table 16–2.

Additional vestibular diagnoses—Other diagnoses involving the vestibular system that should be reviewed in further detail include motion sickness and cervicogenic dizziness.

■ VESTIBULAR FUNCTION TESTS—MEDICAL ASSESSMENT AND MANAGEMENT

Testing for individuals with vestibular dysfunction could involve:

- Electronystagmography/videonystagmography
- Rotational chair testing
- Vestibular-evoked myogenic potential
- Computerized dynamic posturography
- Visual perception tests
- Hearing tests
- Neuroimaging—MRI and/or CT

Pharmacological treatment may be indicated in the acute phases of recovery. See Table 3–24 for a list of common medications.

CEREBELLAR DISORDERS

Disorders of the cerebellum typically involve the clinical presentation of ataxia. Table 3–25 outlines acquired and hereditary cases.

Clinical Manifestations of Cerebellar Damage

The primary sign of cerebellar damage is ataxia, which can be related to gait and balance and/or the limbs themselves. Table 3–26 outlines cerebellar impairments.

TABLE 3–25 Selected causes of cerebellar damage.

Acquired Causes	Hereditary Causes

• Stroke (ischemic, hemorrhagic)
• Toxicity (alcohol, heavy metals [mercury, lead, thallium], medications, organic solvents [toluene, benzene], phencyclidine [PCP])
• Tumor (primary cerebellar tumor, metastatic disease)
• Immune-mediated (multiple sclerosis, celiac disease, vasculitis [Behcet's disease, lupus], paraneoplastic cerebellar degeneration)
• Congenital and developmental (Chiari malformation, agenesis, hypoplasias [Joubert syndrome, Dandy–Walker cyst], dysplasias)
• Infection (cerebellitis, abscess)
• Metabolic (hypothyroidism, acute thiamine [B_1] deficiency, chronic vitamin B_{12} and E deficiencies)
• Trauma
• Degenerative nonhereditary diseases (multiple system atrophy [MSA], idiopathic late-onset cerebellar ataxia [ILOCA])
	• Autosomal recessive:
	  • Friedreich's ataxia (FA)
	  • Early-onset cerebellar ataxia (EOCA)
	  • Ataxia telangiectasia
	• Autosomal dominant:
	  • Spinocerebellar ataxias (SCAs)
	  • Episodic ataxias (EAs)
	  • Dentato-rubral-pallidoluysian atrophy (DRPLA)
	  • Gerstmann–Straussler–Scheinker (GSS) disease
	• X-linked disorders:
	  • Mitochondrial disease
	  • Fragile X–associated tremor/ataxia syndrome

From Nichols-Larsen DS et al. *Neurologic Rehabilitation: Neuroscience and Neuroplasticity in Physical Therapy Practice.* New York, NY: McGraw Hill Professional; 2015. Table 16–10.

TABLE 3–24 Common drugs used to treat acute vertigo and associated nausea and emesis.

Medication	Class	Sedation	Antiemesis	Side Effects
Dimenhydrinate (Dramamine)	Antihistamine; phosphodiesterase inhibitor	+	++	Dry mouth, tinnitus, blurred vision, coordination problems
Diphenhydramine (Benadryl)	Antihistamine	+	++	Tachycardia, urinary retention
Promethazine (Phenergan)	Antihistamine; anticholinergic; phenothiazine	++	++	Dry mouth, constipation, blurred vision
Meclizine (Antivert, Bonine)	Antihistamine; anticholinergic	++	+	Dry mouth, tiredness
Prochlorperazine (Compazine)	Antihistamine; anticholinergic; phenothiazine	+	+++	Dry mouth, blurred vision, constipation
Scopalamine (Transderm Scop)	Anticholinergic (nonselective muscarinic)	+	++	Dry mouth, dilated pupils, blurred vision
Ondansetron (Zofran)	Serotonin 5-hydroxytryp-tamine$_3$ (5-HT$_3$) receptor antagonist		+++	Headache, constipation, blurred vision
Lorazepam	Benzodiazepine	++	+	Addiction, effects increased with other sedative drugs

+, mild; ++, moderate; +++, prominent.
From Nichols-Larsen DS et al. *Neurologic Rehabilitation: Neuroscience and Neuroplasticity in Physical Therapy Practice.* New York, NY: McGraw Hill Professional; 2015. Table 16–4.

TABLE 3-26 Signs and symptoms of cerebellar damage.

Symptom/Sign	Area of Cerebellar Damage	Functional Manifestation	Examination Findings
• Limb ataxia • Dysmetria • Dyssynergia • Dysdiadochokinesia • Decomposition • Rebound	Lateral cerebellum, deep cerebellar nuclei (globose, dentate nuclei)	Uncoordinated movement of ipsilateral arm and/or leg	• Impaired FTN and HTS • Impaired rapid alternating movements • Slow, effortful fine finger movements • Impaired limb rebound
Tremor	Cerebellar efferent pathways to the red nucleus and inferior olivary nucleus, deep cerebellar nuclei	• Postural tremor • Kinetic tremor • Intention tremor (<5 Hz)	• Side-to-side tremor of out-stretched arms or tremor when standing still • End-point tremor on FTN or HTS test
Hypotonia	Vermis, flocculonodular lobe	Decreased ability to maintain a steady force	• Ipsilateral hypotonia of limbs • Pendular deep tendon reflexes
Balance and gait dysfunction	Anterior lobe, vermis, fastigial nucleus	• Wide-based stance • Uncoordinated gait • Difficulty with stopping or turning • Frequent falls	• Impaired sharpened Romberg test • Impaired spatiotemporal/kinematic gait parameters • Unsteady tandem gait • Impaired stopping and turning
Oculomotor dysfunction	Flocculonodular lobe, vermis, fastigial nucleus	• Oscillopsia • Blurred or double vision	• Nystagmus • Impaired slow pursuit • Impaired shift of gaze/saccades • Impaired VOR cancellation
Speech impairments	Rostral paravermal region of the anterior lobes	• Dysarthria • Slurred speech	• Impaired articulation and prosody • May be slow, hesitant, or accentuate some syllables
Cognitive and psychiatric impairments	Bilateral posterior lobes (cognitive), vermis (emotional)	• Memory problems, difficulty functioning at work or in home • Impaired communication skills • Personality changes	• Impaired executive functions • Impaired visuospatial function • Agrammatism, dysprosodia • Blunted affect or disinhibited, inappropriate behavior

FTN, finger-to-nose, HTS, heel-to-shin; VOR, vestibulo-ocular reflex.

From Nichols-Larsen DS et al. *Neurologic Rehabilitation: Neuroscience and Neuroplasticity in Physical Therapy Practice*. New York, NY: McGraw Hill Professional; 2015. Table 16–11.

Medical Management of Cerebellar Damage

There is no cure for patients who suffer from cerebellar damage, and pharmacological interventions to date have had limited success in reducing symptoms or slowing or stopping disease progression.

■ INTERVENTIONS

INTERVENTIONS FOR NEUROMUSCULAR DEFICITS

Stroke

Physical Therapy Management in Acute Care

The rehabilitation team has an early role in assessment and prevention of any additional hospital complications that would affect prognosis. Acute care management typically lasts 24 to 72 hours with a plan for discharge to a skilled nursing facility, inpatient rehabilitation hospital/unit, or home.

Early intervention is essential for long-term improvement in addition to preventing **learned nonuse**. In acute care there is limited time for the physical therapist to return the patient to their highest level of independence, and often there is an emphasis on compensatory interventions which typically encourages the use of the less involved extremities to complete the functional tasks. Research has shown that early compensatory strategies create learned nonuse, and it is the responsibility of the physical therapist to translate the evidence and keep the long-term goals in mind. Interventions shown to be effective focus on the following:

1. Assessment
2. Early intervention and prevention of complications
3. Task-oriented practice
4. Intensive repetitive practice

Assessment

The assessment was previously discussed in the neurologic examination section, and specific to stroke, should utilize standardized outcome measures appropriate for the acute care setting. See the appendices at the end of this chapter to view the ANPT stroke evidence database to guide effectiveness (EDGE) recommendations for stroke and acute care.

Early Intervention and Prevention of Complications

The goal is to minimize acute medical complications so early mobilization and therapy can begin. It is essential for the physical therapist to monitor vital signs during this phase of rehabilitation, and early sessions should focus on preventing contractures and postural hypotension, and minimizing the risk of pneumonia and skin breakdown. Patients, if able, and family members should be trained with ROM techniques to be performed three times a day. Hypertonicity can lead to the development of contractures, thus emphasizing the importance of positioning and ROM, especially with the ankle plantarflexors and hip extensors.

Task-Oriented Practice

Physical therapy should be salient and encourage activities to facilitate the benefits of motor control principles. Acute care interventions should be meaningful and encourage the use of activities or tasks to retrain motor control. Early acute therapy should involve functional mobility in the hospital bed along with exercise to manage fatigue.

Upright Activities

Once the patient is medically stable, interventions should include transfers, gait, and imagery to facilitate mobility. Exercise might start with eccentric activation, depending on the degree of weakness. Box 3–8 provides some suggestions for upright activities in the acute setting.

Assistance Levels

When documenting it is essential to identify the appropriate level of assistance required for patient safety.

Physical Therapy Management in the Rehabilitation Setting

As the inpatient rehabilitation setting begins, the stroke survivor is still in the acute stage of recovery. Interventions need to consider neuroplasticity as a critical component in the recovery process. Inpatient rehabilitation should focus on relearning functional mobility and managing impairments as a component of mobility training.

Intensive practice: upper extremity—The focus of the upper extremity (UE) should be to minimize learned nonuse, as this is associated with a poor long-term outcome. The involved UE should be incorporated with all functional tasks, and hand shaping should be considered. See Box 3–9 for a list of UE rehabilitation suggestions.

Bilateral task training is another successful method for retraining UE function after stroke that is successful in returning function to the UE after CVA.

Both **functional electrical stimulation** (FES) and mirror activities can be beneficial for UE recovery.

Intensive practice: gait—Gait should be practiced with all members of the rehabilitation team in order to ensure the high, intensive practice needed in this stage of recovery. Another treatment modality for intensive gait practice can be through treadmill training. Treadmill training and use of body-weight support systems post-stroke involve starting with an initial velocity of 0.25 meters per second combined with 30% removal of a patient's body weight if the patient is currently nonambulatory, and as soon as it is safe and possible, the speed of the treadmill should be increased and the amount of body-weight support should be decreased.

Gait training, whether over-ground or on the treadmill, should focus on the quality of the gait pattern. Gait needs to include training as a component of the task-oriented approach and involve walking over and around obstacles and on/off of different surfaces, so the patient can begin to utilize problem solving and motor learning at an optimal level. Lastly, as the patient works toward mastery during dynamic gait activities, it is essential to encourage dual-tasking conditions, only if they are safe, so patients practice walking in conditions similar to real-world environments.

Assistive devices—Assistive devices with wheels offer more support for a step-through gait pattern, and unilateral devices unfortunately encourage more of a compensatory gait pattern by permitting patients to spend more time on their stronger or less involved side.

Spasticity: Medical Management in the Chronic Phase

Chronic spasticity, when not responsive to conservative physical therapy interventions, may require the use of pharmaceuticals by the physician. These medications include but are not limited to **botulinum toxin** (**Botox**) as an intramuscular injection and intrathecal or oral baclofen or oral diazepam, dantrolene, and tizanidine.

Physical Therapy Management in the Home Health and Outpatient Environments Following Stroke

In both outpatient and home care environments, it is critical for the physical therapist to engage the patient in an intensive task-specific intervention program. These interventions should include walking on uneven surfaces including stairs and transfers from a variety of surfaces, and should involve functional practice that is specific to the patient's environment. For example, transfer training might include car, toilet, tub, and kitchen chair transfers. Once common tasks and skills have been achieved, physical therapy interventions should include other treatment paradigms such as the use of virtual reality, robotics, circuit and strength training, and constraint-induced movement therapy (CIMT).

BOX 3–8   Techniques for Teaching Transfers and Gait in the Acute Setting

- **Keys to working on transfers**
  - Encourage the individual to be an active participant.
  - The therapist should not provide any more assistance than is absolutely necessary.
  - Positioning of the extremities in positions that lead into the movement can be utilized to help obtain success.
- **Supine to side-lying**
  - Utilize passive positioning to minimize therapist assistance: make sure that the bottom arm is flexed so that it does not end up trapped under the body; if moving onto the non-paretic side, cross the paretic leg over non paretic leg to position for rolling (the client should be encouraged to assist with this positioning, as able).
  - The therapist can then place hands at shoulder and pelvis to assist the client to use momentum to rock twice and then roll over on the third try.
  - Encourage head turning with the roll for additional momentum.
- **Side-lying to sitting edge of bed**
  - Roll to side-lying facing the edge of the bed, using the techniques above.
  - Drop the legs off of the side of the bed from the side-lying position. Encourage the client to use the non-paretic leg to assist in getting the paretic leg off of the bed but with as much active movement of the paretic leg as possible.
  - To make the move from side-lying to sitting easier, the head of the bed may be placed in a slightly elevated position.
  - Instruct to push on the bed with both arms as the legs are dropped over the edge of the bed.
  - The therapist should provide assistance at the shoulder and pelvis only as needed.
  - If the paretic arm is "on top," the therapist may wish to assist by placing the hand in a weight-bearing position.
  - The therapist then places a hand on the client's hand to stabilize it in weight-bearing and places their other hand

on the posterior aspect of the elbow to encourage active weight-bearing through the paretic arm.
- **Sit-to-stand from bed**
  - First, ensure that the feet are both flat on the floor with the hips and knees flexed to 90° (or elevate the bed and place with hips and knees in a less flexed posture to make the transfer easier).
  - Both arms should be placed in a position of weight-bearing during the transfer to encourage active movement and provide proprioceptive input in the early stages of recovery.
  - The bedside table can be utilized to provide a stable surface for weight-bearing through bilateral arms. Bedside tables allow you to start with the table at a lower level and raise the table, as the client comes to standing, and then provide a stable surface for standing activities that allows for use of both arms.
  - If there is reasonable function in the paretic hand, then the client can push off of the bed with bilateral UEs and then place the hands on a walker. Unilateral assistive devices should not be used for standing activities, as they encourage learned nonuse of the involved UE and LE and do not promote equal weight-bearing bilaterally.
- **Early Gait Activities: Acute Care**
  - Equal weight-bearing and use of the paretic leg should be a focus at this stage in rehabilitation.
  - During gait, devices that allow for use of bilateral UEs post-CVA are parallel bars, wheeled walkers with arm trough attached, and the bedside table.
  - Early gait and standing activities should focus on upright trunk control, encouraging use of the paretic limbs during gait, and use of a step-through pattern bilaterally.
  - Therapist assistance with the paretic extremities can be provided as needed to advance the leg and brace the extremities for weight-bearing support.
  - Regardless of ability, the client should attempt to actively take part in all movements to encourage recovery of movement, even in flaccid extremities.

From Nichols-Larsen DS et al. *Neurologic Rehabilitation: Neuroscience and Neuroplasticity in Physical Therapy Practice*. New York, NY: McGraw Hill Professional; 2015.

Physical Therapy Management of Special CVA Syndromes

Neglect syndrome—The goal of physical therapy is to increase the patient's awareness of the "neglected" aspect of their environment and their paretic limb. Treatment involves a variety of interventions that incorporate spatial organization training and increased use of visual scanning and overall sensory awareness.

Pusher syndrome—The goal of physical therapy should be to ensure patients have accurate visual information vertically and to

encourage their own active movements in an attempt to achieve a vertical alignment. The focus should first be on achieving vertical alignment and then progress to practicing other motor tasks while attempting to sustain vertical alignment.

Traumatic Brain Injury

Physical Therapy Management

Physical therapy intervention needs to focus on the three unique aspects of the TBI population: physical, cognitive, and behavioral.

BOX 3–9 Keys to Rehabilitation of the Upper Extremity

1. The hand shapes the activation of the entire upper extremity (UE).
2. Use meaningful tasks.
3. Lower physical demands by
   a. Placing the extremity in a gravity eliminated position for the key musculature
   b. Providing support to the trunk and proximal musculature to minimize degrees of freedom and focus on one joint motion
4. Choose functional tasks that will produce the movements that are the focus for that client's therapy session. Examples:

a. For hand opening, have them reach for a 12-ounce soda can or small ball to encourage finger and wrist extension with a goal of lifting a relatively light object. This activity can also focus on the use of elbow extension in combination with shoulder flexion (moving out of synergy patterns).
b. For coordination, have the individual reach for a small target and push on it.
c. For fine motor control, have the client reach for a small object and remove it and then place it in another location. Example: Remove thumbtack from bulletin board and place in small container for storage.

From Nichols-Larsen DS et al. *Neurologic Rehabilitation: Neuroscience and Neuroplasticity in Physical Therapy Practice*. New York, NY: McGraw Hill Professional; 2015.

Many interventions for CVA are appropriate and evidence-based for TBI, with the additional considerations of possible bilateral involvement, peripheral nerve injuries, and musculoskeletal injuries. The interventions below focus on the cognitive and behavioral aspects of intervention for TBI.

Cognition/Memory—Cognition includes attention, memory, initiation, judgement, and speed of processing. Each of these aspects should be evaluated separately, as all relate to long-term and overall rehabilitation outcomes. It is essential to use standardized outcome measures to quantify the patient's cognition and memory at initial evaluation, during reevaluations, and again at discharge. For full details, see the appendices at the end of this chapter for TBI measures specific to each clinical practice setting.

Early Management—Early care is focused on saving the person's life. After TBI, the patient will be in an intensive care unit (ICU), and the team focuses on determining the severity of the injury, preserving life, and prevention of further damage. As the patient is stabilized, early mobility can occur, including strength and ROM. The physical therapist is monitoring the level of arousal, defining the patient's cognitive state using the RLA stages of cognitive function, and beginning to understand the extent of neuromuscular and musculoskeletal deficits. Table 3–27 describes common behaviors following TBI and suggestions for intervention. While in the ICU, the therapist needs to minimize contractures with splinting, ROM, and/or serial casting.

Assessment and management based on Rancho Los Amigos Levels of Cognitive Functioning—The first three RLA levels are often called the coma levels, as the patient is quite unresponsive. At Level I, the patient does not respond to any stimuli; progression to a generalized response is defined as Level II. Once the responses to stimuli are stimulus-specific, this is defined as Level III. Management in Levels I through III focus

on skin integrity and proper positioning. A variety of stimuli—for example, auditory and tactile—are appropriate components of the intervention, and family members should be educated to communicate with their loved ones, despite their inability to hold a conversation.

As the patient progresses into RLA Level IV, the physical therapist can initiate the motor exam and should utilize standardized outcome measures, as outlined in the appendices of this chapter. In RLA Level IV (Confused and Agitated), the intervention is more about a behavior strategy than a learning strategy, as the patient in this stage is not capable of new learning.

In RLA Levels V and VI, patients continue to have varying levels of agitation as well as other behaviors such as confusion, apathy, lack of initiation, impulsivity, and disinhibition. Physical therapists should offer several options for interventions and engage the patient in positive feedback to reinforce the behavior to participate in therapy sessions.

RLA Levels VII and VIII should focus on return to the community and involve school or work retraining as indicated in the setting of long-term goals and expectations.

Goal setting when working with patients who have sustained a TBI should include body function and structure impairments and activity and participation restrictions, in addition to behavioral and cognitive components.

mTBI and Concussion

Controversy exists in terms of treatment of mTBI and concussion. There is research to support early rest to improve the overall physical and cognitive impairment initially sustained with mTBI, and there is also research that supports moderate physical activity to improve cognitive performance. In addition, there is evidence to support the view that intense physical activity, when introduced too early, will delay recovery. Return to full play in a sport or return to usual physical and cognitive activity should occur only

TABLE 3–27 Common behaviors s/p TBI and their management.

Behavior Description	Key to Management	Management Strategies
Agitation is common s/p TBI and is defined as excesses of behavior. Typical agitated behaviors include restlessness, inability to focus or maintain attention, irritability and, at higher levels of agitation, combativeness.	Prevent escalation of agitation and modify the environment and staff behavior to avoid the use of both physical and medical restraints.	• Be calm both verbally and in your physical and nonverbal actions. • Treatment session goals should be flexible to allow adjustment to the level of agitation. • Treatment environment should be quiet, with minimal external stimuli. • Be aware of tension building up in the client; stop the external stimulation before agitation becomes combative. • Redirect the patient's attention and move them to a location with less stimulating or frustrating activities until agitation is reduced. • Do not attempt to discuss agitation logically or elicit guilt for the behavior. • Do not leave the patient unsupervised or alone during agitation. • Try to maintain consistency in the personnel who interact with the patient so as to promote familiarity and decrease novel stimuli. • To the extent possible, permit moving about or verbalization during periods of increased agitation.
Confusion results from the inability of patients to recall minute-to-minute, hour-to-hour, or day-to-day events in their life. As a result, they are unable to understand their current situation in light of what has or what will occur. Associated problems include diminished attention, learning, and orientation.	Increase and even provide the external structure for the individual, particularly in regard to time, place, and activities.	• Place calendars in client's rooms with a schedule of daily activities posted in their room; also have one that they can take with them throughout the day. • Post the steps for them to follow for their ADLs in their room. • At the start of each treatment session, review your name, what day and date it is, what time of day it is, and where they are. Use calendars, clocks, name tags, and building signage to reinforce this information. • Maximize consistency and establish routines within and between treatment sessions. • To increase client awareness, start each activity with a short and easy-to-understand explanation of what is expected of them. • At the end of the session, use the client's schedule to elicit from him or her the next activity in which he/she will engage.
Impulsivity is a tendency to act without thinking. It is common in people s/p TBI and often seen along with agitation and confusion.	Provide consistency across caregivers and visitors, and have the client verbally rehearse strategies for each treatment activity.	• The entire team should attempt to use the same strategy with a patient; inconsistency will only create confusion. • Verbally review the steps for each activity before allowing the patient to start. • Use a written list of steps that the patient reviews (out loud or to himself) before starting. • The patient verbally rehearses aloud the steps needed to complete the task. • The patient waits a few seconds before beginning a task, and is instructed to think about how to complete the task before doing it. • Aloud, verbal rehearsal should be consistently implemented, in all treatment sessions and throughout the day. As a patient demonstrates increased control, this can be gradually shaped into rehearsing to oneself and then simply pausing before starting the task.
Disinhibition is an inability to stop oneself from acting on one's thoughts. *Sexually inappropriate behavior* is a special case of lack of inhibition.	Remain calm and provide concrete feedback about the behavior.	• Initially, focus on addressing simple situations that may be easiest for the patient to learn to manage. • Identify the issue as "self-control" and use this as the key word for cueing the patient, when they need to be controlling their behaviors. • When delaying gratification is the issue, start with short increments between the behavior and the reward, lengthening the increment as the patient improves. Using a watch or timer for specific cueing may be helpful in this regard. • It is important to provide the patient with feedback on the inappropriateness of sexual behavior in this situation, and not to regard its presence with negative attention. • Avoid emotional responses such as anger or embarrassment; this can reinforce the behavior. • Ignoring the behavior or passing it off with a humorous comment also may reinforce its presence and not provide the patient with the adequate information to understand that the behavior is inappropriate. • The best approach is an immediate, unemotional, straightforward expression of the inappropriateness of the behavior. Be certain the patient knows what behavior is being referred to, such as "your sexual hand gesture is inappropriate and won't be appreciated by most women/men."

(Continued)

TABLE 3–27 Common behaviors s/p TBI and their management. (*Continued*)

Behavior Description	Key to Management	Management Strategies
Perseveration is a person's repetition of certain behaviors, either actions or verbalizations. Some individuals perseverate on a consistent theme, while others repeat external stimuli or their own immediately preceding responses.	Use cueing and pacing to interrupt the repetitive behavior and provide a stimulus to move on to the next step.	• Pace interactions with the client to allow disengagement from one activity before proceeding to the next. • Provide a highly structured environment. • Use cues to redirect the client from the perseverative behavior to the next step. • Do not attempt to use logic to "discuss away" a repetitive theme.
Confabulation is the creation of false memories and is frequent in confused patients, sometimes reflecting the inability to find another explanation for what is happening.	It is important to keep in mind that confabulation may be serving a purpose for the patient, including reducing anxiety.	• For lower functioning, more confused patients, ignore the confabulation and do not challenge its veracity. • For higher functioning patients, provide nonthreatening feedback on the inaccuracy of the memory, then redirect attention to another task.
Inability to self-reflect is due to a lack of insight into the effects of ones behavior on others. The client is not aware of their capabilities or limitations and typically overestimates their ability to perform any given task. These patients will often blame others for their frustration and may exhibit paranoia.	Use concrete goals that are posted within easy access of the person with TBI, and note on the posted goal form as progress is made.	• Include the client in goal setting. • Goals should be concrete and progress should be recorded, where the client can monitor their own progress. • Consistently attempt to elicit the client's insight into their deficits. Be nonjudgmental and express expectations that the deficit will be overcome. • Videotape can provide concrete feedback. • Only make the client aware of deficits that can be worked on in rehabilitation and for which you expect to see improvement. • Continual reinforcement is necessary, after insight is accomplished, to change the behavior.
Apathy can be differentiated from resistance by the presence of lethargy with a bland affect, an absence of agitation, and low motivation. *Depression* is sometimes evident as a patient's self-awareness improves. It may show itself in tears, but also may be evident in social withdrawal, self-degrading comments, anxiety, irritability, and catastrophizing.	Treatment should target choices and acknowledge accomplishments.	• Staff and family should encourage participation. • You may need to remind the patient of the consequences of their injury and the impact of the lack of participation in rehabilitation. • Graphs or other concrete ways of showing progress may be useful to elicit motivation. • Be firm in presenting activities and do not present yes/no choices. Offer two or more alternatives for a given activity. • Working in conjunction with other patients may be motivating. • Activities that the patient spontaneously shows interest in should be used to meet rehabilitation goals. • Ask the client to choose the activity to elicit motivation. • Identify short-term goals and be explicit about the relationship between therapy activities and these goals. • Review progress to date. • Redirect the patient's attention from catastrophic or anxious thoughts. • Inform the psychology staff of the nature of the patient's depressive or anxious thoughts.
Lack of initiation differs from apathy in that the patient is motivated to perform an activity but is unable to determine how to carry it out. Lack of initiation may be evident in problems determining the correct sequence of steps or simply not knowing the first step. It is important to keep in mind that the patient is not always aware of this shortcoming and may provide other excuses for why an activity is not initiated or carried out.	Cueing at the start of or next step in an activity is the key to facilitating initiation.	• Cueing is the primary means of assisting a person who lacks initiation. Cues should be external. • Do not perform or passively assist them to initiate the activity. • Verbal cues should be used initially. Using the same word to cue the same behaviors will assist the patient in moving to the next step. • As independence increases, replace verbal cues with other external cues that do not require another person to present the cue. Examples of external cues are lists posted in the room for ADL routines. External cues should be succinct, readily visible, and free of distracting content. • Clients whose improvement continues should be weaned from external cues to simple verbal statements that can be said aloud or thought to oneself as the patient completes the activity. These self-reminders should be succinct and easy to learn. • While in the inpatient setting, begin to train the patient and family in techniques for establishing a daily routine.

From Nichols-Larsen DS et al. *Neurologic Rehabilitation: Neuroscience and Neuroplasticity in Physical Therapy Practice.* New York, NY: McGraw Hill Professional; 2015. Table 11–6.

after neuropsychological testing has been completed and return to full activity is indicated.

Most individuals will have a resolution of their impairments after a few weeks; however, up to 30% of people will suffer from symptoms that persist for a greater amount of time. This is referred to as post-concussive syndrome, with impairments similar to those outlined with TBI.

Brain Tumor

Physical therapy management of a patient with a brain tumor is similar to those interventions outlined in stroke and/or focal brain injury. Interventions for patients with a brain tumor diagnosis should take additional note of the increased fatigue, cognitive dysfunction with impairments in processing speed, working memory or attention, and diminished respiratory capacity, which often occur after radiation therapy. Physical therapists, along with the rehabilitation team, should consider this specific area of oncology as a specialty area of practice whereby the team should focus on specific body function and body structure impairments, along with activity and participation restrictions related to general physical conditioning. Physical therapy has been found to improve functional outcomes with early intervention as well as to minimize sequelae associated with post radiation therapy.

Spinal Cord Injury

Physical Therapy Management in the Acute Setting

The patient who sustains a SCI will undergo careful observation in the ICU, and team goals are to minimize further medical complication. The physical therapist will begin their assessment once the patient is medically stable. The standardized assessment for the SCI diagnosis is to use the ISNCSCI/AIS exam, which can be completed by many members of the rehabilitation team. The earlier sensory and motor return presents itself, the better the overall prognosis.

Acute Physical Therapy Management

The goal in acute care is to prevent complications such as pneumonia, skin breakdown, and DVT. Patients with tetraplegia are at risk for UE contracture and joint pain so careful consideration should be paid to positioning and ROM.

The patient may have precautions due to spinal stabilization or fracture; however, active exercise should incorporate muscles with partial or full innervation during functional tasks and for basic mobility. Once medically stable, a sitting program should be initiated so the patient can learn to adjust to the cardiovascular changes since the injury. An abdominal binder and/or lower extremity support hose may be indicated to prevent postural hypotension.

Management of the Patient in the Inpatient Rehabilitation Setting

General approach—The focus of inpatient and outpatient therapy for complete SCI focuses on a compensatory approach and seeks to use principles of neuroplasticity when supported by the evidence. Compensatory interventions involve movement strategies such as momentum and muscle substitution and the use of adaptive equipment and bracing to replace the muscles and aspects of the patient's body that are not functioning. There should be a delicate balance between the timing of the compensatory strategies and use of neuroplasticity evidence. Under principles of plasticity, the patient should be encouraged to use maximal effort when performing tasks, should be engaged in making errors to encourage learning, and to involve a high number of repetitions for activity training. Restorative approaches to rehabilitation may replace or supplement compensatory approaches for individuals with incomplete SCI.

Physical therapy intervention needs to be cautious and communicate with and refer to other members of the team regarding spasticity, heterotopic ossification, and osteoporosis.

Physical Therapy Management in the Inpatient Rehabilitation Setting

The level and type of SCI injury predict the expected functional abilities of the patient once spinal shock has resolved. These levels should be reviewed in Table 3–28; note that these levels are simply guidelines, and patients after SCI may have their own unique patterns of recovery.

The goal of inpatient rehabilitation is to prepare the patient to return home. Emphasis is placed on learning how to manage bowel and bladder care, bed mobility, management and protection of the upper extremities, transfers, skin protection, and wheelchair use.

Physical Therapy Management of the Patient in the Outpatient Rehabilitation Setting

In the outpatient setting, emphasis for physical therapy management of SCI is on maximizing patient independence and functional mobility. Continued medical and psychological support may be needed to manage neuropathic pain, spasticity, and to address issues with sexuality, depression, and adjustment to SCI. Research has shown that the greatest changes in motor return occur within the first year after SCI, and recovery seen in the first 6 months is optimal.

Gait training after SCI may follow either a compensatory or restorative approach. The compensatory approach typically involves the use of an assistive device and lower extremity bracing. A restorative approach to locomotor training may the involve the use of a body-weight support system, task training, and overground walking to try approximate normal walking mechanics and speed to promote muscle activation. Individuals with motor incomplete SCI have the best potential for locomotor recovery following a restorative approach.

Multiple Sclerosis Intervention

Physical therapy interventions for MS will depend on the area of deficit and disease stage, and should include further examination of fatigue levels, spasticity, sensory changes and pain complaints, motor deficits, and overall functional losses. Interventions are

TABLE 3-28 Prediction of mobility and outcomes by level of SCI.

SCI Level	Expected Active Muscles	Potential Functional Outcome	Required Equipment
C1–4	Neck and facial muscles Diaphragm–C4	*Bed mobility*: dependent *Transfers*: dependent *Pressure relief*: independent with power WC *Eating*: dependent *Dressing*: dependent *Grooming*: dependent *Bathing*: dependent *WC propulsion*: independent with power WC *Standing*: dependent *Walking*: not expected	Hospital bed Transfer board and/or lift Tilt or recliner WC; WC cushion – – – Rolling shower/commode chair Tilt table; standing frame ventilator
C5	Muscles listed for C1–4 Biceps, brachialis, brachioradialis Deltoid Infraspinatus Subscapularis	*Bed mobility*: min–mod assist *Transfers*: min assist *Pressure relief*: independent with power WC *Eating*: min assist *Dressing*: dependent *Grooming*: min assist *Bathing*: dependent *WC propulsion*: independent with power WC *Standing*: dependent *Walking*: not expected	Hospital bed Transfer board; lift Tilt or recliner WC; WC cushion Splints and equipment to assist eating, dressing, and grooming Rolling shower/commode chair Tilt table; standing frame
C6	Muscles for C1–5 Extensor carpi radialis Serratus anterior	*Bed mobility*: min assist *Transfers*: min assist *Pressure relief*: independent with power WC *Eating*: independent *Dressing*: independent upper body; min–mod assist lower body *Grooming*: independent *Bathing*: independent upper body; min–mod assist lower body *WC propulsion*: independent with power WC; manual: independent indoors; min–mod assist outdoors *Standing*: dependent *Walking*: not expected	Hospital bed Transfer board; lift Tilt or recliner WC; WC cushion Splints Splints Splints Rolling shower/commode chair Tilt table; standing frame
C7–8	Muscles for C1–6 Triceps, flexor carpi ulnaris, finger extensors Finger flexors C8	*Bed mobility*: independent *Transfers*: independent *Pressure relief*: independent with power WC *Eating*: independent *Dressing*: independent *Grooming*: independent *Bathing*: independent upper body; min assist lower body *WC propulsion*: manual independent indoors and outdoors *Standing*: min assist *Walking*: not expected	Hospital bed or standard bed With or without transfer board WC cushion Adaptive devices Adaptive devices Adaptive devices Shower/commode chair Tilt table; standing frame
T1–9	Muscles for C1 to level of injury Intrinsics of hand Intercostals Erector spinae Abdominals T6	*Bed mobility*: independent *Transfers*: independent *Pressure relief*: independent *Eating*: independent *Dressing*: independent *Grooming*: independent *Bathing*: independent *WC propulsion*: manual independent *Standing*: independent *Walking*: not functional	Standard bed With or without transfer board WC cushion Shower/commode chair Standing frame

(Continued)

TABLE 3–28 Prediction of mobility and outcomes by level of SCI. (*Continued*)

SCI Level	Expected Active Muscles	Potential Functional Outcome	Required Equipment
T10–L1	Muscles C1 to level of injury	*Bed mobility*: independent	Standard bed
	Intercostals, external and internal oblique	*Transfers*: independent	
		Pressure relief: independent	WC cushion
	Rectus abdominus	*Eating*: independent	
	L1 partial hip flexor	*Dressing*: independent	
		Grooming: independent	
		Bathing: independent	Padded tub bench
		WC propulsion: manual independent	
		Standing: independent	Standing frame
		Walking: functional; independent to min assist	Walker, forearm crutches, braces
L2–S5	Muscles C1 to level of injury	*Bed mobility*: independent	Standard bed
	Iliopsoas, quadratus lumborum, piriformis, obturators	*Transfers*: independent	
		Pressure relief: independent	WC cushion
		Eating: independent	
		Dressing: independent	
		Grooming: independent	
		Bathing: independent	Padded tub bench
		WC propulsion: manual independent	
		Standing: independent	Standing frame
		Walking: functional; independent to min assist	Forearm crutches, braces

WC, wheelchair.

From Nichols-Larsen DS et al. *Neurologic Rehabilitation: Neuroscience and Neuroplasticity in Physical Therapy Practice.* New York, NY: McGraw Hill Professional; 2015. Table 12–11.

generally presented for relapsing-remitting multiple sclerosis (RRMS), except where otherwise stated.

If a patient is in an acute exacerbation, exercise is not recommended. Often during this time patients are taking high doses of corticosteroids to minimize the inflammatory process; however, these medications have side effects that contraindicate exercise.

Once the patient is past their attack or acute flareup, the physical therapist should monitor blood pressure and check for swelling in the ankles before initiating exercise. Some individuals with MS experience Uhthoff's sign when they become overheated. *Uhthoff's sign* is a temporary worsening of neurologic symptoms, such as increased weakness, spasticity, or blurred vision, when the body gets overheated.

During physical therapy interventions, the therapist should be mindful of fatigue, sensory changes, spasticity, and ataxia.

Interventions should include static and dynamic balance training, and exercises for ataxia and coordination. These are seen in Box 3–10 and are pertinent to supporting patients with MS; however, they are not MS-specific.

Interventions Aimed at Functional Deficits

Interventions to treat changes in functional performance are similar to those identified in the stroke intervention section. Body function and structure impairments should be addressed, and functional training should involve task-specific and task-oriented actives. Physical therapy interventions should include aerobic conditioning because of the connections to improved cognition, strengthening, and balance exercises. Box 3–11 provides exercise progression principles for patients with MS. To manage the fatigue factor with MS, patients need to be educated and take part in energy conservation

techniques. As the disease progresses, functional electrical stimulation (FES) and/or lower extremity bracing may be indicated to address distal weakness. Additionally, assistive devices, adaptive equipment, and wheelchair recommendations may be required.

Parkinson's Disease Management

Physical therapy interventions for individuals with PD may include a variety of treatments to promote motor learning, strength, flexibility and ROM, functional mobility, balance, gait, use of assistive devices, and cardiorespiratory function. Interventions always include patient and family education.

Patients with PD benefit from stretching and ROM activities to minimize the indirect impairments of decreased ROM, stooped posture, and the development of contractures. Stretching and ROM can be targeted for muscle groups frequently affected by rigidity, such as hip flexors, knee flexors, ankle plantarflexors, pectoralis muscles, and cervical flexors. The therapist should promote axial rotation due to the lack of upper and lower trunk disassociation that occurs as a result of PD-associated rigidity. Patients with PD can benefit from strengthening exercises targeting weak extensor muscle groups to try to counteract the active range of motion losses in hip extension, knee extension, ankle dorsiflexion, scapular retraction, and cervical extension. Cardiovascular decline in patients with PD can contribute to decreased functional mobility and participation restrictions. Aerobic training can improve maximal oxygen consumption in individuals with PD.

To address limitations in functional mobility, functional, task-specific training should be incorporated, including repeated

BOX 3–10 Extremity Exercises for Ataxia and Coordination

Instructions: *I want you to copy the motion that I demonstrate, focusing on doing it slowly and smoothly.* Typically these are initially done with the individual in a position to watch what they are doing so that they can use visual feedback. To work on proprioception, they can be progressed to being done without visual feedback.

Upper Extremities

Alternate Flexion and Extension—Flex the right elbow while extending the left elbow and then reverse. Also do this with the wrist and shoulder.

Supination and Pronation—Alternately supinate and pronate the forearm. Difficulty is increased by first going progressively faster, supinating and pronating in sync, and then to make it even harder, do it bilaterally and out of sync (ie, the right forearm is supinated while the left forearm is pronated). This can also be done with shoulder external and internal rotation.

Finger Dexterity—Touch the first digit to the thumb and then extend, touch the second digit to the thumb and extend, and continue to third and fourth digits. Difficulty is increased by going progressively faster.

Rock, Paper Scissors—Make a pattern using the motions of fist to palm of opposite hand, palm to palm of opposite hand, and ulnar side of hand to palm of opposite hand. Start with a combination of two motions then progress to combinations of three motions. Have the individual with MS copy the pattern that you make. You can have them practice doing the pattern repetitively.

Lower Extremities

Flexion and Extension—While in supine slide the heel toward the buttocks and then straighten the leg back out slowly, alternately flexing and then extending the hips and knees. To make this more difficult, place the heel on the shin at knee level and trace the shin bone down to the ankle, then trace it back up. Focus on making a smooth motion.

Dorsiflexion and Plantarflexion—Alternate dorsiflexion and plantarflexion of the ankle.

Bilateral Ankle Dorsi and Plantar Flexion—While seated, first dorsiflex both feet (up on heel), then plantarflex both feet (up on toes) and repeat.

From Nichols-Larsen DS et al. *Neurologic Rehabilitation: Neuroscience and Neuroplasticity in Physical Therapy Practice*. New York, NY: McGraw Hill Professional; 2015.

sit-to-stand from a variety of surfaces, stair climbing, upper extremity overhead reaching activities, and rolling in bed to emphasize trunk disassociation. In addition to functional strength training, patients with PD benefit from education related to restorative and compensatory approaches to functional mobility including bed mobility, transfers, sit-to-stand, gait training, and fall recovery. A therapeutic approach designed to improve movement perception and increase movement scaling in patients with

BOX 3–11 Principles of Exercise Progression in Multiple Sclerosis

1. Exercise should be prescribed on an intermittent basis with a pattern of a brief bout of exercise followed by rest, and then another bout until desired exercise is completed. Training benefits using this type of exercise–rest pattern are similar to the outcomes of continuous exercise with an equal duration.

2. For resistance exercise, the rate of overload progression should be addressed with caution, and full recovery between training sessions should be allowed to prevent musculoskeletal overuse injuries.

3. Resistance can be safely increased by 2% to 5% when 15 repetitions are correctly performed in consecutive training sessions.

4. Cardiorespiratory and resistance programs should alternate training on separate days of the week, with 24 to 48 hours of recovery between training sessions.

5. Watch for Uhthoff's sign, and provide rest and cooling strategies when this occurs.

6. Given the impact of fatigue and weakness on performing activities of daily living, the exercise program progression should:

   • Start by building up participation in activities of daily living

   • Progress to building in inefficiencies to normal daily tasks such as parking a little further away to increase walking distance

   • Move to participation in active recreation that the individual enjoys or typically participates in

   • Finally progress to a structured aerobic training program

From Nichols-Larsen DS et al. *Neurologic Rehabilitation: Neuroscience and Neuroplasticity in Physical Therapy Practice*. New York, NY: McGraw Hill Professional; 2015.

PD is called LSVT* BIG. This exercise approach is based on the Lee Silverman Voice Treatment LSVT LOUD, which is a treatment approach used in increase voice production for patients with PD experiencing hypophonia. The LSVT BIG approach focuses on high-amplitude movements, multiple repetitions, high intensity, and increasing difficulty. This treatment intervention is typically performed for 1 hour, four times per week for 4 weeks.

Gait training and assistive device prescription is an important component of physical therapy management for patients with PD. Common gait deviations include reduced stride length, reduced velocity, cadence abnormalities, increased double limb support time, insufficient dorsiflexion, insufficient hip and knee extension, difficulty turning, festinating gait, freezing of gait, and difficulty with motor and cognitive dual tasking. Gait training in patients with PD can be enhanced with the use of rhythmic auditory stimulation (RAS), visual cues, and body-weight–supported treadmill training.

Patient and family education is an integral part of the physical therapist's role in the care of a patient with PD. Physical therapists provide education to patients, families, and caregivers related to disease progression, symptom management, movement strategies, energy conservation, strategies to perform ADLs and recreational activities, fall prevention strategies, fall recovery strategies, and additional PD resource identification. Individuals with PD often experience psychosocial problems such as depression, anxiety, social isolation, loss of control, and difficulty coping with disability. Physical therapists need to be mindful of medications and their potential side effects. Therapy should be scheduled when medications are optimally dosed.

Huntington's Disease Management

In HD, patients often resort to limited activity and participation due to their apathy and lack of insight into their own deficits. Interventions in the early stages of the disease should include:

- Range of motion and stretching similar to PD
- Transfers with a focus on forward weight shifts

- Gait training similar to PD—research suggests that a rolling walker provides the safest and most organized gait pattern
- Stair training to include definite stops before ascending and descending stairs and use of the railing

Late-stage disease should involve physical therapy interventions for prescribing a custom wheelchair for optimal alignment and supporting a safe home environment with modification as indicated.

Amyotrophic Lateral Sclerosis Management

Creating and supporting interventions for patients with amyotrophic lateral sclerosis (ALS) may be challenging due to the progressive nature of the disease. The research supports individualized interventions and inclusion of exercise and activity at all stages of the disease. The general goals of physical therapy intervention are to maintain optimal independence throughout the disease process. Physical therapy goals should include (1) maintaining safe and independent mobility, (2) maintaining maximal muscle strength and endurance, (3) preventing and minimizing secondary impairments such as skin breakdown and contractures, (4) preventing or managing pain, (5) educating on energy-conservation techniques to prevent unnecessary fatigue and respiratory discomfort, and (6) providing adaptive, assistive, and orthotic equipment to maximize functional independence.

Exercise prescriptions must carefully consider and balance the current level of activity, from disuse atrophy, from overuse activity with continual monitoring of fatigue level. Historically, there is controversy regarding the depth and degree of exercise programs for individuals with ALS. There is a building body of evidence that supports moderate, individualized exercise programs that improve neuronal plasticity and enhance the cardiovascular and pulmonary systems. Box 3–12 displays the current practice and evidence in prescribing exercise programs for persons with ALS.

BOX 3–12 General Exercise Guidelines for Individuals with Amyotrophic Lateral Sclerosis

- Start exercise interventions when individuals are in the early stages of the disease so that they have sufficient strength, respiratory function, and endurance to exercise without excessive fatigue.
- Strengthening exercise programs should emphasize concentric rather than eccentric muscle contractions, at moderate resistance and intensity (eg, 1–2 sets of 8–12 reps or 3 sets of 5 reps), in muscles that have antigravity strength (ie, >3 grade strength) exclusively.
- Endurance exercise programs should emphasize moderate intensity activities (50%–80% peak HR, 11–13 RPE, 3 times per week) as tolerated without inducing excessive fatigue.

- Rest periods are recommended, especially if continuous activity goes beyond 15 minutes.
- Individuals with ALS should be advised to have adequate oxygenation, ventilation, and intake of carbohydrates and fluids before exercising.
- Use available technology (eg, assistive devices, body weight-supported systems) to optimize exercise program effectiveness without causing excessive fatigue.
- Exercise compliance can be improved by integrating enjoyable physical activities along with the formal exercise program, providing opportunities for socialization, and providing rewards for accomplishment of goals.

From Nichols-Larsen DS et al. *Neurologic Rehabilitation: Neuroscience and Neuroplasticity in Physical Therapy Practice.* New York, NY: McGraw Hill Professional; 2015.

TABLE 3-29 ALS disease stages and common intervention strategies.

Stage	Common Impairments and Activity Limitations	Interventions

Early	• Mild to moderate weakness in specific muscle groups
	• Difficulty with ADLs and mobility toward the end of this stage
		• Restorative/Preventative
		  • Strengthening exercises*
		  • Endurance exercises
		  • ROM (active, active-assisted) and stretching exercises
		• Compensatory
		  • Assess potential need for appropriate adaptive and assistive devices
		  • Assess potential need for ergonomic modifications of the home/workplace
		  • Educate patient about the disease process, energy conservation, and support groups

Middle	• Severe muscle weakness in some groups; mild to moderate weakness in other groups
	• Progressive decrease in mobility and ADLs throughout this stage
	• Increasing fatigue throughout this stage
	• Wheelchair needed for long distances; increased wheelchair use toward end of stage
	• Pain (especially shoulders)
		• Compensatory
		  • Support weak muscles (assistive devices, supportive devices, adaptive equipment, slings, orthoses)
		  • Modify the workplace/home (eg, install ramp, move bedroom to first floor)
		  • Prescribe wheelchair
		  • Educate caregivers regarding functional training
		• Preventative
		  • ROM (active, active-assisted, passive) and stretching exercises
		  • Strengthening exercises (early middle)
		  • Endurance exercises (early middle)
		  • Assess need for pressure-relieving devices (eg, pressure distributing mattress)

Late	• Wheelchair dependent or restricted to bed
	• Complete dependence with ADLs
	• Severe weakness of UE, LE, neck, and trunk muscles
	• Dysarthria, dysphagia
	• Respiratory compromise
	• Pain
		• Preventative
		  • Passive ROM
		  • Pulmonary hygiene*
		  • Hospital bed and pressure-relieving devices
		  • Skin care, hygiene*
		  • Educate caregivers on prevention of secondary complications
		• Compensatory
		  • Educate caregivers regarding transfers, positioning, turning, skin care
		  • Mechanical lift

*May be restorative.

From Nichols-Larsen DS et al. *Neurologic Rehabilitation: Neuroscience and Neuroplasticity in Physical Therapy Practice*. New York, NY: McGraw Hill Professional; 2015. Table 15–10.

Physical Therapy Management

Dal Bello-Haas proposed a three-stage model for the progression of ALS as a framework for physical therapy clinical management. See Table 3–29 for details.

Guillain–Barré Syndrome

Physical Therapy Management

Limited evidence exists to support exercise and rehabilitation in people with GBS. However, several studies support the benefits of high-intensity inpatient or outpatient interprofessional rehabilitation to decrease disability and improve overall quality of life.

Acute/progressive stage — Initially, many patients with GBS will be in an intensive care unit (ICU) on ventilation with varying degrees of paralysis and sensory dysfunction. Physical therapy interventions can include education on positioning and prevention of skin breakdown, respiratory care, facilitation of speech and swallowing functions, pain management, bed positioning, ROM exercises, gentle stretching, massage, and initiation of functional activities in sitting and standing as tolerated.

Chronic/recovery stage — Once symptoms have plateaued, strength will begin to return over a period of weeks to months, typically following a descending pattern, with arm function returning prior to leg function. As the patient is recovering, the physical therapist can progress exercise and functional mobility training, while being mindful of fatigue levels. Repetitions should remain low, with a high frequency of short intervals of activity. Most patients require a wheelchair for locomotion for several months. Gait training is often initiated in the parallel bars and eventually progresses to a rolling walker, loftstrand crutches, or a cane. Patients with GBS may also benefit from the use of an ankle-foot orthosis to support distal weakness in the lower extremities. Lastly, energy conservation strategies and being mindful of fatigue levels throughout all stages of rehabilitation should continually guide the intervention.

Postpolio Syndrome

Physical Therapy Management of PPS

Physical therapy interventions need to be mindful of the major complaint from PPS patients of fatigue. Aerobic exercises that

BOX 3–13 General Principles for Designing Exercise Programs

- Use a low to moderate exercise intensity.
- Slowly progress exercise, especially if muscles have not been exercised for a while and/or have obvious chronic weakness from acute poliomyelitis.
- Strengthening exercises should only be attempted with muscles that can move against gravity.
- Pace exercise to avoid fatigue (intermittent periods of rest and exercise).

- Rotate exercise types, such as stretching, general (aerobic) conditioning, strengthening, endurance, or joint range of motion exercises.
- Exercise should not cause muscle soreness or pain.
- Exercise should not lead to fatigue that prevents participation in other activities that day or the days following.

From Nichols-Larsen DS et al. *Neurologic Rehabilitation: Neuroscience and Neuroplasticity in Physical Therapy Practice.* New York, NY: McGraw Hill Professional; 2015.

might include the use of the treadmill, bike, walking, swimming, and resistive activities should be prescribed at a low to moderate intensity. Exercise programs should avoid the overworked muscle groups and should be in alignment with muscle strength testing. Patients with PPS should be encouraged to use the Borg rating of perceived exertion to determine appropriate exercise intensity for aerobic exercise. Programs can be progressed at a slow rate under supervision and direction of the physical therapist. In addition, patients with PPS should be educated in behavior modification related to energy conservation and efficiency. Exercise guidelines are listed in Box 3–13.

Psychosocial Considerations in PPS

Many patients managing their PPS benefit from psychological support to manage their symptoms such as chronic stress, depression, anxiety, compulsiveness, and type A behavior. Referrals to other members of the interprofessional team may be indicated in addition to the physical therapist suggesting a support group.

Peripheral Neuropathy

Physical Therapy Management of Individuals with Peripheral Neuropathies

The best physical therapy intervention is prevention, and for those with prediabetes and diabetes this involves long-term control of blood glucose levels through appropriate diet, oral drugs, or insulin injections to prevent further damage. Exercise can be an effective modality for prevention and treatment. For pain management, medications may be indicated. However, the physical therapist should be mindful of the side effects and potential for variable effectiveness.

Functional training—To support patients with diabetic peripheral neuropathy, research indicates that exercise improves balance, trunk proprioception, strength, 6-minute walk (6MW) distance, and habitual physical activity.

Denervated muscle—The use of electrical stimulation is indicated for patients who are expected to have nerve regrowth after complete denervation. Galvanic current has been used to maintain the connective tissue mobility within the denervated muscle.

There is controversy in the research about the use of electrical stimulation in denervated muscle, as it has been found to slow but does not prevent muscle atrophy.

Sensory impairment—Treatment for sensory impairment should be focused on teaching the client that they are at a high risk of injuring their extremities, since they cannot feel it nor painful stimuli. The physical therapist should teach the patient to perform frequent skin inspections, to avoid tight or restrictive clothing, and to test water temperatures when performing basic ADLs.

Vestibular Disorders

Benign Paroxysmal Positional Vertigo

Physical therapy goals and expected outcomes for patients with BPPV are (1) removal of otoconia from the SCCs, (2) eliminating complaints of vertigo with head movement, (3) improved balance, and (4) independence in all functional activities involving head motions. The greatest efficacy for interventions utilize particle-repositioning head maneuvers that move the displaced otoconia out of the affected SCC. The three main maneuvers used to treat posterior and anterior SCC BPPV are (1) the canalith repositioning maneuver, (2) the liberatory maneuver, and (3) Brandt–Daroff habituation exercises.

The **Canalith repositioning maneuver** (CRM; also called the Epley maneuver) is used to treat canalithiasis, and can be viewed in Figure 3–36.

The **Liberatory maneuver** (also called the Semont maneuver) is the most common maneuver to treat cupulolithiasis, and can be viewed in Figure 3–37.

Brandt–Daroff exercises are repeated movements into and out of positions that cause vertigo, and can be viewed in Figure 3–38.

The **Bar-B-Que roll maneuver** (BBQ roll) is the most common intervention for horizontal SCC cupuolithiasis and canalthiasis. This can be seen in Figure 3–39. Often the BBQ roll is followed by forced prolonged positioning (FPP) when the maneuver is not initially successful. FPP involves lying on the more involved side for 30 to 60 seconds and then slowly rolling into side-lying with the unaffected ear down and remaining in this position overnight.

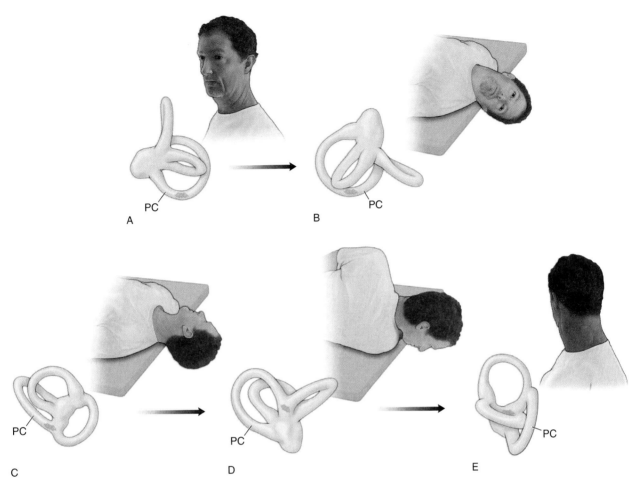

FIGURE 3–36 Canalith repositioning maneuver. The patient is taken through five positions to move the debris through the canal: (A) long-sitting with the head rotated 45 degrees toward the affected side; (B) quickly moved to supine with head extended 30 degrees while maintaining the 45-degree rotation to the affected side, then maintained for 1 to 2 minutes; (C) turn head to the opposite side while maintaining extension over the end of the table; (D) roll to side without moving the head, again maintained for 1 to 2 minutes; (E) return to sitting on the side of the plinth. (From Nichols-Larsen DS, Kegelmeyer DA, Buford JA, Kloos AD, Heathcock JC, Basso D. *Neurologic Rehabilitation: Neuroscience and Neuroplasticity in Physical Therapy Practice.* 2016. Available at: http://accessphysiotherapy.mhmedical.com/content.aspx?bookid=1760 &sectionid=120049508. Accessed March 14, 2018.)

Unilateral Vestibular Hypofunction

Physical therapy goals for patients with UVH and expected outcomes are to (1) improve gaze stability during functional activities (2) decrease the patient's complaints of disequilibrium and oscillopsia with head motions, (3) improve static and dynamic balance, and (4) return the patient to his or her previous level of activity and participation level. Recovery is based on both static and dynamic compensations along the vestibular nerves and firing along the vestibular nuclei. Mechanisms include these compensations and the use of substitution strategies and habituation. Research supports vestibular rehabilitation of UVH for <6 weeks, as long as patients are compliant with their exercise programs.

Gaze stabilization or adaptation exercises—Patients who suffer from visual blurring and dizziness will benefit from individualized exercise that cause retinal slip to create an error signal which in turn causes the brain to adapt to the incoming vestibular input. Exercises that are used to induce adaptation have the patient maintain visual fixation of an object while the head is moving with both a stationary and moving target. See Figure 3–40. These exercises should be progressed in terms of body position, speed of head movement, and overall endurance to continually move the head. Additional adaptation exercises include (1) active eye movements between two targets and (2) between imaginary targets.

Habituation exercises—Habituation exercises can be used to treat patients who report motion-provoked dizziness. These exercises are based on the early Cawthorne and Cooksey exercise and the more recent motion sensitivity quotient. The purpose of the exercises is to provoke symptoms with rests in between to allow the patient's symptoms to return to baseline.

Postural stability exercises—Balance exercise should be a component of the intervention to prevent falls and improve the patient's balance. The physical therapist should consider all balance systems and under both static and dynamic conditions. Box 3–14 provides treatment progressions for balance.

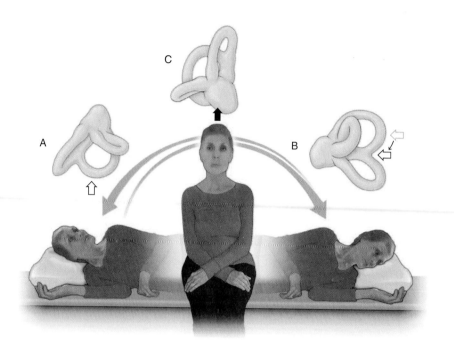

FIGURE 3–37 Liberatory maneuver. The Liberatory maneuver is used to dislodge the debris within the cupula by (A) patient is initially in sidelying; (B) patient is rapidly brought to sitting on the side of the plinth; and (C) patient is rapidly brought to sidelying on the opposite side. This is done by a fluid movement from one side to the other. (From Nichols-Larsen DS, Kegelmeyer DA, Buford JA, Kloos AD, Heathcock JC, Basso D. *Neurologic Rehabilitation: Neuroscience and Neuroplasticity in Physical Therapy Practice.* 2016. Available at: http://accessphysiotherapy .mhmedical.com/content.aspx?bookid=1760&sectionid=120049508. Accessed March 14, 2018.)

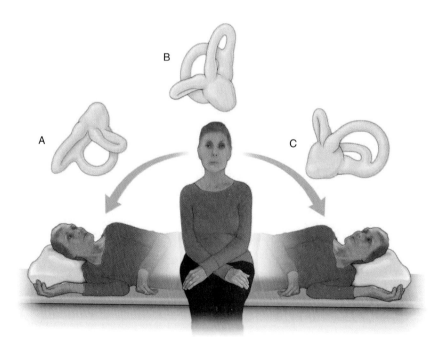

FIGURE 3–38 Brandt–Daroff exercises. The patient begins by sitting sideways on the bed, then quickly lies down on her side with her head turned 45 degrees toward the ceiling. She returns to upright and then quickly lies down on the other side, again with the head turned 45 degrees toward the ceiling. (From Nichols-Larsen DS, Kegelmeyer DA, Buford JA, Kloos AD, Heathcock JC, Basso D. *Neurologic Rehabilitation: Neuroscience and Neuroplasticity in Physical Therapy Practice.* 2016. Available at: http://accessphysiotherapy.mhmedical.com/content.aspx? bookid=1760&sectionid=120049508. Accessed March 14, 2018.)

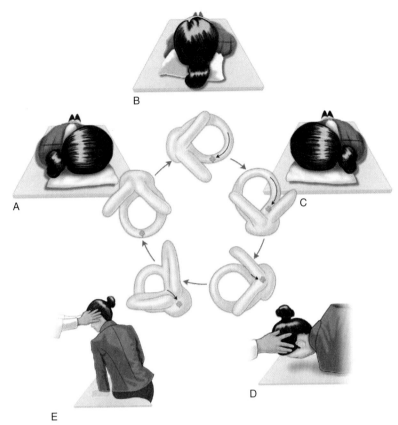

FIGURE 3–39 Bar-B-Que roll maneuver for the treatment of geotropic right horizontal SCC-BPPV. Turn head toward the involved ear while lying supine (A), then turn head 270 degrees toward the unaffected side through a series of stepwise 90-degree turns (B–D); then resume the sitting position (E). Each position should be maintained for at least 1 or 2 minutes, or until the induced nystagmus and vertigo are resolved. The corresponding illustrations demonstrate the orientation of the semicircular canals and the location of the otolithic debris in the horizontal canal. (From Nichols-Larsen DS, Kegelmeyer DA, Buford JA, Kloos AD, Heathcock JC, Basso D. *Neurologic Rehabilitation: Neuroscience and Neuroplasticity in Physical Therapy Practice.* 2016. Available at: http://accessphysiotherapy.mhmedical.com/content.aspx?bookid=1760&sectionid =120049508. Accessed March 14, 2018.)

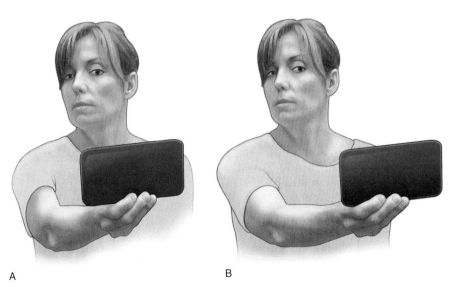

FIGURE 3–40 Gaze stability exercise. A. X1 Paradigm—Patient moves head back and forth while maintaining gaze on stable target. B. X2 Paradigm—Patient moves head back and forth while moving target in the opposite direction. (From Nichols-Larsen DS, Kegelmeyer DA, Buford JA, Kloos AD, Heathcock JC, Basso D. *Neurologic Rehabilitation: Neuroscience and Neuroplasticity in Physical Therapy Practice.* 2016. Available at: http://accessphysiotherapy.mhmedical.com/content.aspx?bookid=1760&sectionid=120049508. Accessed March 14, 2018.)

BOX 3–14 Postural Stability Exercises and Interventions

Static Balance Control

To promote static balance control, the patient can start by maintaining a standing posture on a firm surface. More challenging activities include practice in the tandem and single-leg stance, lunge, and squat positions. Progress these activities by standing on soft surfaces (eg, foam, sand, and grass), narrowing the base of support, moving the head, or closing the eyes. Add a secondary task (ie, catching a ball or mental calculations) to further increase the level of difficulty.

Dynamic Balance Control

To promote dynamic balance control, interventions may involve the following:

- Maintain equal weight distribution and upright trunk postural alignment while standing on a soft surface (eg, carpeting, foam, wobble boards). Progress the activities by superimposing movements such as shifting the body weight, rotating the trunk, rotating the head side to side or up and down.
- Perform standing bends and squats on firm surface. Progress to narrow base of support, eyes closed, soft surface, reaching to touch floor.
- Transitions into and out of chair or on and off floor. Progress to without arm support, eyes closed.
- March in place on a firm surface with eyes open. Progress to marching with eyes closed, on soft surfaces, and with head turns.
- Walk and turn suddenly or walk in a circle while gradually decreasing the circumference of the circle, first in one direction and then in another.

Anticipatory Balance Control

To practice anticipatory balance control the patient can perform the following:

- Reach in all directions to touch or grasp objects, catch a ball, or kick a ball.
- Bend and pick up objects off of lower surfaces.
- Perform step-up and -down exercises or lunges in multiple directions.
- Maneuver through an obstacle course.

Reactive Balance Control

To train reactive balance control the patient can perform the following activities:

- Work to gradually increase the amount of sway in standing in different directions while on a firm, stable surface.
- Practice forward walking with abrupt stops. Progress to backward walking.
- To emphasize training of the *ankle strategy*, practice swaying while standing on one leg with the trunk erect.
- To emphasize training of the *hip strategy*, walk on lines drawn on the floor, perform tandem stance, perform single-leg stance with trunk bending, or stand on a rocker balance board.

- To emphasize the *stepping strategy*, practice stepping up onto a stool or curb or over progressively larger obstacles (ie, electric cord, shoe, phone book) or practice stepping with legs crossed in front or behind the other leg (eg, weaving or braiding).
- To increase the challenge during these activities, add anticipated and unanticipated external forces. For example, have the patient lift boxes that are identical in appearance but of different weights, throw and catch balls of different weights and sizes.

Sensory Organization

Many of the activities previously described can be utilized while varying the reliance on specific sensory systems.

- To reduce or destabilize the *visual inputs*, have the patient close the eyes or practice in low lighting or darkness, or move the eyes and head together during the balance activity.
- To decrease reliance on *somatosensory cues*, patients can narrow the base of support, stand on a soft surface, or stand on an unstable surface (ie, rocker or incline board).

Examples of these types of activities might include the following:

- Walking backward, side-stepping, and braiding performed with the eyes closed.
- Walking while watching a ball being tossed from one hand to the other.
- Walking with head and eye movements.
- Standing or marching in place on foam performed first with eyes open and later with eyes closed.
- Walking across an exercise mat or mattress in the dark.

Balance during Functional Activities

Clinicians should focus on activities similar to the activity limitations identified in the evaluation. For example, if reaching is limited, then the patient should work on activities such as reaching for a glass in the cupboard, reaching behind (as putting arm in a sleeve), or catching a ball off center. Having the patient perform two or more tasks simultaneously increases the level of task complexity. Practicing recreational activities that the patient enjoys, such as golf, increases motivation for practice while challenging balance control.

Safety During Gait, Locomotion, or Balance

To emphasize safety, clinicians should have the patient practice postural sway activities within the person's actual stability limits and progress dynamic activities with emphasis on promoting function. If balance deficits cannot be changed, environmental modifications (eg, better lighting, installation of grab bars, removal of throw rugs), assistive devices, and increased family or external support may be required to ensure safety.

From Nichols-Larsen DS et al. *Neurologic Rehabilitation: Neuroscience and Neuroplasticity in Physical Therapy Practice.* New York, NY: McGraw Hill Professional; 2015.

Bilateral Vestibular Hypofunction

Physical therapy goals for patients with BVH and expected outcomes are to (1) improve the gaze stability, (2) decrease the patient's complaints of disequilibrium and oscillopsia with head motions, (3) improve static and dynamic balance, and (4) prevent physical deconditioning by engaging in an aerobic program.

For patients with BVH who have some remaining function, gaze stability exercises should be used to tolerance and similar to UVH.

Balance exercises for individuals with BVH should enhance the substitution of visual and somatosensory information, as they are at risk of fall. Exercises should aim to improve postural stability and develop compensatory strategies that can be used in situations where balance is compromised.

Patients with BVH may have a significant decrease in their activity, become deconditioned, and have an increased fear of falling. Patients should engage in an aerobic program in the community that could include walking or aquatics.

Central Vestibular Disorders

Physical therapy goals and expected outcomes for patients with central vestibular disorders include (1) fall prevention strategies, (2) compensatory strategies for gaze stability, and (3) prevention of physical deconditioning. Recovery from central vestibular pathologies is often >6 months and may require adaptive mechanisms due to the extent of the damage.

Physical therapy interventions for individuals with central vestibular pathology will depend on the patient's signs and symptoms and the location of the lesion. Treatment interventions will be similar to those for UVH when there is involvement of the vestibular nuclei. When patients have complaints of dizziness, interventions should focus on gaze stability and/or habituation exercises. Lastly, gait and balance exercises that promote the integration of somatosensory, visual, and vestibular inputs are often effective with these patients.

Cerebellar Disorders

Recovery and interventions should depend on the cause and specific regions of the CNS and cerebellum involved. Overall prognosis may be more favorable for causes that involve only a portion or specific location of the cerebellum as compared to a poorer prognosis when the cause is cerebellar degeneration.

Physical therapy goals and expected outcomes for individuals with cerebellar ataxia include (1) improvement of static and dynamic postural stability during functional activities, (2) development of appropriate fall prevention strategies and precautions for safe functioning in daily life, and (3) prevention of physical deconditioning by engaging in aerobic exercise and/or resistance training.

Interventions should focus on stretching, strengthening, aerobic exercise, balance exercises, gait training, and vestibular rehabilitation if the patient is experiencing vertigo, nystagmus, or oculomotor complaints. Examples of static and dynamic balance exercises that are commonly prescribed can be found in Table 3–30.

TABLE 3–30 Exercises for cerebellar ataxia.

Exercise Type	Variations
Static balance activities	Single-limb stance Quadruped weight shift—lift one arm, lift one leg, lift one arm and the opposite leg
Dynamic balance	
Kneeling	• Alternately put one foot in front and then the other (half-kneeling position) • Alternately put one foot to the side and then the other • Alternately come to standing, using a half-kneel position and return to kneeling
Standing	• Swing arms • Step in each direction—front, side, back • Braiding stepping • Stair climbing • Overground walking on different surfaces
Whole body movements	
Quadruped	• Raise one arm and the opposite leg; flex them to touch elbow and knee under the trunk and then extend (repeat multiple times then complete with opposite arm and leg)
Kneeling	• Crouch to floor, bending knees, arms and trunk; then extend back up into a kneeling position • Move into side-sitting to one side, return to kneeling and then to side-sitting on the opposite side
Fall prevention activities	
Standing	• Therapist disturbs balance in forward, backward, and lateral positions • Toe-touches—bends to touch toes and returns to upright; therapist may introduce a balance displacement • Repeatedly move to quadruped from standing and return to upright; therapist may introduce a balance displacement • When pushed in upright, patient practices flexing forward to the floor
Walking	• Therapist provides balance displacement while the patient is walking
Trunk and shoulder mobility	• From prone lying, push up into extended arms position to stretch upper back • Spine rotation: supine lying—bend knees and alternately rotate the knees to the right and left side • Flexion of the shoulder: supine lying—lift the arms in the direction of the head

From Nichols-Larsen DS et al. *Neurologic Rehabilitation: Neuroscience and Neuroplasticity in Physical Therapy Practice*. New York, NY: McGraw Hill Professional; 2015. Table 16–12.

APPENDICES

Academy of Neurologic Physical Therapy Clinical Practice Guidelines

Clinical practice guidelines (CPGs) are recommendations based on the systematic review and evaluation of research evidence used to guide best practice for a specific condition. CPGs are essential

TABLE A-1 Measures of recovery in TBI.

Glasgow Coma Scale Score	JFK Coma Recovery Scale—Revised (Score)	Ranchos Los Amigos Cognitive Scale[*]	Braintree Scale	Disability Rating Scale[**]
3	Unarousable (0); none responsive on all scales (0); may have abnormal posturing (1); total = 0–1	Stage I: Unresponsive	1. Coma—unresponsive	No response on any scale and totally dependent; total score = 29
4–8	Startles to auditory and visual stimuli (1 each); flexor withdrawal to noxious stimulus (2); reflexive oral responses (1); opens eyes to stimulation (1); no communication; total = 6	Stage II: Generalized response—whole-limb or body response to touch, requires complete assistance	2. Vegetative state—begins sleep–wake cycle	Opens eye to pain (2); incomprehensible speech-groans/moans (3); extends (4) or flexes (3) limb to pain or withdraws (2); no awareness for feeding, toileting, grooming (3 each); totally dependent (5) and non-employable (3); total = 24–26
9–10	Localizes sound (1); object fixation—visual pursuit (2–3); localized response to noxious stimulus (3); vocalization/oral movement (2); intentional vocalizing (1); eye opening with or without stimulation (1–2); total = 10–12	Stage III: Localized response—moves part specific to site of touch/pinch, still requires total assistance	3. Minimally conscious—responds inconsistently, no speech	Opens eyes to speech (1) or spontaneously (0); incomprehensible speech (3); localized movement to stimulation (1); no feeding, toileting, or grooming (3 each); totally dependent (5); non-employable (3); total = 21–22
12–14	Moves to command inconsistently/consistently (3–4); reaches to object or recognizes object (4–5); object manipulation or automatic movement or functional object use (4–6); verbalizations understood (3); communication is functional (2); some attention to situation (3); total = 19–23	Stage IV: Confused and agitated, can be abusive and easily provoked, maximal assistance required	4. Post-traumatic amnesia	Spontaneous eye opening (0); confused speech (1); obeying commands to move (0); some awareness of feeding (2); some awareness of toileting needs (2); primitive ability to groom self (2); marked (4) assistance required; not employable (3); total = 17
		Stage V: Confused with less agitation but still inappropriate behavior, requires maximal supervision		Eye opening (0); confused speech (1); moving to commands (0); partial awareness of how to feed self, toileting and grooming (1 each); marked assistance all of the time (4); not employable (3); total = 10
15	Stage VI: Confused but more appropriate behavior; requires moderate supervision Stage VII: Automatic appropriate—can complete ADLs and routine activities if physically able with minimal supervision/assistance, but still have memory problems and difficulty with problem-solving		5. PTA resolution, increased independence	Eye opening (0); oriented speech (0); obeying movement commands (0); full awareness of feeding, toileting, grooming needs (0 each); moderately dependent—needs supervision in the home (3); not employable (3) or able to work in sheltered workshop (2); total = 5 or 6
	Stave VIII: Purposeful, appropriate—independent in many tasks, understands limitations, still some behavioral problems, requires standby assistance		6. Increasing independence and social skills with return to community activity, work, etc.	Same as above but with increasing ability to perform independently with some supervision (1) and likely can work either in a sheltered workshop (2) or selected jobs (1); total = 2 or 3

[*]The Ranchos Scale actually has two more levels: IX, which is associated with increasing ability to maintain focus and switch focus from one task to another but continued mild emotional/behavioral challenges that may require caregiver assistance to refocus, and X, which is associated with good goal-directed function, the ability to multitask, but still with some attentional challenges and the need for more time to complete some activities. Therapists rarely see patients who are at levels VIII–X.

[**]The Disability Rating Scale has a final category of functioning = independent in all skills (0) and work = unrestricted work ability (0).

From Nichols-Larsen DS et al. *Neurologic Rehabilitation: Neuroscience and Neuroplasticity in Physical Therapy Practice.* New York, NY: McGraw Hill Professional; 2015. Table 11–2.

TABLE A-2 ASIA motor scores.

ASIA Key Muscles	Right	Left
C5 elbow flexors	0/5	2/5
C6 wrist extensors	0/5	1/5
C7 elbow extensors	0/5	2/5
C8 finger flexors	0/5	0/5
T1 finger abduction	0/5	0/5
L2 hip flexors	0/5	2/5
L3 knee extensors	1/5	2/5
L4 ankle dorsiflexors	0/5	0/5
L5 long toe extensors	0/5	0/5
S1 ankle plantar flexor	1/5	2/5

From Nichols-Larsen DS et al. *Neurologic Rehabilitation: Neuroscience and Neuroplasticity in Physical Therapy Practice.* New York, NY: McGraw Hill Professional; 2015. Table 12–8.

to bridge the gap between research evidence and clinical practice. CPGs are a dynamic and growing resource.

For further details, please visit the ANPT website and access the professional resources: ANPT Clinical Practice Guidelines (http://neuropt.org/professional-resources/clinical-practice-guidelines and http://neuropt.org/professional-resources/clinical-practice-guidelines/vestibular-hypofunction-cpg).

Resources for Outcome Measures

An outcome measure is one type of test and measure that can be used in the patient management process. Outcome measures are used to assist in the diagnosis and prognosis of patient care in addition to tracking changes in human performance and health status. Many outcome measures, unlike measurement tools such as posture and manual muscle testing, have research evidence that provides psychometric properties for specific patient populations. Understanding the psychometric properties assists in patient-specific clinical decision-making and application of evidence-based practice (EBP).

Two of the most widely used resources are the rehabilitation measures database (RMD) and the ANPT's EDGE documents. Using the RMD, one can search a specific outcome measure and obtain useful information that is clinically applicable, such as a copy of the outcome measure itself, the ICF category, and a wealth of psychometrics. For further details please visit https://www.sralab.org/rehabilitation-measures.

The ANPT has created EDGE documents for the following diagnoses: stroke, multiple sclerosis, traumatic brain injury, spinal cord injury, Parkinson's disease, and vestibular disorders. The EDGE documents within each diagnosis are further categorized for recommended outcome measures in entry-level DPT education, research and a variety of clinical practice settings. For further details please visit http://neuropt.org/professional-resources/neurology-section-outcome-measures-recommendations.

ANPT diagnosis EDGE documents:

- Stroke (http://www.neuropt.org/professional-resources/neurology-section-outcome-measures-recommendations/stroke)
- Multiple sclerosis (http://www.neuropt.org/professional-resources/neurology-section-outcome-measures-recommendations/multiple-sclerosis)
- Spinal cord injury (http://www.neuropt.org/professional-resources/neurology-section-outcome-measures-recommendations/spinal-cord-injury)
- Traumatic brain injury (http://www.neuropt.org/professional-resources/neurology-section-outcome-measures-recommendations/traumatic-brain-injury)
- Parkinson's disease (http://www.neuropt.org/professional-resources/neurology-section-outcome-measures-recommendations/parkinson-disease)
- Vestibular disorders (http://www.neuropt.org/professional-resources/neurology-section-outcome-measures-recommendations/vestibular-disorders)

Resources for Coding and Reimbursement

In clinical practice, coding and reimbursement are highly connected to the use of outcome measures, and when tied to Medicare involve knowledge of G code information. The ANPT has organized support for G codes by diagnosis: stroke, MS, TBI, SCI, PD, and vestibular disorders. For further details, please visit the ANPT's website and access the professional resources for coding and reimbursement at http://neuropt.org/professional-resources/medicare-g-code-information.

BIBLIOGRAPHY

Agrawal Y, Carey JP, Della Santina CC, Schubert MC, Minor LB. Disorders of balance and vestibular function in US adults. *Arch Intern Med.* 2009;169(10):938-944.

Ahire A. Stroke statistics and stroke facts. Available at: http://ezinearticles.com/?expert=Anne_Ahira. Accessed on March 5, 2018.

Akin FW, Davenport MJ. Validity and reliability of the Motion Sensitivity Test. *J Rehabil Res Dev.* 2003;40(5):415-421.

Aksu SK, Ayse Y, Yavuz T, Tan E. The effects of exercise therapy in amyotrophic lateral sclerosis. *Fizyoterapi Rehabilitasyon.* 2002;13:105-112.

Akyuz G, Kenis O. Physical therapy modalities and rehabilitation techniques in the management of neuropathic pain. *Am J Phys Med Rehabil.* 2014;93:253-259.

Albers JW, Pop-Busui R. Diabetic neuropathy: mechanisms, emerging treatments, and subtypes. *Curr Neuro Neurosci Rep.* 2014;473.

Allen NE, Canning CG, Sherrington C, et al. The effects of an exercise program on fall risk factors in people with Parkinson's disease: a randomized controlled trial. *Mov Disord.* 2010;25(9):1217-1225.

Almeida TF, Roizenblatt S, Tufik S. Afferent pain pathways: a neuroanatomical review. *Brain Res.* 2004;1000:40-56.

ALS Functional Rating Scale. Available at: http://www.outcomes-umassmed.org/ALS/alsscale.aspx. Accessed on March 5, 2018.

Amboni M, Barone P, Hausdorff JM. Cognitive contributions to gait and falls: evidence and implications. *Mov Disord.* 2013;28:1520-1533.

Amyotrophic Lateral Sclerosis Association. Available at: http://www.alsa.org/als-care/resources/publications-videos/factsheets/epidemiology.html. Accessed March 5, 2018.

Anderson KD. Targeting recovery: priorities of the spinal cord-injured population. *J Neurotrauma.* 2004;21:1371-1383.

Anderson P. New CNS/AANS guidelines discourage steroids in spinal injury. Medscape Medical News. March 28, 2013. Available at: http://www.medscape.com/viewarticle/781669. Accessed March 5, 20189.

Andriessen TMJC, Jacobs B, Vos PE. Clinical characteristics and pathophysiological mechanisms of focal and diffuse traumatic brain injury. *J Cell Mol Med.* 2014;14(10):2381-2392.

Anthony DC, Couch Y. The systemic response to CNS injury. *Exp Neurol.* 2014;258:105-111.

Arciniegas DB, Wortzel HS. Emotional and behavioral dyscontrol after traumatic brain injury. *Psychiatr Clin N Am.* 2014;37:31-53.

Asia Spinal Injury Association. http://www.asia-spinalinjury.org/elearning/elearning.php. Accessed on March 5, 2018.

Asslander L, Peterka RJ. Sensory reweighting dynamics in human postural control. *J Neurophysiol.* 2014;11(9):1852-1864.

Attarian S, Vedel J-P, Pouget J, Schmied A. Progression of cortical and spinal dysfunction over time in amyotrophic lateral sclerosis. *Muscle Nerve.* 2008;37:364-375.

Aziz NA, van der Marck MA, Rikkert MG, et al. Weight loss in neurodegenerative disorders. *J Neurol.* 2008;255:1872-1880.

Baccini M, Paci M, Rinaldi LA. The scale of contraversive pushing: a reliability and validity study. *Neurorehabil Neural Repair.* 2006;20(4):468-472.

Bach JR. Amyotrophic lateral sclerosis: prolongation of life by noninvasive respiratory aids. *Chest.* 2002;122(1):92-98.

Baier B, Dieterich M. Ocular tilt reaction: a clinical sign of cerebellar infarctions? *Neurology.* 2009;72(6):572-573.

Bakheit AMO, Fedorova NV, Skoromets AA, Timerbaeva SL, Bhakta BB, Coxon L. The beneficial antispasticity effect of botulinum toxin type A is maintained after repeated treatment cycles. *J Neurol Neurosurg Psychiatry.* 2004;75:1558-1561.

Banovac K, Williams JM, Patrick LD, Haniff YM. Prevention of heterotopic ossification after spinal cord injury with indomethacin. *Spinal Cord.* 2001;39:370-374.

Barboi AC, Barkhaus PE. Electrodiagnostic testing in neuromuscular disorders. *Neurol Clin.* 2004;22(3):619-641.

Barone P, Aarsland D, Burn D, Emre M, Kullsevsky J, Weintraub D. Cognitive impairment in nondemented Parkinson's disease. *Mov Disord.* 2011;26(14):2483-2495.

Barrett KM, Meschia JF. Acute ischemic stroke management: medical management. *Semin Neurol.* 2010;30(5):461-468.

Bartolo M, Zucchella C, Pace A, et al. Early rehabilitation after surgery improves functional outcome in inpatients with brain tumors. *J Neurooncol.* 2012;107:537-544.

Bartolomeo P, DeSchotten MT, Chica AB. Brain networks of visuospatial attention and their disruption in visual neglect. *Front Hum Neurosci.* 2012;6(article 10):1-10.

Basso DM, Lang CE. Consideration of dose and timing when applying interventions after stroke and spinal cord injury. *JNPT.* 2017;41:S24-31.

Basso DM, Velozo C, Lorenz D, Suter S, Behrman A. Inter-rater reliability of the Neuromuscular Recovery Scale for spinal cord injury. *Arch Phys Med Rehabil.* 2015;96(8):1397-1403.

Bateni H, Maki BE. Assistive devices for balance and mobility: benefits, demands, and adverse consequences. *Arch Phys Med Rehabil.* 2005;86:134-145.

Bay EJ, Chartier KS. Chronic morbidities after traumatic brain injury: an update for the advanced practice nurse. *J Neurosci Nurs.* 2014;46(3):142-152.

Beekhuizen KS, Field-Fote EC. Massed practice versus massed practice with stimulation: effects on upper extremity function and cortical plasticity in individuals with incomplete cervical spinal cord injury. *Neurorehabil Neural Repair.* 2005;19:33-45.

Beekhuizen KS, Field-Fote EC. Sensory stimulation augments the effects of massed practice training in persons with tetraplegia. *Arch Phys Med Rehabil.* 2008;89:602-608.

Behrman A, Velozo C, Suter S, Lorenz D, Basso DM. Test-retest reliability of the neuromuscular recovery scale. *Arch Phys Med Rehabil.* 2015;96(8):1375-1384.

Behrman AL, Ardolino EM, Harkema S. Activity-based therapy: from basic science to clinical application for recovery after spinal cord injury. *JNPT.* 2017;41:S39-45.

Behrman AL, Harkema SJ. Locomotor training after human spinal cord injury: a series of case studies. *Phys Ther.* 2000;80(7):688-700.

Benarroch EE. Effects of acetylcholine in the striatum. Recent insights and therapeutic implications. *Neurology.* 2012;79(3):274-281.

Beninato M, Portney LG. Applying concepts of responsiveness to patient management in neurologic physical therapy. *JNPT.* 2011;35:75-81.

Ben-Zacharia AB. Therapeutics for multiple sclerosis symptoms. *Mt Sinai J Med.* 2011;78:176-191.

Berg K, Wood-Dauphinee S, Williams JI. The balance scale: reliability assessment with elderly residents and patients with an acute stroke. *Scand J Rehabil Med.* 1995;27(1):27-36.

Berg KO, Wood-Dauphinee SL, Williams JI, Maki B. Measuring balance in the elderly: validation of an instrument. *Can J Public Health.* 1992;83(suppl 2):S7-S11.

Berman JM, Fredrickson JM. Vertigo after head injury—a five year follow-up. *J Otolaryngol.* 1978;7(3):237-245.

Bhattacharyya N, Gubbels SP, Schwartx SR, et al. Clinical practice guideline: benign baroxysmal postional vertigo (update). *Otolaryngol Head Neck Surg.* 2017;156(3S):S1-S47.

Biglan KM, Ross CA, Langbehn DR, et al. PREDICT-HD Investigators of the Huntington Study Group. Motor abnormalities in premanifest persons with Huntington's disease: the PREDICT-HD study. *Mov Disord.* 2009;24:1763-1772.

Blumenfeld H. *Neuroanatomy through Clinical Cases.* 2nd ed. Sunderland, MA: Sinauer Associates; 2010.

Bohannon RW, Smith MB. Interrater reliability of a modified Ashworth scale of muscle spasticity. *Phys Ther.* 1987;67:206-207.

Bohnen NI, Jahn K. Imaging: what can it tell us about parkinsonian gait. *Mov Disord.* 2013;28(11):1492-1500.

Bondon-Guitton E, Perez-Lloret S, Bagheri H, Brefel C, Rascol O, Montastruc JL. Drug-induced parkinsonism: a review of 17 years' experience in a regional pharmacovigilance center in France. *Mov Disord.* 2011;26(12):2226-2231.

Borg GA. Psychophysical bases of perceived exertion. *Med Sci Sports Exerc.* 1982;14:377-381.

Borstad A, Schmalbrock P, Choi S, Nichols-Larsen DS. Neural correlates supporting sensory discrimination after left hemisphere stroke. *Brain Res.* 2012;1460:78-87.

Borstad AL, Bird T, Choi S, Goodman L, Schmalbrock P, Nichols-Larsen DS. Sensorimotor training induced neural reorganization after stroke. *JNPT.* 2013;37(1):27-36.

Bostan AC, Dum RP, Strick PL. Cerebellar networks with the cerebral cortex and basal ganglia. *Trends Cogn Sci.* 2013;17(5):241-254.

Bourbonnais D, Vanden Noven S, Pelletier R. Incoordination in patients with hemiparesis. *Can J Public Health.* 1992;83(Suppl 2):S58-S63.

Bourke SC, Tomlinson M, Williams TL, Bullock RE, Shaw PJ, Gibson GJ. Effects of non-invasive ventilation on survival and quality of life in patients with amyotrophic lateral sclerosis: a randomised controlled trial. *Lancet Neurol.* 2006;5:140-147.

Boyer FC, Tiffreau V, Rapin A, et al. Post-polio syndrome: pathophysiological hypotheses, diagnosis criteria, medication therapeutics. *Annal Phys Rehabil Med.* 2010;53:34-41.

Bracken MB, Shepard MJ, Hellenbrand KG, et al. Methylprednisolone and neurological function 1 year after spinal cord injury. Results of the National Acute Spinal Cord Injury Study. *J Neurosurg.* 1985;63(5):704-713.

Bracken MB, Shepard MJ, Holford TR, et al. Administration of methylprednisolone for 24 or 48 hours or tirilazad mesylate for 48 hours in the treatment of acute spinal cord injury. Results of the Third National Acute Spinal Cord Injury Randomized Controlled Trial. National Acute Spinal Cord Injury Study. *JAMA.* 1997;277(20):1597-1604.

Brainard A, Gresham C. Prevention and treatment of motion sickness. *Am Fam Physician.* 2014;90(1):41-46.

Bramlett HM, Dietrich WD. Long-term consequences of traumatic brain injury: current status of potential mechanisms of injury and neurological outcomes. *J Neurotrauma.* 2015;32:1-15.

Brandt T, Daroff RB. Physical therapy for benign paroxysmal positional vertigo. *Arch Otolaryngol.* 1980;106:484-485.

Bronner G, Vodusek DB. Management of sexual dysfunction in Parkinson's disease. *Ther Adv Neurol Disord.* 2011;4(6):375-383.

Brown KE, Whitney SL, Wrisley DM, Furman JM. Physical therapy outcomes for persons with bilateral vestibular loss. *Laryngoscope.* 2001;111:1812-1817.

Brown LA, de Bruin N, Doan J, Suchowersky O, Hu B. Obstacle crossing among people with Parkinson disease is influenced by concurrent music. *J Rehabil Res Dev.* 2010;47:225-232.

Brown NJ, Mannix RC, O'Brien MJ, Gostine D, Collins MW, Meehan WP. Effect of cognitive activity level on duration of post-concussion symptoms. *Pediatrics.* 2014;133(2): e299-e304.

Brown RG, Dittner A, Findley L, Wessely SC. The Parkinson's fatigue scale. *Parkinsonism Relat Disord.* 2005;11(1):49-55.

Bruno RL, Sapolsky R, Zimmerman JR, Frick NM. Pathophysiology of a central cause of post-polio fatigue. *Ann N Y Acad Sci.* 1995;753:257-275.

Bryce TN, Biering-Sorensen F, Finnerup NB, et al. International Spinal Cord Injury Pain Classification: part I. Background and description. *Spinal Cord.* 2012;50:413-417.

Buchsbaum BR, Baldo J, Okada K, et al. Conduction aphasia, sensory-motor integration, and phonological short-term memory—an aggregate analysis of lesion and fMRI data. *Brain Lang.* 2011;119:119-128.

Buehner JJ, Forrest G, Schmidt-Read, M, White S, Tansey K, Basso DM. Relationship between ASIA exam and functional outcomes in the NeuroRecovery Network Locomotor Training Program. *Arch Phys Med Rehabil.* 2012;93:1530-1540.

Bunge RP, Puckett WR, Becerra JL, et al. Observations on the pathology of human spinal cord injury: a review and classification of 22 new cases with details from a case of chronic cord compression with extensive focal demyelination. *Adv Neurol.* 1993;59:75-89.

Burns S, Biering-Sørensen F, Donovan W, et al. International standards for neurological classification of spinal cord injury (revised 2011). *Top Spinal Cord Inj Rehabil.* 2012;18(1):85-99.

Busse M, Quinn L, Debono K, et al. A randomized feasibility study of a 12-week community-based exercise program for people with Huntington's disease. *J Neurol Phys Ther.* 2013;37(4):149-158.

Busse ME, Wiles CM, Rosser AE. Mobility and falls in people with Huntington's disease. *J Neurol Neurosurg Psychiatry.* 2009;80:88-90.

Byl NN, Pitsch EA, Abrams GM. Functional outcomes can vary by dose: learning-based sensorimotor training for patients stable poststroke. *Neurorehabil Neural Repair.* 2008;22:494-504.

Canning CG, Paul SS, Nieuwboer A. Prevention of falls in Parkinson's disease: a review of fall risk factors and the role of physical interventions. *Neurodegener Dis Manag.* 2014;4(3):203-221.

Caproni S, Muti M, Di Renzo A, et al. Subclinical visuospatial impairment in Parkinson's disease: the role of basal ganglia and limbic system. *Front Neurol.* 2014;5:152.

Cardenas DD, Bryce TN, Shem K, Richards JS, Elhefni H. Gender and minority differences in the pain experience of people with spinal cord injury. *Arch Phys Med Rehabil.* 2004;85:1774-1781.

Casani AP, Vannucci G, Fattori B, Berrettinin S. The treatment of horizontal canal positional vertigo: our experience in 66 cases. *Laryngoscope.* 2002;112:172-178.

Cawthorne T. The physiological basis for head exercises. *J Chart Soc Physiother.* 1944;30:106.

Celik DB, Poyraz EC, Bingol A, Idlman E, Ozakbas S, Kava D. Sexual dysfunction in multiple sclerosis: gender differences. *J Neurol Sci.* 2013;324:17-20.

Centers for Disease Control and Prevention. Available at: http://www.cdc.gov/h1n1flu/vaccination/gbs_qa.htm. Accessed March 5, 2018.

Cernak K, Stevens V, Price R, Shumway-Cook A. Locomotor training using body-weight support on a treadmill in conjunction with ongoing physical therapy in a child with severe cerebellar ataxia. *Phys Ther.* 2008;88:88-97.

Chan MK, Tong RK, Chung KY. Bilateral upper limb training with functional electric stimulation in patients with chronic stroke. *Neurorehab Neural Repair.* 2009;23(4):357-365.

Cheah BC, Boland RA, Brodaty NE, et al. INSPIRATIonAL–INSPIRAtory muscle training in amyotrophic lateral sclerosis. *Amyotroph Lateral Scler.* 2009;10:384-392.

Chen A, Montes J, Mitsumoto H. The role of exercise in amyotrophic lateral sclerosis. *Phys Med Rehabil Clin N Am.* 2008;19:545-557.

Chen D, Guo X, Zheng Z, et al. Depression and anxiety in amyotrophic lateral sclerosis: correlations between the distress of patients and caregivers. *Muscle Nerve.* 2015;51(3): 353-357.

Chiò A, Bottacchi E, Buffa C, Mutani R, Mora G, the PARALS. Positive effects of tertiary centres for amyotrophic lateral sclerosis on outcome and use of hospital facilities. *J Neurol Neurosurg Psychiatry.* 2006;77:948-950.

Chiviacowsky S, Campos T, Domingues MR. Reduced frequency of knowledge of results enhances learning in persons with Parkinson's disease. *Front Psychol.* 2010;16(1);article 226:1-6.

Cholewa J, Boczarska-Jedynak M, Opala G. Influence of physiotherapy on severity of motor symptoms and quality of life in patients with Parkinson disease. *Neurol Neurochir Pol.* 2013;47(3):256-262.

Ciammola A, Sassone J, Sciacco M, et al. Low anaerobic threshold and increased skeletal muscle lactate production in subjects with Huntington's disease. *Mov Disord.* 2011;26:130-136.

Ciccone CD. *Pharmacology in Rehabilitaiton.* 5th ed. Philadelphia, PA: F.A. Davis; 2015.

Citak M, Suero EM, Backhaus M, et al. Risk factors for heterotopic ossification in patients with spinal cord injury: a case-control study of 264 patients. *Spine.* 2012;37(23):1953-1957.

Clendaniel R. The effects of habituation and gaze-stability exercises in the treatment of unilateral vestibular hypofunction – preliminary results. *J Neurol Phys Ther.* 2010;34(2):111-116.

Clendaniel RA, Landel R. Physical therapy management of cervicogenic dizziness. In: Herdman SJ, Clendaniel RA, eds. *Vestibular Rehabilitation.* 4th ed. Philadelphia, PA: F.A. Davis; 2014:590-609.

Cohen H, Blatchly CA, Gombash LL. A study of the clinical test of sensory interaction and balance. *Phys Ther.* 1993;73(6):346-351; discussion 351-344.

Cohen HS, Kimball KT. Development of the vestibular disorders activities of daily living scale. *Arch Otolaryngol Head Neck Surg.* 2000;126:881-887.

Cohen HS, Wells J, Kimball KT, Owsley C. Driving disability and dizziness. *J Safety Res.* 2003;34(4):361-369.

Connoly SJ, McIntyre A, Mehta S, Foulon BL, Teasell RW. Upper limb rehabilitation following spinal cord injury. In: Eng JJ, Teasell RW, Miller WC, et al., eds. *Spinal Cord Injury Rehabilitation Evidence.* Version 5.0. Vancouver; 2014:1-74.

Conroy BE, DeJong G, Horn SD. Hospital-based stroke rehabilitation in the United States. *Top Stroke Rehabil.* 2009;16(1):34-43.

Consortium for Spinal Cord Medicine. Pressure ulcer prevention and treatment following spinal cord injury: a clinical practice guideline for health-care professionals. *J Spinal Cord Med.* 2001;24(Suppl 1):S40-101.

Cooke DL. Central vestibular disorders. *Neurol Rep.* 1996; 20:22-29.

Cooksey FS. Rehabilitation in vestibular injuries. *Proc Royal Soc Med.* 1946;39:273-278.

Cossu, G. Therapeutic options to enhance coma arousal after traumatic brain injury: state of the art of current treatments to improve coma recovery. *Br J Neurosurg.* 2014;28(2):187.

Courtney AM, Castro-Borrero W, Davis SL, Frohman TC, Frohman EM. Functional treatments in multiple sclerosis. *Curr Opin Neurol.* 2011;24(3):250-254.

Coward JL, Wrisley DM, Walker M, Strasnick B, Jacobson JT. Efficacy of vestibular rehabilitation. *Otolaryngol Head Neck Surg.* 1998;118(1):49-54.

Crozier KS, Graziani V, Ditunno JF, Herbison GJ. Spinal cord injury: prognosis for ambulation based on sensory examination in patients who are initially motor complete. *Arch Phys Med Rehabil.* 1991;72(2):119 121.

Curthoys IA, Halmagyi GM. Vestibular compensation-recovery after unilateral vestibular loss. In: Herdman SJ, Clendaniel RA, eds. *Vestibular Rehabilitation.* 4th ed. Philadelphia, PA: F.A. Davis; 2014:121-150.

Czaplinski A, Yen AA, Appel SH. Amyotrophic lateral sclerosis: early predictors of prolonged survival. *J Neurol.* 2006b;253:1428-1436.

Dal Bello-Haas V. A framework for rehabilitation in degenerative diseases: planning care and maximizing quality of life. *Neurol Rep.* 2002;26(3):115-129.

Dal Bello-Haas V, Florence JM, Kloos AD, et al. A randomized controlled trial of resistance exercises in individuals with ALS. *Neurology.* 2007;68:2003-2007.

Dal Bello-Haas V, Kloos AD, Mitsumoto H. Physical therapy for a patient through six stages of amyotrophic lateral sclerosis. *Phys Ther.* 1998;78:1312-1324.

Dalrymple-Alford JC, MacAskill MR, Nakas CT, et al. The MoCA well-suited screen for cognitive impairment in Parkinson disease. *Neurology.* 2010;75(19):1717-1725.

Daly JJ, Ruff Rl. Construction of efficacious gait and upper limb functional interventions based on brain plasticity evidence and model-based measures for stroke patients. *Sci World J.* 2006;7:2031-2045.

Dauer W, Przedborski S. Parkinson's disease: mechanisms and models. *Neuron.* 2003;39:889-909.

Dawes H, Collett J, Debono K, et al. Exercise testing and training in people with Huntington's disease. *Clin Rehabil.* 2014.

de Almeida JP, Silvestre R, Pinto AC, de Carvalho M. Exercise and amyotrophic lateral sclerosis. *Neurol Sci.* 2012;33(1):9-15.

De Leon RD, See PA, Chow CH. Differential effects of low versus high amounts of weight supported treadmill training in spinally transected rats. *J Neurotrauma.* 2011;28(6): 1021-1033.

de Vries JM, Hagemanns MLC, Bussmann JBJ, van der Ploeg AT, van Doorn PA. Fatigue in neuromuscular disorders: focus on Guillain-Barré and Pompe disease. *Cell Mol Life Sci.* 2010;67(5):701-713.

DeAngelis LM, Wen PY. Primary and metastatic tumors of the nervous system. In: *Harrison's Neurology in Clinical Medicine.* Chicago, IL: McGraw Hill; 2013.

DeKroon JR, IIzerman MJ, Chae J, Lankhorst GJ, Zilvoid G. Relation between stimulation characteristics and clinical outcome in studies using electrical stimulation to improve motor control of the upper extremity in stroke. *J Rehabil Med.* 2005;37(2):65-74.

Del Pozo-Cruz B, Adsuar JC, del Pozo Cruz JA, Olivares PR, Gusi N. Using whole-body vibration training in patients affected with common neurological diseases: a systematic literature review. *J Altern Complement Med.* 2012;18(1):29-41.

Deli G, Bosnyak E, Pusch G, Komoly S, Feher G. Diabetic neuropathies: diagnosis and management. *Neuroendocrinology.* 2013;98(4):267-280.

Delval A, Krystkowiak P, Delliaux M, et al. Role of attentional resources on gait performance in Huntington's disease. *Mov Disord.* 2008;23(5):684-689.

Detloff MR, Smith EJ, Quiros Molina D, Ganzer PD, Houle JD. Acute exercise prevents the development of neuropathic pain and the sprouting of non-peptidergic (GDNF-and artemin-responsive) c-fibers after spinal cord injury. *Exp Neurol.* 2014;255:38-48.

Dibble LE, Hale TF, Marcus RL, Droge J, Gerber JP, LaStayo PC. High-intensity resistance training amplifies muscle hypertrophy and functional gains in persons with Parkinson's disease. *Mov Disord.* 2006;21(9):1444-1452.

Dieterich M. Central vestibular disorders. *J Neurol.* 2007;254:559-568.

Dieterich M, Brandt T. Ocular torsion and tilt of subjective visual vertical are sensitive brainstem signs. *Ann Neurol.* 1993;33(3):292-299.

Dieterich M, Brandt T. Vestibular lesions of the central vestibular pathways. In: Herdman SJ, Clendaniel RA, eds. *Vestibular Rehabilitation.* 4th ed. Philadelphia, PA: F.A. Davis; 2014:59-84.

Dillingham TR, Lauder TD, Andary M, et al. Identification of cervical radiculopathies: optimizing the electromyographic screen. *Am J Phys Med Rehabil.* 2001;80(2):84-91.

Ditunno JF, Little JW, Tester A, Burns AS. Spinal shock revisited: a four-phase model. *Spinal Cord.* 2004;42:383-395.

DiVita MA, Granger CV, Goldstein R, Niewczyk P, Freudenheim JL. Risk factors for development of new or worsened pressure ulcers among patients in inpatient rehabilitation facilities in the United States: data from the uniform data system for medical rehabilitation. *Phys Med Rehabil.* 2015;7(6):599-612.

Djousse L, Knowlton B, Cupples LA, Marder K, Shoulson I, Myers RH. Weight loss in the early stages of Huntington's disease. *Neurology.* 2002;59:1325-1330.

Dobkin B, Apple D, Barbeau H, et al. Weight-supported treadmill vs over-ground training for walking after acute incomplete SCI. *Neurology.* 2006;66:484-493.

Docherty MJ, Burn DJ. Parkinson's dementia. *Curr Neurol Neurosci Rep.* 2010;10(4):292-298.

Duncan PW, Sullivan KJ, Behrman AL, et al. Body-weight-supported treadmill rehabilitation after stroke. *N Engl J Med.* 2011;364:2026-2036.

Duncan PW, Weiner DK, Chandler J, Studenski S. Functional reach: a new clinical measure of balance. *J Gerontol.* 1990;45(6):M192-M197.

Dunn W, Griffith J, Morrison MT, et al. Somatosensation assessment using the NIH Toolbox. *Neurology.* 2013;80(11 suppl 3): S41-S44.

Dupont SA, Wijdicks EFM, Lanzino G, Rabinstein AA. Aneurysmal subarachnoid hemorrhage: an overview for the practicing neurologist. *Semin Neurol.* 2010;30(5):545-554.

Dvorak EM, Ketchum NC, McGuire JR. The underutilization of intrathecal baclofen in poststroke spasticity. *Top Stroke Rehabil.* 2011;18(3):195-202.

Ebersbach G, Ebersbach A, Edler D, et al. Comparing exercise in Parkinson's disease – the Berlin LSVT®BIG study. *Mov Disord.* 2010;25(12):1902-1908. doi:10.1002/mds.23212. Erratum in: *Mov Disord.* 2010;25(14):2478.

Ebersbach G, Moreau C, Gandor F, Defebvre L, Devos D. Clinical syndromes: parkinsonian gait. *Mov Disord.* 2013;28(11): 1552-1559.

Edgerton VR, Roy RR. A new age for rehabilitation. *Eur J Phys Rehabil Med.* 2012;48(1):99-109.

Edgerton VR, Roy RR. Activity-dependent plasticity of spinal locomotion: implications for sensory processing. *Exer Sport Sci Rev.* 2009;37(4):171-178.

EFNS Task Force on Diagnosis and Management of Amyotrophic Lateral Sclerosis, Andersen PM, Abrahams S, Borasio GD, et al. EFNS guidelines on the clinical management of amyotrophic lateral sclerosis (MALS) – revised report of an EFNS task force. *Eur J Neurol.* 2012;19(3):360-375.

Elliott J, Smith M. The acute management of intracerebral hemorrhage: a clinical review. *Anesth Analg.* 2010;110: 1419-1427.

Ellis T, Boudreau JK, DeAngelis TR, et al. Barriers to exercise in people with Parkinson disease. *Phys Ther.* 2013;93(5):628-636.

Ellis T, Motl RW. Physical activity behavior change in persons with neurologic disorders: overview and examples from Parkinson disease and multiple sclerosis. *J Neurol Phys Ther.* 2013;37(2):85-90.

Fabbrini G, Latorre A, Suppa A, Bloise M, Frontoni M, Berardelli A. Fatigue in Parkinson's disease: motor or non-motor symptom? *Parkinsonism Relat Disord.* 2013;19:148-152.

Falvo MJ, Schilling BK, Earhart GM. Parkinson's disease and resistive exercise: rationale, review, and recommendations. *Mov Disord.* 2008;23(1):1-11.

Farbu E, Gilhus NE, Barnes MP, et al. EFNS guideline on diagnosis and management of post-polio syndrome. Report of an EFNS task force. *Eur J Neurol.* 2006;13:795-801.

Farley BG, Koshland GF. Training BIG to move faster: the application of the speed-amplitude relation as a rehabilitation strategy for people with Parkinson's disease. *Exp Brain Res.* 2005;167(3):462-467.

Faulkner MA. Safety overview of FDA-approved medications for the treatment of the motor symptoms of Parkinson's disease. *Expert Opin Drug Safety.* 2014;13(8):1055-1069.

Féasson L, Camdessanché JP, El Mandhi L, Calmels P, Millet GY. Fatigue and neuromuscular diseases. *Ann Readapt Med Phys.* 2006;49:375-384.

Feigin A, Ghilardi M-F, Huang C, et al. Preclinical Huntington's disease: compensatory brain responses during learning. *Ann Neurol.* 2006;59:53-59.

Fetter M. Vestibular system disorders. In: Herdman SJ, Clendaniel RA, eds. *Vestibular Rehabilitation.* 4th ed. Philadelphia, PA: F.A. Davis; 2014:50-58.

Field-fote EC, Roach KE. Influence of a locomotor training approach on walking speed and distance in people with chronic spinal cord injury: a randomized clinical trial. *Physical Ther.* 2011;1(1):48-60.

Fife TD, Iverson DJ, Lempert T, et al. Practice parameter: therapies for benign paroxysmal positional vertigo (an evidence-based review): report of the Quality Standards Subcommittee of the American Academy of Neurology. *Neurology.* 2008;70:2067-2074.

Fife TD, Tusa RJ, Furman JM. Assessment: vestibular testing techniques in adults and children: report of the Therapeutics and Technology Assessment Subcommittee of the American Academy of Neurology. *Neurology*. 2000;55:1431-1441.

Finnerup NB, Baastrup C, Jensen TS. Neuropathic pain following spinal cord injury pain: mechanisms and treatment. *Scand J Pain*. 2009;51:S3-S11.

Fisher BE, Li Q, Nacca A, et al. Treadmill exercise elevates striatal dopamine D2 receptor binding potential in patients with early Parkinson's disease. *Neuroreport*. 2013;24(10):509-514.

Flaherty-Craig C, Brothers A, Dearman B, Eslinger P, Simmons Z. Penn State screen exam for the detection of frontal and temporal dysfunction syndromes: application to ALS. *Amyotroph Lateral Scler*. 2009;10(2):107-112.

Flannery J. Using the levels of cognitive functioning assessment scale with patients with traumatic brain injury in an acute care setting. *Rehabil Nurs*. 1998;23(2):88-94.

Fokke C, van den Berg B, Drenthen J, Walgaard C, van Doorn PA, Jacobs BC. Diagnosis of Guillain-Barré syndrome and validation of Brighton criteria. *Brain*. 2014;137:33-43.

Folstein MJ, Folstein SE, McHugh PR. Mini-mental state: a practical method for grading the cognitive state of patients for the clinician. *J Psychiatr Res*. 1975;12(3):189-198.

Forrest GF, Hutchinson K, Lorenz DJ, et al. Are the 10 meter and 6 minute walk tests redundant in patients with spinal cord injury? *PLoS One*. 2014;9(5):e94108.

Forsberg A, Press R, Einarsson U, de Pedro-Cuesta J, Widén Holmqvist L, Swedish Epidemiological Study Group. Impairment in Guillain-Barré syndrome during the first 2 years after onset: a prospective study. *J Neurol Sci*. 2004;227:131-138.

Forsting M, Jansen O. *MR Neuroimaging*. New York, NY: Thieme, 2017.

Fortis P, Ronchi R, Senna I, et al. Rehabilitating patients with left spatial neglect by prism exposure during a visuomotor activity. *Neuropsychology*. 2010;24(6):681-697.

Fritz S, Lusardi M. White paper: "walking speed: the sixth vital sign." *J Geriatr Phys Ther*. 2009;32(2):46-49.

Fugl-Meyer AR, Jääskö L, Leyman I, Olsson S, Steglind S. The post-stroke hemiplegic patient: a method for evaluation of physical performance. *Scand J Rehabil Med*. 1975;7(1):13-31.

Fukuda T. The stepping test: two phases of the labyrinthine reflex. *Acta Otolaryngol*. 1959;50(2):95-108.

Furlan JD, Fehlings MG. Cardiovascular complications after acute spinal cord injury: pathophysiology, diagnosis and management. *Neurosurg Focus*. 2008;25(5):e13.

Furman JM, Whitney SL. Central causes of dizziness. *Phys Ther*. 2000;80(2):179-187.

Galveston Orientation and Amnesia Test (GOAT). Available at: http://scale-library.com/pdf/Galveston_Orientation_Amnesia_Test.pdf. Accessed March 5, 2018.

Garssen MP, Bussmann JB, Schmitz PI, et al. Physical training and fatigue, fitness, and quality of life in Guillain-Barré syndrome and CIDP. *Neurology*. 2004;63(12):2393-2395.

Gauthier LV, Taub E, Perkins C, Ortmann M, Mark VW, Uswatte G. Remodeling the brain: plastic structural brain changes produced by different motor therapies after stroke. *Stroke*. 2008;39(5):1520-1525.

Gelb DJ. Diagnostic criteria for Parkinson disease. *Arch Neurol*. 1999;56:33-39.

Gélis A, Dupeyron A, Legros P, Benaïm C, Pelissier J, Fattal C. Pressure ulcer risk factors in persons with spinal cord injury part 1: the acute and rehabilitation stages. *Spinal Cord*. 2009;47:99-107.

Gibbons ZC, Richardson A, Neary D, Snowden JS. Behaviour in amyotrophic lateral sclerosis. *Amyotroph Lateral Scler*. 2008;9:67-74.

Gibson-Horn C. Balance-based torso-weighting in a patient with ataxia and multiple sclerosis: a case report. *J Neurol Phys Ther*. 2008;32:139-146.

Gigo-Benato D, Russo TL, Geuna S, Domingues NR, Salvini TF, Parizotto NA. Electrical stimulation impairs early functional recovery and accentuates skeletal muscle atrophy after sciatic nerve crush injury in rats. *Muscle Nerve*. 2010;41(5):685-693.

Giladi N, Azulay TJ, Rascol O, et al. Validation of the freezing of gait questionnaire in patients with Parkinson's disease. *Mov Disord*. 2009;24(5):655-661.

Giladi N, Shabtai H, Simon ES, Biran S, Tal J, Korczyn AD. Construction of freezing of gait questionnaire for patients with Parkonsonism. *Parkinsonism Relat Disord*. 2000;6:165-170.

Gilbert MR, Armstrong TS, Pope WB, van den Bent MJ, Wen PY. Facing the future of brain tumor clinical research. *Clin Cancer Res*. 2014;20(22):5591-5600.

Gill DJ, Freshman A, Blender JA, Ravina B. The Montreal cognitive assessment as a screening tool for cognitive impairment in Parkinson's disease. *Mov Disord*. 2008;23(7):1043-1046.

Gill-Body KM. Current Concepts in the Management of Individuals With Vestibular Dysfunction. Monograph published by the American Physical Therapy Association, Alexandria, VA.

Giray M, Kirazli Y, Karapolat H, Celebisoy N, Bilgen C, Kirazli T. Short-term effects of vestibular rehabilitation in patients with chronic unilateral vestibular dysfunction: a randomized controlled study. *Arch Phys Med Rehabil*. 2009;90(8):1325-1331.

Giuffrida CG, Demery JA, Reyes LR, Lebowitz BK, Hanlon RE. Functional skill learning in men with traumatic brain injury. *Am J Occup Ther*. 2009;63(4):398-407.

Giulioni M, Marucci G, Martinoni M, et al. Epilepsy associated tumors. *World J Clin Cases*. 2014;2(1):623-641.

Glendinning DS, Enoka RM. Motor unit behavior in Parkinson's disease. *Phys Ther*. 1994;74:61-70.

Goetz CG, Poewe W, Rascol O, et al. Movement Disorder Society Task Force Report on the Hoehn and Yahr Staging Scale: status and recommendations. The Movement Disorder Society Task Force on Rating Scales for Parkinson's Disease. *Mov Disord*. 2004;19(9):1020-1028.

Goetz CG, Tilley BC, Shaftman SR, et al. and Movement Disorder Society UPDRS Revision Task Force. Movement Disorder Society-sponsored revision of the Unified Parkinson's Disease Rating Scale (MDS-UPDRS): scale presentation and clinimetric testing results. *Mov Disord*. 2008;23(15):2129-2170.

Gołąb-Janowska M, Honczarenko K, Stankiewicz J. Usefulness of the ALSAQ-5 scale in evaluation of quality of life in amyotrophic lateral sclerosis. *Neurol Neurochir Pol*. 2010;44(6):560-566.

Gonzalez H, Olsson T, Borg K. Management of postpolio syndrome. *Lancet Neurol*. 2010;9:634-642.

Goodwin VA, Richards SH, Henley W, Ewings P, Taylor AH, Campbell JL. An exercise intervention to prevent falls in people with Parkinson's disease: a pragmatic randomised controlled trial. *J Neurol Neurosurg Psychiatry*. 2011;82(11):1232-1238.

Gourraud P-A, Harbo HF, Hauser SL, Baranzini SE. The genetics of multiple sclerosis: an up-to-date review. *Immunol Rev.* 2012;248:87-103.

Gouvier WD, Blanton PD, LaPorte KK, Nepomuceno C. Reliability and validity of the Disability Rating Scale and the Levels of Cognitive Functioning Scale in monitoring recovery from severe head injury. *Arch Phys Med Rehabil.* 1987;68(2):94-97.

Grauwmeijer E, Heijenbrok-Kal MH, Haitsma IK, Ribbers GM. A prospective study on employment outcome 3 years after moderate to severe traumatic brain injury. *Arch Phys Med Rehabil.* 2012;93(6):993-999.

Great Lakes ALS Study Group. A comparison of muscle strength testing techniques in amyotrophic lateral sclerosis. *Neurology.* 2003;61:1503-1507.

Gregg M, Hall C, Butler A. The MIQ-RS: a suitable option for examining movement imagery ability. *eCAM.* 2010;7(2):249-257.

Griffin JW, Hogan MV, Chhabra AB, Deal DN. Peripheral nerve repair and reconstruction. *J Bone Joint Surg Am.* 2013;95(23):2144-2151.

Grimbergen YA, Knol MJ, Bloem BR, Kremer BP, Roos RA, Munneke M. Falls and gait disturbances in Huntington's disease. *Mov Disord.* 2008;23(7):970-976.

Grobelny TJ. Brain aneurysms: epidemiology, treatment options, and milestones of endovascular treatment evolution. *Dis Mon.* 2011;567:647-655.

Guide to Physical Therapy Practice, Edition 3.0. Available at: http://guidetopractice.apta.org. Accessed on March 5, 2018.

Hackney ME, Earhart GM. Effects of dance on gait and balance in Parkinson's disease: a comparison of partnered and nonpartnered dance movement. *Neurorehabil Neural Repair.* 2010;24(4):384-392.

Hain TC, Helminski JO. Anatomy and physiology of the normal vestibular system. In: Herdman SJ, ed. *Vestibular Rehabilitation.* 4th ed. Philadelphia, PA: FA Davis; 2014.

Haines D. *Neuroanatomy in Clinical Context: An Atlas of Structures, Sections, and Systems.* 9th ed. Baltimore: Lippincott Williams and Wilkins; 2015.

Hall CD, Herdnan SJ, Whitney SL, et al. Vestibular rehabilitaiton for peripheral vestibular hypofunction: an evidence-based clinical practice guideline. *J Neurol Phys Ther.* 2016;40:124-154.

Halsband U, Lange RK. Motor learning in man: a review of functional and clinical studies. *J Physiol Paris.* 2006;99(4-6):414-424.

Hansen RB, Staun M, Kalhauge A, Langholz E, Biering-Sorensen F. Bowel function and quality of life after colostomy in individuals with spinal cord injury. *J Spinal Cord Med.* 2015;39(3):281-289.

Hanson RW, Franklin MR. Sexual loss in relation to other functional losses for spinal cord injured males. *Arch Phys Med Rehabil.* 1979;57:291-293.

Harkema SJ, Hurley SL, Patel UK, Requejo PS, Dobkin BH, Edgerton VR. Human lumbosacral spinal cord interprets loading during stepping. *J Neurophysiol.* 1997;77(2):797-811.

Harkema SJ, Schmidt-Read M, Lorenz DJ, Edgerton R, Behrman AL. Balance and ambulation improvements in individuals with chronic incomplete spinal cord injury using locomotor training-based rehabilitation. *Arch Phys Med Rehabil.* 2012;93:1508-1517.

Hasegawa T, Shintai K, Kato T, Iizuka H. Stereotactic radiosurgery as the initial treatment for patients with nonfunctioning pituitary adenomas. *World Neurosurg.* 2015;83(6):1173-1179.

Hausdorff JM, Cudkowicz ME, Firtion R, Wei JY, Goldberger AL. Gait variability and basal ganglia disorders: stride-to-stride variations of gait cycle timing in Parkinson's disease and Huntington's disease. *Mov Disord.* 1998;13(3):428-437.

Heemskerk A-W, Roos RAC. Dysphagia in Huntington's disease: a review. *Dysphagia.* 2011;26:62-66.

Hendricks HT, Heeren AH, Vos PE. Dysautonomia after severe traumatic brain injury. *Eur J Neurol.* 2001;17:1172-1177.

Herbison GJ, Isaac Z, Cohen ME, Ditunno JF. Strength post-spinal cord injury: myometer vs manual muscle test. *Spinal Cord.* 1996;34(9):543-548.

Herdman SJ, Clendaniel RA. Physical therapy management of bilateral vestibular hypofunction and loss. In: Herdman SJ, Clendaniel RA, eds. *Vestibular Rehabilitation.* 4th ed. Philadelphia, PA: F.A. Davis; 2014:432-456.

Herdman SJ, Hall CD, Schubert MC, Das VE, Tusa RJ. Recovery of dynamic visual acuity in bilateral vestibular hypofunction. *Arch Otolaryngol Head Neck Surg.* 2007;133(4):383-389.

Herdman SJ, Hoder JM. Physical therapy management of benign paroxysmal positional vertigo. In: Herdman SJ, Clendaniel RA, eds. *Vestibular Rehabilitation.* 4th ed. Philadelphia, PA: F.A. Davis; 2014:324-354.

Herdman SJ, Whitney SL. Physical therapy treatment of vestibular hypofunction. In: Herdman SJ, Clendaniel RA, eds. *Vestibular Rehabilitation.* 4th ed. Philadelphia, PA: F.A. Davis; 2014:394-431.

Hesse S. Treadmill training with partial body weight support after stroke: a review. *NeuroRehabilitation.* 2008;23(1):55-65.

Hillier SL, Hollohan V. Vestibular rehabilitation for unilateral peripheral vestibular dysfunction. *Cochrane Database Syst Rev.* 2007;(4):CD005397.

Hillier SL, McDonnell M. Vestibular rehabilitation for unilateral peripheral vestibular dysfunction. *Cochrane Database Syst Rev.* 2011;(2):CD005397.

Hislop H, Avers D, Brown M. *Daniels and Worthingham's Muscle Testing.* 9th ed. Philadelphia, PA: Elsevier/Saunders; 2013.

Hoffman LR, Field-Fote EC. Cortical reorganization following bimanual training and somatosensory stimulation in cervical spinal cord injury: a case report. *Phys Ther.* 2007;87:208-223.

Honaker JA, Shepard NT. Performance of Fukuda Stepping Test as a function of the severity of caloric weakness in chronic dizzy patients. *J Am Acad Audiol.* 2012;23(8):616-622.

Horak FB. Postural compensation for vestibular loss. *Ann N Y Acad Sci.* 2009;1164:76-81.

Horak FB, Henry SM, Shumway-Cook A. Postural perturbations: new insights for treatment of balance disorders. *Phys Ther.* 1997;77(5):517-533.

Horkova D, Kalincik T, Dusankova JB, Dolezai O. Clinical correlates of grey matter pathology in multiple sclerosis. *BMC Neurol.* 2012;12:10-20.

Hornby GT, Campbell DD, Zemon DH, Kahn JH. Clinical and quantitative evaluation of robotic-assisted treadmill walking to retrain ambulation after spinal cord injury. *Top Spinal Cord Injury Rehabil.* 2005;11:1-17.

Horner RD, Kamins KG, Feussner JR, Grambow SC, Hoff-Lindquist J, Harati Y. Occurrence of amyotrophic lateral sclerosis among Gulf War veterans. *Neurology.* 2003;61:742-749.

Hubli M, Dietz V. The physiological basis of neurorehabilitation—locomotor training after spinal cord injury. *J Neuroeng Rehabil.* 2013;10:5-8.

Hughes RA, Swan AV, van Doorn PA. Intravenous immunoglobulin for Guillain-Barré syndrome. *Cochrane Database Syst Rev.* 2014;19(9):CD002063.

Hughes RA, Wijdicks EF, Barohn R, et al. Practice parameter: immunotherapy for Guillain-Barré syndrome: report of the Quality Standards Subcommittee of the American Academy of Neurology. *Neurology.* 2003;61(6):736-740.

Huntington's Disease Society of America's Fast Facts. Available at: http://www.hdsa.org/images/content/2/2/v2/22556/HDSA-FastFacts-2-7-14-final.pdf. Accessed March 5, 2018.

Hutchinson KJ, Gomez-Pinilla F, Crowe MJ, Ying Z, Basso DM. Three exercise paradigms differentially improve sensory recovery after spinal cord contusion in rats. *Brain.* 2004;127:1403-1414.

Induruwa I, Constantinescu CS, Gran B. Fatigue in multiple sclerosis – a brief review. *J Neurol Sci.* 2012;323:9-15.

Ingels PL, Rosenfeld J, Frick SL, Bryan WJ. Adhesive capsulitis: a common occurrence in patients with ALS. *Amyotroph Lateral Scler Other Motor Neuron Disord.* 2001;2(S2):60.

Inkster LM, Eng JJ. Postural control during a sit-to-stand task in individuals with mild Parkinson's disease. *Exp Brain Res.* 2004;154(1):33-38.

Inkster LM, Eng JJ, MacIntyre DL, Stoessl AJ. Leg muscle strength is reduced in Parkinson's disease and related to the ability to rise from a chair. *Mov Disord.* 2003;18:157-162.

International Spinal Cord Society. http://www.iscos.org.uk/international-sci-pain-data-sets. Accessed on March 5, 2018.

Jacobson GP, Newman CW. The development of the Dizziness Handicap Inventory. *Arch Otolaryngol Head Neck Surg.* 1990;116(4):424-427.

Jacobson GP, Newman CW, Hunter L, Balzer GK. Balance function test correlates of the Dizziness Handicap Inventory. *J Am Acad Audiol.* 1991;2(4):253-260.

Jankovic J. Parkinson's disease: clinical features and diagnosis. *J Neurol Neurosurg Psychiatry.* 2008;79;368-376.

Javalkar V, Khan M, Davis DE. Clinical manifestations of cerebellar disease. *Neurol Clin.* 2014;32:871-879.

Jeffcoat B, Shelukhin A, Fong A, Mustain W, Zhou W. Alexander's law revisited. *J Neurophysiol.* 2008;100(1):154-159.

Jenkinson C, Fitzpatrick R. Reduced item set for the amyotrophic lateral sclerosis assessment questionnaire: development and validation of the ALSAQ-5. *J Neurol Neurosurg Psychiatry.* 2001;70:70-73.

Jenkinson C, Fitzpatrick R, Brennan C, Swash M. Evidence for the validity and reliability of the ALS assessment questionnaire: the ALSAQ-40. *Amyotroph Lateral Scler Other Motor Neuron Disord.* 1999b;1:33-40.

Jette DU, Slavin MD, Andres PL, Munsat TL. The relationship of lower-limb muscle force to walking ability in patients with amyotrophic lateral sclerosis. *Phys Ther.* 1999;79:672-681.

Jubelt B, Agre JC. Characteristics and management of postpolio syndrome. *JAMA.* 2000;284:412-414.

Julia PE, Sa'ari MY, Hasnan N. Benefit of triple strap abdominal binder on voluntary cough in patients with spinal cord injury. *Spinal Cord.* 2011;49:1138-1142.

Kadivar Z, Corcos DM, Foto J, Hondzinski JM. Effect of step-training and rhythmic auditory stimulation on functional performance in Parkinson patients. *Neurorehabil Neural Repair.* 2011;25(7):626-635.

Kalmar K, Giacino JT. The JFK Coma Recovery Scale—revised. *Neuropsychol Rehabil.* 2005;15:454-460.

Kalron A, Dvir Z, Achiron A. Effect of a cognitive task on postural control in patients with a clinically isolated syndrome suggestive of multiple sclerosis. *Eur J Phys Rehabil Med.* 2011;47(4):579-586.

Kamide N, Asakawa T, Shibasaki N, et al. Identification of the type of exercise therapy that affects functioning in patients with early-stage amyotrophic lateral sclerosis: a multicenter, collaborative study. *Neurol Clinical Neurosci.* 2014;2:135-139.

Kandel S, Schwartz JH, Jessell TM, Siegelbaum SA, Hudspeth AJ. *Principles of Neural Science.* 5th ed. New York, NY: McGraw-Hill; 2013.

Kanno H, Pearse DD, Ozawa H, Itoi E, Bunge MB. Schwann cell transplantation for spinal cord injury repair: its significant therapeutic potential and prospectus. *Rev Neurosci.* 2015;26(2):121-128.

Karnath HO, Broetz D. Understanding and treating "pusher syndrome". *Phys Ther.* 2003;83:1119-1125.

Karr JE, Areshenkoff CN, Garcia-Barrera MA. The neuropsychological outcomes of concussion: a systematic review of meta-analyses on the cognitive sequelae of mild traumatic brain injury. *Neuropsychology.* 2014;28(3):321-336.

Katz DI, Polyak M, Coughlan D, Nichols M, Roche A. Natural history of recovery from brain injury after prolonged disorders of consciousness: outcome of patients admitted to inpatient rehabilitation with 1-4 year follow-up. *Prog Brain Res.* 2009;177:73-88.

Kaufmann P, Levy G, Montes J, QALS Study Group, et al. Excellent inter-rater, intra-rater, and telephone-administered reliability of the ALSFRS-R in a multicenter clinical trial. *Amyotroph Lateral Scler.* 2007;8:42-46.

Kegelmeyer DA, Parthasarathy S, Kostyk SK, White SE, Kloos AD. Assistive devices alter gait patterns in Parkinson disease: advantages of the four-wheeled walker. *Gait Posture.* 2013;38(1):20-24.

Kehagia AA, Barker RA, Robbins TW. Neuropsychological and clinical heterogeneity of cognitive impairment and dementia in patients with Parkinson's disease. *Lancet Neurol.* 2010;9(12):1200-2013.

Kelly NA, Ford MP, Standaert DG, et al. Novel, high-intensity exercise prescription improves muscle mass, mitochondrial function, and physical capacity in individuals with Parkinson's disease. *J Appl Physiol.* 2014;116(5):582-592.

Kerr GK, Worringham CJ, Cole MH, Lacherez PF, Wood JM, Silburn PA. Predictors of future falls in Parkinson disease. *Neurology.* 2010;75(2):116-124.

Keshner EA, Galgon AK. Postural abnormalities in vestibular disorders. In: Herdman SJ, Clendaniel RA, eds. *Vestibular Rehabilitation.* 4th ed. Philadelphia, PA: F.A. Davis; 2014:85-109.

Khan F, Amatya B. Rehabilitation interventions in patients with acute demyelinating inflammatory polyneuropathy: a systematic review. *Eur J Phys Rehabil Med.* 2012;48(3):507-522.

Khan F, Ng L, Amatya B, Brand C, Turner-Stokes L. Multidisciplinary care for Guillain-Barre syndrome. *Cochrane Database Syst Rev.* 2010;10:CD008505.

Khan F, Pallant JF, Amatya B, Ng L, Gorelik A, Brand C. Outcomes of high-and low-intensity rehabilitation programme for persons in chronic phase after Guillain-Barré syndrome: a randomized controlled trial. *J Rehabil Med.* 2011;43(7):638-646.

Kheirollahi M, Dashti S, Khalaj Z, Nazemroaia F, Mahzouni P. Brain tumors: special characters for research and banking. *Adv Biomed Res.* 2015;4:4.

Kim JS, Oh SY, Lee SH, et al. Randomized clinical trial for geotropic horizontal canal benign paroxysmal positional vertigo. *Neurology.* 2012;79(7):700-707.

Kim SD, Allen NE, Canning CG, Fung VS. Postural instability in patients with Parkinson's disease. Epidemiology, pathophysiology and management. *CNS Drugs.* 2013;27(2):97-112.

Kimberly TJ, Samargia S, Moore LG, Shakya JK, Lang CE. Comparison of amounts and types of practice during rehabilitation of traumatic brain injury and stroke. *J Rehabil Res Dev.* 2010;47(9):851-862.

Kirkwood SC, Su JL, Connealy P, Faoroud T. Progression of symptoms in the early and middle stages of Huntington's disease. *Arch Neurol.* 2001;58:273-278.

Kirshblum S, Millis S, McKinley W, Tulsky D. Late neurologic recovery after traumatic spinal cord injury. *Arch Phys Med Rehabil.* 2004;85(11):1811-1817.

Kleim JA, Barbay S, Nudo RJ. Functional reorganization of the rat motor cortex following motor skill learning. *J Neurophysiol.* 1998;80:3321-3325.

Kleim JA, Jones TA. Principles of experience-dependent neural plasticity: implications for rehabilitation after brain damage. *J Speech Lang Hear Res.* 2008;51:S225-S239.

Kloos AD, Dal Bello-Haas V, Proch C, Mitsomoto H. Validity of the Tinetti Assessment Tool in individuals with ALS. In: *Proceedings of the 9th International Symposium on Amyotrophic Lateral Sclerosis/Motor Neuron Disease Conference.* Munich, Germany; 1998:149.

Kloos AD, Dal Bello-Haas V, Thome R, et al. Interrater and intrarater reliability of the Tinetti Balance Test for individuals with amyotrophic lateral sclerosis. *J Neurol Phys Ther.* 2004;28(1):12-19.

Kloos AD, Fritz NE, Kostyk SK, Young GS, Kegelmeyer DA. Video game play (Dance Dance Revolution) as a potential exercise therapy in Huntington's disease: a controlled clinical trial. *Clin Rehabil.* 2013;27(11):972-982.

Kloos AD, Kegelmeyer DK, White S, Kostyk S. The impact of different types of assistive devices on gait measures and safety in Huntington's disease. *PLoS One.* 2012;7(2):e30903.

Konczak J, Corcos DM, Horak F, et al. Proprioception and motor control in Parkinson's disease. *J Mot Behav.* 2009;41(6):543-552.

Kondziolka D, Shin SM, Brunswick A, Kim I, Silverman JS. The biology of radiosurgery and its clinical applications for brain tumors. *Neuro Oncol.* 2015;17(1):29-44.

Koob M, Girard N. Cerebral tumors: specific features in children. *Diagn Interv Imaging.* 2014;95:965-983.

Kose G, Hatipoglu S. Effect of head and body positioning on cerebral blood flow velocity in patients who underwent cranial surgery. *J Clin Nurs.* 2012;21(13-14):1859-1867.

Kraft GH. The electromyographer's guide to the motor unit. *Phys Med Rehabil Clin N Am.* 2007;8(4):711-732.

Krassioukov A, Eng JJ, Claxton G, Sakakibara BM, Shum S. Neurogenic bowel management after spinal cord injury: a systematic review of the evidence. *Spinal Cord.* 2010;48:718-733.

Krause JS, Kemp B, Coker J. Depression after spinal cord injury: relation to gender, ethnicity, aging and socioeconomic indicators. *Arch Phys Med Rehabil.* 2000;81:1099-1109.

Krause JS, Vines CL, Farley TL, Sniezek J, Coker J. An exploratory study of pressure ulcers after spinal cord injury: relationship to protective behaviors and risk factors. *Arch Phys Med Rehabil.* 2001;82:107-113.

Krebs DE, Gill-Body KM, Parker SW, Ramirez JV, Wernick-Robinson M. Vestibular rehabilitation: useful but not universally so. *Otolaryngol Head Neck Surg.* 2003;128(2):240-250.

Krebs DE, Gill-Body KM, Riley PO, Parker SW. Double-blind, placebo-controlled trial of rehabilitation for bilateral vestibular hypofunction: preliminary report. *Otolaryngol Head Neck Surg.* 1993;109(4):735-741.

Kubler A, Winter S, Kaiser J, Birbaumer N, Hautzinger M. The ALS Depression Inventory (ADI): a questionnaire to measure depression in degenerative neurological diseases. *Z Klin Psychol Psychother.* 2005;31:19-26.

Kuypers HG. Anatomy of descending pathways. *Handbook of Physiology. Sect. I. The Nervous System. Vol. II. Motor Control, pt 1.* Bethesda, MD: The American Physiological Society; 1981:597-666.

Lai JM, Francisco GE, Willis FB. Dynamic splinting after treatment with botulinum toxin type-A: a randomized controlled pilot study. *Adv Ther.* 2009;26(2):241-248.

Lam T, Wolfe DL, Domingo A, Eng JJ, Sproule S. Lower limb rehabilitation following spinal cord injury. In: Eng JJ, Teasell RW, Miller WC, et al., eds. *Spinal Cord Injury Rehabilitation Evidence.* Version 5.0. Vancouver; 2014:1-73.

Lance, JW. Symposium synopsis. In: Feldman RG, Young RR, Koella WP, eds. *Spasticity: Disordered Motor Control.* Chicago, IL: Year Book Medical Publishers; 1980:485-494.

Langley FA, Mackintosh SF. Timed Up and Go test (TUG), the Tinetti Mobility Test (TMT), the Dynamic Gait Index (DGI) and the BEST test or mini-BEST test. *J Allied Health Sci Pract.* 2007;5(4):1-11.

Latt MD, Lors SR, Morris JG, Fung VS. Clinical and physiological assessments for elucidating falls risk in Parkinson's disease. *Mov Disord.* 2009;24(9):1280-1289.

Lau KW, Mak MK. Speed-dependent treadmill training is effective to improve gait and balance performance in patients with sub-acute stroke. *J Rehabil Med.* 2011;43(8):709-713.

Laub M, Midgren B. Survival of patients on home mechanical ventilation: a nationwide prospective study. *Respir Med.* 2007;101:1074-1078.

Laxe S, Terre R, Leon D, Bernabeu M. How does dysautonomia influence the outcome of traumatic brain injured patients admitted in a neurorehabilitation unit? *Brain Inj.* 2013;27(12):1383-1387.

Lee H. Neuro-otological aspects of cerebellar stroke syndrome. *J Clin Neurol.* 2009;5:65-73.

Lee-Kubli CA, Lu P. Induced pluripotent stem cell-derived neural stem cell therapies for spinal cord injury. *Neural Regen Res.* 2015;10:10-16.

Lemay V, Routhier F, Noreau L, Phang SH, Ginis KA. Relationships between wheelchair skills, wheelchair mobility and level of injury in individuals with spinal cord injury. *Spinal Cord.* 2012;50(1):37-41.

Lemon RN. Descending pathways in motor control. *Ann Rev Neurosci.* 2008;31(1):195-218.

Lerche S, Seppi K, Behnke S, et al. Risk factors and prodromal markers and the development of Parkinson's disease. *J Neurol.* 2014;261:180-187.

Lezak MD. Psychological implications of traumatic brain damage for the patient's family. *Rehabil Psychol.* 1986;3(4):241-250.

Li F, Harmer P, Fitzgerald K, et al. Tai chi and postural stability in patients with Parkinson's disease. *N Engl J Med.* 2012;366(6):511-519.

Lim I, Van Wegen E, de Goede C, et al. Effects of external rhythmical cueing on gait in patients with Parkinson's disease: a systematic review. *Clin Rehabil.* 2005;19(7):695-713.

Lima LO, Scianni A, Rodrigues-de-Paula F. Progressive resistance exercise improves strength and physical performance in people with mild to moderate Parkinson's disease: a systematic review. *J Physiother.* 2013;59(1):7-13.

Lin CH, Sullivan KJ, Wu AD, Kantak S, Winstein CJ. Effect of task practice order on motor skill learning in adults with Parkinson disease: a pilot study. *Phys Ther.* 2007;87(9):1120-1131.

Lindvall O, Bjorklund A. Cell therapy in Parkinson's disease. *NeuroRx.* 2004;1(4):382-393.

Logroscino G, Traynor BJ, Hardiman O, et al. EURALS. Descriptive epidemiology of amyotrophic lateral sclerosis: new evidence and unsolved issues. *J Neurol Neurosurg Psychiatry.* 2008;79:6-11.

Lord S, Allen G, Williams P, Gandevia S. Risk of falling: predictors based on reduced strength in persons previously affected by polio. *Arch Phys Med Rehabil.* 2002;83:757-763.

Lou JS. Fatigue in amyotrophic lateral sclerosis. *Phys Med Rehabil N Am.* 2008;19(3):533-543.

Lowenstein DH. Epilepsy after head injury: an overview. *Epilepsy.* 50(suppl 2):4-9.

Lu J, Goh SJ, Tng PYL, Deng YY, Ling EA, Moochhala S. Systemic inflammatory response following acute traumatic brain injury. *Front Biosci.* 2009;14:3795-3813.

Lui AJ, Byl NN. A systematic review of the effect of moderate intensity exercise on function and disease progression in amyotrophic lateral sclerosis. *J Neurol Phys Ther.* 2009;33(2):68-87.

Lulé D, Diekmann V, Müller HP, Kassubek J, Ludolph AC, Birbaumer N. Neuroimaging of multimodal sensory stimulation in amyotrophic lateral sclerosis. *J Neurol Neurosurg Psychiatry.* 2010;81(8):899-906.

MacGregor EA, Brandes J, Eikermann A. Migraine prevalence and treatment patterns: the global Migraine and Zolmitriptan Evaluation survey. *Headache.* 2003;43(1):19-26.

Maier MA, Armand J, Kirkwood PA, Yang HW, Davis JN, Lemon RN. Differences in the corticospinal projection from primary motor cortex and supplementary motor area to macaque upper limb motoneurons: an anatomical and electrophysiological study. *Cereb Cortex.* 2002;12(3):281-296.

Maloni HW. Multiple sclerosis: managing patients in primary care. *Nurse Pract.* 2013;38:25-35.

Mancini M, Horak FB, Zampieri C, Carlson-Kuhta P, Nutt JG, Chiari L. Trunk accelerometry reveals postural instability in untreated Parkinson's disease. *Parkinsonism Relat Disord.* 2011;17(7):557-562.

Mancini M, Rocchi L, Horak FB, Chiari L. Effects of Parkinson's disease and levodopa on functional limits of stability. *Clin Biomech.* 2008;23(4):450-458.

Mancuso M, Orsucci D, Siciliano G, Bonuccelli U. The genetics of ataxia: through the labyrinth of the Minotaur, looking for Ariadne's thread. *J Neurol.* 2014;261(suppl 2):S528-S541.

Mandalà M, Pepponi E, Santoro GP, et al. Double-blind randomized trial on the efficacy of the Gufoni maneuver for treatment of lateral canal BPPV. *Laryngoscope.* 2013;123(7):1782-1786.

Mandioli J, Faglioni P, Nichelli P, Sola P. Amyotrophic lateral sclerosis: prognostic indicators of survival. *Amyotroph Lateral Scler.* 2006;7:217-220.

Mari S, Serrao M, Casali C, et al. Turning strategies in patients with cerebellar ataxia. *Exp Brain Res.* 2012;222(1-2):65-75.

Marmolino D, Manto M. Past, present, and future therapeutics for cerebellar ataxias. *Curr Neuropharmacol.* 2010;8:41-61.

Marquer A, Barbieri G, Perennou D. The assessment and treatment of postural disorders in cerebellar ataxia: a systematic review. *Ann Phys Rehabil Med.* 2014;57:67-78.

Marsden J, Harris C. Cerebellar ataxia: pathophysiology and rehabilitation. *Clin Rehabil.* 2011;25:195-216.

Martin JH. *Neuroanatomy Text and Atlas.* 4th ed. New York, NY: McGraw-Hill; 2012.

Mason SL, Barker RA. Emerging drug therapies in Huntington's disease. *Expert Opin Emerg Drugs.* 2009;14(2):273-297.

Mayadev AS, Weiss MD, Distad BJ, Krivickas LS, Carter GT. The amyotrophic lateral sclerosis center: a model of multidisciplinary management. *Phys Med Rehabil Clin N Am.* 2008;19:619-631.

McCain KJ, Smith PS, Polo FE, Coleman SC, Baker S. Excellent outcomes for adults who experienced early standardized treadmill training during acute phase of recovery from stroke: a case series. *Top Stroke Rehabil.* 2011;18(4):428-436.

McCrory P, Collie A, Anderson V, Davis G. Can we manage sport related concussion in children the same as adults? *Br J Sports Med.* 2004;38(5):516-519.

McDonald-Williams MF. Exercise and postpolio. *Neurol Rep.* 1996;20(2):31-36.

McElhiney MC, Rabkin JG, Gordon PH, Goetz R, Mitsumoto H. Prevalence of fatigue and depression in ALS patients and change over time. *J Neurol Neurosurg Psychiatry.* 2009;80:1146-1149.

McKee AC, Daneshvar DH, Alvarez VE, Stein TD. The neuropathology of sport. *Acta Neuropathol.* 2014;127(1):29-51.

McKinley WO, Tewksbury MA, Mujteba NM. Spinal stenosis vs traumatic spinal cord injury: a rehabilitation outcome comparison. *J Spinal Cord Med.* 2002;25(1):28-32.

Megna J. The differential diagnosis of dizziness in the older adult. In: Hardage J, ed. *Topics in Geriatrics. Volume 6, Issue 3. An Independent Study Course Designed for Individual Continuing Education.* Alexandria, VA: Geriatric Section, American Physical Therapy Association; 2010 .

Mehanna R, Jankovic J. Respiratory problems in neurologic movement disorders. *Parkinsonism Relat Disord.* 2010;16:626-638.

Mehrholz J, Friis R, Kugler J, Twork S, Storch A, Pohl M. Treadmill training for patients with Parkinson's disease. *Cochrane Database Syst Rev.* 2010;(1):CD007830.

Meijer R, Ihnenfeldt DS, van Limbeek J, Vermeulen M, de Haan RJ. Prognostic factors in the subacute phase after stroke for the future residence after six months to one year. A systematic review of the literature. *Clin Rehabil.* 2003;17(5):512-520.

Mejerske CW, Mihalik JP, Ren D, et al. Concussion in sports: postconcussive activity levels, symptoms, and neurocognitive performance. *J Athl Train.* 2008;43(3):265-274.

Mentes BB, Yuksel O, Aydin A, Tezcaner T, Leventoglu A, Aytac B. Posterior tibial nerve stimulation for fecal incontinence after partial spinal injury: preliminary report. *Tech Coloproctol.* 2007;11:115-119.

Merkelbach S, Haensch C-A, Hemmer B, Koehler J, Konig NH, Ziemsscn T. Multiple sclerosis and the autonomic nervous system. *J Neurol.* 2006;253:1/21-1/25, online.

Messinis L, Kosmidis MH, Lyros E, Panathanasopoulos P. Assessment and rehabilitation of cognitive impairment in multiple sclerosis. *Int Rev Psychiatry.* 2010;22:22-34.

Meyer BC, Hemmen TM, Jackson CM, Lyden PD. Modified national institutes of health stroke scale for use in stroke clinical trials: prospective reliability and validity. *Stroke.* 2002;33:1261-1266.

Meythaler JM, Peduzzi JD, Eleftheriou E, Novack TA. Current concepts: diffuse axonal injury-associated traumatic brain injury. *Arch Phys Med Rehabil.* 2001;82:1461-1471.

Mhatre PV, Vilares I, Stibb SM, et al. Wii Fit balance board playing improves balances and gait in Parkinson disease. *PM R.* 2013;4(9):769-777.

Miller R, DeCandio ML, Dixon-Mah Y, et al. Molecular targets and treatment of meningioma. *J Neurol Neurosurg.* 2014;1(1):1-15.

Miller RG, Mitchell JD, Lyon M, Moore DH. Riluzole for amyotrophic lateral sclerosis (ALS)/motor neuron disease (MND). *Cochrane Database Syst Rev.* 2007;1:CD001447.

Min KK, Jong S, Kim MJ, Cho CH, Cha HE, Lee JH. Clinical use of subjective visual horizontal and vertical in patients of unilateral vestibular neuritis. *Otol Neurotol.* 2007;28(4):520-525.

Mink JW. The basal ganglia and involuntary movements: impaired inhibition of competing motor patterns. *Arch Neurol.* 2003;60(10):1365-1368.

Minkel JL. Seating and mobility considerations for people with spinal cord injury. *Phys Ther.* 2000;80(7):701-709.

Missaoui B, Thoumie P. How far do patients with sensory ataxia benefit from so-called "proprioceptive rehabilitation"? *Neurophysiol Clin.* 2009;39(4-5):229-233.

Mitchell JD, Borasio GD. Amyotrophic lateral sclerosis. *Lancet.* 2007;369:2031-2041.

Mitiguy JS. Coping with survival. Headlines. 1990:228. In: Power PW, Dell Orto AE, eds. *Families Living with Chronic Illness and Disability: Interventions, Challenges, and Opportunities.* New York, NY: Springer; 2004.

Miyai I, Ito M, Hattori N, et al. Cerebellar ataxia rehabilitation trial in degenerative cerebellar diseases. *Neurorehabil Neural Repair.* 2012;(5):515-522.

Montes J, Cheng B, Diamond B, Doorish C, Mitsumoto H, Gordon PH. The Timed Up and Go Test: predicting falls in ALS. *Amyotroph Lateral Scler.* 2007;8:292-295.

Morris AE, Lutman ME, Yardley L. Measuring outcome from vestibular rehabilitation, PART II: refinement and validation of a new self-report measure. *Int J Audiol.* 2009;48(1):24-37.

Morris JH, Van Wijck F. Responses of the less affected arm to bilateral upper limb task training in early rehabilitation after stroke: a randomized controlled trial. *Arch Phys Med Rehabil.* 2012;93(7):1129-1137.

Morton AJ. Circadian and sleep disorder in Huntington's disease. *Exp Neurol.* 2013;243:34-44.

Morton SM, Bastian AJ. Relative contributions of balance and voluntary leg-coordination deficits to cerebellar gait ataxia. *J Neurophysiol.* 2003;89:1844-1856.

Moseley AM, Hassett LM, Leung J, Clare JS, Herbert RD, Harvey LA. Serial casting versus positioning for the treatment of elbow contractures in adults with traumatic brain injury: a randomized controlled trial. *Clin Rehabil.* 2008;22(5):406-417.

Motl RW, Smith DC, Elliott J, Weikert M, Diugonski D, Sosnoff JJ. Combined training improves walking mobility in persons with significant disability from multiple sclerosis: a pilot study. *J Neurol Phys Ther.* 2012;36(1):32-37.

Munger KL, Zhang SM, O'Reilly E. Vitamin D intake and incidence of multiple sclerosis. *Neurology.* 2004;62:60-65.

Munhoz RP, Li JY, Kurtinecz M, et al. Evaluation of the pull test technique in assessing postural instability in Parkinson's disease. *Neurology.* 2004;62(1):125-127.

Murdin L, Davies RA, Bronstein AM. Vertigo as a migraine trigger. *Neurology.* 2009;73(8):638-642.

Murphy J, Henry R, Lomen-Hoerth C. Establishing subtypes of the continuum of frontal lobe impairment in amyotrophic lateral sclerosis. *Arch Neurol.* 2007;64:330-334.

Murphy MP, Carmine H. Long-term health implications of individuals with TBI: a rehabilitation perspective. *NeuroRehabilitation.* 2012;31:85-94.

Myers J, Kirati J, Jaramillo J. The cardiometabolic benefits of routine physical activity in persons living with spinal cord injury. *Curr Cardiovasc Risk Rep.* 2012;6:323-330.

Nakamura T, Hirayama M, Hara T, Hama T, Watanabe H, Sobue G. Does cardiovascular autonomic dysfunction contribute to fatigue in Parkinson's disease? *Mov Disord.* 2011;26(10):1869-1874.

Nance MA, Myers RH. Juvenile onset Huntington's disease – clinical and research perspectives. *Ment Retard Dev Disabil Res Rev.* 2001;7:153-157.

Nardone A, Galante M, Lucas B, Schieppati M. Stance control is not affected by paresis and reflex hyperexcitability: the case of spastic patients. *J Neurol Neurosurg Psychiatry.* 2001;70(5):635-643.

Nashner LM. Sensory neuromuscular and biomechanical contributions to human balance. In Duncan PW, ed. *Balance Proceedings of the APTA Forum.* Alexandria, VA: American Physical Therapy Association; 1990.

Nasreddine ZS, Phillips NA, Bedirian V, et al. The Montreal Cognitive Assessment, MoCA: a brief screening tool for mild cognitive impairment. *J Geriatr Soc.* 2005;53:695-699.

Natale A, Taylor S, LaBarbera J, et al. SCIRehab Project series: the physical therapy taxonomy. *J Spinal Cord Med.* 2009;32(3):270-282.

National Stroke Association's Stroke 101 Fact Sheet. Available at: http://www.stroke.org/site/DocServer/STROKE_101_Fact_Sheet.pdf?docID=4541. Accessed March 5, 2018.

Newton RA. Validity of the multi-directional reach test: a practical measure for limits of stability in older adults. *J Gerontol A Biol Sci Med Sci.* 2001;56(4):M248-M252.

Ng YS, Stein J, Ning M, Black-Schaffer RM. Comparison of clinical characteristics and functional outcomes of ischemic stroke in different vascular territories. *Stroke.* 2007;38:2309-2314.

Nichols-Larsen D, Kegelmeyer D, Buford J, Kloos A, Heathcock J, Basso DM. *Neurologic Rehabilitation: Neuroscience and Neuroplasticity in Physical Therapy Practice.* New York, NY: McGraw-Hill; 2016. http://accessphysiotherapy.mhmedical.com/book.aspx?bookid=1760.

Nieuwboer A, Rochester L, Muncks L, Swinnen SP. Motor learning in Parkinson's disease: limitations and potential for rehabilitation. *Parkinsonism Relat Disord.* 2009;15(suppl 3):S53-S58.

NIOSH. Performing motor and sensory neuronal conduction studies in humans: a NIOSH technical manual (NIOSH) Publication No. 90-113. Washington, DC: National Institute for Occupational Safety and Health, 1990.

Nordon-Craft A, Moss M, Quan D, Schenkman M. Intensive care unit-acquired weakness: implications for physical therapist management. *Phys Ther.* 2012;92(12):1494-1506.

Noyce AJ, Bestwick JP, Silveira-Moriyama L, et al. Meta-analysis of early nonmotor features and risk factors for Parkinson disease. *Ann Neurol.* 2012;72:893-901.

NPUAP. Available at: http://www.npuap.org/wp-content/uploads/2012/02/Final_Quick_Prevention_for_web_2010.pdf. Accessed on March 5, 2018.

Nunez RA, Cass SP, Furman JM. Short and long-term outcomes of canalith repositioning for benign paroxysmal positional vertigo. *Arch Otolaryngol Head Neck Surg.* 2000;122:647-652.

Nuti D, Nati C, Passali D. Treatment of benign paroxysmal positional vertigo: no need for postmaneuver restrictions. *Otol Head Neck Surg.* 2000;122:440-444.

O'Sullivan SB, Schmitz TJ. *Improving Functional Outcomes in Physical Rehabilitation.* 2nd ed. Philadelphia, PA: F.A. Davis; 2016.

O'Sullivan SB, Schmitz TJ. *Physical Rehabilitation.* 6th ed. Philadelphia, PA: F.A. Davis; 2014.

Olvey EL, Armstrong EP, Grizzle AJ. Contemporary pharmacologic treatments for spasticity of the upper limb after stroke: a systematic review. *Clin Ther.* 2010;32(4):2282-2303.

Oncu J, Durmaz B, Karapolat H. Short-term effects of aerobic exercise on functional capacity, fatigue, and quality of life in patients with post-polio syndrome. *Clin Rehabil.* 2009;23(2):155-163.

Owens GP, Bennett JL. Trigger, pathogen, or bystander: the complex nexus linking Epstein-Barr virus and multiple sclerosis. *Mult Scler J.* 2012;18(9):1204-1208.

Paltamaa J, Sjogren T, Peurala SH, Heinonen A. Effects of physiotherapy interventions on balance in multiple sclerosis: a systematic review and meta-analysis of randomized controlled trials. *J Rehabil Med.* 2012;44(10):811-823.

Pape HC, Lehmann U, van GM, Gansslen A, von GS, Krettek C. Heterotopic ossifications in patients after severe blunt trauma with and without head trauma: incidence and patterns of distribution. *J Orthop Trauma.* 2001;15:229-237.

Parent A, Carpenter MB. *Carpenter's Human Neuroanatomy.* Baltimore: Williams and Wilkins; 1996.

Park CK, Phi JH, Park SH. Glial tumors with neuronal differentiation. *Neurosurg Clin N Am.* 2015;26:117-138.

Park E, Ai J, Baker AJ. Cerebellar injury: clinical relevance and potential in traumatic brain injury research. *Prog Brain Res.* 2007;161:327-338.

Parkinson's Disease Backgrounder. National Institute of Neurological Disorders and Stroke. Available at: http://www.ninds.nih.gov/disorders/parkinsons_disease/parkinsons_disease_backgrounder.htmed. Accessed March 5, 2018.

Parkinson's Disease Foundation. Statistics on Parkinson's. Available at: http://www.pdf.org/en/parkinson_statistics. Accessed March 5, 2018.

Pasquina P, Kirtley R, Ling G. Moderate-to-severe traumatic brain injury. *Semin Neurol.* 2014;34:572-583.

Patten C, Horak FB, Krebs DE. Head and body center of gravity control strategies: adaptations following vestibular rehabilitation. *Acta Otolaryngol.* 2003;123(1):32-40.

Paulsen JS. Cognitive impairment in Huntington's disease: diagnosis and treatment. *Neurol Neurosci Rep.* 2011;11(5):474-483.

Peach PE. Overwork weakness with evidence of muscle damage in a patient with residual paralysis from polio. *Arch Phys Med Rehabil.* 1990;71:248-250.

Pepe JL, Barba CA. The metabolic response to acute traumatic brain injury and implications for nutritional support. *J Head Trauma Rehabil.* 1999;14(5):462-474.

Pergolizzi J, Ahlbeck K, Aldington D, et al. The development of chronic pain: physiological CHANGE necessitates a multidisciplinary approach to treatment. *Curr Med Res Opin.* 2013;1-9.

Pernet L, Jughters A, Kerckhofs E. The effectiveness of different treatment modalities for the rehabilitation of unilateral neglect in stroke patients: a systematic review. *NeuroRehabilitation.* 2013;33:611-620.

Perry J, Burnfield JM. Gait Analysis: *Normal and Abnormal Function.* 2nd ed. Thorofare, NJ: Slack; 2010.

Peurala SH, Kantanen MP, Sjogren T, Paltamaa J, Karhula M, Heinonen A. Effectiveness of constraint-induced movement therapy on activity and participation after stroke: a systematic review and meta-analysis of randomized controlled trials. *Clin Rehabil.* 2011;26(3):209-223.

Picelli A, Melotti C, Origano F, Neri R, Waldner A, Smania N. Robot-assisted gait training versus equal intensity treadmill training in patients with mild to moderate Parkinson's disease: a randomized controlled trial. *Parkinsonism Relat Disord.* 2013;19(6):605-610.

Pickering RM, Grimbergen YA, Rigney U, et al. A meta-analysis of six prospective studies of falling in Parkinson's disease. *Mov Disord.* 2007;22(13):1892-1900.

Pilutti LA, Greenlee TA, Motl RW, Nickrent MS, Petruzzello SJ. Effects of exercise training on fatigue in multiple sclerosis: a meta-analysis. *Psychosom Med.* 2013;75(6):575-580.

Pinto S, Swash M, de Carvalho M. Respiratory exercise in amyotrophic lateral sclerosis. *Amyotroph Lateral Scler.* 2012;13(1):33-43.

Pirko I, Lucchinetti CF, Sriram S, Bakshi R. Gray matter involvement in multiple sclerosis. *Neurology.* 2007;68:634-642.

Podsiadlo D, Richardson S. The timed "Up & Go": a test of basic functional mobility for frail elderly persons. *J Am Geriatr Soc.* 1991;9:142-148.

Poewe W, Wenning G. The differential diagnosis of Parkinson's disease. *Eur J Neurol.* 2002;9(S3):23-30.

Pompeu JE, Mendes FA, Silva KG, et al. Effect of Nintendo Wii™-based motor and cognitive training on activities of daily living in patients with Parkinson's disease: a randomized clinical trial. *Physiotherapy.* 2012;98(3):196-204.

Potter K, Fulk, GD, Salem Y, Sullivan J. Outcome measures in neurological physical therapy practice: part I. Making sound decisions. *J Neurol Phys Ther.* 2011;35(2):57-64.

Potts MB, Adwanikar H, Noble-Haeusslein LJ. Models of traumatic cerebellar injury. *Cerebellum.* 2009;8(3):211-221.

Powell LE, Myers AM. The Activities-specific Balance Confidence (ABC) Scale. *J Gerontol A Biol Sci Med Sci.* 1995;50:28-34.

Prakash RS, Snook EM, Motl RW, Kramer AF. Aerobic fitness is associated with gray matter volume and white matter integrity in multiple sclerosis. *Brain Res.* 2010;1341:41-51.

Profyris C, Cheema SS, Zang D, Azari MF, Boyle K, Petratos S. Degenerative and regenerative mechanisms governing spinal cord injury. *Neurobiol Dis.* 2004;15:415-436.

Purtilo R, Haddad A. *Health Professional and Patient Interaction.* 7th ed. Philadelphia, PA: WB Saunders; 2007.

Quinn L, Busse M. On behalf of the members of the European Huntington's Disease Network Physiotherapy Working Group. Physiotherapy clinical guidelines for Huntington's disease. *Neurodegener Dis Manag.* 2012;2(1):21-31.

Quinn L, Khalil H, Dawes H, et al. Reliability and minimal detectable change of physical performance measures in individuals with pre-manifest and manifest Huntington's disease. *Phys Ther.* 2013;93(7):942-956.

Rabinowitz AR, Levin HS. Cognitive sequelae of traumatic brain injury. *Psychiatr Clin N Am.* 2014;37(1):1-11.

Radtke A, von Brevern M, Neuhauser H, Hottenrott T, Lempert T. Vestibular migraine: long-term follow-up of clinical symptoms and vestibulo-cochlear findings. *Neurology.* 2012;79(15):1607-1614.

Radunovic A, Mitsumoto H, Leigh PN. Clinical care of patients with amyotrophic lateral sclerosis. *Lancet Neurol.* 2007;6:913-925.

Rajabally YA, Uncini A. Outcome and its predictors in Guillain-Barré syndrome. *J Neurol Neurosurg Psychiatry.* 2012;83:711-718.

Rancho Los Amigos Cognitive Recovery Scale. Available at: https://www.neuroskills.com/resources/rancho-los-amigos-revised.php. Accessed March 5, 2018.

Rao AK, Mazzoni P, Wasserman P, Marder K. Longitudinal change in gait and motor function in pre-manifest Huntington's disease. *PLoS Curr.* 2011;3:RRN1268.

Rao AK, Muratori L, Louis ED, Moskowitz CB, Marder KS. Spectrum of gait impairments in presymptomatic and symptomatic Huntington's disease. *Mov Disord.* 2008;23(8):1100-1107.

Rasquin SM, Lodder J, Ponds RW, Winkens I, Jolles J, Verhey FR. Cognitive functioning after stroke: a one-year follow-up study. *Dement Geriatr Cogn Disord.* 2004;18:138-144.

Ray AD, Udhoji S, Mashtare TL, Fisher NM. A combined inspiratory and expiratory muscle training program improves respiratory muscle strength and fatigue in multiple sclerosis. *Arch Phys Med Rehabil.* 2013;94(10):1964-1970.

Rehabilitation Measures Database. Available at: www.rehabmeasures.org. Accessed on March 5, 2018.

Riederer P, Laux G. MAO-inhibitors in Parkinson's disease. *Exp Neurobiol.* 2011;20(1):1-17.

Rietberg MB, Brooks D, Uitdehaag BM, Kwakkel G. Exercise therapy for multiple sclerosis. *Cochrane Database Syst Rev.* 2005;1:CD003980.

Rinaldi S. Update on Guillain-Barré syndrome. *J Peripher Nerv Syst.* 2013;18(2):99-112.

Rincon F, Ghosh S, Dey S, et al. Impact of acute lung injury and acute respiratory distress syndrome after traumatic brain injury in the United States. *Neurosurgery.* 2012;71:795-803.

Rine RM, Schubert MC, Balkany TJ. Visual-vestibular habituation and balance training for motion sickness. *Phys Ther.* 1999;79:949-957.

Robberecht W, Philips T. The changing scene of amyotrophic lateral sclerosis. *Nat Rev Neurosci.* 2013;14(4):248-264.

Robinson CJ, Kett NA, Bolam JM. Spasticity in spinal cord injured patients: 2: initial measures and long-term effects of surface electrical stimulation. *Arch Phys Med Rehabil.* 1988;69(10):862-868.

Rocco A, Pasquini M, Cecconi E, et al. Monitoring after the acute stage of stroke: a prospective study. *Stroke.* 2007;38(4):1225-1228.

Rodriguez-Oroz MC, Jahanshahi M, Krack P, et al. Initial clinical manifestations of Parkinson's disease: features and pathophysiological mechanisms. *Lancet Neurol.* 2009;8:1128-1139.

Rodriquez AA, Agre JC. Electrophysiologic study of the quadriceps muscles during fatiguing exercise and recovery: a comparison of symptomatic and asymptomatic postpolio patients and controls. *Arch Phys Med Rehabil.* 1991;72:993-997.

Roland PE, Larsen B, Lassen NA, Skinhoj E. Supplementary motor area and other cortical areas in organization of voluntary movements in man. *J Neurophysiol.* 1980;43(1):118-136.

Romo R, Lemus L, de Lafuente V. Sense, memory, and decision-making in the somatosensory cortical network. *Curr Opin Neurol.* 2012;22:914-919.

Ropper AH, Brown RH. *Adams and Victor's Principles of Neurology.* 10th ed. New York, NY: Mc Graw Hill; 2017.

Rose D, Paris T, Crews E, Wu SS, Sun A, Behrman AL, Duncan P. Feasibility and effectiveness of circuit training in acute stroke rehabilitation. *Neurorehabil Neural Repair.* 2011;25(2):140-148.

Rose DJ. *FallProof! A Comprehensive Balance and Mobility Program.* Champaign, IL: Human Kinetics; 2003.

Rosenblatt A. Neuropsychiatry of Huntington's disease. *Dialogues Clin Neurosci.* 2007;9(2):191-197.

Rosenfield J, Paksima N. Peripheral nerve injuries and repair in the upper extremity. *Bull Hosp Jt Dis.* 2002;60(3-4):155-161.

Rossi FH, Franco MC, Estevez AG. Pathophysiology of amyotrophic lateral sclerosis. In: Estévez AG, ed. *Current Advances in Amyotrophic Lateral Sclerosis.* 2013.

Rosti-Otajarvi E, Hamalainen P. Behavioural symptoms and impairments in multiple sclerosis: a systematic review and meta-analysis. *Mult Scler J.* 2012;19:31-45.

Ruts L, Drenthen J, Jongen JL, et al. Dutch GBS Study Group. Pain in Guillain-Barré syndrome: a long-term follow-up study. *Neurology.* 2010;75:1439-1447.

Saeys W, Vereeck L, Truijen S, Lafosse C, Wuyts FP, Heyning PV. Randomized controlled trial of truncal exercises early after stroke to improve balance and mobility. *Neurorehabil Neural Repair.* 2012;26(3):231-238.

Said G. Diabetic neuropathy. *Handb Clin Neurol.* 2013;115:579-589.

Sakaida M, Takeuchi K, Ishinaga H, Adachi M, Majima Y. Long-term outcome of benign paroxysmal positional vertigo. *Neurology.* 2003;60(9):1532-1534.

Sanaya K, Douglas A. Neuroimaging in amyotrophic lateral sclerosis. *Amyotroph Lateral Scler Other Motor Neuron Disord.* 2003;4:243-248.

Sandberg A, Stalberg E. Changes in macro electromyography over time in patients with a history of polio: a comparison of two muscles. *Arch Phys Med Rehabil.* 2004;85:1174-1182.

Sanjak M, Bravver E, Bockenek WL, Norton J, Brooks BR. Supported treadmill ambulation for amyotrophic lateral sclerosis: a pilot study. *Arch Phys Med Rehabil.* 2010;91:1920-1929.

Santamato A, Panza F, Ranieri M, Fiore P. Effect of botulinum toxin type A and modified constraint-induced movement therapy on motor function of upper limb in children with obstetrical brachial plexus palsy. *Childs Nerv Syst.* 2011;27:2187-2192.

Santangelo G, Barone P, Cuoco S, et al. Apathy in untreated, de novo patients with Parkinson's disease: validation study of Apathy Evaluation Scale. *J Neurol.* 2014;261(12):2319-2328.

Saracchi E, Fermi S, Brighina L. Emerging candidate biomarkers for Parkinson's disease: a review. *Aging Dis.* 2014;5(1):27-34.

Saute JA, Donis KC, Serrano-Munuera C, et al. Iberoamerican Multidisciplinary Network for the Study of Movement Disorders (RIBERMOV) Study Group. Ataxia rating scales – psychometric profiles, natural history and their application in clinical trials. *Cerebellum.* 2012;11(2):488-504.

Schaechter JD, Moore CK, Connell BD, Rosen BR, Dijkhuizen RM. Structural and functional plasticity in the somatosensory cortex of chronic stroke patients. *Brain.* 2006;129:2722-2733.

Scherder E, Statema M. Huntington's disease. *Lancet.* 2010; 376:1464.

Schiemanck SK, Post MM, Kwakkel G, Witkamp TD, Kappelle LJ, Prevo AJH. Ischemic lesion volume correlates with long-term functional outcome and quality of life of middle cerebral artery stroke survivors. *Restor Neurol Neurosci.* 2005;23:257-263.

Schiess MC, Oh IJ, Stimming EF, et al. Prospective 12-month study of intrathecal baclofen therapy for poststroke spastic upper and lower extremity motor control and functional improvement. *Neuromodulation.* 2011;14:38-45.

Schjolberg A, Sunnerhagen KS. Unlocking the locked in: a need for team approach in rehabilitation of survivors with locked-in syndrome. *Acta Neurol Scand.* 2012;125:192-198.

Schmidt EP, Drachman DB, Wiener CM, Clawson L, Kimball R, Lechtzin N. Pulmonary predictors of survival in amyotrophic lateral sclerosis: use in clinical trial design. *Muscle Nerve.* 2006;33:127-132.

Schneider R, Leigh RJ. Pharmacological and optical methods to treat vestibular disorders and nystagmus. In: Herdman SJ, Clendaniel RA, eds. *Vestibular Rehabilitation.* 4th ed. Philadelphia, PA: F.A. Davis; 2014:250-265.

Schneider SA, Wilkinson L, Bhatia KP, et al. Abnormal explicit but normal implicit sequence learning in premanifest and early Huntington's disease. *Mov Disord.* 2010;25:1343-1349.

Schniepp R, Wuehr M, Schlick C, et al. Increased gait variability is associated with the history of falls in patients with cerebellar ataxia. *J Neurol.* 2014;261(1):213-223.

Schoneburg B, Mancini M, Horak F, Nutt JG. Framework for understanding balance dysfunction in Parkinson's disease. *Mov Disord.* 2013;11:1474-1482.

Schubert MC. Vestibular function tests. In: Herdman SJ, Clendaniel RA, eds. *Vestibular Rehabilitation.* 4th ed. Philadelphia, PA: F.A. Davis; 2014:178-194.

Schubert MC, Tusa RJ, Grine LE, Herdman SJ. Optimizing the sensitivity of the head thrust test for identifying vestibular hypofunction. *Phys Ther.* 2004;84(2):151-158.

Schwartz S, Cohen ME, Herbison GJ, Shah A. Relationship between two measures of upper extremity strength: manual muscle test compared to hand-held myometry. *Arch Phys Med Rehabil.* 1992;73(11):1063-1068.

Seidler RD, Bo J, Anguera JA. Neurocognitive contributions to motor skill learning: the role of working memory. *J Mot Behav.* 2012;44(6):445-453.

Sejvar JJ, Baughman AL, Wise M, Morgan OW. Population incidence of Guillain-Barré syndrome: a systematic review and meta-analysis. *Neuroepidemiology.* 2011;36:123-133.

Serrao M, Conte C, Casali C, et al. Sudden stopping in patients with cerebellar ataxia. *Cerebellum.* 2013;12(5):607-616.

Serrao M, Mari S, Conte C, et al. Strategies adopted by cerebellar ataxia patients to perform U-turns. *Cerebellum.* 2013;12(4):460 468.

Seung-Han L, Kim JS. Benign paroxysmal positional vertigo. *J Clin Neurol.* 2010;6:51-63.

Shabbott B, Ravindran R, Schumacher JW, Wasserman PB, Marder KS, Mazzoni P. Learning fast accurate movements requires intact frontostriatal circuits. *Front Hum Neurosci.* 2013;7:752.

Shadmehr R, Smith MA, Krakauer JW. Error correction, sensory prediction, and adaptation in motor control. *Ann Rev Neurosci.* 2010;33:89-108.

Shaia WT, Zappia JJ, Bojrab DI, LaRouere ML, Sargent EW, Diaz RC. Success of posterior semicircular canal occlusion and application of the Dizziness Handicap Inventory. *Otolaryngol Head Neck Surg.* 2006;134(3):424-430.

Sharma KR, Cross J, Farronay O, Ayyar DR, Shebert RT, Bradley WG. Demyelinating neuropathy in diabetes mellitus. *Arch Neurol.* 2002;59(5):758-765.

Shehab D, Elgazzar AH, Collier BD. Heterotopic ossification. *J Nucl Med.* 2002;43(3):346-353.

Shen-Ting L, Dendi R, Holmes C, Goldstein DS. Progressive loss of cardiac sympathetic innervation in Parkinson's disease. *Ann Neurol.* 2002;52:220-223.

Sherer M, Yablon SA, Nakase-Richardson R. Patterns of recovery of posttraumatic confusional state in neurorehabilitation admissions after traumatic brain injury. *Arch Phys Med Rehabil.* 2009;96:1749-1754.

Shulman LM, Katzel LI, Ivey FM, et al. Randomized clinical trial of 3 types of physical exercise for patients with Parkinson disease. *JAMA Neurol.* 2013;70(2):183-190.

Shumway-Cook A, Horak FB. Assessing the influence of sensory interaction of balance. Suggestion from the field. *Phys Ther.* 1986;66(10):1548-1550.

Shumway-Cook A, Woollacott MH. *Motor Control Translating Research into Clinical Practice.* 5th ed. Philadelphia, PA: Wolters and Kluwer; 2017.

Shupak A, Gordon CR. Motion sickness: advances in pathogenesis, prediction, prevention, and treatment. *Aviat Space Environ Med.* 2006;77(12):1213-1223.

Siderowf A, Lang AE. Premotor Parkinson's disease: concepts and definitions. *Mov Disord.* 2012;27(5):608-616.

Siegel A, Sapru H. *Essential Neuroscience Revised.* Philadelphia, PA: Lippincott Williams & Wilkins; 2006.

Simmons Z, Felgoise SH, Bremer BA, et al. The ALSSQOL: balancing physical and nonphysical factors in assessing quality of life in ALS. *Neurology.* 2006;67:1659-1664.

Sinemet. Available at: www.drugs.com/pro/sinemet.html. Accessed March 3, 2018.

Singer BJ, Jegasothy GM, Singer KP, Allison GT. Evaluation of serial casting to correct equinovarus deformity of the ankle after acquired brain injury in adults. *Arch Phys Med Rehabil.* 2003;84(4):483-491.

Singh R, Rohilla RK, Sangwa K, Siwach R, Magu NK, Sangwan SS. Bladder management methods and urological complications in spinal cord injury patients. *Indian J Orthop.* 2011;45(2):141-147.

Sitek EJ, Soltan W, Woeczorek D, et al. Unawareness of deficits in Huntington's disease. *J Int Neuropsychol Soc.* 2011;17:788-795.

Skodda S, Schlegel U, Hoffmann R, Saft C. Impaired motor speech performance in Huntington's disease. *J Neural Transm.* 2014;121:399-407.

Skorvanek M, Nagyova I, Rosenberger J, et al. Clinical determinants of primary and secondary fatigue in patients with Parkinson's disease. *J Neurol.* 2013;260(6):1554-1561.

Skough K, Krossén C, Heiwe S, Theorell H, Borg K. Effects of resistance training in combination with coenzyme Q10 supplementation in patients with post-polio: a pilot study. *J Rehabil Med.* 2008;40(9):773-775.

Slattery EL, Sinks BC, Goebel JA. Vestibular tests for rehabilitation: applications and interpretation. *NeuroRehabilitation.* 2011;29:143-151.

Smania N, Corato E, Tinazzi M, et al. Effect of balance training on postural instability in patients with idiopathic Parkinson's disease. *Neurorehabil Neural Repair.* 2010;24(9):826-834.

Smets EM, Garssen B, Bonke B, De Haes JC. The Multidimensional Fatigue Inventory (MFI): psychometric qualities of an instrument to assess fatigue. *J Psychosom Res.* 1995;39(3):315-325.

Smith-Wheelock M, Shepard NT, Telian SA. Physical therapy program for vestibular rehabilitation. *Am J Otol.* 1991;12:218-225.

Snaphaan L, Rijpkema M, van Uden I, Fernandez G, de Leeuw FE. Reduced medial temporal lobe functionality in stroke patients: a functional magnetic resonance imaging study. *Brain.* 2009;132:1882-1888.

Snijders AH, Haaxma CA, Hagen YJ, Munneke M, Bloem BR. Freezer or non-freezer: clinical assessment of freezing of gait. *Parkinsonism Relat Disord.* 2012;18(2):149-154.

Snoek GJ, Ijzerman MJ, Hermens HJ, Biering-Sorensen F. Survey of the needs of patients with spinal cord injury: impact and priority for improvement in hand function in tetraplegics. *Spinal Cord.* 2004;42:526-532.

Somers MF. *Spinal Cord Injury: Functional Rehabilitaiton.* 3rd ed. Upper Saddle River, NJ: Pearson; 2010.

Sommerfeld DK, Gripenstedt UK, Welmer AK. Spasticity after stroke: an overview of prevalence, test instruments, and treatments. *Am J Phys Med Rehabil.* 2012;91(9):814-820.

Song CH, Petrofsky JS, Lee SW, Lee KJ, Yim JE. Effects of an exercise program on balance and trunk proprioception in older adults with diabetic neuropathies. *Diabetes Tech Ther.* 2011;13:803-811.

Spiess MR, Müller RM, Rupp R, Schuld C, EM-SCI Study Group, van Hedel HJ. Conversion in ASIA impairment scale during the first year after traumatic spinal cord injury. *J Neurotrauma.* 2009;26(11):2027-2036.

Spinal Cord Medicine Consortium. Clinical practice guidelines: neurogenic bowel management in adults with spinal cord injury. *J Spinal Cord Med.* 1998;21(3):248-293.

Steinlin M. A clinical approach to arterial ischemic childhood stroke; increasing knowledge over the last decade. *Neuropediatrics.* 2012;43:1-9.

Stocchetti N, Maas AIR. Traumatic intracranial hypertension. *N Engl J Med.* 2014;370:2121-2130.

Stocchi F, Jenner P, Obeso JA. When do levodopa motor fluctuations first appear in Parkinson's disease? *Eur Neurol.* 2010;63(5):257-266.

Streckmann F, Zopf EM, Lehmann HC, et al. Exercise intervention studies in patients with peripheral neuropathy: a systematic review. *Sports Med.* 2014;44(9):1289-1304.

Strupp M, Brandt T. Diagnosis and treatment of vertigo and dizziness. *Dtsch Arztebl Int.* 2008;105(10):173-180.

Strupp M, Kalla R, Glasauer S, et al. Aminopyridines for the treatment of cerebellar and ocular motor disorders. *Prog Brain Res.* 2008;171:535-541.

Stuifbergen AK, Blozis SA, Harrison TC, Becker HA. Exercise, functional limitations, and quality of life: a longitudinal study of persons with multiple sclerosis. *Arch Phys Med Rehabil.* 2006;87(7):935-943.

Sullivan EV, Rose J, Pfefferbaum A. Effect of vision, touch and stance on cerebellar vermian-related sway and tremor: a quantitative physiological and MRI study. *Cereb Cortex.* 2006;16:1077-1086.

Sullivan J, Williams A, Lanzino D, Peron A, Potter K. Outcome measures in neurological physical therapy practice: part ii. a patient-centered process. *J Neurol Phys Ther.* 2011;35:65-74.

Sundman MH, Hail EE, Chen NK. Examining the relationship between head trauma and neurodegenerative disease: a review of epidemiology, pathology, and neuroimaging techniques. *J Alzheimers Dis Parkinsonism.* 2014;4. pii:137.

Swartling FJ, Cancer M, Frantz A, Weishaupt H, Persson AI. Deregulated proliferation and differentiation in brain tumors. *Cell Tissue Res.* 2015;359:225-254.

Tam SL, Archibald V, Jassar B, Tyreman N, Gordon T. Increased neuromuscular activity reduces sprouting in partially denervated muscles. *J Neurosci.* 2001;21:654-667.

Tam SL, Archibald V, Tyreman N, Gordon T. Effect of exercise on stability of chronically enlarged motor units. *Muscle Nerve.* 2002;25:359-369.

Taub E. Somatosensory deafferentation search with monkeys: implications for rehabilitation medicine. In: Ince LP, ed. *Behavioral Psychology in Rehabilitation Medicine: Clinical Applications.* New York, NY: Williams & Wilkins; 1980:316-401.

Taub E, Crago JE, Burgio LD, et al. An operant approach to rehabilitation medicine: overcoming learned nonuse by shaping. *J Exp Anal Behav.* 1994;61(2):281-293.

Taub E, Uswatte G, Bowman MH, et al. Constraint-induced movement therapy combined with conventional neurorehabilitation techniques in chronic stroke patients with plegic hands: a case series. *Arch Phys Med Rehabil.* 2013;94:86-94.

Taylor P, Humphreys L, Swain I. The long-term cost-effectiveness of the use of Functional Electric Stimulation for the correction of dropped foot due to upper motor neuron lesion. *J Rehabil Med.* 2013;45(2):154-160.

Taylor-Schroeder S, LaBarbera J, McDowell S, et al. Physical therapy treatment time during inpatient spinal cord injury rehabilitation. *J Spinal Cord Med.* 2011;34:149-161.

Teasdale G, Maas A, Lecky F, Manley G, Stocchetti N, Murray G. The Glasgow Coma Scale at 4 years: standing the test of time. *Lancet Neurol.* 2014;18:844-854.

Tee LH, Chee NWC. Vestibular rehabilitation therapy for the dizzy patient. *Ann Acad Med Singapore.* 2005;34:289-294.

Teeter L, Gassaway J, Taylor S, et al. Relationship of physical therapy inpatient rehabilitation interventions and patient characteristics to outcomes following spinal cord injury: the SCIRehab project. *J Spinal Cord Med.* 2012;35(6):503-526.

Thacker EL, Ascherio A. Familial aggregation of Parkinson's disease: a meta-analysis. *Mov Disord.* 2008;23:1174-1183.

Thanvi B, Lo N, Robinson T. Levodopa-induced dyskinesia in Parkinson's disease: clinical features, pathogenesis, prevention and treatment. *Postgrad Med J.* 2007;83(980):384-388.

Thompson AK, Wolpaw JR. Operant conditioning of spinal reflexes: from basic science to clinical therapy. *Front Integr Neurosci.* 2014;8:25.

Thompson TL, Amadee R. Vertigo: a review of common peripheral and central vestibular disorders. *Ochsner J.* 2009;9(1):20-26.

Tiffreau V, Rapin A, Serafi R, et al. Post-polio syndrome and rehabilitation. *Ann Phys Rehabil Med.* 2010;53(1):42-50.

Tillakaratne NJ, de Leon RD, Hoang TX, Roy RR, Edgerton VR, Tobin AJ. Use-dependent modulation of inhibitory capacity in the feline lumbar spinal cord. *J Neurosci.* 2002;22(8):3130-3143.

Tinetti ME. Performance-oriented assessment of mobility problems in elderly patients. *J Am Geriatr Soc.* 1986;34:119-126.

Tolosa E, Compta Y. Dystonia in Parkinson's disease. *J Neurol.* 2006;253(suppl 7):VII7-VII13.

Tomaszczyk JC, Green NL, Frasca D, et al. Negative neuroplasticity in chronic traumatic brain injury and implications for neurorehabilitation. *Neuropsychol Rev.* 2014;24:409-427.

Traynor BJ, Alexander M, Corr B, Frost E, Hardiman O. Effect of a multidisciplinary amyotrophic lateral sclerosis (ALS) clinic on ALS survival: a population based study, 1996-2000. *J Neurol Neurosurg Psychiatry.* 2003;74:1258-1261.

Trujillo-Martin MM, Serrano-Aguilar P, Monton-Alvarez F, Carrillo-Fumero R. Effectiveness and safety of treatments for degenerative ataxias: a systematic review. *Mov Disord.* 2009;24(8):1111-1124.

Tuckey J, Greenwood R. Rehabilitation after severe Guillain-Barré syndrome: the use of partial body weight support. *Physiother Res Int.* 2004;9(2):96-103.

Umphred, DA. *Neurological Rehabiltation.* 6th ed. St. Louis, MO: Mosby Elsevier, 2012.

Uncini A, Kuwabara S. Electrodiagnostic criteria for Guillain-Barrè syndrome: a critical revision and the need for an update. *Clin Neurophysiol.* 2012;123(8):1487-1495.

United Kingdom Parkinson's Disease Society Brain Bank Clinical Diagnostic Criteria. Available at: http://www.ncbi.nlm.nih.gov/projects/gap/cgi-bin/GetPdf.cgi?id=phd000042. Accessed March 5, 2018.

Urban PP. Speech motor deficits in cerebellar infarctions. *Brain Lang.* 2013;127(3):323-326.

Vakhnina NV, Nikitina YL, Parfenov VA, Yakhno NN. Post-stroke cognitive impairments. *Neurosci Behav Physiol.* 2009;39(8):16-21.

Van de Port IGL, Wevers LEG, Lindeman E, Kwakkel G. Effects of circuit training as alternative to usual physiotherapy after stroke: randomized controlled trial. *BMJ.* 2012;344:e2672.

Van Den Eeden SK, Tanner CM, Bernstein AL, et al. Incidence of Parkinson's disease: variation by age, gender, and race/ethnicity. *Am J Epidemiol.* 2003;157(11):1015-1022.

van der Warrenberg BP, Steijens JA, Muneke M, Kremer PB, Bloem BR. Falls in degenerative cerebellar ataxias. *Mov Disord.* 2005;20:497-500.

van Hedel HJ, Dietz V, European Multicenter Study on Human Spinal Cord Injury (EM-SCI) Study Group. Walking during daily life can be validly and responsively assessed in subjects with a spinal cord injury. *Neurorehabil Neural Repair.* 2009;23(2):117-124.

van Kuijk AA, Geurts AC, van Kuppevelt HJ. Neurogenic ossification in spinal cord injury. *Spinal Cord.* 2002;40:313-326.

van Middendorp JJ, Hosman AJ, Pouw MH, EM-SCI Study Group, Van de Meent H. ASIA impairment scale conversion in traumatic SCI: is it related with the ability to walk? A descriptive comparison with functional ambulation outcome measures in 273 patients. *Spinal Cord.* 2009;47(7):555-560.

Vanderah T, Gould D. *Nolte's The Human Brain.* 7th ed. Philadelphia, PA: Elsevier; 2015.

Vaney C, Gattlen B, Lugon-Moulin V, et al. Robotic-assisted step training (lokomat) not superior to equal intensity of over-ground rehabilitation in patients with multiple sclerosis. *Neurorehabil Neural Rep.* 2012;26(3):212-221.

Vaseghi B, Zoghi M, Jaberzadeh S. Does anodal transcranial direct current stimulation modulate sensory perception and pain? A meta-analysis study. *Clin Neurophysiol.* 2014;125(9):1847-1858.

Vasudevan EV, Glass RN, Packel AT. Effects of traumatic brain injury on locomotor adaptation. *J Neurol Phys Ther.* 2014;38(3):172-182.

Vaugoyeau M, Azulay JP. Sensory information in the control of postural orientation in Parkinson's disease. *J Neurol Sci.* 2010;289:66-68.

Vazques RG, Sedes PR, Farina MM, Marques AM, Velasco MEF. Respiratory management in the patient with spinal cord injury. *Biomed Res Int.* 2013;2013:12.

Velozo C, Moorhouse M, Ardolino E, et al. Validity of the Neuromuscular Recovery Scale: a measurement model approach. *Arch Phys Med Rehabil.* 2015;96(8):1385-1396.

Visintin M, Barbeau H. The effects of body weight support on the locomotor pattern of spastic paretic patients. *Can J Neurol Sci.* 1989;16:315-325.

Voulgari C, Pagoni S, Vinik A, Poirier P. Exercise improves cardiac autonomic function in obesity and diabetes. *Metabolism.* 2013;62(5):609-621.

Wakerley BR, Yuki N. Pharyngeal-cervical-brachial variant of Guillain-Barre syndrome. *J Neurol Neurosurg Psychiatry.* 2014;85(3):339-344.

Walgaard C, Lingsma HF, Ruts L, et al. Prediction of respiratory insufficiency in Guillain-Barre syndrome. *Ann Neurol.* 2010;67:781-787.

Walgaard C, Lingsma HF, Ruts L, van Doorn PA, Steyerberg EW, Jacobs BC. Early recognition of poor prognosis in Guillain-Barre syndrome. *Neurology.* 2011;76:968-975.

Walker FO. Huntington's disease. *Lancet.* 2007;369:218-228.

Walling AD, Dickson G. Guillain-Barré syndrome. *Am Fam Physician*. 2013;87(3):191-197.

Warburton DER, Krassiokov A, Sproule S, Eng JJ. Cardiovascular health and exercise following spinal cord injury. In: Eng JJ, Teasell RW, Miller WC, et al., eds. *Spinal Cord Injury Rehabilitation Evidence*. Version 5.0. Vancouver; 2014:1-48.

Waters RL, Adkins RH, Yakua JS, Sie I. Motor and sensory recovery following incomplete tetraplegia. *Arch Phys Med Rehabil*. 1994;75(3):306-311.

Weintraub D, Koester J, Potenza MN, et al. Impulse control disorders in Parkinson disease: a cross-sectional study of 3090 patients. *Arch Neurol*. 2006;63:969-973.

West TW. Transverse myelitis – a review of the initial presentation, diagnosis, and initial management. *Discov Med*. 2013;16(88):167-177.

Whitney SL, Herdman SJ. Physical therapy assessment of vestibular hypofunction. In: Herdman SJ, Clendaniel RA, eds. *Vestibular Rehabilitation*. 4th ed. Philadelphia, PA: F.A. Davis; 2014:359-393.

Whitney SL, Hudak MT, Marchetti GF. The dynamic gait index relates to self-reported fall history in individuals with vestibular dysfunction. *J Vestib Res*. 2000;10(2):99-105.

Whitney SL, Wrisley DM, Marchetti GF, Gee MA, Redfern MS, Furman JM. Clinical measurement of sit-to-stand performance in people with balance disorders: validity of data for the Five-Times-Sit-to-Stand Test. *Phys Ther*. 2005;85(10):1034-1045.

Widener GL, Allen DD, Gibson-Horn C. Randomized clinical trial of balance-based torso weighting for improving upright mobility in people with multiple sclerosis. *Neurorehabil Neural Repair*. 2009;23:784-791.

Widerstrom-Noga E, Biering-Sorensen F, Bryce TN, et al. The international spinal cord injury pain data set. *Spinal Cord*. 2008;46(12):818-823.

Widerstrom-Noga E, Turk DC. Types and effectiveness of treatments used by people with chronic pain associated with spinal cord injuries: influence of pain and psychosocial characteristics. *Spinal Cord*. 2003;41:600-609.

Winser SJ, Smith C, Hale LA, Claydon LS, Whitney SL. Balance outcome measures in cerebellar ataxia: a Delphi survey. *Disabil Rehabil*. 2015;37(2):165-170.

Winser SJ, Smith C, Hale LA, Claydon LS, Whitney SL, Mehta P. Systematic review of the psychometric properties of balance measures for cerebellar ataxia. *Clin Rehabil*. 2015;29(1):69-79.

Wirdefeldt K, Adami H-O, Cole P, Trichopoulos D, Mandel J. Epidemiology and etiology of Parkinson's disease: a review of the evidence. *Eur J Epidemiol*. 2011;26:S1-S58.

Witgert M, Salamone AR, Strutt AM, et al. Frontal-lobe mediated behavioural dysfunction in amyotrophic lateral sclerosis. *Eur J Neurol*. 2010;17:103-110.

Wolf SL, Lecraw DE, Barton LA, Jann BB. Forced use of hemiplegic upper extremities to reverse the effect of learned nonuse among chronic stroke and head injured patients. *Exp Neurol*. 1989;104(2):125-132.

Wolf SL, Winstein CJ, Miller JP, et al. Effect of constraint-induced movement therapy on upper extremity function 3 to 9 months after stroke: the EXCITE randomized clinical trial. *JAMA*. 2006;296(17):2095-2104.

Woolley SC, York MK, Moore DH, et al. Detecting fronto-temporal dysfunction in ALS: utility of the ALS Cognitive Behavioral Screen (ALS-CBS). *Amyotroph Lateral Scler*. 2010;11(3):303-311.

World Health Organization. Does polio still exist? Is it curable? Available at: http://www.who.int/features/qa/07/en. Accessed March 5, 2018.

Wrisley DM, Marchetti GF, Kuharsky DK, Whitney SL. Reliability, internal consistency, and validity of data obtained with the functional gait assessment. *Phys Ther*. 2004;84(10):906-918.

Wrisley DM, Sparto PJ, Whitney SL, Furman JM. Cervicogenic dizziness: a review of diagnosis and treatment. *J Orthop Sports Phys Ther*. 2000;30(12):755-766.

Wrisley DM, Whitney SL, Furman JM. Vestibular rehabilitation outcomes in patients with a history of migraine. *Otol Neurotol*. 2002;23(4):483-487.

Wu C, Chuang L, Lin K, Chen H, Tsay P. Randomized trial of distributed constraint-induced therapy versus bilateral arm training for the rehabilitation of upper-limb motor control and function after stroke. *Neurorehabil Neural Repair*. 2011;24(2):130-139.

Wu T, Hallett M. A functional MRI study of automatic movements in patients with Parkinson's disease. *Brain*. 2005;128:2250-2259. www.NRS.com.

Yaguez L, Canavan A, Lange HW, Homberg V. Motor learning by imagery is differentially affected in Parkinson's and Huntington's diseases. *Behav Brain Res*. 1999;102:115-127.

Yuki N, Hartung H-P. Guillain-Barre syndrome. *N Engl J Med*. 2012;366(24):2294-2304.

Zia S, Cody F, O'Boyle D. Joint position sense is impaired by Parkinson's disease. *Ann Neurol*. 2000;47(2):218-228.

Ziegler MD, Zhong H, Roy RR, Edgerton VR. Why variability facilitates spinal learning. *J Neurosci*. 2010;30(32):10720-10726.

Zimmermann-Schlatter A, Schuster C, Puhan MA, Siekierka E, Steurer J. Efficacy of motor imagery in post-stroke rehabilitation: a systematic review. *J Neuroeng Rehabil*. 2008;5:8.

Zinzi P, Salmaso D, DeGrandis R, et al. Effects of an intensive rehabilitation programme on patients with Huntington's disease: a pilot study. *Clin Rehabil*. 2007;21(7):602-613.

QUESTIONS

Neuroscience/Neuroanatomy

1. A 65-year-old man is evaluated by a physical therapist following a diagnosis of a cerebrovascular accident (CVA). During the examination the patient demonstrates ataxic movements during reaching and gait activities. Which region of the brain was most likely affected by the CVA?
   A. Brainstem
   B. Cerebellum
   C. Frontal lobe
   D. Parietal lobe

2. Damage to the basal ganglia is likely to result in what clinical signs and symptoms?
   A. Unilateral sensory and motor loss
   B. Bilateral sensory and motor loss
   C. Rigidity, bradykinesia, postural instability, and tremor
   D. Spasticity, hyperkinesia, postural instability, and tremor

3. A physical therapist is testing a patient's ability to move the eye medially during cranial nerve testing. Which cranial nerve is the therapist testing?
  A. Abducens nerve
  B. Optic nerve
  C. Oculomotor nerve
  D. Trochlear nerve

4. A 68-year-old woman presents to the ER with signs and symptoms of a CVA. She has complaints of a left frontal headache and right foot drag. Muscle tone and reflexes were slightly hyper-reflexive upon testing. She has a history of HTN and diabetes. The most likely location of the lesion is:
  A. L Middle cerebral artery
  B. L Anterior cerebral artery
  C. R Anterior cerebral artery
  D. R Middle cerebral artery

5. A patient with amyotrophic lateral sclerosis (ALS) presents to physical therapy. Cranial nerve testing reveals motor impairments of the tongue including wasting and deviation on protrusion. Which cranial nerve is likely damaged based on these results?
  A. IX
  B. X
  C. XI
  D. XII

6. Which of the following is a clinical manifestation of an upper motor neuron lesion?
  A. Spasticity
  B. Flaccidity
  C. Hypotonicity
  D. Areflexia

Stroke

7. A patient presents to physical therapy following a cerebrovascular accident (CVA). During the examination you ask the patient to reach for a glass of water. The patient is unable to do the skill when requested. However, later during the examination the patient reaches for the glass and takes a drink of water. What impairment is the patient likely exhibiting?
  A. Ideomotor apraxia
  B. Ideational apraxia
  C. Unilateral neglect
  D. Visual agnosia

8. A patient presents to outpatient physical therapy 2 weeks following a left cerebrovascular accident (CVA). When attempting to reach for an item using her right upper extremity she can initiate the movement voluntarily; however, she is unable to move out of an abnormal synergistic pattern. Muscle tone testing reveals spasticity in the flexor muscles of the upper extremity. According to Brunnstrom's stages of motor recovery, which stage of recovery is this patient in?
  A. Stage 1
  B. Stage 2
  C. Stage 3
  D. Stage 4

Spinal Cord Injury

9. An individual with a complete spinal cord injury (SCI) presents with sensory and motor loss affecting all four extremities. Which area of the spinal cord was likely damaged?
  A. Cervical
  B. Thoracic
  C. Lumbar
  D. Sacral

10. Autonomic dysreflexia typically occurs in spinal cord injuries (SCI) at what levels?
  A. T6 and above
  B. T12 and above
  C. L1 and above
  D. L5 and above

11. A patient sustained an incomplete T12 spinal cord injury (SCI) from a stabbing injury. The patient has absent proprioception and motor function below T12 on the ipsilateral side and absent pain and temperature on the contralateral side below T12. These examination findings describe which syndrome?
  A. Brown-Sequard syndrome
  B. Anterior cord syndrome
  C. Central cord syndrome
  D. Cauda equina syndrome

12. A patient with an incomplete spinal cord injury (SCI) presents to inpatient rehabilitation with paralysis and sensory loss to the upper extremities with normal sensory and motor function in the lower extremities. What SCI clinical syndrome is most likely for this patient?
  A. Brown-Sequard syndrome
  B. Anterior cord syndrome
  C. Central cord syndrome
  D. Cauda equina syndrome

Parkinson's Disease

13. A patient with Parkinson's disease presents with complaints of dizziness and lightheadedness immediately after standing. What is the most likely cause of these symptoms?
  A. Benign paroxysmal positional vertigo (BPPV)
  B. Vestibulopathy
  C. Decreased proprioception in the lower extremities
  D. Orthostatic hypotension

14. Which of the following is a cardinal sign of Parkinson's disease?
  A. Intention tremor
  B. Hypophonia
  C. Postural instability
  D. Decreased cognition

15. Tremor in early Parkinson's disease is:
  A. Typically bilateral
  B. Increased with activity
  C. Present at rest
  D. Usually improved with levodopa

16. A physical therapist is working with a patient with advanced Parkinson's disease. The patient has lost weight and his family is concerned with his ability to swallow. Which of the following would be the appropriate referral for additional services?

A. Speech therapy
B. Social work
C. Occupational therapy
D. Dietitian

Outcome Measures

17. Which of the following outcome measures would be the most appropriate to test a patient's ability to shift and adapt between the three sensory systems important for postural control?
A. Berg Balance Test
B. Tinetti Balance and Gait Test
C. Clinical Test of Sensory Integration of Balance
D. Romberg Test

18. Which of the following assessment tools would be the most appropriate to measure the participation restrictions in an individual with Parkinson's disease?
A. Berg Balance Scale (BBS)
B. Six-Minute-Walk Test (6MWT)
C. Medical Outcomes Study 36-Item Short-Form Health Survey (SF-36)
D. Functional Reach Test (FRT)

Intervention

19. A patient is having difficulty with maintaining upright sitting posture following a CVA. The patient sits forward-flexed and leaning to the non-hemiplegic side. Which body segment should the physical therapist align FIRST?
A. Scapula and ribcage
B. Thoracic spine
C. Pelvis
D. Lower extremities

20. Which of the following PNF bilateral UE patterns is the BEST to improve upright posture for a patient with Parkinson's disease who has an increase in thoracic kyphosis in sitting and standing?
A. Bilateral symmetrical UE Flex/Add/ER pattern
B. Bilateral symmetrical reciprocal UE Flex/Add/ER & UE Ext/Abd/IR UE pattern
C. Bilateral symmetrical reciprocal UE Flex/Abd/ER & UE Ext/Add/IR UE pattern
D. Performing bilateral symmetrical UE Flex/Abd/ER pattern

21. A patient with a diagnosis of multiple sclerosis requires moderate assist with sit to stand due to bilateral quad weakness. Which of the following is the BEST intervention to improve this patient's independent performance of sit to stand?
A. Partial squats performed against the wall
B. Partial lunges bilaterally
C. Repetitive sit to stand from a raised treatment table
D. Long arc quads with cuff weights seated edge of mat

22. A patient with a traumatic brain injury has difficulty ascending stairs due to weak lower extremity extensors. Which of the following would be the BEST treatment strategy to address the patient's deficit?
A. Alternating high-knee marching exercises with unilateral UE support
B. Alternating 4″ step-ups with unilateral UE support
C. Alternating quadruped hip extension exercises
D. Alternating prone hip extension exercises

23. Which of the following statements is TRUE regarding compensatory and restorative approaches to rehabilitation?
A. A compensatory approach focuses on regaining strength and resuming the performance of functional abilities.
B. A restorative strategy focuses on restoring the individual's ability to perform a task with the use of adaptive equipment using different movement strategies than the individual used before his/her injury.
C. A restorative approach is always the most appropriate approach.
D. A compensatory approach uses a variety of substitution movement strategies and/or adaptive equipment to accomplish desired tasks.

ICF

24. Following a traumatic brain injury, which of the following would be an example of a restriction in the participation domain of the ICF model?
A. Inability to walk on the beach with a spouse
B. Inability to stand from her couch without assistance
C. Inability to load the step out of the shower without assistance
D. Inability to walk without an assistive device

Assistive Device and Wheelchair Prescription

25. An individual has a complete spinal cord injury C3 (ASIA A) from a motor vehicle accident. What equipment will this patient likely require?
A. Power tilt and recline, joystick-controlled wheelchair and a universal cuff
B. Power tilt and recline, joystick-controlled wheelchair and a mechanical ventilator
C. Power tilt and recline, breath-controlled wheelchair and a universal cuff
D. Power tilt and recline, breath-controlled wheelchair and a mechanical ventilator

26. A physical therapist is evaluating a patient with Parkinson's disease. The patient and his caregivers report the patient has begun falling and they would like to know what the best assistive device is for this patient. During your evaluation, you note that he requires moderate assistance for losses of balance and demonstrates freezing of gait. He does not demonstrate festinating gait. Which assistive device would be the MOST appropriate for this patient?
A. Front-wheeled walker
B. Single-point cane
C. Standard four-point walker
D. Inverted cane

Gait

27. A patient with multiple sclerosis is referred to physical therapy for difficulty walking. During initial contact to loading response, the patient's foot "slaps" the floor. The most likely cause of this gait deviation is:
A. Flaccid plantar flexors
B. Tight plantar flexors
C. Spastic dorsiflexors
D. Weak dorsiflexors

Multiple Sclerosis

28. A patient with multiple sclerosis presents to physical therapy with reports of a sudden worsening in her symptoms since her move from New York to Miami. What could this change be attributed to?
A. Fatigue
B. Natural disease progression
C. CNS plaque formation
D. Uthoff's phenomenon

ALS

29. A patient reports difficulty picking up small items and writing with the left hand, but denies difficulty when using the right hand. Physical examination reveals fasciculations and a positive Babinski sign in the left upper extremity. Which of the following is the MOST likely diagnosis?
A. Amyotrophic lateral sclerosis
B. Guillain-Barré syndrome
C. Multiple sclerosis
D. Stroke

Guillain-Barré

30. A patient presents with a rapid onset of extreme fatigue and bilateral, symmetrical flaccid paralysis. The onset of muscle weakness occurred in a distal-to-proximal pattern. Patient reports an upper respiratory disorder approximately 2 weeks prior to symptom onset. What is the most likely diagnosis?
A. Multiple sclerosis
B. Amyotrophic lateral sclerosis
C. Guillain-Barré syndrome
D. Poliomyelitis

31. A physical therapist is working with a patient who has difficulty with sit-to-stand transfers. The therapist decides to teach the patient the skill by breaking it down into smaller components, having the patient practice these components, then putting the components together in one complete movement. What is this type of practice called?
A. Distributed practice
B. Part-to-whole task practice
C. Random practice
D. Massed practice

32. The use of sit-to-stand practice as a method of strengthening the lower extremities is an example of what type of intervention?
A. Knowledge of performance
B. Results-based
C. Task-oriented
D. Impairment-based

33. A physical therapist is evaluating a patient with suspected BPPV involving the posterior semicircular canal. The maneuver with the best diagnostic accuracy for this condition is the:
A. Dix-Hallpike maneuver
B. Supine roll test
C. Epley maneuver
D. Semont liberatory maneuver

34. If a patient with BPPV is taking a vestibular suppressant medication such as meclizine, the evidence suggests that the physical therapist should:
A. Collaborate with the prescribing physician recommending the continued use of vestibular suppressant medications
B. Advise the patient to continue with the plan as initially determined by the physician for an additional 6 weeks
C. Collaborate with the prescribing physician recommending the discontinuation of vestibular suppressant medications
D. Advise the patient to immediately discontinue the use of vestibular suppressant medications

35. A physical therapist is evaluating a patient with suspected BPPV involving the lateral semicircular canal. The maneuver with the best diagnostic accuracy for this condition is:
A. Dix-Hallpike maneuver
B. Supine roll test
C. Epley maneuver
D. Semont liberatory maneuver

36. Current evidence-based practice involves which maneuver to treat lateral semicircular canal BPPV?
A. Barbecue roll
B. Dix-Hallpike maneuver
C. Epley maneuver
D. Semont liberatory maneuver

37. Which standardized outcome measures is the most comprehensive and sensitive to change when assessing gait and balance dysfunction in a community-dwelling older adult with a vestibular pathology?
A. Functional Gait Assessment (FGA)
B. Dynamic Gait Index (DGI)
C. Berg Balance Scale (BBS)
D. Performance Oriented Mobility Assessment (POMA)

38. Which of the following descriptions of nystagmus is most consistent with an acute (4 days) left unilateral peripheral vestibular disorder?
A. Nystagmus that is purely vertical, observable in room light and with fixation blocked, and increases with upward gaze
B. Nystagmus that is mixed right horizontal and torsional, not observable in room light, observable with fixation blocked, and increases with right gaze
C. Nystagmus that is mixed left horizontal and torsional, not observable in room light, observable with fixation blocked, and increases with left gaze
D. Nystagmus that is mixed left horizontal and torsional, observable in room light and with fixation blocked, and does not increase with gaze in any direction

39. Habituation exercises are a component of vestibular rehabilitation. The premise behind these exercises is to:
    A. Avoid head movement until the symptoms are alleviated.
    B. Perform rapid and repeated head motions to induce severe symptoms until the symptoms are alleviated.
    C. Gradually perform head and body movements that induce mild to moderate symptoms until the symptoms are alleviated.
    D. Take vestibular suppressants to desensitize the nervous system over time until the symptoms are alleviated.

40. A physical therapist is asked to evaluate a patient diagnosed with Guillain-Barré syndrome at an acute care hospital. The patient was diagnosed 3 days ago and is currently experiencing a gradual loss of strength and sensation. What is the most appropriate treatment plan for this patient at this time?
    A. Initiate an exercise program of supine therapeutic exercise including straight leg raises, gluteal squeezes, hip abduction, and ankle pumps to improve strength.
    B. Defer the evaluation now and educate the patient to limit all movement in bed and out of bed.
    C. Educate the patient and family on proper positioning in bed and gentle passive range of motion for ankles, knees, and hips to decrease risk of skin breakdown and development of joint contractures.
    D. Gradually progress the patient daily from sitting at the edge of the bed to eventually ambulating with appropriate assistive device to decrease his potential for losing functional mobility.

41. A physical therapist is treating a patient with Guillain-Barré syndrome in an outpatient clinic 3 times per week. On arrival for his second treatment session the patient reports that he felt weaker and less stable when ambulating. What is the most appropriate course of action for this scheduled therapy session?
    A. Hold his therapy session for the day and recommend he visit his physician for an assessment and blood work.
    B. Perform fewer repetitions and lower intensity of the already established exercises.
    C. Educate the patient that this is a normal part of muscle strengthening and continue the current treatment plan.
    D. Eliminate any eccentric exercises and train muscles only concentrically for the remainder of rehabilitation.

ANSWERS

1. The answer is **B**. The cerebellum has a major role in the coordination of voluntary movement. Damage to the cerebellum often results in ataxia.

2. The answer is **C**. Damage to the basal ganglia is implicated in Parkinson's disease; the four cardinal features of Parkinson's disease are rigidity, bradykinesia, postural instability, and tremor.

3. The answer is **C**. The oculomotor nerve (CN III) is responsible for up, down, and medial eye movements. The oculomotor nerve is also responsible for pupillary constriction.

4. The answer is **B**. The left anterior cerebral artery is the most likely location of the lesion based on area of headache (left) and the contralateral hemiparesis involving the right lower extremity. The middle cerebral artery provides circulation to the area of the brain controlling contralateral upper extremity motor function, and the anterior cerebral artery provides circulation to the area of the brain controlling the contralateral lower extremity.

5. The answer is **D**. Cranial nerve XII is the hypoglossal nerve which innervates the muscles of the tongue.

6. The answer is **A**. Upper motor neuron signs include hypertonicity, including spasticity and hyperreflexia.

7. The answer is **A**. Ideomotor apraxia is a neurological deficit represented by the inability to perform a motor function on request or imitate a motor activity while the ability to spontaneously perform the motor task remains intact.

8. The answer is **C**. Brunnstrom's stages of motor recovery describe typical recovery of motor function following a stroke. There are six stages, from flaccidity and no voluntary movement immediately after a stroke (Stage 1) to full voluntary movement and minimal to no spasticity (Stage 6). The patient in this case has spasticity and voluntary limb control but is unable to move out of an abnormal muscle synergy pattern, which represents Stage 3 of Brunnstrom's motor recovery scale.

9. The answer is **A**. The cervical spinal cord controls sensory and motor function for the upper extremities. A spinal cord injury at the cervical level will disrupt communication to all levels of the spinal cord caudal to the area of injury, which will result in sensory and motor loss affecting all four extremities and the trunk.

10. The answer is **A**. Autonomic dysreflexia is a phenomenon typically occurring in spinal cord injuries (SCI) above the T6 level. Signs and symptoms of autonomic dysreflexia include a sudden increase in blood pressure, pounding headache, flushing, and profuse sweating above the level of the SCI. It is due to disruption in the connection between the brain and the sympathetic neurons in the thoracolumbar spine.

11. The answer is **A**. The incomplete SCI clinical syndrome represented by proprioception and motor loss below the level of injury ipsilaterally and absent pain and temperature contralaterally below the level of injury is Brown-Sequard syndrome.

12. The answer is **C**. The incomplete SCI clinical syndrome represented by greater upper extremity motor and sensory loss than lower extremity motor and sensory loss is the central cord syndrome.

13. The answer is **D**. Orthostatic hypotension is a common side effect of the medication carbidopa-levodopa (Sinemet) used to treat Parkinson's disease, and is characterized by a drop in blood pressure that occurs when changing positions causing dizziness, lightheadedness, and can cause syncope.

14. The answer is **C**. The cardinal signs of Parkinson's disease include the direct impairments of tremor, bradykinesia, postural instability, and rigidity.

15. The answer is **C**. Unilateral tremor is often an early sign of Parkinson's disease (PD). Tremor associated with PD is usually present at rest and is diminished with activity. Levodopa is more effective at improving bradykinesia and rigidity and less effective in reducing tremor and postural instability.

16. The answer is **A**. A referral to speech therapy to evaluate this patient's swallowing abilities is appropriate. Speech therapy can address the possibility of dysphagia, which could be potentially life-threatening, as it can lead to aspiration

pneumonia. The speech therapist can also evaluate the patient's ability to speak clearly. Patients with Parkinson's disease frequently have difficulty related to speech production related to hypophonia and/or dysarthria.

17. The answer is **C**. The Clinical Test of Sensory Integration of Balance (CTSIB) is commonly referred to as the foam and dome test. This assessment measures the effectiveness of the three sensory systems for postural control with the ability to stand with eyes open and closed, on and off a compliant surface, and with inadequate visual cues with the use of a dome. The modified CTSIB does not use the dome.

18. The answer is **C**. The tool that measures participation restrictions is the Medical Outcomes Study 36-Item Short-Form Health Survey (SF-36), which assesses quality of life (including physical and mental domains) from the patient's point of view. The BBS, 6MWT, and FRT measure the direct impairments common in patients with PD: functional mobility, gait, balance, and postural stability.

19. The answer is **C**. In sitting, the pelvis should always be aligned first to provide a stable base from which to build.

20. The answer is **D**. To improve thoracic kyphosis the bilateral UE PNF pattern that promotes the most thoracic extension is bilateral symmetrical UE Flex/Abd/ER.

21. The answer is **C**. Task-specific functional mobility training to improve sit-to-stand can be done with repetitive sit-to-stand training.

22. The answer is **B**. Alternating 4″ step-ups with unilateral UE support is the most task-specific activity of the provided choices to improve ascending stairs.

23. The answer is **D**. Rehabilitation approaches may include teaching the individual compensatory strategies to allow them to perform tasks using substitution strategies and/or adaptive equipment to accomplish desired tasks. A restorative approach to rehabilitation is typically used in rehabilitation with the goal of recovery of normal movement and minimal compensations.

24. The answer is **A**. The inability to walk on the beach with a spouse is a participation restriction because it represents a social activity or an activity that is meaningful to the individual's life satisfaction. The other options all represent activity limitations.

25. The answer is **D**. An individual with a complete spinal cord injury at the C3 level will require mechanical assistance with ventilation due to the lack of innervation at the diaphragm and accessory breathing musculature. The breath-controlled (also referred to as a sip-and-puff) power tilt and recline wheelchair will allow the individual to be independent with wheelchair locomotion and pressure reliefs.

26. The answer is **A**. A single-point cane will likely be insufficient to prevent falls in a patient with balance impairments requiring moderate assistance for recovery of balance. An inverted cane is used to provide a visual cue for a patient with freezing gait, but will likely also be insufficient to prevent a fall for this patient. A standard walker can worsen freezing episodes and will not help with retropulsion related falls. A front-wheeled walker can be used in patients with freezing of gait effectively to prevent falls but may be unsafe for patients with festinating gait, which this patient does not have.

27. The answer is **D**. In initial contact to loading response, the dorsiflexors work eccentrically to slow the progression of the foot from a dorsiflexed position to a plantarflexed position. Weak dorsiflexors cause this change in position to happen with less control, causing the foot to slap on the floor.

28. The answer is **D**. Uthoff's phenomenon is characterized by a decline in neurologic symptoms caused by overheating of the body for individuals with MS. This overheating may be due to hot weather, exercise, body fever, saunas, hot tubs, or other heat-inducing environments. The patient in this case recently moved from a cooler to warmer climate, which may explain the sudden worsening of her symptoms.

29. The answer is **A**. Amyotrophic lateral sclerosis (ALS) is a degenerative neurological condition which causes both upper motor and lower motor nerve degeneration. Muscle twitching, called fasciculations, are commonly seen in individuals with ALS and is a lower motor neuron sign. Babinski's sign is an abnormal response of the foot to extend, typically seen in the great toe in response to stimulation on the plantar surface of the foot. A normal response to this is for the foot to plantarflex. An abnormal response in adults may be as sign of an upper motor neuron disfunction.

30. The answer is **C**. Guillain-Barré syndrome presents with bilateral, symmetrical flaccid paralysis progressing in a distal to proximal pattern.

31. The answer is **B**. Part-to-whole task practice was used in this example. The patient practiced the component tasks first, then practiced the entire task.

32. The answer is **C**. Using a functional task that is specific, both in regard to the task and the context, is the hallmark of the task-oriented approach.

33. The answer is **A**. The Dix-Hallpike maneuver should be used to diagnose posterior canal BPPV. The Epley maneuver is used to treat posterior canal BPPV once this is determined with a positive Dix-Hallpike maneuver. The roll test should be used to diagnose lateral canal BPPV, and the Semon liberatory is used to treat lateral canal BPPV.

34. The answer is **C**. Clinical practice guidelines for BPPV recommend against the use of vestibular suppressant medications. The physical therapist should make recommendations to the prescribing physician regarding these guidelines.

35. The answer is **B**. The supine roll test should be used to diagnose lateral canal BPPV.

36. The answer is **A**. The barbecue roll maneuver is an effective maneuver to treat lateral canal BPPV. Forced prolonged positioning can also be used to treat lateral canal BPPV.

37. The answer is **A**. Although moderate correlations exist between all the options listed, the FGA is the most comprehensive and sensitive to change when assessing gait and balance dysfunction in community-dwelling elderly and in individuals with vestibular dysfunction. An FGA score of ≤22/30 is predictive of increased fall risk.

38. The answer is **B**. With a unilateral peripheral vestibular disorder, the patient may be able to suppress the nystagmus in room light after 3 days following symptom onset. Nystagmus is less likely to be suppressed with fixation blocked using Frenzel goggles. The direction of nystagmus will be mixed horizonal and torsional in the direction of the intact ear.

According to Alexander's law, nystagmus will also increase when the patient looks toward the fast phase.

39. The answer is **B**. Habituation exercises involve repeated, gradual, and graded performance of exercises or activities that induce dizziness, with the goal of getting the nervous system accustomed to the stimuli without symptom provocation.

40. The answer is **C**. The patient has recently been diagnosed and is in a phase of decline, with progressive muscular weakness and sensation loss. It is important to educate the patient and family on proper positioning techniques and gentle range of motion to decrease risks of skin breakdown and joint contractures. This will reduce additional complications in his recovery once he is cleared for mobilization.

41. The answer is **A**. The patient may be experiencing overwork weakness, which is a serious contraindication to therapy. The patient needs to be evaluated by his physician and have lab work done to check for increased serum levels of creatine kinase. He must be cleared by his physician to resume exercise.

CHECKLIST

When you complete this chapter, you should be able to:

❏ Outline neuroanatomy and neurophysiology principles for clinical practice.

❏ Outline various neurologic pathologies.

❏ Compare neurologic interventions across different pathologies.

❏ Outline standardized outcome measures for various neurologic pathologies across practice settings.

Integumentary System

Annie Burke-Doe and Rolando Lazaro

■ CLINICAL APPLICATION OF FOUNDATIONAL SCIENCES

The integumentary system is the largest organ in the body and is important to our survival in many ways. The skin is a membranous barrier between our internal system and the environment, and responds to external and internal changes. Examination requires understanding of the structures and function of the system. Understanding of healthy and disease states of skin, hair, nails, mucous membranes, circulation, and sensory structures is essential to examination.

The integumentary system has two major components, the cutaneous membrane (skin), and accessory structures (Figure 4–1).

High-Yield Terms to Learn

Capillary refill	Press down on one of the patient's nails until it pales. Release the nail and observe for the pink color to return. The normal color should return in less than 3 seconds. *Note:* Capillary refill can be affected by room and body temperature, vasoconstriction from smoking, or peripheral edema.
Clubbing	Normal concave nail bases will create a small, diamond-shaped space when the nails of the index fingers of each hand are placed together. Clubbed fingers are convex at the bases and will touch without leaving a space. *Note:* Finger clubbing, a sign of chronic tissue hypoxia, occurs when the angle between the fingernail and where the nail enters the skin increases.
Cyanosis	Dark bluish or purplish discoloration of the integument and mucous membranes. *Note:* May indicate hypoxia or hematologic pathology.
Hyperthermia	Increased temperature. *Note:* May indicate localized or systemic infection, inflammation, thermal injury; hyperthyroidism or fever is generalized.
Hypothermia	Decreased temperature. *Note:* May indicate arterial insufficiency or shock.
Jaundice	Yellowish discoloration of skin and sclera. *Note:* May indicate liver disease or hemolytic pathology.
Tzanck smear	Scraping of an ulcer base to look for Tzanck cells (acantholytic cells). It is sometimes also called the chickenpox skin test or the herpes skin test.
Dermatitis	Inflammation of the skin.
Total body surface area	Used to estimate the total fluid and caloric requirements, and is a predictor of mortality.
Hypertrophic scar	A raised scar that stays within the boundaries of the burn wound; characteristically red, raised, firm.
Keloid scar	A raised scar that extends beyond the boundaries of the original burn wound; red, raised, firm.
Pruritus	Itching.
Exudate	Also known as drainage, exudate is a liquid produced by the body in response to tissue damage.

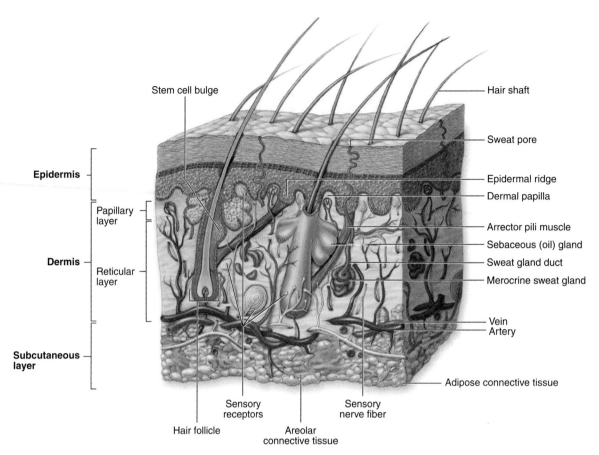

FIGURE 4–1 Anatomy of the skin. (From Hamm RL. *Text and Atlas of Wound Diagnosis and Treatment*. https://accessphysiotherapy.mhmedical.com/content.aspx?bookid=1334&sectionid=77259853. Copyright © McGraw-Hill Education. All rights reserved.)

The skin is divided into three layers: the epidermis, the dermis, and subcutaneous tissue. The accessory structures include the hair, nails, vascular supply, sweat glands, and sebaceous glands. The skin is the site of many complex and dynamic processes, which include being a protective barrier, having immunologic functions for first-line defenses, and functions of melanin production, vitamin D synthesis, sensation, temperature regulation, protection from trauma, and aesthetics.[1]

EXAMINATION

The physical therapist's examination includes taking the individual's history, conducting a standardized system review, and performing selected tests and measures to identify potential and existing movement-related disorders. During the history-gathering phase, the physical therapist may seek information on integumentary symptoms and complaints that may warrant referral for additional medical evaluation. Key points for the integumentary history may include history of present illness, symptoms, date of onset, severity, medications, history of a previous problem, changes in size or appearance of a lesion, bleeding from the lesion, and sunscreen use. The physical therapist may decide to use one, more than one, or portions of several specific tests and measures as part of the examination, based on the purpose of the visit, the complexity of the condition, and the direction taken in the clinical decision-making process.

Signs and symptoms of integumentary disorders may include but are not limited to:

- Lesions of the skin (primary [Table 4–1] and secondary [Table 4–2])
- Pigment changes (changes in color, eg, cyanosis, redness, paleness, yellowing)
- Rash/pruritus (itching, length of time present)
- Blisters
- Bruising/bleeding
- Nevi/moles/nodules/cysts (changes in area, border, color, diameter)
- Dryness/sweating (xerosis)
- Presence of edema
- Changes in appearance of nails
- Changes in skin turgor, texture

Tests, measures (Table 4–2), and screening that may be relevant to the integumentary system may include but are not limited to:

- Inspection of skin and changes (eg, color, temperature, turgor, moisture, odor, scars, masses, moles, nails, skin mobility)
- Capillary refill
- Palpation (eg, lesion tenderness, firmness, depth)
- Measurement (length, width, depth, subcutaneous extension) using perpendicular, clock, tracing, and photographic methods
- Location/color/shape/size (Table 4–3)

TABLE 4–1 Primary lesions and their morphology.

Terminology	Morphology	Examples
Macule	A flat, level with surface of skin (≤1 cm) lesion with color change	Rubeola, rubella, scarlet fever, roseola infantum
Papule	A solid, elevated lesion, sharply circumscribed, small (1 cm) colored lesion (pink, tan, red, or any variation)	Dermatitis, ringworm, psoriasis
Wheal	An elevated white to pink edematous lesion that is unstable and associated with pruritus that lasts <24 hours	Mosquito bites and hives (urticaria)
Nodule	Dermal or subcutaneous solid, elevated lesion	Amelanotic melanoma
Vesicle	A bulging, small (<1 cm) blister containing clear fluid	Herpes simplex, varicella, poison ivy, herpes zoster
Pustule	An elevated, sharply circumscribed (<1 cm) cavity filled with pus	Impetigo, acne, *Staphylococcus* infections
Cyst	Cavity filled with pus or keratin	Epidermal cyst
Petechiae	Tiny, reddish purple, sharply circumscribed spots of hemorrhage in the superficial layers of the skin or epidermis	Meningococcemia, bacterial endocarditis, nonthrombocytopenia purpura

TABLE 4–2 Secondary lesions and their morphology.

Terminology	Morphology	Examples
Crust	Dried blood, serum, scales, and pus from corrosive lesions	Infectious dermatitis
Excoriation	Mechanical removal of the epidermis leaving dermis exposed	Scratch, scrape of original lesion
Scales	Dried fragments of sloughed dead epidermis	Seborrhea and tinea capitis
Ulcer	Destruction and loss of epidermis, dermis, and possibly subcutaneous layers	Decubitus ulceration
Fissure	A vertical, linear crack through the epidermis and dermis	
Scar	Formation of dense connective tissue resulting from destruction of skin	

- Presence and type of exudate (Table 4–4)
- Temperature (hypothermia, hyperthermia)
- Sensation
- Nail inspection (clubbing, discoloration, brittleness, ridging, cleanliness)
- Functional status

TABLE 4–3 Documentation characteristics (location/color/shape/size).

Description	Examples
Characteristics	• Size • Shape • Color • Texture • Elevation or depression
Type	• Abrasion: A wearing away of the upper layer of skin as a result of applied friction force. • Contusion (bruise): Caused when blood vessels are damaged or broken as the result of a direct blow to the skin. • Ecchymosis: The skin discoloration caused by the escape of blood into the tissues from ruptured blood vessels. • Hematoma: A localized collection of blood, usually clotted, in a tissue or organ. • Excoriation: Lesion of a traumatic nature with epidermal loss in a generally linear shape. • Laceration: An injury involving penetration of the skin, in which the wound is deeper than the superficial skin level. • Penetrating wound: A wound accompanied by disruption of the body surface that extends into the underlying tissue or a body cavity. • Petechiae: Tiny red spots in the skin that do not blanch when pressed upon. Petechiae result from red blood leaking from capillaries into the skin (intradermal hemorrhages). Petechiae are <3 mm in diameter. • Puncture: A wound made by a pointed object (like a nail). • Ulcer: A lesion on the surface of the skin or the surface of the mucous membrane, produced by the sloughing of inflammatory, necrotic tissue.
Exudates (see Table 4–4)	• Color • Odor • Amount • Consistency
Pattern of arrangement	• Annular • Grouped • Linear • Diffuse
Location and distribution	• Generalized or localized • Region of the body • Discrete or confluent

From Dutton M. *McGraw-Hill's NPTE (National Physical Therapy Examination)*. 2nd ed. New York, NY: McGraw-Hill; 2012: Table 13–2.

TABLE 4–4 Exudate classification.

Type of Exudate	Description
Serous	Presents as clear, light color with a thin, watery consistency. Serous exudate is considered to be normal in a healthy healing wound.
Sanguinous	Presents as red with a thin, watery consistency. Sanguinous exudate appears to be red due to the presence of blood or may be brown if allowed to dehydrate. This type of exudate may be indicative of new blood vessel growth or the disruption of blood vessels.
Serosanguinous	Presents as light red or pink, with a thin, watery consistency. Serosanguinous exudate can be normal in a healthy healing wound.
Seropurulent	Presents as an opaque, yellow or tan color, with a thin, watery consistency. Seropurulent exudate may be an early warning sign of an impending infection.
Purulent	Presents as a yellow or green color with a thick, viscous consistency. This type of exudate is generally an indicator of wound infection.

From Dutton M. *McGraw-Hill's NPTE (National Physical Therapy Examination)*. 2nd ed. New York, NY: McGraw-Hill; 2012: Table 13–3.

■ FOUNDATIONS FOR EVALUATION, DIFFERENTIAL DIAGNOSIS, PROGNOSIS, AND INTERVENTIONS

Herpes Zoster[2] (Shingles)

Herpes zoster (shingles) represents reactivation of latent varicella (chicken pox) infection. Persons with a history of primary varicella have a 20% to 30% lifetime risk of developing herpes zoster. Following a varicella infection, varicella-zoster virus may be retained in dorsal root ganglia in a latent form. Reactivation of the virus, leading to cutaneous eruption in the distribution of the affected sensory nerve(s), may be induced by trauma, stress, fever, radiation therapy, or immunosuppression. Direct contact with vesicular fluid can result in varicella in a susceptible person. It is reported that there are 1 million cases of shingles every year, and one out of three individuals in the United States will develop shingles in their lifetime.[3]

Clinical Significance

Disturbances include:

1. Painful skin rash with blisters in a dermatome. These blisters will typically scab in 7 to 10 days and will clear within 2 to 4 weeks.[3]
2. Persistent postherpetic neuralgia can have a negative impact on a patient's health and quality of life. It is associated with insomnia, anorexia, and depression, especially in the elderly.

3. Fever, headache, or chills.
4. Upset stomach.

Diagnostic Tests and Measures

The key diagnostic clinical features of herpes zoster are grouped painful vesicles within a dermatome.

Other Tests

- Tzanck smear
- Viral cultures
- Polymerized chain reaction (PCR) testing (used to reproduce [amplify] selected sections of DNA and RNA for analysis)

Clinical Findings, Secondary Effects, Complications

1. Intense pain in a dermatome
2. Pain may precede the eruption by one or a few days
3. Pruritus, tingling, tenderness, or hyperesthesia may also develop
4. Eruption presents as grouped vesicles within the dermatome of the affected nerves, usually within a single unilateral dermatome (trunk and trigeminal nerve)
5. Any area of the body may be affected, but it is seen most frequently on the trunk

Interventions/Treatment

Medical—Oral antiviral medications, if given early, may reduce the duration of the eruption and may reduce the risk and severity of acute pain and perhaps postherpetic neuralgia. The treatments should be started within 72 hours of onset of symptoms. Appropriate treatment for acute pain may be needed. Vaccination with live zoster vaccine (Zostavax) may reduce the risk of development of herpes zoster.

Pharmacological—Acyclovir (Zovirax), famciclovir (Famvir), valacyclovir 1000 mg (Valtrex). Treatments may include topical lidocaine or capsaicin, antidepressants (such as amitriptyline, desipramine, and nortriptyline), and anticonvulsants (such as carbamazepine and gabapentin). Acupuncture and biofeedback may also be helpful.

Physical therapy—As mentioned previously, the patient may complain of intense pain in a dermatomal pattern. The physical therapist must correlate the signs and symptoms to identify that this pain is nonmusculoskeletal in origin. If the patient is part of the therapist's caseload, appropriate universal precautions should be used, especially during the blister phase of the condition.

Differential Diagnosis

- Herpes simplex
- Impetigo
- Contact dermatitis[4]
- Headaches
- Myocardial infarction
- Pleuritic chest pain

Neuropathic Foot Ulcer/Pressure Ulcers

Neuropathic foot ulcers are sequelae of peripheral neuropathy, often in persons with diabetes. In areas of the foot with sustained increased pressure, absence of sensation in the area inhibits the body to relieve pressure, thereby resulting in microtrauma, which over time will lead to tissue damage and ulceration. Groups of patients most susceptible include those with diabetes, but ulceration can occur in the elderly, neurologically involved, and acutely hospitalized. Motor neuron damage is common as well.

Pressure areas in the foot include the plantar surface of the foot, the big toe, and the metatarsophalangeal joints.[5] In addition, cuts and bruises on the foot may lead to ulceration due to decreased circulation in the area and decreased healing secondary to diabetes. Complications from neuropathic foot ulcers include infections/sepsis and amputation. Clinical features of various types of ulcerations are presented in Table 4–5.

In general, pressure against the skin over a body prominence increases risk for development of necrosis and ulceration in any area of the body. Contributing factors for ulceration can include infection, improper skincare, shear, friction, heat, maceration (softening associated with excessive moisture), medication, malnutrition, and muscle atrophy.

Clinical Significance

Disturbances include the following:[6]

1. Symmetrical distal polyneuropathy in a stocking (lower leg and feet) distribution. The sensory loss is chronic and progressive.
2. Common complaints are persistent numbness and tingling that worsens at night.
3. Ophthalmoplegia affecting cranial nerve III (oculomotor) and less frequently, cranial nerve VI (abducens) on one side.
4. Mononeuropathy of limbs or trunk, including painful lumbar radiculopathy.
5. Diabetic amyotrophy can be present with motor neuropathy of the lower limbs.
6. Symmetrical proximal weakness and atrophy.
7. Autonomic impairment.
8. Fall risk.

Diagnostic Tests and Measures

Skin assessment is vital for signs and symptoms of pressure ulcerations, as is evaluation for risk factors, which may include emaciation, obesity, increased age, immobilization, decreased activity, diabetes, circulatory disorders, incontinence, and decreased mental status. Pressure ulcers are graded using a four-stage system (Table 4–6).

TABLE 4–5 Clinical features of ulcers.

Clinical Features	Venous Ulcer	Arterial Ulcer	Diabetic Ulcer	Pressure Ulcer
Pulses	Normal	Poor or absent	May be present or diminished	
Pain	None to aching (in dependent position)	Often severe, intermittent claudication, progressing to pain at rest	Typically not painful; sensory loss usually present	Can be painful if sensation is intact
Color	Normal or cyanotic May see dark pigmentation (thick, tender, indurated, fibrous tissue)	Pale on elevation: dusky rubor on dependency		Red, brown/black, or yellow
Temperature	Normal	Cool		May be warm if localized infection present (associated fever)
Edema	Often marked	Usually absent		
Skin changes	Pigmentation, stasis dermatitis, thickening of skin as scarring develops	Trophic changes (thin, shiny, atrophic skin); loss of hair on foot and toes; nails thicken		Inflammatory response with necrotic tissue
Ulceration	May develop, especially on the medial ankle; wet, with large amount of exudate	On toes or feet; can be deep	May develop due to trauma to insensitive skin	Typically occurs over bony prominences, ie, sacrum, heels, trochanter, lateral malleolus, ischial areas, elbows
Gangrene	Absent	Black gangrenous skin adjacent to ulcer can develop	May develop if left untreated	May develop if left untreated

TABLE 4–6 Pressure ulcer stages.

Stage	Characteristics	Preferred Practice Pattern According to the Guide[a]
Stage I	An observable pressure-related alteration of intact skin whose indicators as compared to an adjacent or opposite area of the body may include changes in skin color, skin temperature (warm or cool), tissue consistency (firm or boggy), and/or sensation (pain, itching).	7B: Impaired integumentary integrity associated with superficial skin involvement
Stage II	A partial-thickness skin loss that involves the epidermis and/or dermis. The ulcer is superficial and presents clinically as an abrasion, blister, or shallow crater.	7C: Impaired integumentary integrity associated with partial-thickness skin involvement and scar formation
Stage III	A full-thickness skin loss that involves damage or necrosis of subcutaneous tissue that may extend down to, but not through, underlying fascia. The ulcer presents clinically as a deep crater with or without undermining adjacent tissue.	7D: Impaired integumentary integrity associated with full-thickness skin involvement and scar formation
Stage IV	A full-thickness skin low with extensive destruction, tissue necrosis, or damage to muscle, bone, or supporting structures (eg, tendon, joint capsule). Undermining or sinus tracts may be present.	7E: Impaired integumentary integrity associated with skin involvement extending into fascia, muscle, or bone, and scar formation

[a]American Physical Therapy Association. Guide to Physical Therapist Practice. Second Edition. American Physical Therapy Association. *Phys Ther.* 2001;81(1):9-746.

Data from Pressure ulcer prevention and treatment following spinal cord injury: a clinical practice guideline for health-care professionals. *J Spinal Cord Med.* 2001;24 (suppl 1):S40–S101.

Blood test—Infection is a major risk factor with ulcers, including neuropathic foot ulcers. Blood tests, including white blood cell (WBC) count, erythrocyte[7] sedimentation rate, and C-reactive protein level, may aid in differentially diagnosing an infection. Nutritional assessment can made by testing for serum proteins (albumin) and hemoglobin (anemia).

Imaging—Radiography can be helpful in diagnosing bone infections. Gas in soft tissues may also be detected by radiography; gas may indicate soft tissue infection due to anaerobic organisms.[7] Nerve conduction studies and electromyography can also be useful.

Clinical Findings, Secondary Effects, Complications

1. Decreased sensation (touch, vibration, proprioception)
2. Unpleasant odor
3. Presence of pus or exudate
4. A wound that is slow to heal

5. Infection
6. Poor arterial flow
7. Charcot deformity
8. Pain (rare, due to lack of sensation)
9. Ulcerations with prominent callus rim, with good granulation tissue and little drainage
10. Wound skin appears dry or cracked
11. Distal limb appears shiny and cool to touch
12. Diminished pedal pulses
13. Gangrene
14. Amputation
15. Weakness with muscle atrophy
16. Decreased deep tendon reflexes
17. Impaired vision
18. Impaired balance

Interventions/Treatment

Medical—The most direct treatment for neuropathic foot ulcers is debridement of dead tissue around the wound. Wound dressings should also be applied to assist in healing.

Pharmacological—Antibiotics may be administered to control infection. Diabetic medications may include insulin (short acting, long acting), sulfonylureas to increase insulin production by beta cells of the pancreas (glyburide), biguanides to decrease liver glucose production and increase insulin sensitivity (metformin), alpha-glucosidase inhibitors, which prevent digestion of carbohydrates, and meglitinides, which lower glucose rise after a meal.

Physical therapy—Physical therapists play a vital role as members of the wound care team. Wounds are constantly changing as they heal, and the physical therapist may be actively involved in treatment. Primary wound care principles include wound cleansing, management of edema and exudate, reduction of necrotic tissue, and control of microorganisms. Table 4–7 describes wound debridement techniques. Dressing selection is based on optimal healing in the changing wound environment; it is rare that a single treatment plan for any given wound will remain the same throughout the healing process. Specific wound and patient characteristics will drive treatment decisions, and include wound

TABLE 4–7 Methods of wound debridement.

Wound debridement can be accomplished in a number of ways:
- Mechanically: Whirlpool, pulsatile lavage, other forms of spray irrigation, and the traditional wet-to-dry dressing.
- Surgically: Performed by a physician with the patient anesthetized. Sharp debridement removes necrotic tissue by means of a scalpel or other sharp instrument with the patient alert.
- Chemically: The use of enzymes or other topical agents, such as Dakin's solution (weak bleach).
- Autolytically: The body does its own cleaning. This type of debridement is the least traumatic to healthy tissue but may take longer than enzymes or more invasive forms of debridement.

From Dutton M. *McGraw-Hill's NPTE (National Physical Therapy Examination).* 2nd ed. New York, NY: McGraw-Hill; 2012: Chapter 13.

TABLE 4-8 Bates-Jensen wound assessment tool.

Instructions for Use

General Guidelines

Fill out the attached rating sheet to assess a wound's status after reading the definitions and methods of assessment described below. Evaluate once a week and whenever a change occurs in the wound. Rate according to each item by picking the response that best describes the wound and entering that score in the item score column for the appropriate date. When you have rated the wound on all items, determine the total score by adding together the 13-item scores. The HIGHER the total score, the more severe the wound status. Plot total score on the Wound Status Continuum to determine progress. If the wound has healed/resolved, score items 1,2,3 and 4 as =0.

Specific Instructions

1. **Size:** Use ruler to measure the longest and widest aspect of the wound surface in centimeters; multiply length by width. Score as = 0 if wound healed/resolved.

2. **Depth:** Pick the depth and thickness most appropriate to the wound using these additional descriptions, score as =0 if wound healed/resolved:

   1 = Tissues damaged but no break in skin surface

   2 = Superficial abrasion, blister, or shallow crater; even with and/or elevated above skin surface (eg, hyperplasia)

   3 = Deep crater with or without undermining of adjacent tissue

   4 = Visualization of tissue layers not possible due to necrosis

   5 = Supporting structures include tendon, joint capsule

3. **Edges:** Score as = 0 if wound healed/resolved. Use this guide:

Indistinct, diffuse	=	unable to clearly distinguish wound outline
Attached	=	even or flush with wound base, no sides or walls present; flat
Not attached	=	sides or walls are present; floor or base of wound is deeper than edge
Rolled under, thickened	=	soft to firm, and flexible to touch
Hyperkeratosis	=	callous-like tissue formation around wound and at edges
Fibrotic, scarred	=	hard, rigid to touch

4. **Undermining:** Score as = 0 if wound healed/resolved. Assess by inserting a cotton-tipped applicator under the wound edge; advance it as far as it will go without using undue force; raise the tip of the applicator so it may be seen or felt on the surface of the skin; mark the surface with a pen; measure the distance from the mark on the skin to the edge of the wound. Continue process around the wound. Then use a transparent metric measuring guide with concentric circles divided into four (25%) pie-shaped quadrants to help determine percent of wound involved.

5. **Necrotic Tissue Type:** Pick the type of necrotic tissue that is predominant in the wound according to color, consistency, and adherence using this guide:

White/gray nonviable tissue	=	may appear prior to wound opening; skin surface is white or gray
Nonadherent, yellow slough	=	thin, mucinous substance; scattered throughout wound bed; easily separated from wound tissue
Loosely adherent, yellow slough	=	thick, stringy, clumps of debris; attached to wound tissue
Adherent, soft, black eschar	=	soggy tissue; strongly attached to tissue in center or base of wound
Firmly adherent, hard/black eschar	=	firm, crusty tissue; strongly attached to wound base and edges (like a hard scab)

6. **Necrotic Tissue Amount:** Use a transparent metric measuring guide with concentric circles divided into four (25%) pie-shaped quadrants to help determine percent of wound involved.

7. **Exudate Type:** Some dressings interact with wound drainage to produce a gel or trap liquid. Before assessing exudate type, gently cleanse wound with normal saline or water. Pick the exudate type that is predominant in the wound according to color and consistency, using this guide:

Bloody	=	thin, bright red
Serosanguineous	=	thin, watery pale red to pink
Serous	=	thin, watery, clear
Purulent	=	thin or thick, opaque tan to yellow or green may have offensive odor

8. **Exudate Amount:** Use a transparent metric measuring guide with concentric circles divided into four (25%) pie-shaped quadrants to determine percent of dressing involved with exudate. Use this guide:

   None = wound tissues dry

   Scant = wound tissues moist; no measurable exudate

   Small = wound tissues wet; moisture evenly distributed in wound; drainage involves <25% dressing

   Moderate = wound tissues saturated; drainage may or may not be evenly distributed in wound; drainage involves >25%–<75% dressing

   Large = wound tissues bathed in fluid; drainage freely expressed; may or may not be evenly distributed in wound; drainage involves >75% of dressing

9. **Skin Color Surrounding Wound:** Assess tissues within 4 cm of wound edge. Dark-skinned persons show the colors "bright red" and "dark red" as a deepening of normal ethnic skin color or a purple hue. As healing occurs in dark-skinned persons, the new skin is pink and may never darken.

(Continued)

TABLE 4–8 Bates-Jensen wound assessment tool. (*Continued*)

10. **Peripheral Tissue Edema and Induration:** Assess tissues within 4 cm of wound edge. Nonpitting edema appears as skin that is shiny and taut. Identify pitting edema by firmly pressing a finger down into the tissues and waiting for 5 seconds; on release of pressure, tissues fail to resume previous position and an indentation appears. Induration is abnormal firmness of tissues with margins. Assess by gently pinching the tissues. Induration results in an inability to pinch the tissues. Use a transparent metric measuring guide to determine how far edema or induration extends beyond wound.

11. **Granulation Tissue:** Granulation tissue is the growth of small blood vessels and connective tissue to fill in full-thickness wounds. Tissue is healthy when bright, beefy red, shiny, and granular with a velvety appearance. Poor vascular supply appears as pale pink or blanched to dull, dusky red color.

12. **Epithelialization:** Epithelialization is the process of epidermal resurfacing and appears as pink or red skin. In partial-thickness wounds, it can occur throughout the wound bed as well as from the wound edges. In full-thickness wounds, it occurs from the edges only. Use a transparent metric measuring guide with concentric circles divided into four (25%) pie-shaped quadrants to help determine percent of wound involved and to measure the distance the epithelial tissue extends into the wound.

BATES-JENSEN WOUND ASSESSMENT TOOL   NAME

Complete the rating sheet to assess wound status. Evaluate each item by picking the response that best describes the wound and entering the score in the item score column for the appropriate date. If the wound has healed/resolved, score items 1,2,3, & 4 as =0.

Location: Anatomic site. Circle, identify right **(R)** or left **(L)**, and use **"X"** to mark site on body diagrams:

_____	Sacrum and coccyx	_____	Lateral ankle		
_____	Trochanter	_____	Medial ankle		
_____	Ischial tuberosity	_____	Heel	Other site:	_____
_____	Buttock				

Shape: Overall wound pattern; assess by observing perimeter and depth.

Circle and date appropriate description:

_____	Irregular	_____	Linear or elongated		
_____	Round/oval	_____	Bowl/boat		
_____	Square/rectangle	_____	Butterfly	Other shape:	_____

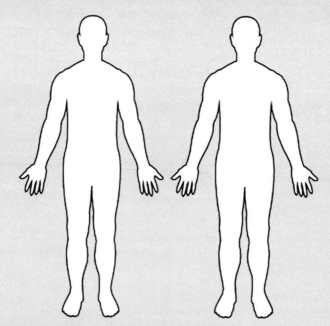

Item	Assessment	Date Score	Date Score	Date Score
1. Size*	*0 = Healed, resolved wound 1 = Length × width <4 sq cm 2 = Length × width 4–<16 sq cm 3 = Length × width 16.1–<36 sq cm 4 = Length × width 36.1–<80 sq cm 5 = Length × width >80 sq cm			

(*Continued*)

TABLE 4–8 Bates-Jensen wound assessment tool. (*Continued*)

2. Depth*	*0 = Healed, resolved wound 1 = Nonblanchable erythema on intact skin 2 = Partial-thickness skin loss involving epidermis and/or dermis 3 = Full-thickness skin loss involving damage or necrosis of subcutaneous tissue; may extend down to but not through underlying fascia; and/or mixed partial- and full-thickness and/or tissue layers obscured by granulation tissue 4 = Obscured by necrosis 5 = Full-thickness skin loss with extensive destruction, tissue necrosis, or damage to muscle, bone, or supporting structures			
3. Edges*	*0 = Healed, resolved wound 1 = Indistinct, diffuse, none clearly visible 2 = Distinct, outline clearly visible, attached, even with wound base 3 = Well defined not attached to wound base 4 = Well defined not attached to base, rolled under, thickened 5 = Well defined fibrotic, scarred, or hyperkeratotic			
4. Undermining*	*0 = Healed, resolved wound 1 = None present 2 = Undermining <2 cm in any area 3 = Undermining 2–4 cm involving <50% wound margins 4 = Undermining 2–4 cm involving >50% wound margins 5 = Undermining >4 cm or tunneling in any area			
5. Necrotic Tissue Type	1 = None visible 2 = White/gray nonviable tissue and/or nonadherent yellow slough 3 = Loosely adherent yellow slough 4 = Adherent, soft, black eschar 5 = Firmly adherent, hard, black eschar			
6. Necrotic Tissue Amount	1 = None visible 2 = <25% of wound bed covered 3 = 25%–50% of wound covered 4 = >50% and <75% of wound covered 5 = 75%–100% of wound covered			
7. Exudate Type	1 = None 2 = Bloody 3 = Serosanguinous: thin, watery, pale red/pink 4 = Serous: thin, watery, clear 5 = Purulent: thin or thick, opaque, tan/yellow, with or without odor			
8. Exudate Amount	1 = None, dry wound 2 = Scant, wound moist but no observable exudate 3 = Small 4 = Moderate 5 = Large			
9. Skin Color Surrounding Wound	1 = Pink or normal for ethnic group 2 = Bright red and/or blanches to touch 3 = White or gray pallor or hypopigmented 4 = Dark red or purple and/or nonblanchable 5 = Black or hyperpigmented			

TABLE 4–8 Bates-Jensen wound assessment tool. (*Continued*)

10. Peripheral Tissue Edema	1 = No swelling or edema 2 = Nonpitting edema extends <4 cm around wound 3 = Nonpitting edema extends >4 cm around wound 4 = Pitting edema extends <4 cm around wound 5 = Crepitus and/or pitting edema extends >4 cm around wound			
11. Peripheral Tissue Induration	1 = None present 2 = Induration <2 cm around wound 3 = Induration 2–4 cm extending <50% around wound 4 = Induration 2–4 cm extending >50% around wound 5 = Induration >4 cm in any area around wound			
12. Granulation Tissue	1 = Skin intact or partial-thickness wound 2 = Bright, beefy red; 75%–100% of wound filled and/or tissue overgrowth 3 = Bright, beefy red; <75% and >25% of wound filled 4 = Pink, and/or dull, dusky red and/or fills <25% of wound 5 = No granulation tissue present			
13. Epithelialization	1 = 100% wound covered, surface intact 2 = 75%–<100% wound covered and/or epithelial tissue extends >0.5 cm into wound bed 3 = 50%–<75% wound covered and/or epithelial tissue extends to <0.5 cm into wound bed 4 = 25%–<50% wound covered 5 = <25% wound covered			
TOTAL SCORE				
SIGNATURE				

Wound Status Continuum

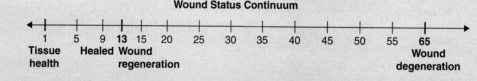

1 — 5 — 9 — **13** 15 — 20 — 25 — 30 — 35 — 40 — 45 — 50 — 55 — **65**

Tissue health   Healed Wound regeneration   Wound degeneration

Plot the total score on the Wound Status Continuum by putting an **"X"** on the line and the date beneath the line. Plot multiple scores with their dates to see regeneration or degeneration of the wound at a glance.

location, size, tissue type, exudate, peri-wound condition, bacterial burden, pain, support needs, and quality of life (Tables 4–8 to 4–11). Optimal dressing selection (Table 4–12) depends on a thorough assessment of the wound, especially for the primary dressing that will interact with the wound bed to facilitate healing, as well as assessment of the patient. Dressing choice can vary (Table 4–12), but ideally the dressing should create a moist environment without maceration or desiccation. Two key terms used to describe dressings are *occlusion* and *moisture*. Occlusion refers the ability of a dressing to transmit moisture, vapor, or gases from the wound bed to the atmosphere. Occlusive dressings are completely impermeable, while nonocclusive dressings are completely permeable. The following dressings are arranged from most occlusive to nonocclusive: hydrocolloids, hydrogels, semipermeable

TABLE 4–9 Wound colors.

Color	Wound Description	Intervention Goals
Red	Healthy, pink granular tissue with absence of necrotic tissue	Protect wound; maintain moist environment
Yellow	Presence of adherent fibrinous exudates and debris (moist yellow slough)	Debride necrotic tissue; absorb drainage
Black	Presence of black, thick eschar (dried necrotic tissue), firmly adhered	Debride necrotic tissue

Data from Cozzell J. The new red, yellow, black color code. *Am J Nurs.* 1989;10:1014.

TABLE 4–10 Wound and patient characteristics assessed for treatment decisions.

Location	The location of the wound helps determine the secondary dressing that will best secure the primary dressing.
Size	The wound size determines the size and amount of the primary dressing that is required to adequately fill and cover the wound surface.
Tissue type	The tissue appearance and predominant tissue type as well as the presence of any exposed structures are key determinants of primary dressing selection.
Exudate	The amount and type of exudate is a fundamental consideration in both primary and secondary dressing selection.
Periwound condition	A key goal of the total dressing is to maintain the periwound skin integrity, which reduces pain and risk of infection.
Bacterial burden	The use of topical agents and dressings to reduce local bioburden can reduce the number of bacteria before they replicate to a critical level.
Support needs	Compression for venous wounds, off-loading for diabetic foot ulcers, and visualization for infected wounds are examples of needs that may require special dressings.

foam, semipermeable film, impregnated gauze, alginates, and traditional gauze. Moisture dressings can be classified according to the ability to retain moisture. The following dressings are arranged from most moisture retentive to least moisture retentive: alginates, semipermeable foam, hydrocolloids, hydrogels, and semipermeable films. Activity levels and patient goals are important for selection of the secondary dressings and interventions such as negative pressure wound therapy that may affect activities of daily living and work demands.

Physical therapists can administer interventions that help the healing process, which may include negative pressure wound therapy, selective debridement (sharp, enzymatic autolytic), and nonselective debridement (wet to dry, wound irrigation, hydrotherapy). In addition, the physical therapist can provide educational intervention to prevent development of new ulcers (Table 4–13). The use of orthotics and splints may also assist in preventing development of ulcers. Physical therapy documentation of wounds assists in monitoring healing progression Table 4–13. Functional activities such as bed mobility, transfers, gait, and stairs to improve mobility and reduce fall risk are essential in this patient population.

Differential Diagnosis[8,9]

- Lumbar radiculopathy
- Squamous cell carcinoma
- Superficial thrombophlebitis
- Vascular lesions
- Syphilis

Cellulitis

Cellulitis is an acute infection of the dermis and subcutaneous tissue. Most cases of cellulitis are caused by *Staphylococcus aureus* and group A *Streptococcus*. However, in certain situations other organisms may be involved, such as gram-negative organisms or *Haemophilus influenzae* in young infants. Cellulitis typically presents with rubor (erythema), dolor (pain), calor (warmth), and tumor (edema), and may begin with the acute onset of localized erythema and tenderness. The borders may be ill defined, and surface crusts may develop. Other symptoms include fever, malaise, and chills. Less common findings include ascending lymphangitis and regional lymphadenopathy. Cellulitis usually presents in a unilateral distribution.

Clinical Significance

Disturbances include the following:[6]

1. Involved site is red, hot, swollen, and tender, with the lower extremity being the most common site.
2. Borders of the involved area are not elevated or sharply demarcated.
3. Regional lymphadenopathy is present with malaise, chills, fever, and toxicity.
4. Skin infection without underlying drainage, penetrating trauma, eschar, or abscess is likely caused by streptococci; however, community-acquired methicillin-resistant *S. aureus* (CA-MRSA) is the most likely pathogen when these factors are present.[10]
5. Cellulitis characterized by violaceous color and bullae suggests more serious or systemic infection with organisms such as *Vibrio vulnificus* or *Streptococcus pneumoniae*.
6. Lymphangitic spread (red lines streaking away from the area of infection), crepitus, and hemodynamic instability are indications of severe infection, requiring more aggressive treatment.
7. Circumferential cellulitis or pain that is disproportional to examination findings should prompt consideration of severe soft-tissue infection.

Diagnostic Tests and Measures

The key diagnostic clinical feature of cellulitis is a painful, warm, red, edematous plaque.

Laboratory tests—If indicated, cultures from exudate or blistered areas can be taken with a swab or cultures can be obtained by aspirating the affected skin. A skin punch biopsy of affected skin may also be cultured.

Imaging—Imaging studies may be needed if crepitant or necrotic cellulitis is suspected.

Clinical Findings, Secondary Effects, Complications

1. Cellulitis typically presents with rubor (erythema), dolor (pain), calor (warmth), and tumor (edema)
2. Malaise, chills, fever, and toxicity
3. Lymphangitic spread (red lines streaking away from the area of infection)
4. Circumferential cellulitis
5. Pain disproportionate to examination findings

TABLE 4-11 Characteristics of the ideal wound dressing.

Provides a moist wound environment	By either donating or removing moisture from the wound bed, the dressing maintains the optimal moisture level, thereby preventing desiccation of the cells.
Manages exudate appropriately	The dressing adequately absorbs or manages the wound exudate so that it is sequestered in the dressing and does not exude onto the intact periwound skin, thus causing maceration or denudation.
Facilitates autolytic debridement	In the presence of necrotic tissue, the dressing creates an environment so that ambient wound fluid containing phagocytic cells and endogenous enzymes is in contact with the tissue, thus facilitating autolysis.
Provides antimicrobial properties if needed	If a wound is highly colonized or infected, the antimicrobial dressing will aid in sequestering wound fluid or providing active antimicrobial activity to reduce or eliminate bacteria.
Minimizes pain	The selected dressing material does not adhere to the wound bed and cause disruption of the surface, thus harming healthy cells. By not adhering, the dressing lifts from the wound and periwound easily, and as a result does not cause the patient undue discomfort.
Prevents contamination by being impermeable to environmental bacteria	On all wounds (especially those in the sacral, coccyx, and ischial area where contamination is likely), the dressing surface is impermeable to bacteria and contamination from the environment. This is especially important for the patient who is incontinent.
Is compatible with support needs	The dressing can be used under support treatments such as contact casts and compression wraps that are often left in place for a full week.
Insulates and maintains optimal temperature	The dressing allows maintenance of constant temperature without frequent cooling of the tissue that can impact healing. Frequent dressing changes can negatively impact wound healing more than the dressing selection itself.
Prevents particulate contamination or allergens from coming in contact with the wound surface	The dressing does not leave threads or pieces of adherent dressing in the wound bed, which could act as a foreign body in the tissue. Also, the dressing does not contain common allergens such as latex.
Is easily applied and removed (user friendly)	The dressing can be used by the care providers in the patient's setting, including by family members at home.
Is available and cost-effective	The dressing must be available in the healthcare setting in which the patient resides. Choices available in a hospital or clinic may not be reimbursable for the patient at home, or they may not be on the formulary of a particular home care agency or skilled nursing facility. Flexibility in dressing selection by the prescriber is required as long as the selection meets the needs of the wound.

Hamm RL. Anatomy and physiology of the integumentary system. In: Hamm RL. *Text and Atlas of Wound Diagnosis and Treatment.* McGraw-Hill; 2015. Available at: http://accessphysiotherapy.mhmedical.com/content.aspx?bookid=1334&sectionid=77259853. Accessed January 10, 2018.

Indications for emergent surgical evaluation are as follows:

1. Violaceous bullae
2. Cutaneous hemorrhage
3. Skin sloughing
4. Skin anesthesia
5. Rapid progression
6. Gas in the tissue
7. Hypotension

Interventions/Treatment

Medical—The most direct treatment for cellulitis is an oral antibiotic.[11] Treatment for the most common forms of cellulitis that are likely caused by methicillin-sensitive *S. aureus* includes use of penicillinase-resistant penicillin, first-generation cephalosporin, amoxicillin-clavulanate, a macrolide, or a fluoroquinolone antibiotic. Extensive disease may require IV antibiotics.

Pharmacological—Culture of the infection may be necessary to determine the best pharmacologic treatment. Mild cases can be treated with antibiotics such as dicloxacillin, amoxicillin, and cephalexin. Resistant strains may need alternatives such as fluoroquinolones.

Physical therapy—Physical therapists need to understand the signs and symptoms of cellulitis to be able to refer to appropriate individuals if a patient presentation is consistent with this diagnosis. Treatment measures may include elevation and immobilization of the involved limb to reduce swelling as well as functional activities as appropriate. Physical therapists are also integral members of the wound care team.

Differential Diagnosis[12-14]

- Allergic contact dermatitis
- Stasis dermatitis
- Necrotizing fasciitis
- Inflammatory carcinoma of the breast or other cutaneous malignancy
- Neutrophilic eccrine hidradenitis
- Sweet syndrome
- Tumor necrosis factor receptor–associated syndrome
- Thrombophlebitis/deep vein thrombosis

TABLE 4–12 Dressing choices.

Dressing Types	Examples	Advantages	Disadvantages	Indications	Contraindications
Semipermeable—thin, adhesive, transparent polyurethane film	OpSite, Tegaderm	Some moisture evaporation. Reduces pain. Barrier to external contamination. Allows inspection.	Exudate may pool, may be traumatic to remove.	Superficial wounds. As a secondary dressing.	Highly exudative wounds
Nonadherent, moist (Tulle Gras dressing)—gauze impregnated with paraffin or similar May be impregnated with antiseptics or antibiotics	Jelonet, Unitulle, Bactigras, Sofra-Tulle	Reduces adhesion to wound. Moist environment aids healing.	Does not absorb exudate. Requires secondary dressing. May induce allergy or delay healing when impregnated.	Burns. Wounds healing by secondary intention.	Allergy
Nonadherent, dry—thin perforated plastic film coating attached to absorbent pad	Melolin, Melolite, Tricose	Low wound adherence. May absorb light exudate.	Not suitable in high exudate. Can dry out and stick to wound. May require secondary dressing.	Wounds with moderate exudate.	Dry wounds (may cause tissue dehydration)
Fixation sheet—porous polyester fabric with adhesive backing	Fixomull, Hypafix, Mefix	Can be used directly on wound site. Conforms to body contours. Good pain relief and controls edema. Remains permeable, allowing exudate to escape and be washed and dried off wound. Dressing changes can be left for 5–7 days.	Dressing needs washing with soap and water, pat-dried twice daily. Requires application of oil prior to removal—ideally soaked in oil and wrapped in cling film overnight.	Wounds with mild exudate, not needing frequent review.	Infected wounds; allergy to adhesives
Calcium alginate—natural polysaccharide from seaweed	Kaltostat	Forms gel on wound and hence moist environment. Reduces pain. Can pack cavities. Absorbent in exudative wounds. Promotes hemostasis. Low allergenic.	May require secondary dressing. Not recommended in anaerobic infections. Gel can be confused with slough or pus in wound.	Moderately or highly exudative wounds. Need for hemostasis.	Dry wounds or hard eschar
Foam dressings—polyurethane foam dressing with adhesive layer incorporated	PolyMem	Moist, highly absorbent, and protective.	Set size of foam may be limited by wound size.	Wounds with mild to moderate exudate.	Dry wounds; wounds that need frequent review
Hydrocolloid dressings—polyurethane film coated with adhesive mass	Duoderm	Retains moisture, painless removal.	Avoid on high-exudate wounds.	Burns (small); abrasions.	Dry wounds; infection
Paper adhesive tapes—adhesive tape may be applied directly to healing laceration	Micropore	Nonallergenic. Provides wound support.	Nonabsorbent.	Small wounds.	Exudative or large wounds

From https://www.rch.org.au/clinicalguide/guideline_index/Wound_dressings_acute_traumatic_wounds/.

TABLE 4–13 Pressure ulcer prevention.

Prevention Technique	Suggested Strategies
Proper positioning in bed and in wheelchair	Bony prominences protected and pressure distributed equally over large surface areas Use of pressure distribution equipment such as wheelchair cushions, custom mattresses, and alternating pressure mattress pads
Frequent changes in position	Every 2 hours when in bed Every 15–20 minutes when seated
Keep skin clean and dry	Good bowel and bladder care with immediate cleansing after episode of incontinence Current cleansing and drying of skin at least once daily Inspect skin for areas of redness in a.m. and p.m.
Nutrition	Diet with adequate calories, protein, vitamins, and minerals Sufficient water intake
Clothing	Avoid clothes that are either too tight or too loose fitting Avoid clothes with thick seams, buttons, or zippers in areas of pressure
Activity	Regular cardiovascular exercise Gradual buildup of skin tolerance for new activities, equipment, and positions Avoid movements that rub, drag, or scratch the skin

Data from Spangler LL. Nonprogressive spinal cord disorders. In: Cameron MH, Monroe LG, eds. *Physical Rehabilitation: Evidence-Based Examination, Evaluation, and Intervention.* St. Louis, MO: Saunders/Elsevier; 2007:538-579.

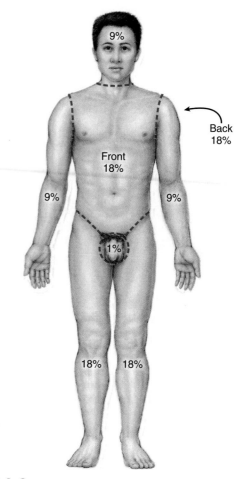

FIGURE 4–2 TBSA determination by rule of nines. (From Hamm RL. *Text and Atlas of Wound Diagnosis and Treatment.* https://accessphysiotherapy.mhmedical.com/content.aspx?bookid=1334&sectionid=77261714. Copyright 2018 McGraw-Hill Education. All rights reserved.)

Burns[15]

Thermal injury to the skin is the result of the direct energy to the tissue in relation to temperature and contact time. Transfer of heat to cellular structures of the skin results in denaturation of proteins, vaporization of water, and thrombosis of cutaneous blood vessels, resulting in tissue and cell death. This process may be immediate in the case of high temperature and/or prolonged contact time, but may also be potentiated by the patient's premorbid condition, injury status, and local inflammatory factors.

The severity of a burn injury is determined by depth of penetration and surface area of the injured skin in relationship to total body surface area (TBSA) of the patient. Determination of TBSA in relation to burn size for the adult can be generalized utilizing the rule of nines (Figure 4–2). More specific charts have been developed to estimate the body surface in relation to age, which is more useful in the pediatric population. Burns were previously classified as first, second, and third degree, but this classification has been replaced by the designations of superficial, partial thickness, and full thickness.

Clinical Significance

Disturbances include the following:[6]

1. Superficial burns are limited to the epidermis without disruption of epithelial integrity. The skin's appearance includes erythema because of the inflammatory process.

2. Superficial partial-thickness burns involve the epidermis and the superficial dermis. They are characterized by intense pain (sensate), blanching with pressure, and blistering because of the local inflammatory process between the dermis and epidermis.

3. Deep partial-thickness injuries extend into the reticular dermis and are insensate, have a mottled white appearance, and do not blanch with pressure as the result of impaired vascularity and capillary refill.

4. Full-thickness burns extend through the entire dermis and into the subcutaneous tissue. The appearance is leathery brown or black eschar with no capillary refill.

Diagnostic Tests and Measures

Indicators of depth of injury include biopsy, ultrasound, or perfusion. None are as reliable as physical examination at 48 to 72 hours. Burn infection is diagnosed by a quantitative biopsy.

Blood test—Complete blood counts should be monitored throughout treatment, including protein status.

Imaging—Ultrasound.

Clinical Findings, Secondary Effects, Complications

1. Mechanisms of burn injuries may include scalding, flame, electrical, chemical, and radiation
2. Keloid scarring
3. Hypertrophic scarring
4. Pain
5. Infection
6. Peripheral hypoperfusion
7. Cardiac complications (arrhythmia, hypoxia, acidosis, hyperkalemia)
8. Pulmonary complications (inhalation difficulty, distress, abnormal breath sounds)
9. Metabolic complications (hemoglobinuria, myoglobinuria)
10. Heterotrophic scarring
11. Wound contracture

Interventions/Treatment

Medical—Surgical management for removal of nonviable tissue, restoration of the immunologic barrier, and restoration of normal esthetics as required in sensitive areas (skin grafting). Fluid resuscitation to prevent organ damage. Nutritional requirements will need to be managed for proper healing progression. Pain control for all pain types (breakthrough, background, procedural) to assist in comfortable engaging in dressing changes and participation in rehabilitation exercises.

Pharmacological—Analgesics, anti-inflammatories, topical antimicrobial medications, silver sulfadiazine (Silvadene), mafenide acetate (Sulfamylon), silver nitrate, silver-impregnated gauze.

Physical therapy[16]—Treatment of the burn patient must always consider the psychosocial aspects of the patient during this traumatic event. Gentle conversation, encouragement, and an unhurried approach to therapy sessions may be beneficial. Early phases of treatment will focus on minimizing edema, promotion of venous return, passive range of motion for all joints in all cardinal planes, and splinting to prevent wound contracture and functional limitations. To assist with extremity edema reduction, the therapist may employ tubular elastic dressings, elastic wrap dressings, elevation, and retrograde massage. Proper antideformity positioning (Figure 4–3) minimizes shortening of tendons, collateral ligaments, and joint capsules; it also reduces extremity and facial edema. Positioning techniques may include removal

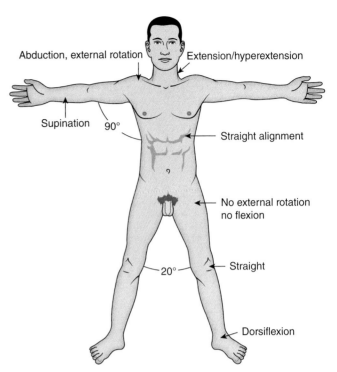

FIGURE 4–3 Burn patient positions. (Modified from McCulloch JM, Kloth LC. *Wound Healing: Evidence-Based Management.* 4th ed. Philadelphia, PA: FA Davis, 2010.)

of pillows, splints, web spacers, prone position, and padded footboards. Performance of activity of daily living tasks and the impending return to play/school/work are important considerations. Scar management may be favorably influenced using pressure garments and topical silicone. Active range of motion (ROM) may be increased, progressing to strengthening with resistive exercises. Resisted ROM, isometric exercises, active strengthening, and gait training are important objectives.

Differential Diagnosis

- Rash
- Toxic epidermal necrolysis
- Staphylococcal scalded skin syndrome

Dermatitis

Dermatitis pertains to the inflammation of the skin caused by exposure to irritants, allergy, or genetic predisposition. Examples of disorders related to dermatitis include eczema, contact dermatitis, and seborrheic dermatitis. Eczema, or atopic dermatitis, denotes the reaction of the skin to various diseases or conditions. Eczema can be accompanied by hay fever or asthma. It can be a long-lasting condition with flareups. Contact dermatitis results from the skin's reaction to exposure to specific substances such as metals, drugs, or poison ivy. Seborrheic dermatitis affects the oily areas of the body such as the scalp, face, sides of the nose, or ears.

Clinical Significance

1. Diagnosis is based on medical history and examination of the integument.
2. Contact dermatitis: Diagnosis is based on medical history, the appearance of the skin, and a history of exposure to irritants or allergens.
3. Seborrheic dermatitis: Diagnosis is based on history, appearance of the skin, physical examination, and skin biopsy.
4. Atopic dermatitis (eczema): Diagnosis is based on history and appearance of the skin.
5. Eczema and dermatitis have three primary stages: acute, subacute, and chronic.

Diagnostic Tests and Measures

Blood tests and laboratory tests—No blood test is necessary to diagnose this condition unless complications such as infections arise, in which case blood work may be necessary to diagnose the infection and identify the best course of action. Skin lesion biopsies or skin cultures may be used to rule out other causes.

Imaging—No imaging is needed to diagnose this condition.

Clinical Findings, Secondary Effects, Complications

1. Redness or inflammation
2. Dry skin
3. Pruritus
4. Itching that may be severe at night
5. Elevated bumps that may ooze and crust over when scratched
6. Localized edema
7. Burning or tenderness
8. Flakes on the scalp, greasy skin with yellow or white flakes (seborrheic dermatitis)

Interventions/Treatment

Medical—Dermatitis is a common skin condition that is treated based on the cause. Lifestyle changes are often recommended such as applying corticosteroid creams, anti-itching products (such as calamine lotion), and oral antihistamines. Applying cool compresses, taking baths, avoiding scratching, wearing cotton clothing, moisturizing the skin, and reducing stress are recommended. Exposing the skin to controlled amounts of natural and artificial light may assist in healing.

Pharmacological—Pharmacologic management may include shampoos, creams, or gels to control inflammation.

- Antifungal medications
- Dupilumab (Dupixent) for eczema from allergies
- Steroid creams or ointments
- Oral corticosteroids
- Antihistamines
- Anti-inflammatories

Physical therapy—Physical therapists need to be aware of the signs and symptoms of these conditions to be able to refer these patients to appropriate medical professionals if needed. If the patient has already been diagnosed with the condition, the therapist must also be aware of any signs and symptoms of infection, and refer the patient accordingly.

Differential Diagnosis

- Psoriasis
- Scabies
- Fungal infections
- Impetigo
- Tinea versicolor
- Rosacea

■ SUMMARY

The integumentary system is a key area of physical therapy practice. Physical therapists identify skin involvement related to common lesions and prevention of wounds as well as conditions that are secondary to pathology and sequelae of other conditions.

REFERENCES

1. Bohjanen K. Structure and functions of the skin. In: Soutor C, Hordinsky MK, eds. *Clinical Dermatology*. New York, NY: McGraw-Hill. http://accessmedicine.mhmedical.com/content.aspx?bookid=2184&sectionid=165458458. Accessed March 1, 2018.
2. Bart B. Viral Infections of the skin. In: Soutor C, Hordinsky MK, eds. *Clinical Dermatology*. New York, NY: McGraw-Hill. http://accessmedicine.mhmedical.com/content.aspx?bookid=2184&sectionid=165459445. Accessed March 16, 2018.
3. Centers for Disease Control. Shingles (herpes zoster). Available at: https://www.cdc.gov/shingles/index.html. Accessed March 20, 2018.
4. Sampathkumar P, Drage LA, Martin DP. Herpes zoster (shingles) and postherpetic neuralgia. *Mayo Clin Proc*. 2009;84(3):274-280.
5. Wound Source. Neuropathic ulcers and wound care: symptoms, causes, and treatments. Wound Source. Available at: http://www.woundsource.com/blog/neuropathic-ulcers-and-wound-care-symptoms-causes-and-treatments. Accessed March 20, 2018.
6. Venglar M. Diabetic neuropathy. In: Shamus E, ed. *The Color Atlas of Physical Therapy*. New York, NY: McGraw-Hill. http://accessphysiotherapy.mhmedical.com/content.aspx?bookid=1491&sectionid=90315949. Accessed March 14, 2018.
7. Williams DT, Hilton JR, Harding KG. Diagnosing foot infection in diabetes. *Clin Infect Dis*. 2004;1:39(Suppl 2):S83-86.
8. Medscape. Diabetic foot infections differential diagnoses. Available at: https://emedicine.medscape.com/article/237378-differential. Accessed March 20, 2018.
9. Wheeless CR. Differential diagnosis of neuropathic ulceration. *Wheeless' Textbook of Orthopedics*. Available at: http://www.wheelessonline.com/ortho/differential_diagnosis_of_neuropathic_ulceration. Accessed March 20, 2018.

10. Busch BA, Ahern MT, Topinka M, Jenkins JJ 2nd, Weiser MA. Eschar with cellulitis as a clinical predictor of community acquired MRSA skin abscess. *J Emerg Med.* 2010;38(5):563-566.

11. Mayo Clinic. Cellulitis. Available at: https://www.mayoclinic.org/diseases-conditions/cellulitis/diagnosis-treatment/drc-20370766. Accessed March 20, 2018.

12. Swartz MN. Clinical practice. Cellulitis. *N Engl J Med.* 2004;350(9):904-912.

13. Schmid MR, Kossmann T, Duewell S. Differentiation of necrotizing fasciitis and cellulitis using MR imaging. *AJR Am J Roentgenol.* 1998;170(3):615-620.

14. Cellulitis differential diagnoses. emedicine.medscape.com. Accessed March 24, 2018.

15. Davis GB, Carey JN, Wong AK. Burn wound management. In: Hamm RL, ed. *Text and Atlas of Wound Diagnosis and Treatment.* New York, NY: McGraw-Hill; 2015. http://accessphysiotherapy.mhmedical.com/content.aspx?bookid=1334&sectionid=77261714. Accessed March 24, 2018.

16. Chapter 13. Integumentary physical therapy. In: Dutton M, ed. *McGraw-Hill's NPTE (National Physical Therapy Examination).* 2nd ed. New York, NY: McGraw-Hill; 2012. http://accessphysiotherapy.mhmedical.com/content.aspx?bookid=478&sectionid=40174792. Accessed March 24, 2018.

QUESTIONS

1. A physical therapist inspects and palpates the skin of a patient with peripheral vascular disease. The therapist notices a dark purplish-blue discoloration of the skin. This finding may indicate a
   A. Normal response to pressure on the skin
   B. Reflex vasoconstriction due to cold response
   C. Pathology involving the liver
   D. Tissue hypoxia or hematologic pathology

2. On observation, a physical therapist notes yellowish discoloration of the skin and sclera. What medical screening question is most appropriate to identify a possible underlying pathology based on the observation?
   A. Have you previously experienced difficulty in breathing or other problems affecting your lungs or respiration?
   B. Have you experienced instances where you feel that your heart is racing and your pulse is fast?
   C. Have you been diagnosed with or been told that you have a liver problem?
   D. Do you have any difficulty urinating?

3. Which of the following statements is TRUE regarding checking the nail bed for possible pathology?
   A. Finger clubbing is a normal age-related change affecting the nails.
   B. Normal nail bases should look convex and will create a oval-shaped space when nails of opposite hands are placed together.
   C. Finger clubbing refers to an increased angle between the fingernail and where the nail enters the skin.
   D. Abnormalities seen on the nail beds are not sensitive tests to indicate any systemic pathology.

4. A physical therapist notes a solid, elevated, sharply circumscribed, small (1 cm) colored lesion (pink, tan, red, or any variation) on the patient's lower extremities. The appropriate term to denote this lesion is a
   A. Macule
   B. Papule
   C. Pustule
   D. Cyst

5. A therapist inspects the skin of a patient who was referred for low back pain. The therapist notes yellowish and whitish crust on the scalp, face, sides of nose, and ears. The therapist also notes that these areas appear oily. The appropriate diagnosis for the condition is:
   A. Contact dermatitis
   B. Psoriasis
   C. Seborrheic dermatitis
   D. Eczema

ANSWERS

1. The answer is **D**. A dark bluish or purplish discoloration of the integument and mucous membranes is termed cyanosis, and may indicate hypoxia or hematologic pathology.

2. The answer is **C**. Jaundice, or yellowish discoloration of the skin, may be indicative of an underlying liver pathology.

3. The answer is **C**. Finger clubbing refers to an increased angle between the fingernail and where the nails enters the skin, and may indicate chronic tissue hypoxia.

4. The answer is **B**. A papule refers to a solid, elevated lesion, sharply circumscribed, small (1 cm) colored lesion (pink, tan, red, or any variation), commonly seen in dermatitis, ringworm, or psoriasis.

5. The answer is **C**. Seborrheic dermatitis refers to yellowish and whitish flaky crust affecting the oily areas of the body such as the scalp, nose, ears, or face.

CHECKLIST

When you complete this chapter, you should be able to:

❑ Outline signs and symptoms of selected integumentary conditions.

❑ List general classifications of signs and symptoms associated with integumentary disease.

❑ Identify specific clinical findings of selected pathologies affecting the integumentary system.

❑ Identify pertinent diagnostic tests and measures to confirm the presence of selected integumentary pathologies.

❑ Select pertinent medical imaging modalities to confirm the diagnosis of selected integumentary conditions.

❑ Discuss the medical and pharmacological management of selected integumentary conditions.

❑ Describe techniques for wound measurement.

❑ Compare dressing types for wounds with increased exudate.

❑ Compare selective and non-selective debridement.

❑ List wound staging classifications.

❑ Compare necrotic and granulation tissue.

❑ Discuss the role of physical therapy in the management of selected integumentary conditions.

Metabolic and Endocrine Systems

5

Annie Burke-Doe and Rolando Lazaro

■ CLINICAL APPLICATION OF FOUNDATIONAL SCIENCES

The endocrine system is a collection of cells, tissues, glands, and organs that work together to produce and regulate signaling molecules called **hormones**. Hormones are released into the bloodstream where they bind to receptors, or in target cells, and function to regulate their activity to maintain homeostasis. The locations of selected endocrine glands and hormones released are shown in Figure 5–1. This system overlaps with the nervous system, and its responsibilities include the regulation of blood pressure, **metabolism**, growth and development, and reproduction. Hormone secretion itself is highly regulated by various mechanisms, including hormonal signals from the **hypothalamus**

High-Yield Terms to Learn	
Addison disease	A rare disease marked by deficient secretion of adrenocortical hormones (such as cortisol) that is characterized by fatigue, muscle weakness, weight loss, low blood pressure, irritability or depression, and brownish pigmentation of the skin, and is caused by progressive destruction of the adrenal glands (as by an autoimmune response or infection).
Addisonian crisis	Low levels of cortisol can cause weakness, fatigue, and low blood pressure. There may be more symptoms with untreated Addison disease or damaged adrenal glands due to severe stress, such as from a car accident or an infection. These symptoms may include sudden dizziness, vomiting, and loss of consciousness.
Aldosterone	A steroid hormone $C_{21}H_{28}O_5$ of the adrenal cortex that functions in the regulation of the salt and water balance of the body.
Anabolism	The constructive part of metabolism concerned especially with macromolecular synthesis.
Androgens	A male sex hormone (as testosterone).
Buffalo torso	Extra fat around the torso; is a symptom of Cushing syndrome.
Catabolism	Destructive metabolism involving the release of energy and resulting in the breakdown of complex materials within the organism.
Cretinism	A usually congenital abnormal condition marked by physical stunting and mental retardation and caused by severe thyroid deficiency—called also *infantile myxedema.*
Cushing syndrome	An abnormal condition caused by excess levels of corticosteroids, especially cortisol, in the body due to either hyperfunction of the adrenal gland (as from adrenal adenoma or hypersecretion of ACTH by the pituitary gland) or to prolonged use of corticosteroid medications (as prednisone) and that is characterized by a variety of signs and symptoms including a change in appearance marked by moon face with plethora and truncal obesity, easy bruising, fatigue, muscle weakness, and hypertension.
Diabetes mellitus	A variable disorder of carbohydrate metabolism caused by a combination of hereditary and environmental factors and usually characterized by inadequate secretion or utilization of insulin, excessive urine production, excessive amounts of sugar in the blood and urine, and thirst, hunger, and loss of weight.

High-Yield Terms to Learn (*continued*)

Diabetic coma	A life-threatening diabetes complication that causes unconsciousness. In persons with diabetes, dangerously high blood sugar (hyperglycemia) or dangerously low blood sugar (hypoglycemia) can lead to a diabetic coma.
End-stage renal disease	The final stage of chronic kidney disease in which the kidneys no longer function adequately to meet the needs of daily life.
Exophthalmos	Abnormal protrusion of the eyeball.
Fragility fracture	Any fall from a standing height or less, that results in a fracture.
Graves disease	A common form of hyperthyroidism that is an autoimmune disease characterized by goiter, rapid and irregular heartbeat, weight loss, irritability, anxiety, and often a slight protrusion of the eyeballs—caused by the production of thyroid-stimulating immunoglobins (antibody) against the thyroid-stimulation hormone (TSH) receptor.
Glucocorticoids	Any of a group of corticosteroids (as cortisol or dexamethasone) that are involved especially in carbohydrate, protein, and fat metabolism, that tend to increase liver glycogen and blood sugar by increasing gluconeogenesis, that are anti-inflammatory and immunosuppressive, and that are used widely in medicine (as in the alleviation of the symptoms of rheumatoid arthritis).
Goiter	An enlargement of the thyroid gland that is commonly visible as a swelling of the anterior part of the neck, that often results from insufficient intake of iodine and then is usually accompanied by hypothyroidism, and in other cases is associated with hyperthyroidism usually together with toxic symptoms and exophthalmos.
Hashimoto disease	Also known as chronic lymphocytic thyroiditis; an autoimmune disease in which the thyroid gland is gradually destroyed.
Hirsutism	Excessive growth of hair of normal or abnormal distribution.
Hormone	A product of living cells that circulates in body fluids and produces a specific, often stimulatory, effect on the activity of cells, usually a distance from its point of synthesis.
Hyperadrenalism	The presence of an excess of adrenal hormones (as epinephrine) in the blood.
Hyperinsulinemia	The presence of excess insulin in the blood.
Hyperparathyroidism	The presence of excess parathyroid hormone in the body, resulting in disturbance of calcium metabolism with increase in serum calcium and decrease in inorganic phosphorus, loss of calcium from bone, and renal damage, with frequent kidney stone formation.
Hyperthyroidism	Excessive functional activity of the thyroid gland; *also*, the resulting condition marked especially by increased metabolic rate, enlargement of the thyroid gland, rapid heart rate, and high blood pressure; called also *thyrotoxicosis*.
Hypoadrenalism	Abnormally decreased activity of the adrenal glands.
Hypothyroidism	Deficient activity of the thyroid gland; *also*, a resultant bodily condition characterized by lowered metabolic rate and general loss of vigor.
Hypoparathyroidism	Deficiency of parathyroid hormone in the body; *also*, the resultant abnormal state marked by low serum calcium and a tendency to chronic tetany.
Hypothalamus	A basal part of the diencephalon that lies beneath the thalamus on each side, forms the floor of the third ventricle, and includes vital autonomic regulatory centers (as for the control of food intake).
Insulin resistance	Reduced sensitivity to insulin by the body's insulin-dependent processes (as glucose uptake, lipolysis, and inhibition of glucose production by the liver) that results in decreased activity of these processes or an increase in insulin production or both, and that is typical of type II diabetes but often occurs in the absence of diabetes.
Ischemia	Deficient supply of blood to a body part (as the heart or brain) that is due to obstruction of the inflow of arterial blood (as by the narrowing of arteries by spasm or disease).
Metabolic acidosis	Acidosis resulting from excess acid due to abnormal metabolism, excessive acid intake, or renal retention or from excessive loss of bicarbonate (as in diarrhea).
Metabolic syndrome	A syndrome marked by the presence of usually three or more of a group of factors (as high blood pressure, abdominal obesity, high triglyceride levels, low high-density lipoprotein [HDL] levels, and high fasting levels of blood sugar) that are linked to an increased risk of cardiovascular disease and type II diabetes—also called *insulin resistance syndrome*, *syndrome X*.

High-Yield Terms to Learn (*continued*)

Metabolism	The sum of the processes in the buildup and destruction of protoplasm; specifically, the chemical changes in living cells by which energy is provided for vital processes and activities and new material is assimilated.
Mineralocorticoid	A corticosteroid (as aldosterone) that affects chiefly the electrolyte and fluid balance in the body.
Moon face	The full rounded facies characteristic especially of Cushing syndrome and typically associated with deposition of fat.
Myocardial infarction	An acute episode of coronary heart disease marked by the death or damage of heart muscle due to insufficient blood supply to the heart muscle, usually as a result of a coronary artery becoming blocked by a blood clot formed in response to a ruptured or torn fatty arterial deposit.
Myxedema	Severe hypothyroidism characterized by firm inelastic edema, dry skin and hair, and loss of mental and physical vigor.
Negative feedback	Feedback that tends to stabilize a process by reducing its rate or output when its effects are too great.
Osmotic diuresis	Increased urination due to the presence of certain substances in the fluid filtered by the kidneys. This fluid eventually becomes urine. These substances cause additional water to come into the urine, increasing its amount.
Osteoblast	A bone-forming cell.
Osteoclast	Any of the large multinucleate cells closely associated with areas of bone resorption (as in a fracture that is healing).
Osteomalacia	A disease of adults that is characterized by softening of the bones and is analogous to rickets in the young.
Osteoporosis	A condition that affects especially older women and is characterized by decrease in bone mass with decreased density and enlargement of bone spaces producing porosity and brittleness.
Periarthritis	Inflammation of the structures (as the muscles, tendons, and bursa of the shoulder) around a joint.
Pituitary	Relating to the pituitary gland.
Polydipsia	Excessive or abnormal thirst.
Polyphagia	Excessive appetite or eating.
Polyuria	Excessive secretion of urine.
Positive feedback	A process that occurs in a feedback loop in which the effects of a small disturbance on a system include an increase in the magnitude of the perturbation (childbirth, blood clotting).
Retinopathy	Any of various noninflammatory disorders of the retina, including some that cause blindness.
Rickets	A deficiency disease that affects the young during the period of skeletal growth, is characterized especially by soft and deformed bones, and is caused by failure to assimilate and use calcium and phosphorus, normally due to inadequate sunlight or vitamin D.
Stroke	Sudden impairment or loss of consciousness, sensation, and voluntary motion that is caused by rupture or obstruction (as by a clot) of a blood vessel supplying the brain and is accompanied by permanent damage of brain tissue.
Thyroid storm	A sudden life-threatening exacerbation of the symptoms (as high fever, tachycardia, weakness, or extreme restlessness) of hyperthyroidism that is brought on by various causes (as infection, surgery, or stress).

and the **pituitary gland**, and by **positive** and **negative feedback** from target cells.

Initiation of synthesis, secretion, and biologic activity of most hormones is caused by a regulated cascade of events that begins in the hypothalamus of the brain and ends at the target tissue, with some exceptions (pancreatic and adrenal medulla hormones). The hypothalamus and the pituitary in the brain control many other endocrine glands. The hypothalamus receives signals from diverse sources such as the thalamus, reticular activating system, and limbic system, which it collects, integrates, and creates releasing hormones. The secretion of pituitary hormones is controlled by releasing factors or neurosecretory cells from the hypothalamus, giving rise to the concept of the **hypothalamic–pituitary axis** (Figure 5–2). Hormonal balance must be maintained within a narrow range. Too little or too much of a hormone may produce profound changes in the body systemically, including abnormalities of the central nervous system, joints, and integumentary systems, gastrointestinal and genitourinary systems, cardiopulmonary system,

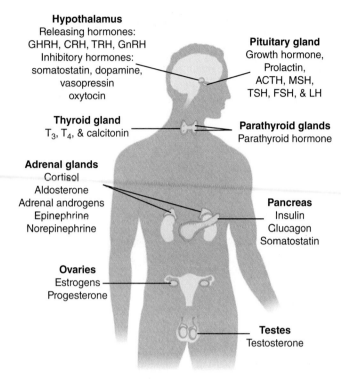

FIGURE 5-1 The endocrine system. (From General principles of endocrine physiology. In: Molina PE. *Endocrine Physiology.* 5th ed. New York, NY: McGraw-Hill; 2018. Chapter 1. https://accessmedicine.mhmedical.com/content.aspx?bookid=2343&sectionid=183487986#1150880483.)

and the reproductive system. Table 5–1 provides an overview of selected hormone systems and their most important actions.

The metabolic and neuroendocrine systems work together to maintain and control storage and mobilization of energy reserves required for cellular work for basic life functions (metabolism). Metabolism includes a range of biochemical processes that occur within the cell, and consists of building up cells/tissues (**anabolism**) and breaking down cells/tissues (**catabolism**). The basic functions of cellular metabolism are presented in Figure 5–3. Many of these functions require an energy source. Carbohydrates, fats, and proteins can all be utilized by cells to synthesize adenosine triphosphate (ATP), which is used as an energy source for almost all cellular functions (metabolism). Hormones, digestion, exercise, and temperature alter cell function by altering the activity of enzymes and thus altering the cells' metabolism. ATP energizes cellular synthesis and growth, muscle contraction, membrane transport, glandular secretion, nerve conduction, and active absorption. If greater amounts of energy are needed for cellular activities, it can be provided by oxidative aerobic metabolism and anaerobic breakdown of glucose. Alterations in metabolism can lead to bone, neuronal, and fluid and electrolyte disorders. Exercise can stimulate the release of several main hormones that will lead to muscle, fat, bone, and tissue responses outlined in Table 5–2.

EXAMINATION

The physical therapist's examination includes taking the individual's history, conducting a standardized systems review, and performing selected tests and measures to identify potential and existing movement-related disorders. The physical therapist may

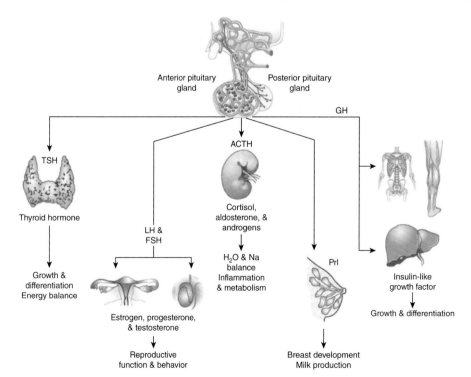

FIGURE 5-2 The hypothalamic pituitary axis. (From Molina PE. *Endocrine Physiology, 5e*; 2018. Available at: https://accessmedicine.mhmedical.com/content.aspx?bookid=2343&sectionid=183488163 Accessed: August 09, 2018. Copyright (c) 2018 McGraw-Hill Education. All rights reserved.)

decide to use one, more than one, or portions of several specific tests and measures as part of the examination, based on the purpose of the visit, the complexity of the condition, and the directions taken in the clinical decision-making process. Tests and measures that may be relevant to endocrine and metabolic disorders include but are not limited to:

- Aerobic capacity and endurance (eg, osteoporosis, diabetes)
- Anthropometric characteristics (eg, weight gain, weight loss)
- Balance (eg, diabetes mellitus with peripheral neuropathy)
- Circulation (arterial, venous, lymphatic) (eg, diabetes)
- Cranial and nerve integrity (eg, Ménière disease, viral encephalitis)
- Joint integrity and mobility (eg, gout, osteoporosis)
- Muscle performance (eg, diabetes)
- Neuromotor development and sensory processing (eg, fetal alcohol syndrome, lead poisoning)
- Pain (eg, osteoporosis, rheumatologic disease)
- Integumentary integrity (eg, diabetes, liver disease, kidney disease)

TABLE 5–1 Endocrine hormones.

Location/ Endocrine Gland	Hormone(s)	Target Tissue/Organ	Function
Pineal gland	Melatonin	Brain, other tissue	Circadian rhythm immune function antioxidant
Hypothalamus	Growth hormone–releasing hormone (GHRH), growth hormone inhibitor hormone (IH) (somatostatin), thyrotropin-releasing hormone (TRH), corticotropin-releasing hormone (CRH), gonadotropin-releasing hormone (GRH)	Anterior and posterior pituitary	Stimulation of hormones released from the posterior pituitary and hormones that regulate the anterior pituitary
Posterior pituitary	Antidiuretic hormone (ADH); also called vasopressin	Kidney	Increases water reabsorption by kidneys and causes vasoconstriction and increased blood pressure
	Oxytocin	Myoepithelial muscle of breast; uterus	Stimulates milk ejection from breasts and uterine contractions
Anterior pituitary	Growth hormone (GH)	Liver, bone, muscle, kidney, and others	Stimulates the liver to produce growth factors that stimulate bone and cartilage growth
	Thyroid-stimulating hormone (TSH)	Thyroid	Stimulates synthesis and secretion of thyroid hormones
	Adrenocorticotropic hormone (ACTH)	Adrenal cortex	Stimulates synthesis and secretion of adrenal cortical hormones
	Follicle-stimulating hormone (FSH)	Gonads	Causes growth of follicles in ovaries and sperm maturation in testes
	Leutinizing hormone (LH)		Stimulates testosterone synthesis in testes, stimulates ovulation, formation of corpus luteum and estrogen and progesterone synthesis in ovaries
	Prolactin	Breast	Stimulates mammary gland growth and milk production
Thyroid	Thyroxine (T4) and triiodothyronine (T3)	Most cells	Increases rate of chemical reaction in most cells, thus increasing metabolic rate
	Calcitonin		Promotes deposition of calcium in bone and decreased extracellular fluid calcium ion concentration
Adrenal cortex	Cortisol		Multiple metabolic functions for controlling metabolism of proteins, carbohydrates, and fate; also, anti-inflammatory effects
	Aldosterone		Increased renal sodium reabsorption, potassium secretion and hydrogen ion secretion
Adrenal medulla	Norepinephrine, epinephrine	Heart, lungs	Same effects as sympathetic stimulation
Pancreas	Insulin (beta cells)	Many cells	Promotes glucose entry into many cells; in this way controls carbohydrate metabolism
	Glucagon (alpha cells)		Increases the synthesis and release of glucose from the liver into the body fluids
Parathyroid	Parathyroid hormone (PTH)	Gut, kidneys, bone	Controls serum calcium ion concentration by increasing calcium absorption by the gut and kidneys and releasing calcium from bone

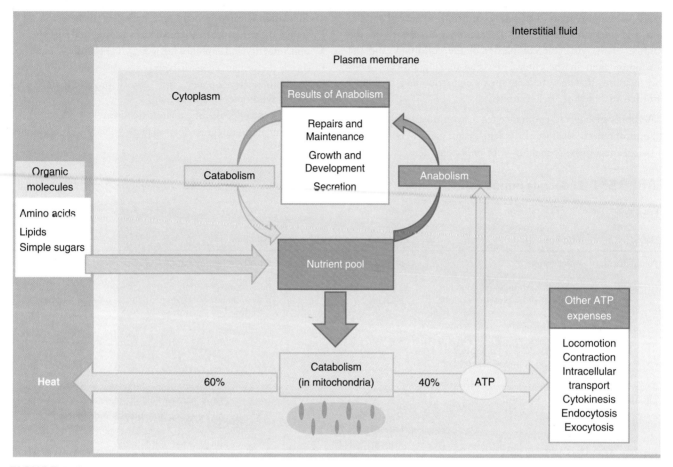

FIGURE 5–3 The basic functions of cellular metabolism.

TABLE 5–2 Hormones released during acute exercise.

Hormone	Stimulant for Release	Target Tissue	Response
Epinephrine	Moderate to intense exercise, stress, hypotension	Skeletal muscle	↑ Glycogenolysis (breakdown of glycogen), vasoconstriction
Norepinephrine	Moderate to intense exercise, hypoglycemia	Adipose tissue, liver	↑ Lipolysis (breakdown of fat), ↑ heart rate, ↑ glycogenolysis
Growth hormone (GH)	Exercise, hypoglycemia	Skeletal tissue, bone, adipose tissue, liver	Stimulation of growth, FFA mobilization, ↑ gluconeogenesis, ↓ glucose uptake
Testosterone	↑ FSH, ↑ LH, exercise, stress	Skeletal muscle, bone	Protein synthesis, sperm production, sex drive
Estrogen	↑ FSH, ↑ LH, light to moderate exercise	Skeletal muscle, adipose tissue	Inhibition of glucose uptake, fat deposition
Cortisol	↑ ACTH, intense prolonged exercise	Skeletal muscle, adipose tissue, liver	↑ Gluconeogenesis, ↑ protein synthesis, ↓ glucose uptake
Insulin-like growth factor (IGF-1)	↑ GH	Almost all cells	Stimulation of growth

FSH, follicle-stimulating hormone; LH, leutinizing hormone; ACTH, adrenocorticotropic hormone; GH, growth hormone.

■ FOUNDATIONS FOR EVALUATION, DIFFERENTIAL DIAGNOSIS, PROGNOSIS, AND INTERVENTIONS

ABNORMALITIES OF THE THYROID

Hyperthyroid

Hyperthyroidism (overactive thyroid; also called thyrotoxicosis) is a condition in which the thyroid gland is overactive and makes excessive amounts of thyroid. When the thyroid gland is overactive, the body's metabolism speeds up and patients experience nervousness, anxiety, weight loss, sweating, rapid heartbeat (tachycardia), and hand tremor (Table 5–3). **Graves disease** is the most common form of hyperthyroidism and is an autoimmune disease in which antibodies form against the thyroid-stimulation hormone (TSH) receptor to induce continual activation. **Thyroid storm** is a condition associated with inadequately treated hyperthyroidism. This is an acute episode of thyroid overactivity characterized by high fever, severe tachycardia, delirium, dehydration, and extreme irritability.

TABLE 5–3 Key features of hyperthyroid and hypothyroid.

Hyperthyroid (Thyrotoxicosis)	Hypothyroid
Warm, moist skin due to capillary dilation	Pale, cool puffy yellowish skin, face, and hands Brittle hair and nails
Sweating, heat intolerance	Sensation of being cold
Tachycardia, increased stroke volume, cardiac output and pulse pressure	Bradycardia, decreased stroke volume, cardiac output, and pulse pressure
Dyspnea, weakness of respiratory muscles, hypoventilation	Pleural effusions, hypoventilation, and CO_2 retention
Increased appetite	Reduced appetite
Nervousness, irritability, hyperkinesia, tremor	Lethargy, general slowing for mental processes, depression
Weakness, atrophy, increased deep tendon reflexes, periarthritis	Stiffness, decreased deep tendon reflexes, carpal tunnel syndrome, muscle and joint edema
Menstrual irregularity, decreased fertility	Infertility, decreased libido, impotence, oligospermia
Weight loss	Weight gain
Reaction of upper lid with wide stare, exophthalmos (Graves disease)	Drooping eyelids

Clinical Significance

Disturbances include the following:

1. In hyperthyroidism, the thyroid gland is increased to two to three times its normal size (goiter), with tremendous hyperplasia and infoldings of the follicular cell lining in the follicles so the number of cells is increased.
2. With increased cells, an increased production of thyroid hormone occurs.
3. In Graves disease, antibodies called thyroid-stimulating immunoglobulins (TSIs) form against the TSH receptor in the thyroid gland. The TSI antibody binds the TSH receptors and increases the activation of cyclic adenosine monophosphate (cAMP), with the resultant development of hyperthyroid.
4. Hyperthyroid can occasionally occur because of a localized adenoma (tumor) that secretes large quantities of thyroid hormone.

Diagnostic Tests and Measures
Blood tests

- Thyroid function tests
  - Concentration of "free" thyroxine in plasma
  - Concentration of TSH
  - Concentration of TSI
- Basal metabolic rate (BMR)

Imaging

- Magnetic resonance imaging (MRI)
- Computed tomography (CT)

Clinical Findings, Secondary Effects, Complications

1. High state of excitability with nervousness or other psychic disorders
2. Extreme fatigue but inability to sleep
3. Impaired cardiopulmonary function (increased heart and respiratory rates)
4. Intolerance of heat and increased sweating
5. Hyper metabolism
6. Mild to extreme weight loss (sometimes as much as 100 lb)
7. Varying degrees of diarrhea
8. Muscle weakness (proximal)
9. Tremor of the hands
10. **Exophthalmos**
11. **Periarthritis**
12. Osteoporosis

Interventions/Treatment

Medical—The most direct treatment for hyperthyroid is partial or complete surgical removal of the thyroid gland. Antithyroid medications and radioactive iodine are also used for treatment.

Pharmacological—Prior to surgery, the gland is prepared with propylthiouracil to assist in BMR reduction. High concentrations of iodides are administered 1 to 2 weeks prior to surgery to cause the gland to recede in size and diminish its blood supply.

Radioactive iodine therapy can destroy most of the secretory cells of the thyroid gland.

Propylthiouracil and methimazole directly inhibit thyroid hormone synthesis.

Beta blockers can be a helpful adjuvant for symptoms of tachycardia, palpitations, and restlessness.

Physical therapy—Physical therapists will potentially treat patients with endocrine dysfunction as a comorbidity or due to the clinical findings of the pathology itself. Physical therapists will address impairments and activity limitations such as exercise intolerance and decreased exercise capacity, proximal weakness, atrophy, arthralgia, gait abnormalities, balance impairment, fatigue, poor endurance, and self-care.

Physical therapy interventions should address the underlying findings from the physical therapy evaluation targeting movement abnormalities. Activities may include pain management, strengthening, therapeutic exercise, balance training, functional training, energy conservation techniques, and activities of daily living training.

Differential Diagnosis

- Endocrine disorders
- Cancer
- Autoimmune disorders
- Blood disorders
- Gastrointestinal disorders

Hypothyroid

Hypothyroidism (underactive thyroid; also called myxedema) is a condition in which the thyroid gland does not produce enough thyroid hormones. Hypothyroidism is characterized by slowed metabolic rate, fatigue, extreme muscle sluggishness, and cardiac abnormalities (Table 5–3). Hypothyroidism is often initiated by autoimmunity against the thyroid gland, known as **Hashimoto disease**.

Cretinism is caused by extreme hypothyroid during fetal life, infancy, or childhood. This condition is characterized especially by failure of body growth and by intellectual disability.

Clinical Significance

Disturbances include the following:

1. Hypothyroidism is caused by autoimmune thyroiditis that destroys the gland, causing progressive deterioration and finally fibrosis of the gland.
2. Hypothyroidism results in diminished or absent secretion of thyroid hormone.
3. Goiter (enlargement of the thyroid) can be caused by dietary iodide and iodine deficiency.

Diagnostic Tests and Measures
Blood tests

- Thyroid function tests
  - Concentration of "free" thyroxine in plasma
  - Concentration of TSH
- BMR

Imaging

- MRI
- CT
- Ultrasound
- Chest x-ray
- Dual-energy x-ray absorptiometry (DEXA) for medication use

Clinical Findings, Secondary Effects, Complications

1. Goiter
2. Fatigue
3. Extreme somnolence, with sleeping up to 12 to 14 hours a day
4. Extreme muscular sluggishness
5. Cold sensitivity
6. Slowed heart rate, decreased cardiac output, decreased blood volume
7. Increased body weight
8. Constipation
9. Mental sluggishness
10. Depression
11. Failure of many trophic functions in the body (hair, skin)
12. Myxedema (edematous appearance throughout the body)
13. Cardiac abnormalities
14. Poor circulation
15. Atherosclerosis
16. Joint edema
17. Carpal tunnel syndrome
18. Back pain

Interventions/Treatment

Medical—Hormone replacement therapy; reverse symptoms, prevent progression.

Pharmacological—Thyroxine (levothyroxine, liothyronine) daily.

Physical therapy—Physical therapists will potentially treat patients with endocrine dysfunction as a comorbidity or due to the clinical findings of the pathology itself. Physical therapists will address functional impairments such as activity intolerance, weakness, atrophy, gait abnormalities, balance impairment, poor endurance, and weight gain.

Physical therapy interventions should address the underlying findings from the physical therapy evaluation targeting movement abnormalities. Activities may include strengthening, therapeutic exercise, balance training, functional training, energy conservation techniques, and activities of daily living training.

Differential Diagnosis

- Endocrine disorders
- Cancer
- Nonmalignant tumors
- Cardiac disorders
- Autoimmune disorders
- Gastrointestinal disorders
- Renal disorders

ABNORMALITIES OF ADRENAL CORTICAL SECRETION

Addison Disease

Hypoadrenalism (adrenal insufficiency)—insufficient production or release of glucocorticoids (cortisol), mineralocorticoids (aldosterone), and androgens (testosterone, estrogen). Most frequently caused by primary atrophy or injury of the adrenal cortices. Because half of all people with idiopathic Addison disease have circulating autoantibodies that react against adrenal tissue, this condition can also have an autoimmune basis. These hormones have key roles in response to stress, electrolyte and fluid balance for maintenance of blood pressure, conversion of food to energy, and the inflammatory response. An acute form of the disease is called **Addisonian crisis**, in which patients have severe abdominal pain, back and leg pain, severe vomiting, and hypotension due to low levels of cortisol.

Clinical Significance

Disturbances include:

1. Mineralocorticoid (aldosterone) deficiency due to lack of sodium reabsorption, allowing sodium, chloride, and water to be lost in urine, leading to decreased extracellular fluid volume with hyponatremia, hyperkalemia, and mild acidosis. As the extracellular fluid becomes depleted, plasma volume falls, red blood cell concentration increases, and cardiac output and blood pressure decrease.
2. Glucocorticoid (cortisol) deficiency makes it difficult for the person with Addison disease to maintain normal blood glucose, protein and fat mobilization between meals. This depresses metabolism including muscle function.
3. Melanin pigmentation increases in the mucous membranes and skin of persons with Addison disease, which is thought to be linked to the lack of negative feedback of adrenocorticotropic hormone (ACTH), leading to increased melatonin-stimulating hormone.

Diagnostic Tests and Measures
Blood tests

- Hormone levels (ACTH, cortisol)
- Electrolyte levels (Na^+, K^+)

Imaging

- CT scans

Selected Clinical Findings, Secondary Effects, Complications

1. Muscle weakness
2. Fatigue, decreased activity tolerance
3. Poor endurance
4. Loss of appetite, weight loss
5. Hypoglycemia
6. Hypotension
7. Hyperpigmentation
8. Metabolic derangement
9. Pain (joints, lower back, leg)

Interventions/Treatment

Medical—Address the cause (impaired pituitary function, impaired adrenal gland, other).

Pharmacological—Hormone replacement, electrolyte replacement.

Physical therapy—Physical therapists will potentially treat patients with endocrine dysfunction as a comorbidity or due to the clinical findings of the pathology itself. Physical therapists will address functional impairments such as weakness, atrophy, gait abnormalities, balance impairment, and poor endurance.

Physical therapy interventions should address the underlying findings from the physical therapy evaluation targeting movement abnormalities. Activities may include strengthening, therapeutic exercise, balance training, functional training, energy conservation techniques, and activities of daily living training.

The clinical setting should have carbohydrates available if needed secondary to a drop in blood sugar, ability to monitor blood pressure, or response to treatment.

Differential Diagnosis

- Endocrine disorders
- Autoimmune disease
- Gastrointestinal disorders
- Gynecologic disorders
- Tuberculosis
- Cancer

Cushing Syndrome

Hyperadrenalism is most commonly due to excess secretion of ACTH by the anterior pituitary, leading to excessive production and release of **glucocorticoids** (**cortisol**), mineral corticoids (**aldosterone**), and **androgens**. Hypersecretion can lead to Cushing syndrome with abnormalities ascribable to increased amounts of cortisol and androgens. Hypercortisolism can also occur with administration of large amounts of glucocorticoids over prolonged periods for therapeutic purposes (such as chronic inflammation). A unique characterization of Cushing syndrome is the mobilization of fat from the lower part of the body, with deposition of the fat in the thoracic and upper abdominal regions (**buffalo torso**). Excess secretion of steroids also leads to an edematous appearance of the face (**moon face**), and the androgenic potency of some hormones can cause acne and **hirsutism** (excess growth of facial hair).

Clinical Significance

Disturbances include the following:

1. The abundance of cortisol can cause increased blood sugar concentration, sometimes to levels twice normal after meals (hyperglycemia, diabetes).
2. The effect of increased glucocorticoids on protein metabolism causes greatly reduced tissue proteins almost everywhere in the body except the liver.
3. The loss of proteins from muscle can cause fatigue, severe weakness, and paralysis, and can lead to tendon rupture.
4. The loss of protein from the lymphatic tissue impairs immune function, leading to infections, with increased mortality due to infections.
5. Mobilization of fat from the lower body with deposition in the thoracic and upper abdominal regions can occur.
6. The skin has decreased protein collagen fibers so that the subcutaneous tissue tears easily, resulting in the development of large purplish striae (stretch marks). The skin is at risk for bruising and poor wound healing.
7. Severely diminished protein deposition in bone leads to severe osteoporosis.

Diagnostic Tests and Measures
Blood tests

- Plasma levels of ACTH and cortisol
- Dexamethasone test

Imaging

- CT scan
- MRI
- X-ray

Clinical Findings, Secondary Effects, Complications

1. Fatigue
2. Severe muscle weakness
3. Paralysis
4. Tendon rupture
5. Excess body fat
6. Round face (moon face)
7. Weight loss/gain
8. Osteoporosis
9. Hyperglycemia
10. Diabetes
11. Low back pain
12. Cardiac abnormalities
13. Gastrointestinal abnormalities

Interventions

Medical—Address the cause of the syndrome (tumor removal, partial adrenalectomy, radiation). Administration of adrenal steroids to make up for any insufficiency that develops.

Pharmacological—Medications that block steroidogenesis (metyrapone, ketoconazole) or inhibit ACTH secretion (serotonin agonists and GABA transaminase inhibitors). If removal of the adrenal gland is necessary, adrenal should be administered. Medications for cardiac dysfunction and diabetes may also be indicated.

Physical therapy—Physical therapists will potentially treat patients with endocrine dysfunction as a comorbidity or due to the clinical findings of the pathology itself. Physical therapists will address functional impairments such as weakness, gait abnormalities, balance impairment, poor endurance, and wound healing.

Differential Diagnosis

- Other corticoadrenal hyperactivity
- Autoimmune dysfunction
- Cardiovascular disease
- Pituitary dysfunction
- Gastrointestinal dysfunction

ABNORMALITIES OF THE PANCREAS

Diabetes Mellitus

Diabetes mellitus (DM) is a syndrome of impaired metabolism of carbohydrate, fat, and proteins caused by either a lack of insulin production by the pancreas or decreased sensitivity of the tissues to insulin. The two general types are diabetes type I, caused by a lack of insulin secretion in the pancreas, and diabetes type II, initially caused by decreased sensitivity of target tissues to the metabolic effect of insulin. This reduced sensitivity to insulin is often called **"insulin resistance."** **"Metabolic syndrome"**—a cluster of conditions including increased blood pressure, high blood sugar, excess body fat around the waist and abdomen, increased cholesterol and triglyceride levels, increasing risk for heart disease, stroke, and diabetes—typically precedes type II diabetes.

In both types of DM, metabolism of all the main foodstuffs is altered. The basic effect of insulin lack or insulin resistance on glucose metabolism is to prevent efficient uptake and utilization of glucose by most cells of the body. As a result, blood glucose concentration increases, cell utilization of glucose falls increasingly lower, and utilization of fats and proteins increases.

Clinical Significance

Disturbances include the following:
Type I

1. Injury to beta cells of the pancreas or diseases that impair insulin production lead to diabetes type I. Type I may develop abruptly, over a period of a few days or weeks, with three principal sequelae: increased blood glucose, increased utilization of fats for energy (formation of cholesterol by the liver), and depletion of the body's proteins.
2. Blood glucose levels are increased, causing loss in urine (**polyuria**). Increased blood glucose causes dehydration due to osmotic transfer of water out of the cells and loss of water in the kidney (**osmotic diuresis**). Dehydration leads to excessive thirst (**polydipsia**).

3. Chronic high blood sugar causes tissue damage. Blood vessels in multiple tissues in the body begin to function abnormally and undergo structural changes that result in inadequate blood flow to the tissues (**ischemia**). This in turn leads to risk of **myocardial infarction, stroke, end-stage renal disease, retinopathy,** and blindness. In addition, chronically high glucose levels damage peripheral nerves (polyneuropathy) and cause autonomic nervous system dysfunction (impaired cardiac reflexes).

4. DM causes increased utilization of fats and **metabolic acidosis**. The shift from carbohydrate to fat metabolism increases the release of keto acids. As a result, patients develop severe metabolic acidosis from the excess keto acids, which is associated with dehydration due to excessive urine formation. This rapidly leads to **diabetic coma** if untreated. Excess fat utilization in the liver causes large amounts of cholesterol in the blood, leading to atherosclerosis and other vascular lesions.

5. DM can deplete the body of proteins. Failure to use glucose for energy leads to increased utilization and decreased storage of proteins and fats. Therefore, a person with DM suffers rapid weight loss and lack of energy despite eating large amounts of food (**polyphagia**). Without treatment, metabolic abnormalities cause severe body wasting and mortality in weeks.

Type II

1. Obesity (increase of visceral fat), insulin resistance, and "metabolic syndrome" usually precede the development of diabetes type II. Type II diabetes is associated with increased plasma insulin concentration (**hyperinsulinemia**). This occurs as a compensatory response by the beta cells of the pancreas for diminished sensitivity of target tissues to the metabolic effects of insulin (insulin resistance).

2. "Insulin resistance" is part of a cascade of disorders that is often called "metabolic syndrome," which often precedes DM type II. Features of metabolic syndrome include obesity, insulin resistance, fasting hyperglycemia, lipid abnormalities, and hypertension. Several of these metabolic abnormalities increase the risk of cardiovascular disease.

Clinical Findings, Secondary Effects, Complications

1. Hyperglycemia
2. Glycosuria
3. Polyuria
4. Polydipsia
5. Polyphagia
6. Atherosclerosis
7. Arteriosclerosis
8. Severe coronary heart disease
9. Hypertension
10. Susceptibility to infection
11. Retinopathy
12. Cataracts
13. Polyneuropathy
14. Chronic renal disease
15. Polyuria
16. Fatigue
17. Weight loss/gain
18. Weakness
19. Poor endurance
20. Metabolic syndrome
21. Hyperlipidemia

Diagnostic Tests and Measures
Blood tests

- Glucose (plasma glucose concentrations ≥200 mg/dL)
- HbA1c (≥6.5%)
- Urinary glucose
- Fasting blood glucose (>126 mg/dL) and insulin levels
- Glucose tolerance test
- Acetone breath
- Kidney function

Imaging

- Ultrasound
- CT scan
- MRI

Interventions/Treatment

Medical—Effective treatment of type I DM requires administration of insulin so that the patient will have enough insulin for normal metabolism of carbohydrates, fats, and proteins. In persons with type II diabetes, dieting and exercise are recommended to induce weight loss and reverse the insulin resistance. Drugs may also be administered to increase insulin sensitivity or to simulate increased production of insulin by the pancreas, or exogenous insulin will be provided to metabolize foodstuff.

Pharmacological—Drugs may also be administered (pump, oral, injection) to increase insulin sensitivity or to simulate increased production of insulin by the pancreas, or exogenous insulin will be provided to metabolize foodstuff.

Physical therapy—Physical therapists will potentially treat patients with endocrine dysfunction as a comorbidity or due to the clinical findings of the pathology itself. The physical therapy examination should include vital signs, vascular (peripheral pulses) and neurologic examination (sensory neuropathy), and a foot assessment. Physical therapists will educate the patient on diabetic foot care, control of risk factors (obesity, physical inactivity), and disease management. The physical therapist will address functional impairments such as weakness, gait abnormalities, balance impairment, poor endurance, polyneuropathy, amputation, and wound healing. Physical therapists should monitor blood glucose levels, as this relates to when and how the patient has taken medication, if they have eaten, and response to exercise. If blood glucose levels are high (at or near 250 mg/dL) or if blood glucose levels are poorly controlled, exercise is contraindicated. Clinics should have carbohydrates available for low blood sugar. Interventions may include therapeutic exercise, self-care management for skin integrity, peripheral neuropathy risk, stump care, prosthetic use, and generalized fitness for life. Patients may require wound management.

Differential Diagnosis

- Autoimmune disorders
- Endocrine disorders
- Gastrointestinal disorders
- Cancer

ABNORMALITIES OF THE PARATHYROID

Hyperparathyroidism

Hyperparathyroidism is an abnormality of the parathyroid gland leading to excess secretion of parathyroid hormone (PTH), which may be due to an impairment of the parathyroid (primary) or due to lack of vitamin D or chronic renal disease (secondary). Hyperparathyroidism causes extreme **osteoclastic** activity in the bones. This elevates the calcium ion concentration in the extracellular fluid while depressing the concentration of phosphate ions because of increased renal excretion of phosphate.

Clinical Significance

Disturbances include the following:

1. Bone disease in hyperparathyroidism can occur in severe cases because osteoclastic resorption of bone occurs at a faster rate than **osteoblastic** deposition, and the bone may be eaten away almost entirely. The person with severe hyperparathyroidism often seeks medical treatment due to bone fractures.
2. Hyperparathyroidism can cause the plasma calcium level to rise significantly. The effects of elevated calcium can lead to depression of the central and peripheral nervous systems, muscle weakness, constipation, abdominal pain, peptic ulcer, lack of appetite, and depressed relaxation of the heart during diastole. Hyperparathyroidism can also lead to **osteoporosis**, which diminishes bone through excess osteoclastic activity. Osteoporosis can also be caused by lack of physical stress on bone due to inactivity, malnutrition, lack of vitamin C, postmenopausal lack of estrogen, increased age, and Cushing syndrome. Thus many deficiencies of protein metabolism can cause osteoporosis.
3. When increased quantities of PTH are secreted, the level of calcium in the body fluids rises. Phosphate rises as well because the kidneys cannot excrete it rapidly enough. This causes both calcium and phosphate in the blood to become supersaturated so that calcium phosphate crystals ($CaHPO_4$) begin to deposit in the alveoli of the lungs, tubules of the kidneys, thyroid gland, stomach mucosa, and arteriole walls. This extensive metastatic deposition can occur over a few days. Many clients with hyperparathyroid will develop kidney stones.
4. Secondary hyperparathyroidism can be caused by vitamin D deficiency or chronic renal disease. The vitamin D deficiency leads to **osteomalacia** (inadequate mineralization of bone in adults), and high levels of PTH cause absorption of bones.
5. **Rickets** (a form of vitamin D deficiency) occurs mainly in children and results from calcium or phosphate deficiency in the extracellular fluid, usually due to a lack of vitamin D. Plasma concentrations of vitamin D and phosphate decrease with the phosphate being excreted in urine. During prolonged rickets, the marked compensatory increase in PTH secretion causes extreme osteoclastic absorption of the bone, which causes the bone to become progressively weaker.
6. If the bones finally become exhausted of calcium, the level of calcium may fall rapidly. As the blood levels of calcium fall below 7 mg/dL, the usual signs of tetani develop (muscle spasm).

Diagnostic Tests and Measures

Blood tests

- Thyroid function tests
- Elevated calcium
- Elevated parathyroid
- Plasma alkaline phosphatase
- Vitamin D deficiency
- Urinalysis

Imaging

- X-ray
- Ultrasound
- MRI
- CT scan
- DEXA scan

Clinical Findings, Secondary Effects, Complications

1. Fatigue
2. Depression
3. Forgetfulness
4. Hypercalcemia
5. Hypertension
6. Depression of the central and peripheral nervous systems
7. Muscle weakness (proximal)
8. Muscle spasms
9. Poor endurance
10. Constipation
11. Abdominal pain
12. Bone pain
13. Arthralgias
14. Gout
15. Joint hypermobility
16. Pathologic fractures
17. Peptic ulcer, lack of appetite
18. Kidney stones
19. Depressed relaxation of the heart during diastole

Interventions/Treatment

Medical—Effective treatment of parathyroid disorders may involve surgery to remove the glands and medications to address the cause, as well as lifestyle changes related to diet and exposure to sunlight.

Pharmacological—Medication may include vitamin D to assist with gastrointestinal absorption of calcium, calcium supplements, calcium mimetics, bisphosphonates, and hormone replacement therapy.

Physical therapy—Physical therapists will potentially treat patients with endocrine dysfunction as a comorbidity or due to the clinical findings of the pathology itself. Physical therapists will address functional impairments such as weakness, gait abnormalities, balance impairment, poor endurance, neuropathy, osteoporosis, and increased risk for falls. Patients with hyperparathyroid hormone may sustain pathological and fragility fractures that will require physical therapy interventions for improved functional ability.

Differential Diagnosis

- Autoimmune disorders
- Gastrointestinal dysfunction
- Endocrine disorders
- Renal impairment
- Vitamin D deficiency
- Rickets
- Osteomalacia
- Osteoporosis
- Osteopenia
- Kidney stones

Hypoparathyroidism

Hypoparathyroidism occurs when the parathyroid does not secrete sufficient parathyroid hormone, leading to depressed calcium reabsorption from the bone and osteoclasts becoming almost totally inactive. As a result, the calcium level in body fluids decreases. Yet because calcium and phosphate are not being absorbed from the bone, the bone usually remains strong. When low calcium levels are reached, signs of muscle tetany develop. Laryngeal musculature is especially sensitive to low calcium levels, and spasms can lead to obstruction of respiration.

Clinical Significance

Disturbances include:

1. Depressed calcium resorption from bone leading to decreased calcium levels in body fluids.
2. Muscle spasms (tetany) and neuromuscular problems due to low calcium.
3. Breathing difficulties may arise due to laryngeal spasms.

Diagnostic Tests and Measures
Blood tests

- Hypocalcemia
- Hypophosphatemia
- Hypomagnesemia
- Urinalysis
- Thyroid function tests

Imaging

- Ultrasound
- X-rays
- CT scans
- MRI
- DEXA

Clinical Findings, Secondary Effects, Complications

1. Muscle weakness
2. Neuroexcitability
3. Muscle spasm
4. Abdominal pain
5. Breathing difficulties
6. Cardiac abnormalities
7. Dry, scaly skin
8. Nausea, vomiting
9. Constipation, diarrhea
10. Irritability, depression, anxiety

Interventions/Treatment

Medical—Treatment for hypoparathyroid may include PTH and vitamin D replacement. PTH is only used occasionally because of the expense, the short half-life, and the tendency of the body to develop antibodies against it. In most patients with hypoparathyroidism, administration of extremely large doses of vitamin D keeps the calcium ion concentration in a normal range.

Pharmacological—Medication may include PTH, vitamin D replacement, and recommendation for dietary changes.

Physical therapy—Physical therapists will potentially treat patients with endocrine dysfunction as a comorbidity or due to the clinical findings of the pathology itself. Physical therapists will address functional impairments such as weakness, gait abnormalities, balance impairment, poor endurance, neuropathy, and increased risk for falls.

Differential Diagnosis

- Autoimmune disorders
- Gastrointestinal dysfunction
- Endocrine disorders
- Renal impairment

ABNORMALITIES OF BONE METABOLISM

Osteoporosis

Osteoporosis is the most common bone disease in adults, especially with increased age. Osteoporosis is characterized by decrease in bone mass resulting in weak or brittle bones. Bones that are weakened come with an increased risk for fractures, including **fragility fractures** (fall from standing height that results in fracture). Osteoporosis can be a primary bone disorder or secondary to many other disorders. Primary osteoporosis occurs with increased age and after menopause in women. Secondary osteoporosis can be caused through dietary alterations, medications, endocrine dysfunction, and lifestyle choices (sedentary lifestyle, alcohol consumption, smoking). Osteoporosis can be contrasted with osteomalacia (bone softening), osteopenia (low bone mass), and osteopetrosis (increased bone density).

Clinical Significance

Disturbances include:

1. Decreased bone matrix due to reduced osteoblast activity, increased osteoclastic activity, or both. As a result, the rate of bone osteoid deposition is diminished.
2. Destruction of bone mass and density, especially cortical bone thickness and cancellous bone trabeculae. Weakened bone can lead to increased fractures, fragility fractures, and bone deformity.
3. In primary osteoporosis, bone weakness occurs as one ages and accelerates during menopause. Etiology is considered to be multifactorial (age, gender, race, family history).
4. In secondary osteoporosis, reduction in hormone levels (estrogen, testosterone), thyroid and parathyroid overactivity, dietary factors (low calcium, food restrictions, changes in intestinal surface area), medications (steroid use), and medical conditions such as inflammatory bowel disease, rheumatoid arthritis, and cancer can all lead to increased risk.

Diagnostic Tests and Measures

Imaging

- DEXA (bone density testing T score of −2.5 or lower)
- Ultrasound
- CT
- MRI

Clinical Findings, Secondary Effects, Complications

1. Back pain due to vertebral compression fractures
2. Loss of height
3. Stooped or flex posture
4. Bone fracture from a standing height or less
5. Decreased physical activity

Interventions/Treatment

Medical—Nutrition to improve calcium, vitamin D, magnesium, and vitamin K levels. Medications to slow the breakdown of bone. Medical procedures may include kyphoplasty, vertebroplasty, and surgery for fractures.

Pharmacological—Medications can include bisphosphonates to slow bone breakdown, hormone replacement therapy, and hormone-like medications. Pain medications for pain management. Calcium and vitamin D (cholecalciferol).

Physical therapy—Physical therapists will potentially treat patients with osteoporosis to improve muscle strength, posture, the need for weight-bearing activities, balance activities, and pain management.

Treatment may be after surgery for fractures or for prevention and wellness. Physical therapists will address functional impairments such as weakness, atrophy, gait abnormalities, balance impairment, posture, and poor endurance. Physical therapy interventions should address the underlying findings from the physical therapy evaluation targeting movement abnormalities. Activities may include strengthening, therapeutic exercise, balance training, functional training, activities of daily living training, pain education, and need for assistive devices and/or home modifications. Calcium intake and vitamin D in conjunction with exercise should be discussed.

Differential Diagnosis

- Autoimmune disorders
- Endocrine/hormonal disorders
- Gastrointestinal disorders
- Bone disorders
- Cancer

■ SUMMARY

The endocrine and nervous systems work closely to coordinate a variety of physiologic functions to keep our body in homeostasis through the release and action of specific hormones. The combined efforts regulate metabolism, water and salt balance, blood pressure, response to stress, and sexual reproduction. As physical therapists, we must consider the body's hormonal, environmental, and energy requirements during rest and exercise conditions. Understanding physiology, pathology, and the medications to treat abnormalities is a prerequisite to determination of the best treatment interventions, progression, and care.

BIBLIOGRAPHY

Bauer DC, McPhee SJ. Thyroid disease. In: Hammer GD, McPhee SJ, eds. *Pathophysiology of Disease: An Introduction to Clinical Medicine.* 7th ed. New York, NY: McGraw-Hill; 2013: Chapter 20. http://accessphysiotherapy.mhmedical.com/content.aspx?bookid=961&sectionid=53555701. Accessed October 27, 2017.

Burke-Doe A. Screening for endocrine and metabolic disease. In: Goodman CC, Heick J, Lazaro RT, eds. *Differential Diagnosis for Physical Therapists: Screening for Referral.* 6th ed. St. Louis, MO: Elsevier; 2018: Chapter 11.

Ciccone CD. *Pharmacology in Rehabilitation.* 5th ed. Philadelphia, PA: F.A. Davis; 2015.

Else T, Hammer GD. Disorders of the Hypothalamus & Pituitary Gland. In: Hammer GD, McPhee SJ, eds. *Pathophysiology of Disease: An Introduction to Clinical Medicine.* 7th ed. New York, NY: McGraw-Hill; 2013: Chapter 19. http://accessphysiotherapy.mhmedical.com/content.aspx?bookid=961&sectionid=53555700. Accessed October 27, 2017.

Endocrine physiology. In: Kibble JD, Halsey CR, eds. *Medical Physiology: The Big Picture.* New York, NY: McGraw-Hill; 2014: Chapter 8. http://accessphysiotherapy.mhmedical.com/content.aspx?bookid=1291&sectionid=75577697. Accessed October 27, 2017.

Garcia AS, Shamus E. Osteoporosis. In: Shamus E, ed. *The Color Atlas of Physical Therapy.* New York, NY: McGraw-Hill;

2015: Chapter 135. http://accessphysiotherapy.mhmedical.com/content.aspx?bookid=1491&sectionid=90322411. Accessed October 28, 2017.

General principles of endocrine physiology. In: Molina PE. *Endocrine Physiology*. 4th ed. New York, NY: McGraw-Hill; 2013: Chapter 1. http://accessmedicine.mhmedical.com/content.aspx?bookid=507&sectionid=42540501. Accessed August 7, 2017.

Goodman CC, Pariser G. The endocrine and metabolic systems. In: Goodman CC, Fuller KS, eds. *Pathology: Implications for the Physical Therapist*. 4th ed. St. Louis, MO: Elsevier; 2015: Chapter 11.

Guide to Physical Therapist Practice 3.0. American Physical Therapy Association. ISBN: 978-1-931369-85-5, DOI: 10.2522/ptguide3.0_978-1-931369-85-5.

Hall JE. Thermoregulation. In: Hall JE, ed. *Guyton and Hall Textbook of Medical Physiology*. 13th ed. Philadelphia, PA: Saunders Elsevier; 2016.

Hypothyroidism. In: Shamus E, ed. *Quick Answers: Physiotherapy*. New York, NY: McGraw-Hill; 2012. http://accessphysiotherapy.mhmedical.com/content.aspx?bookid=855&sectionid=49734685. Accessed January 15, 2018.

MedlinePlus Medical Dictionary. https://medlineplus.gov/mplusdictionary.html. Accessed January 15, 2018.

Pathology of the bones and joints. In: Kemp WL, Burns DK, Brown TG, eds. *Pathology: The Big Picture*. New York, NY: McGraw-Hill; 2008: Chapter 19. http://accessphysiotherapy.mhmedical.com/content.aspx?bookid=499&sectionid=41568302. Accessed October 28, 2017.

Taylor JM, Thompson HS, Clarkson PM, Miles MP, De Souza MJ. Growth hormone response to an acute bout of resistance exercise in weight-trained and non-weight-trained women. *J Strength Cond Res*. 2000;14(2):220-227.

QUESTIONS

1. In Graves disease, the cause of hyperthyroidism is the production antibody that does which of the following?
   A. Activates the pituitary thyrotropin-releasing hormone (TRH) receptor and stimulates TSH release
   B. Activates the thyroid gland TSH receptor and stimulates thyroid hormone synthesis and release
   C. Activates thyroid hormone receptors in peripheral tissues
   D. Binds to thyroid gland thyroglobulin and accelerates the release of T4 and T3

2. A 54-year-old woman presents to the emergency room with tachycardia, shortness of breath, and chest pain. She has had shortness of breath and diarrhea for the last 2 days and is sweating and anxious. A TSH measurement reveals a value of <0.01 mIU/L (normal 0.4–4.0 mIU/L). The diagnosis of thyroid storm is made. Which of the following is a drug that is a useful adjuvant in the treatment of thyroid storm?
   A. Amiodarone (antiarrhythmic)
   B. Betamethasone (glucocorticoid)
   C. Epinephrine (sympathomimetic)
   D. Propranolol (beta blocker)

3. Which of the following is a sign or symptom that would be expected to occur in the event of chronic overdose with exogenous T4?
   A. Bradycardia
   B. Dry, puffy skin
   C. Drooping of the eyelids
   D. Weight loss

4. When initiating T4 therapy for an elderly patient with long-standing hypothyroidism, it is important to monitor cardiovascular response at rest and with activity to identify which of following?
   A. A flareup of exophthalmos
   B. Acute renal failure
   C. Hemolysis
   D. Overstimulation of the heart

5. A 64-year-old woman presents with complaints of fatigue, sluggishness, and weight gain. She needs to nap several times a day, which is unusual for her. She complains of being cold and has had difficulty with dry skin. What is the most likely diagnosis of her current condition?
   A. Hyperthyroid
   B. Hypothyroid
   C. Hypoparathyroid
   D. Hyperparathyroid

6. A 25-year-old woman presents with insomnia and fears she may have "something wrong with [her] heart." She describes her "heart jumping out of [her] chest." She feels healthy otherwise and reports she has lots of energy and has enjoyed her recent weight loss even thought her appetite has increased. Which of the following is the most likely diagnosis?
   A. Hyperthyroid
   B. Hypothyroid
   C. Hypoparathyroid
   D. Hyperparathyroid

7. A 50-year-old man, a known asthmatic for the past 30 years, presents to the emergency department with a 2-day history of worsening breathlessness and cough. Chest auscultation reveals bilateral polyphonic inspiratory and expiratory wheeze. Supplemental oxygen, nebulized albuterol (bronchodilator), and ipratropium (bronchodilator) as well as intravenous methyl prednisolone (glucocorticoid) are administered. Which of the following is a pharmacologic effect of exogenous glucocorticoids?
   A. Increased muscle mass
   B. Hypoglycemia
   C. Inhibition of leukotriene synthesis
   D. Improved wound healing

8. A 36-year-old woman with ulcerative colitis has required long-term treatment with pharmacologic doses of a glucocorticoid agonist. Which of the following is a toxic effect associated with long-term glucocorticoid treatment that would impact physical therapy?
   A. Fluid and electrolyte imbalance
   B. Adrenal gland neoplasm
   C. Hepatotoxicity
   D. Osteoporosis

9. A patient presents to the emergency department with hypotension, tachycardia, and loss of consciousness. The family reports a diagnosis of Addison disease and says that over the last few days the patient has had severe abdominal pain with vomiting and leg and back pain, which they thought was due to an infection. The patient is diagnosed with Addisonian crisis. What is the hormone deficiency mostly likely to cause this crisis?
   A. ACTH
   B. Aldosterone
   C. Testosterone
   D. Cortisol

10. Cushing syndrome occurs because of excess cortisol release from the adrenal glands or from exogenously administered glucocorticoids. Cortisol release would be implicated in which of the following physiologic responses?
   A. Dehydration
   B. Diabetes
   C. Increased ACTH secretion
   D. Hypotension

11. The pancreas is involved with the regulation of blood sugar. The alpha cells release_____, while the beta cells release _____.
   A. Cortisol; aldosterone
   B. Epinephrine; norepinephrine
   C. Glucagon; insulin
   D. Aldosterone; cortisol

12. The primary glucocorticoid produced by the adrenal cortex is _____, and the primary mineralocorticoid produced by the adrenal cortex is _____.
   A. Cortisol; aldosterone
   B. Progesterone; testosterone
   C. Estrogen; testosterone
   D. Testosterone; aldosterone

13. The cardinal signs of type I diabetes mellitus include which of the following?
   A. Hypodipsia
   B. Oliguria
   C. Ketonuria
   D. Hyperphagia

14. Which of the following is routinely added to calcium supplements and milk for preventing rickets in children and osteomalacia in adults?
   A. Cholecalciferol
   B. Calcitriol
   C. Gallium nitrate
   D. Vitamin C

15. A 60-year-old postmenopausal woman was sent for DEXA to evaluate the bone mineral density of her lumbar spine, femoral neck, and total hip. The test results (T = –2.5) revealed low bone mineral density in all sites. The appropriate diagnosis would be:
   A. Osteopenia
   B. Osteomalacia
   C. Paget disease
   D. Osteoporosis

16. Parathyroid hormone _____ plasma calcium levels by _____ calcium resorption from bone.
   A. Increases; increasing
   B. Increases; decreasing
   C. Decreases; decreasing
   D. Decreases; decreasing

17. Upon physical examination you note that the patient presents what appears to be extra fat around the trunk (buffalo torso). What condition is associated with this symptom?
   A. Addison disease
   B. Graves disease
   C. Hashimoto syndrome
   D. Cushing syndrome

18. In patients with diabetes, a life-threatening complication due to severe hyperglycemia or hypoglycemia is called
   A. Diabetic coma
   B. Hyperlipidemia
   C. Metabolic syndrome
   D. Polyneuropathy

19. A physical therapist is treating a patient with diabetes. On review of the medical chart, the patient was noted to have polydipsia. This means that the patient
   A. Perspires excessively
   B. Has excessive abnormal thirst
   C. Tires easily
   D. Is unable to follow multistep commands

20. A deficiency that affects the young during skeletal growth characterized by soft and deformed bones due to inadequate sunlight or vitamin D is:
   A. Chagas disease
   B. Osteogenesis imperfecta
   C. Fifth disease
   D. Rickets

21. A syndrome indicated by group of factors that are linked to increased risk of cardiovascular disease and type II diabetes is also called
   A. Hashimoto disease
   B. Addison syndrome
   C. Graves disease
   D. Metabolic syndrome

22. An autoimmune disease in which the thyroid gland is gradually destroyed is called
   A. Hashimoto disease
   B. Addison syndrome
   C. Graves disease
   D. Metabolic syndrome

23. A physical therapist is treating a patient whose medical diagnosis includes thyrotoxicosis. Which of the following are signs or symptoms of this condition?
   A. Brittle hair and nails
   B. Pleural effusion, hypoventilation, and carbon dioxide retention
   C. Bradycardia, deceased stroke volume, and cardiac output
   D. Sweating or heat intolerance

24. A patient with hypothyroidism will more likely demonstrate which sign/symptom below?
   A. Pale, cool, puffy, yellowish skin, face, and hands
   B. Dyspnea, weakness of respiratory muscles
   C. Nervousness or irritability
   D. Exophthalmos

25. A patient being treated in physical therapy demonstrates exophthalmos, which is the bulging of the eye anteriorly out of the orbit. Which of the following endocrine/metabolic conditions is associated with exophthalmos?
   A. Hashimoto disease
   B. Addison syndrome
   C. Graves disease
   D. Metabolic syndrome

ANSWERS

1. The answer is **B**. The antibodies produced in Graves disease activate thyroid gland TSH receptors. Their effects mimic those of TSH.

2. The answer is **D**. In thyroid storm, beta blockers such as propranolol are useful in controlling the tachycardia and other cardiac abnormalities, and propranolol also inhibits peripheral conversion of T4 to T3.

3. The answer is **D**. In hyperthyroidism, the metabolic rate increases and even though there is increased appetite, weight loss often occurs. The other choices are symptoms seen in hypothyroidism.

4. The answer is **D**. Patients with longstanding hypothyroidism, especially those who are elderly, are highly sensitive to the stimulatory effects of T4 on cardiac function, which can cause overstimulation of the heart and cardiac collapse.

5. The answer is **B**. Patients with early hypothyroidism have clinical features of vague and ordinary fatigue, mild sensitivity to cold, mild weight gain, forgetfulness, depression, and dry skin and hair.

6. The answer is **A**. Patients with early hyperthyroidism have clinical features that include goiter, nervousness, heat intolerance, increased heart rate and tachycardia, tremors, and weight loss.

7. The answer is **C**. Glucocorticoids inhibit the production of both leukotrienes and prostaglandins via inhibition of phospholipase A2. This is a key component of their anti-inflammatory action.

8. The answer is **D**. One of the adverse metabolic effects of long-term glucocorticoid therapy is a net loss of bone, which can result in osteoporosis.

9. The answer is **D**. Addisonian crisis is due to low levels of cortisol, which cause weakness, fatigue, and low blood pressure. Symptoms may include sudden dizziness, vomiting, and loss of consciousness.

10. The answer is **B**. Excess cortisol would cause steroid diabetes, weakness due to muscle wasting, potassium depletion, sodium and water retention, hypertension, abnormal fat distribution, increased susceptibility to infection, and mental changes.

11. The answer is **C**. The pancreas is involved with the regulation of blood sugar. The alpha cells release glucagon, while the beta cells release insulin.

12. The answer is **A**. The primary glucocorticoid produced by the adrenal cortex is cortisol, and the primary mineralocorticoid produced by the adrenal cortex is aldosterone.

13. The answer is **C**. Ketonuria occurs with type I diabetes because fatty acids are broken down, so ketones are present in the urine.

14. The answer is **A**. The two forms of vitamin D—cholecalciferol and ergocalciferol—are commonly added to calcium supplements and dairy products. Calcitriol, the active 1,25-dihydroxy vitamin D3 metabolite, would prevent vitamin D deficiency and is available as an oral formulation.

15. The answer is **D**. Osteoporosis is diagnosed with a DEXA T score of –2.5 or lower. Osteopenia is a T score of –1.0 to –2.4.

16. The answer is **A**. Parathyroid hormone increases plasma calcium levels by increasing calcium resorption from bone.

17. The answer is **D**. Buffalo torso is a typical symptom of Cushing syndrome.

18. The answer is **A**. Diabetic coma is a serious and life-threatening complication of diabetes.

19. The answer is **B**. Polydipsia is excessive or abnormal thirst, which is a symptom of diabetes.

20. The answer is **D**. Rickets is a deficiency disease that affects the young during the period of skeletal growth, is characterized especially by soft and deformed bones, and is caused by failure to assimilate and use calcium and phosphorus, normally due to inadequate sunlight or vitamin D.

21. The answer is **D**. Metabolic syndrome is marked by the presence of usually three or more of a group of factors (as high blood pressure, abdominal obesity, high triglyceride levels, low HDL levels, and high fasting levels of blood sugar) that are linked to an increased risk of cardiovascular disease and type II diabetes. This is also called insulin-resistance syndrome or syndrome X.

22. The answer is **A**. Hashimoto disease, also known as chronic lymphocytic thyroiditis, is an autoimmune disease in which the thyroid gland is gradually destroyed.

23. The answer is **D**. Sweating or heat intolerance is a symptom associated with thyrotoxicosis or hyperthyroidism. The other choices are signs or symptoms of hypothyroidism.

24. The answer is **A**. Pale, cool, puffy, yellowish skin, face, and hands is associated with hypothyroidism. The other choices are signs and symptoms of thyrotoxicosis or hyperthyroidism.

25. The answer is **C**. Exophthalmos, which is the bulging of the eye anteriorly out of the orbit, can be noted in patients with Graves disease.

CHECKLIST

When you complete this chapter, you should be able to:

❑ Outline signs and symptoms of various endocrine pathologies.

❑ Compare hyperthyroidism and hypothyroidism.

❑ Compare hyperadrenalism and hypoadrenalism.

❑ Compare diabetes and metabolic syndrome.

❑ Compare hyperparathyroid and hypoparathyroid.

Gastrointestinal System

6

Annie Burke-Doe and Rolando Lazaro

■ CLINICAL APPLICATION OF FOUNDATIONAL SCIENCE

The gastrointestinal (GI) tract serves to transport food and absorb nutrients to sustain life. The main functions of the GI tract include the digestion of food, absorption of nutrients, and elimination of waste. Pathologic conditions affecting the GI system result from the impairment of these functions. Malignancies in the GI tract, specifically the colon, are common conditions that affect this system. The most common signs and symptoms associated with GI disease include the following: (1) chest and/or abdominal pain, (2) disturbances in food ingestion (possibly due to vomiting, nausea, difficulty or painful swallowing, or anorexia),[1] (3) alterations in bowel movements (constipation or diarrhea), and (4) bleeding in the GI tract. The anatomy of the GI system is shown in Figure 6–1. Table 6–1 summarizes the selected GI pathologies discussed in this chapter. Table 6–2 identifies organs associated with abdominal quadrants.

EXAMINATION

The physical therapist's examination includes taking the individual's history, conducting a standardized system review, and performing selected tests and measures to identify potential and existing movement-related disorders. During the history-gathering phase, the physical therapist may seek and receive information on GI symptoms and complaints that may warrant referral for additional medical evaluation. The physical therapist may decide to use one, more than one, or portions of several specific tests and measures as part of the examination, based on the purpose of the visit, the complexity of the condition, and the directions taken in the clinical decision-making process. Signs and symptoms of GI disorders may include but are not limited to:

- Referred pain (eg, to abdomen, shoulder, neck, sternum, scapula, back, pelvis, sacrum)
- Dysphagia (eg, difficulty swallowing)
- Odynophagia (eg, pain with swallowing)

High-Yield Terms to Learn

Gastroesophageal reflux disease (GERD)	Condition resulting from a weak lower esophageal sphincter that allows the stomach contents, including acidic digestive juices, to go back (reflux) into the esophagus.
Dysphagia	Difficulty swallowing.
Borborygmi	High-pitched bowel sounds that may be due to hyperactivity of the intestines.
Esophageal achalasia	Condition in which the lower sphincter of the esophagus is unable to relax properly, causing a functional obstruction resulting in dysphagia, regurgitation, and chest pain.
Diverticulosis versus diverticulitis	Diverticulosis is a benign condition in which the weakened areas in the lining of the mucosa of the colon balloon out. Diverticulitis refers to the inflammation and infection of the perforation of the diverticula.
McBurney's sign	Tenderness on palpation of the McBurney's point (right side of the lower abdomen); a sign of appendicitis.
Steatorrhea	Fatty stools, which can be a sign of chronic pancreatitis.
Crohn's disease	Chronic inflammatory disease affecting the distal portion of the ileum and the colon.
Rebound tenderness	Pain elicited during abdominal examination when the examiner removes pressure suddenly during palpation. This clinical sign is associated with peritoneal inflammation (eg, peritonitis, appendicitis).

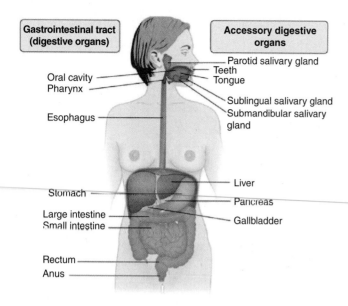

FIGURE 6–1 Gastrointestinal system. (From Ash R, Morton DA, Scott SA. *The Big Picture: Histology.* McGraw-Hill; 2013.)

- Acid reflux (eg, burning sensation)
- Early satiety (eg, full sensation with eating)
- Melena (eg, black stool)
- Symptoms during or after eating
- Abdominal cramping
- Bloody diarrhea
- Increased urgency
- Constipation
- Weight loss
- Nausea
- Vomiting
- Guarding (eg, muscle cramping)

Tests, measures, and screening that may be relevant to the GI system include but are not limited to:

- Abdominal inspection by quadrant (for distension, redness, scars, lumps, herniation)
- Palpation (for herniation, McBurney's point for acute appendicitis, lymph node swelling)
- Check for rebound tenderness (eg, peritonitis, appendicitis)
- Percussion
- Auscultation (for bowel sounds)

TABLE 6–1 Selected gastrointestinal pathologies.

- Gastroesophageal reflux disease (GERD)
- Gastroenteritis
- Diverticular disease
- Appendicitis
- Pancreatitis
- Pancreatic cancer
- Crohn's disease
- Colorectal cancer

TABLE 6–2 Organs associated with abdominal quadrants.

Right Abdominal Quadrants	Left Abdominal Quadrants
Right Upper Quadrant (RUQ)	**Left Upper Quadrant (LUQ)**
RUQ extends from the median plane, superior to the transumbilical plane	*LUQ extends from the median plane, superior to the transumbilical plane*
• Liver	• Liver (left lobe)
• Gallbladder	• Pancreas (body and tail)
• Pancreas (head)	• Left suprarenal gland
• Right suprarenal gland	• Left kidney (upper lobe)
• Right kidney (upper lobe)	• Descending colon (proximal)
• Ascending colon (distal)	• Splenic flexure
• Hepatic flexure	• Transverse colon (distal)
• Transverse colon (proximal)	
Right Lower Quadrant (RLQ)	**Left Lower Quadrant (LLQ)**
RLQ extends from the median plane, inferior to the transumbilical plane	*LLQ extends from the median plane, inferior to the transumbilical plane*
• Right kidney (lower lobe)	• Left kidney (lower lobe)
• Cecum	• Most of jejunum
• Appendix	• Descending colon
• Most of ileum	• Sigmoid colon
• Ascending colon (proximal)	• Left uterine tube
• Right uterine tube	• Left ovary
• Right ovary	• Left ureter
• Right ureter	• Uterus (if enlarged)
• Uterus (if enlarged)	• Urinary bladder (if full)
• Urinary bladder (if full)	

From Hankin MH, Morse DE, Bennett-Clarke CA, eds. *Clinical Anatomy: A Case Study Approach.* New York, NY: McGraw-Hill; 2013, Table 3.4.1.

■ FOUNDATIONS FOR EVALUATION, DIFFERENTIAL DIAGNOSIS, PROGNOSIS, AND INTERVENTIONS FOR SELECTED GASTROINTESTINAL PATHOLOGIES

Gastroesophageal Reflux Disease

Clinical Significance

Gastroesophageal reflux disease (GERD) is the result of a weak lower esophageal sphincter (LES) that allows the stomach contents, including acidic digestive juices, to go back (reflux) to the esophagus.[2] Of all the GI disorders, GERD is noted to be most common and most costly.[3] Table 6–2 summarizes the causes of LES dysfunction.[3] The mucosal lining of the esophagus is not able to withstand the strong acidity of the refluxed material, causing ulcerations in the esophagus. Repeated trauma to this area results in metaplasia, which is a change in the cellular type lining this structure. Dysplastic changes seen at the gastroesophageal junction (Barrett's esophagus) could be a precancerous lesion in the structure, hence the need for periodic endoscopic examination in a person with GERD.[3]

Diagnostic Tests and Measures

Blood tests

- pH monitoring[4]
- Biopsy of lower esophageal cells if metaplastic changes are suspected[3]

Imaging

- Barium radiography (swallow)
- Esophageal manometry

Clinical Findings, Secondary Effects, Complications[5,6]

- Persistent heartburn (burning sensation in the chest) due to acid reflux
- Chest pain (may increase when lying flat)
- Sensation of lump in throat
- Dysphagia (difficulty swallowing)
- Coughing

Disturbance of sleep from coughing and heartburn at night can lead to fatigue and decreased functioning during the day.

Chronic GERD is a risk factor for adenocarcinoma.

Interventions/Treatment[7]

Medical—Surgical treatment, changes in positioning or eating patterns.

Pharmacological

- Antacids
- H2 receptor blockers
- Proton pump inhibitors (PPIs)

Physical therapy—Therapists should be aware of side effects of medications such as headaches, constipation or diarrhea, dizziness, or abdominal pain.

Differential Diagnosis

- Esophageal[4] motor disorders
- Non-ulcer dyspepsia
- Esophageal cancer

Gastroenteritis

Clinical Significance

Gastroenteritis is also called stomach flu. The condition is due to inflammation of the intestinal lining due to offending organisms such as virus, bacteria, chemical toxins, or parasites.[8] This is a highly common and contagious condition affecting millions every year. The duration of the illness may be short (acute viral infection) or long (in chronic gastroenteritis due to food allergies).[9]

TABLE 6–3 Common organisms that cause gastroenteritis.

Viral, bacterial, and parasitic microorganisms most commonly cause gastroenteritis.

Viral (approximately 70% of cases of gastroenteritis)
- Adenovirus
- Coronavirus
- Norovirus
- Parvovirus
- Rotavirus

Bacterial (15%-20% of cases of gastroenteritis)
- *Bacillus cereus*
- *Campylobacter jejuni*
- *Clostridium difficile*
- *Clostridium perfringens*
- *Escherichia coli*—enterohemorrhagic O157:H7
- Enterotoxigenic, enteroadherent, enteroinvasive
- *Listeria*
- *Micobacterium avium-intracellulare*, immunocompromised
- *Providencia*
- *Salmonella*
- *Shigella*
- *Vibrio cholera*
- *Vibrio parahaemolyticus*
- *Vibrio vulnificus*
- *Yersinia enterocolitica*

Parasitic (10%-15%)
- *Amebiasis*
- *Cryptosporidium*
- *Cyclospora*
- *Giardia lamblia*

Foodborne toxigenic diarrhea
- Performed toxin: *Staphylococcus aureus, B. cereus*
- Postcolonization: *V. cholera, C. perfringens, enterotoxigenic E. coli, Aeromonas*

From Capriotti T, Frizzell JP. *Pathophysiology. Introductory Concepts and Clinical Perspectives*. Philadelphia, PA: FA Davis Co; 2016, Box 29-2.

Table 6–3 shows the common organisms that cause gastroenteritis. Noroviruses are extremely contagious and are commonly transmitted through close contact or fecal–oral medium.[3] For children, rotaviruses are the more common offending pathogen, and follow the fecal–oral route of transmission. Dehydration often occurs with continuous diarrhea and vomiting. Children and the elderly are particularly susceptible to dehydration, and hospitalization may be necessary to replenish lost fluids and electrolytes. In acute diarrhea, symptoms can persist for 12 to 72 hours.[3]

Diagnostic Tests and Measures

Blood tests—In most cases where the clinical findings are consistent with a diagnosis of gastroenteritis, no laboratory tests are needed. However, blood cultures may be needed if the patient appears to be seriously ill or with very high fevers.[10] In patients who present with severe dehydration, laboratory tests such as blood urea nitrogen (BUN) and electrolyte levels may be needed.[11]

Imaging—If conditions such as bowel obstruction or perforation are suspected, an acute abdominal series may be necessary.[12]

Clinical Findings, Secondary Effects, Complications

- Watery diarrhea
- Nausea
- Vomiting
- Lower abdominal stomach pain and cramps
- Hyperactivity of the intestinal tract causes cramping and high-pitched bowel sounds called borborygmi[3]

Interventions/Treatment

Medical—Identification of the etiology.

Pharmacological—Antibiotics are prescribed in bacterial gastroenteritis.

Physical therapy—Physical therapists must be able to identify signs and symptoms of dehydration (fainting, rapid heartbeat or breathing, dry skin, confusion or irritability) and report these to the members of the medical team so the patient can be given immediate care.

Differential Diagnosis

- Other infections
- Pseudomembranous colitis
- Toxins
- Hormonal (vasoactive intestinal peptides)
- Drugs (eg, sorbitol, cholinergics, caffeine)
- Postsurgical complications

Esophageal Achalasia

Clinical Significance

Condition in which the lower sphincter of the esophagus is unable to relax properly, causing a functional obstruction resulting in dysphagia, regurgitation, and chest pain.[1]

Diagnostic Tests and Measures

Blood tests—None.

Imaging

- Endoscopy
- Video esophagram
- Barium will stay longer in the esophagus during barium swallow testing

Clinical Findings, Secondary Effects, Complications

As the condition progresses, the esophagus will enlarge and contain a large quantity of infected material, also resulting in

increased risk of aspiration pneumonia.[1] In the absence of medical intervention, progressive weight loss will occur.

Interventions/Treatment

Surgery, dilation, or stretching of the esophagus.

Medical—Oral medications.

Pharmacological—Injection of medications to relax the muscles of the esophagus (botulism toxin).

Physical therapy—Therapists should be aware that patients with this condition may not be getting adequate nutrition and may demonstrate general weakness or muscle wasting.

Differential Diagnosis

- Esophageal cancer
- Chagas disease[13]

Diverticular Disease

Clinical Significance

Diverticular disease is a generic term that describes the development of small bulges, sacs, or pouches (diverticula) in the wall of the large intestine[14] (sigmoid colon). *Diverticulosis* is a benign condition in which the weakened areas in the lining of the mucosa of the colon balloon out. *Diverticulitis* refers to the inflammation and infection of the perforation of the diverticula. Complications may include abscess formation with peritonitis, rectal bleeding, formation of a stricture (narrowing of the colon, causing difficulty in the passage of stool), or formation of a fistula (a tunnel to the skin or another organ). In the case of a fistula, it most commonly connects the colon to the bladder.[14]

Diagnostic Tests and Measures

Blood tests—May be indicated to identify the presence of infection or extent of bleeding.[15]

Imaging

- Colonoscopy
- Abdominal and pelvic computed tomography (CT) scan may confirm the diagnosis

Clinical Findings, Secondary Effects, Complications

Most patients demonstrate no symptoms; patients with diverticulitis will complain of lower abdominal pain and may have rectal bleeding.[14]

Interventions/Treatment

Medical—Patients may be advised to maintain a high-fiber diet, with more fruits and vegetables, and to limit consumption of red meat. Surgical interventions may be indicated to remove the diseased colon. The extent of the surgical intervention and the need for a colostomy or ileostomy is dependent on the extent of the damaged colon.

Pharmacological—In patients with diverticulitis, antibiotic therapy either orally or intravenously is the treatment of choice; in patients with abscesses, a drain may be placed.[14]

Physical therapy—Physical therapists must be aware of the signs and symptoms of this condition, including the referred pain patterns from this condition, so that appropriate medical referrals can be made.

Differential Diagnosis
- Acute gastritis
- Acute pancreatitis
- Irritable bowel disease

Appendicitis
Clinical Significance
Appendicitis refers to the inflammation of the appendix. It is a medical emergency that requires surgery to remove the inflamed appendix. If left untreated, the appendix could become obstructed and inflamed and could eventually burst, with the contents spreading to the abdominal cavity, which may cause peritonitis.[7,16]

Diagnostic Tests and Measures
Blood tests—WBC count to identify infection.

Imaging
- Abdominal radiographs
- Abdominal ultrasound
- CT

Clinical Findings, Secondary Effects, Complications
1. Positive McBurney's sign
2. Umbilical or upper abdominal pain that becomes sharp toward the right side of the lower abdomen[17]
3. Nausea and vomiting
4. Fever
5. Severe cramps
6. Loss of appetite
7. Abdominal distention

Interventions/Treatment
Medical—Surgical treatment—appendectomy; laparoscopic surgery may lead to a faster healing process.[18]

Abscess may need to be drained via insertion of a tube.

Pharmacological—Antibiotic treatment to control the infection.

Physical therapy—Physical therapists must be aware of possible systemic origins of hip or thigh pain.

Physical therapists must be aware of McBurney's sign (tenderness on palpation of McBurney's point, located in the right side

of the lower abdomen, one-third of the distance between the anterior superior iliac spine and the navel).[19,20] Deep tenderness at McBurney's is indicative of a positive result. This sign is a clinical indication of acute appendicitis with inflammation that is no longer limited to the appendix and is irritating the parietal peritoneum.

Differential Diagnosis[7]
- Crohn's disease
- Perforated duodenal ulcers
- Cholecystitis
- Urinary tract infection[21]

Pancreatitis
Clinical Significance
Refers to inflammation of the pancreas. The inflammation could be acute, with sudden onset and lasting for days, or chronic, which is longstanding.[22] Repeated occurrences of acute pancreatitis will damage the pancreas, causing formation of scar tissue and affecting pancreatic function.[22]

Diagnostic Tests and Measures
Blood tests—To detect increased levels of pancreatic enzymes.

Imaging
- CT and abdominal ultrasound to identify extent of pancreatic inflammation and the presence of gallstones
- Endoscopic ultrasound to identify inflammation and possible pancreatic or bile duct blockages

Clinical Findings, Secondary Effects, Complications
Patients with acute pancreatitis may complain of upper abdominal pain that may be more severe after a meal. This pain may also radiate to the back. Patients may also suffer from nausea and vomiting.

Patients with chronic pancreatitis may complain of upper abdominal pain, weight loss, and steatorrhea (fatty stools).[23] Pancreatitis can be caused by many conditions, including chronic alcoholism, gallstones, cigarette smoking, pancreatic cancer, or high triglyceride levels in the blood.[22]

Interventions/Treatment
Medical
- Surgical interventions such as gallbladder or pancreatic surgeries may be needed to remove diseased tissues or repair blockages.[22]
- Treatment for alcohol dependence if primary cause of pancreatitis is excessive consumption of alcohol.
- Low-fat and high-nutrient diet.

Pharmacological—Pain medications and intravenous fluids.

Physical therapy—Physical therapists must recognize possible systemic causes of abdominal or lower back pain.

Differential Diagnosis[24,25]

- Cholecystitis
- Colon cancer
- Gallstones
- Irritable bowel syndrome
- Crohn's disease
- Pancreatic cancer

Pancreatic Cancer

Clinical Significance

According to the American Cancer Society, pancreatic cancer accounts for 7% of all cancer deaths and 3% of all cancers in the United States.[26] It is thought of as an aggressive form of cancer, with absence of significant symptoms until the later stages of the condition,[7,27] when the bile ducts are obstructed, or the malignancy is of significant size to press on neighboring structures. Risk factors include chronic pancreatitis, diabetes, smoking, obesity, old age, or family history of pancreatic cancer.[28]

Diagnostic Tests and Measures

Blood tests—Blood tests for specific tumor markers to diagnose the cancer.

Imaging—CT, magnetic resonance imaging (MRI), and positron emission tomography (PET) will visualize the location and extent of the malignancy.

Clinical Findings, Secondary Effects, Complications[28]

1. Upper abdominal pain with radiation to low back
2. Nausea and vomiting
3. Fatigue

Pain manifestation is dependent on the location of the malignancy. Affectation of the pancreatic head may cause epigastric and mid-thoracic pain, while involvement of the tail of the pancreas may refer pain to the left shoulder.[7] Radiation of pain to the low back is also possible.

Complications include weight loss, jaundice, pain, or bowel obstruction.

Interventions/Treatment

Medical/Pharmacological—Treatment is dependent on the location and extent of the malignancy. If the cancer involves the head of the pancreas, pancreaticoduodenectomy (Whipple procedure) may be performed. Removal of the entire pancreas (total pancreatectomy) may be performed. Chemotherapy, either alone or in combination with radiation, may be utilized to kill the malignancy and control growth.[29]

Physical therapy—Physical therapists must be aware of the possible systemic causes of shoulder or low back pain. Physical therapists must also screen for cancers and refer individuals to appropriate medical professionals if presenting signs and symptoms fall outside the physical therapy scope of practice.

Differential Diagnosis[30]

- Chronic pancreatitis
- Bile duct stones
- Autoimmune pancreatitis

Crohn's Disease

Clinical Significance

Crohn's disease is a chronic inflammatory disease affecting the distal portion of the ileum and the colon.[7] It is thought to be part of a group of conditions diagnosed as inflammatory bowel disease (IBD).[31] Twenty-five percent of people diagnosed with the condition have also been found to have arthritis or joint pain.[7]

Diagnostic Tests and Measures
Blood tests

- Red blood cell/white blood cell (RBC/WBC) count to detect infection
- Determine levels of iron, proteins, or minerals
- Erythrocyte sedimentation rate

Imaging[32]

- Upper and lower GI series to identify problem areas
- CT scans to detect abscesses
- Colonoscopy/sigmoidoscopy to identify small ulcers or inflammation
- Video capsule endoscopy (in which a small capsule that contains a small video camera is ingested by the patient, and the camera captures images as it travels through the digestive system to provide detailed images of the digestive tract)[33]

Clinical Findings, Secondary Effects, Complications[7,31,34]

- Persistent diarrhea
- Abdominal pain and cramps
- Constipation
- Rectal bleeding
- Fever
- Nausea

Secondary effects include fissures in the anus, fistulas, or thickening of intestinal walls, causing partial or total intestinal blockage and malnutrition.

Interventions/Treatment

Medical—Management priorities for Crohn's disease should be focused on reducing inflammation, relieving symptoms such as pain and diarrhea, and replenishing nutritional deficits caused by impairments in the digestive system.

Pharmacological

- Medications that reduce inflammation (sulfasalazine or mesalamine)[35]
- Corticosteroids to decrease inflammation
- Immunomodulators

Physical therapy—Physical therapists need to be aware that patients diagnosed with Crohn's disease could also present with arthralgias or arthritis, so it is very important to be able to differentiate musculoskeletal and nonmusculoskeletal reasons for pain.

Differential Diagnosis[36]

- Ulcerative colitis
- Incidental chronic colitis

Gastric Ulcer[1]

Clinical Significance

A gastric ulcer (ulceration) is a lesion in the lining of the stomach caused by acidic digestive juices. Gastric ulceration is distinguished from erosive gastritis by the depth of the lesion, which penetrates through the mucosal lining and is believed to be related to impaired mucosal defenses, because acid and pepsin secretory capacity is affected in some patients. Ulcerations are often located in the stomach and duodenum. The most common causes of peptic ulcer include infection with the bacterium *Helicobacter pylori* and long-term use of aspirin and certain other pain medications. Stress and diets that include spicy foods do not cause peptic ulcers, but they can increase symptomology.

Diagnostic Tests and Measures
Blood tests

- Complete blood count (erythrocytes, leukocytes, hemoglobin)
- *Helicobacter pylori* antibodies
- Fecal occult blood test (FOBT)

The urea breath test is a noninvasive method for identifying *H. pylori* infection. It is based on the ability of *H. pylori* to convert urea to ammonia and carbon dioxide. The results of this test can be confounded by the patient's medications.

Imaging

- Barium swallow
- Chest radiographs
- CT
- Esophagogastroduodenoscopy (EGD)

Clinical Findings, Secondary Effects, Complications

1. Burning stomach pain (stabbing pain in inferior sternum, left upper abdomen)
2. Heartburn
3. Bloating
4. Fatty food intolerance
5. Left shoulder pain
6. Nausea
7. Hypoactive bowel sounds
8. Internal bleeding
9. Vomiting (coffee ground emesis is indication blood)
10. Melena (dark blood in stools, or stools that are black or tarry)
11. Guarding of the superior and anterolateral abdominal wall
12. Epigastric and left upper quadrant tenderness during deep palpation
13. Obstruction
14. Infection

Interventions/Treatment
Medical[37]—Identification of the etiology, changes in medications, and changes in diet will most likely be recommended.

Pharmacological[38]—Antibiotics, acid-reducing medications (esomeprazole [Nexium], dexlansoprazole [Dexilant], omeprazole [Zegerid]).

Physical therapy—Physical therapists need to screen for signs and symptoms of gastric ulcer. Clients may need referral for further medical treatment.

Differential Diagnosis[39]

- Differential diagnosis
- Esophageal cancer
- Celiac disease
- Irritable bowel syndrome
- GERD

Colorectal Cancer

Clinical Significance

Colorectal cancer affects the large intestine. It ranks as the third most common cancer diagnosed in the United States.[7] This type of cancer often begins as a small, noncancerous growth (polyp) that forms in the inner wall of the rectum or colon and becomes malignant over time.[40] Patients with colon cancer are mostly asymptomatic in the early stages of the condition. Intensity of symptoms varies according to the size of the malignancy and location within the large intestine.[7,41] Studies have shown a relationship between a high-fat, low-fiber diet and colon cancer. Risk factors include old age, African-American race, personal history of colorectal cancer and polyps, family history of colon cancer, sedentary lifestyle, obesity, and diabetes.[41]

Diagnostic Tests and Measures
Blood tests

- Kidney and liver function tests
- Tests to identify carcinoembryonic antigen (CEA)

Imaging—MRI with contrast.

Clinical Findings, Secondary Effects, Complications

1. Rectal bleeding
2. Hemorrhoids
3. Back pain that may radiate to the legs
4. Constipation
5. Diarrhea
6. Nausea, vomiting

Interventions/Treatment

Medical[42]

- Surgery to remove polyps in early stages
- Endoscopic mucosal resection
- Surgery to remove malignancy in later stages
- Lymph node removal
- Chemotherapy with or without radiation

Pharmacological[40]

- Chemotherapeutic drug therapy including bevacizumab (Avastin), cetuximab (Erbitux), or panitumumab (Vectibix)
- Immunotherapy such as pembrolizumab (Keytruda) or nivolumab (Opdivo)

Physical therapy—Physical therapists need to screen for signs and symptoms of malignancy. Also, physical therapy interventions that improve range of motion and strength may be needed to mitigate chemotherapy-related secondary impairments.

Differential Diagnosis[43]

- Crohn's disease
- Ulcerative colitis
- Small intestinal diverticulosis

■ SUMMARY

Screening of the GI system is key to identification of further need for medical referral. Understanding signs, symptoms, and pathologies related to GI dysfunction will assist the physical therapist in identification of GI structures that can cause pain that is referred to the abdomen, shoulder, neck, sternum, scapula, back, pelvis, and sacrum.

REFERENCES

1. Mills JC, Stappenbeck TS. Gastrointestinal disease. In: *Pathophysiology of Disease: An Introduction to Clinical Medicine*. 7th ed. McGraw-Hill; 2014.

2. WebMD. Gastroesophageal reflux disease. Available at: https://www.webmd.com/heartburn-gerd/guide/reflux-disease-gerd-1#1. Accessed March 10, 2018.

3. Capriotti T, Frizzell JP. *Pathophysiology. Introductory Concepts and Clinical Perspectives*. St. Louis, MO: Elsevier; 2016.

4. Laine C, Goodman D. Gastroesophageal reflux disease. Available at: https://www.med.unc.edu/medselect/resources/course%20reading/ITC%20GERD.full.pdf. Accessed March 10, 2018.

5. Mayo Clinic. Gastroesophageal reflux disease. Available at: https://www.mayoclinic.org/diseases-conditions/gerd/symptoms-causes/syc-20361940. Accessed March 10, 2018.

6. National Institute of Diabetes and Digestive and Kidney Diseases. Acid reflux (GER & GERD) in adults. Available at: https://www.niddk.nih.gov/health-information/digestive-diseases/acid-reflux-ger-gerd-adults. Accessed March 10, 2018.

7. Goodman CC, Heick J, Lazaro R. *Differential Diagnosis for Physical Therapists*. 6th ed. St. Louis, MO: Elsevier; 2017.

8. Medline Plus. Gastroenteritis. Available at: https://medlineplus.gov/gastroenteritis.html. Accessed March 12, 2018.

9. Medicine.net. Stomach flu (gastroenteritis) symptoms, signs treatment remedies, diet. Available at: https://www.medicinenet.com/gastroenteritis_stomach_flu/article.htm. Accessed March 12, 2018.

10. Medscape. Viral gastroenteritis workup. Available at: https://emedicine.medscape.com/article/176515-workup. Accessed March 12, 2018.

11. Medscape. Emergent treatment of gastroenteritis workup. Available at: https://emedicine.medscape.com/article/775277-workup. Accessed March 12, 2018.

12. Medscape. Emergent treatment of gastroenteritis workup. Available at: https://emedicine.medscape.com/article/775277-workup#c6. Accessed March 12, 2018.

13. Medicine.net. Achalasia. Available at: https://www.medicinenet.com/achalasia/article.htm#how_is_achalasia_diagnosed. Accessed March 10, 2018.

14. American Society of Colon and Rectal Surgeons. Diverticular disease. Available at: https://www.fascrs.org/patients/disease-condition/diverticular-disease. Accessed March 10, 2018.

15. WebMD. Diverticular disease. Available at: https://www.webmd.com/digestive-disorders/diverticular-disease#1. Accessed March 10, 2018.

16. WebMD. Appendicitis. Available at: https://www.webmd.com/digestive-disorders/digestive-diseases-appendicitis#1. Accessed March 10, 2018.

17. Mayo Clinic. Appendicitis symptoms. Available at: https://www.mayoclinic.org/diseases-conditions/appendicitis/symptoms-causes/syc-20369543. Accessed March 10, 2018.

18. Mayo Clinic. Appendicitis diagnosis and treatment. Available at: https://www.mayoclinic.org/diseases-conditions/appendicitis/diagnosis-treatment/drc-20369549. Accessed March 10, 2018.

19. Wikipedia. McBurney's point. Available at: https://en.wikipedia.org/wiki/McBurney%27s_point. Accessed March 10, 2018.

20. Abdomen. In: Hankin MH, Morse DE, Bennett-Clarke CA, eds. *Clinical Anatomy: A Case Study Approach*. New York, NY: McGraw-Hill. http://accessphysiotherapy.mhmedical.com/content.aspx?bookid=2215&sectionid=169757343. Accessed March 13, 2018.

21. Medscape. Appendicitis. Differential diagnosis. Available at: https://emedicine.medscape.com/article/773895-differential. Accessed March 10, 2018.

22. Mayo Clinic. Pancreatitis. Available at: https://www.mayoclinic.org/diseases-conditions/pancreatitis/symptoms-causes/syc-20360227. Accessed March 10, 2018.

23. Wikipedia. Steatorrhea. Available at: https://en.wikipedia.org/wiki/Steatorrhea. Accessed March 10, 2018.

24. Medscape. Acute pancreatitis differential diagnosis. Available at: https://emedicine.medscape.com/article/181364-differential. Accessed March 10, 2018.

25. Medscape. Chronic pancreatitis differential diagnosis. Available at: https://emedicine.staging.medscape.com/article/181554-differential. Accessed March 10, 2018.

26. American Cancer Society. Key statistics for pancreatic cancer. Available at: https://www.cancer.org/cancer/pancreatic-cancer/about/key-statistics.html. Accessed March 10, 2018.

27. WebMD. Pancreatic Cancer Health Center. Available at: https://www.webmd.com/cancer/pancreatic-cancer/default.htm. Accessed March 10, 2018.

28. Mayo Clinic. Pancreatic cancer. Available at: https://www.mayoclinic.org/diseases-conditions/pancreatic-cancer/symptoms-causes/syc-20355421. Accessed March 10, 2018.

29. Mayo Clinic. Pancreatic cancer diagnosis. Available at: https://www.mayoclinic.org/diseases-conditions/pancreatic-cancer/diagnosis-treatment/drc-20355427. Accessed March 10, 2018.

30. Epocrates. Pancreatic cancer. Available at: https://online.epocrates.com/diseases/26535/Pancreatic-cancer/Differential-Diagnosis. Accessed March 10, 2018.

31. Crohn's and Colitis Foundation. What is Crohn's disease. Available at: http://www.crohnscolitisfoundation.org/what-are-crohns-and-colitis/what-is-crohns-disease/. Accessed March 10, 2017.

32. WebMD. Diagnosing Crohn's disease. Available at: https://www.webmd.com/ibd-crohns-disease/crohns-disease/crohns-disease-diagnosis#1. Accessed March 10, 2018.

33. WebMD. Diagnosing Crohn's disease. CT scans. Available at: https://www.webmd.com/ibd-crohns-disease/crohns-disease/crohns-disease-diagnosis#2. Accessed March 10, 2018.

34. WebMD. What are the symptoms of Crohn's disease? Available at: https://www.webmd.com/ibd-crohns-disease/crohns-disease/symptoms-crohns-disease. Accessed March 10, 2018.

35. WebMD. Crohn's disease treatment: common medications for treating Crohn's. Available at: https://www.webmd.com/ibd-crohns-disease/crohns-disease/crohns-disease-treatment-common-medications-for-treating-crohns#3. Accessed March 10, 2018.

36. Stanford Medicine. Crohn's disease. Available at: http://surgpathcriteria.stanford.edu/gi/crohn-disease/differential-diagnosis.html. Accessed March 10, 2018.

37. Mayo Clinic. Peptic ulcer diagnosis. Available at: https://www.mayoclinic.org/diseases-conditions/peptic-ulcer/diagnosis-treatment/drc-20354229. Accessed August 17, 2018.

38. Medscape. Peptic Ulcer Medications. Available at: https://emedicine.medscape.com/article/181753-medication. Accessed Aug 17, 2018.

39. Epocrates. Peptic ulcer disease differential diagnosis. Available at: https://accessphysiotherapy.mhmedical.com/content.aspx?sectionid=53555694&bookid=961&Resultclick=2#1100860733. Accessed August 17, 2018.

40. National Cancer Institute. Colorectal cancer. Available at: https://www.cancer.gov/types/colorectal. Accessed March 10, 2018.

41. Mayo Clinic. Colon cancer. Available at: https://www.mayoclinic.org/diseases-conditions/colon-cancer/symptoms-causes/syc-20353669. Accessed March 10, 2018.

42. Mayo Clinic. Colon cancer diagnosis. Available at: https://www.mayoclinic.org/diseases-conditions/colon-cancer/diagnosis-treatment/drc-20353674. Accessed March 10, 2018.

43. Medscape. Colon cancer differential diagnosis. Available at: https://emedicine.staging.medscape.com/article/277496-differential. Accessed March 10, 2018.

QUESTIONS

1. This condition results from a weak esophageal sphincter that allows the stomach contents to go back into the esophagus.
   A. Irritable esophageal syndrome (IES)
   B. Gastroesophageal reflux disease (GERD)
   C. Esophageal achalasia
   D. Diverticulosis

2. The most common symptom of GERD due to the reflux of stomach acid and contents into the esophagus is
   A. Chest pain
   B. Abdominal pain
   C. Heartburn
   D. Dysphagia

3. Esophageal achalasia occurs because of
   A. Inability of the lower esophageal sphincter to relax
   B. Development of sacs in the lining of the esophagus
   C. Inflammation of the esophageal walls
   D. Abnormal distention of the esophageal tract

4. A medical condition resulting from inflammation and infection in the weakened areas of the esophageal lining is
   A. Diverticulosis
   B. Esophageal peritonitis
   C. Diverticulitis
   D. Gastroesophageal reflux disease

5. Which of the following positive signs may be indicative of appendicitis?
   A. Lhermitte sign
   B. Iliopsoas sign
   C. McBurney's test
   D. Thomas test

6. This term indicates fatty stools, which could be due to decreased function of the pancreas.
   A. Jaundice
   B. Steatorrhea
   C. Hematochezia
   D. Melena

7. In cases of pancreatic cancer affecting the pancreatic head, the patient may complain of referred pain to which of the following areas?
   A. Left shoulder
   B. Midscapular area
   C. Low back
   D. Epigastric and midthoracic regions

8. This condition refers to the inflammatory disease affecting the distal portion of the ileum and the colon.
   A. Crohn's disease
   B. Irritable bowel syndrome
   C. Leaky gut syndrome
   D. Degenerative colitis

9. A major risk factor to consider in children and elderly individuals with vomiting and diarrhea due to gastroenteritis is
   A. Orthostatic hypotension
   B. Tension headache
   C. Dehydration
   D. Dysphagia

10. Changes in cellular structure at this junction may be an indication of malignancy in patients with GERD.
    A. Barrett's esophagus
    B. McBurney's point
    C. Diverticular junction
    D. Biliopancreatic cleft

ANSWERS

1. The answer is **B**. Gastroesophageal reflux disease (GERD) occurs when there is backup (reflux) of stomach contents into the esophagus due to a weak esophageal sphincter.

2. The answer is **C**. Heartburn is caused by the backup of digestive acids and content into the esophagus.

3. The answer is **A**. In esophageal achalasia, the lower sphincter of the esophagus is unable to relax properly, causing a functional obstruction in the esophagus.

4. The answer is **C**. Diverticulitis is the inflammation and infection of perforations in the diverticula.

5. The answer is **C**. A positive McBurney's test (tenderness to palpation of the McBurney's point) may be indicative of appendicitis.

6. The answer is **B**. Steatorrhea refers to increased fatty content in the stool.

7. The answer is **D**. Cancer affecting the pancreatic head will likely refer pain in the epigastric and midthoracic regions. Cancer affecting the tail of the pancreas may refer pain to the left shoulder.

8. The answer is **A**. Crohn's disease refers to the inflammatory disease affecting the distal portion of the ileum and the colon.

9. The answer is **C**. Dehydration is a risk factor in children and elderly who are having vomiting and diarrhea due to gastroenteritis. Hospitalization may be necessary to replenish lost fluids and electrolytes.

10. The answer is **A**. Changes in the cellular structure in the Barrett's esophagus may indicate early malignancy. Regular endoscopy may be indicated to monitor the condition.

CHECKLIST

When you complete this chapter, you should be able to:

❑ Identify the main functions of the GI tract.

❑ List general classifications of signs and symptoms associated with GI disease.

❑ Identify specific clinical findings of selected pathologies affecting the GI tract.

❑ Identify pertinent diagnostic tests and measures to confirm the presence of selected GI pathologies.

❑ Discuss pertinent medical imaging modalities to confirm the presence of selected GI pathologies.

❑ Identify appropriate pharmacological management of selected GI conditions.

❑ List most common malignancies affecting the GI system.

❑ Discuss the role of physical therapy in the medical management of selected GI pathologies.

Genitourinary System

7

Annie Burke-Doe and Rolando Lazaro

■ CLINICAL APPLICATION OF FOUNDATIONAL SCIENCES

The genitourinary system is comprised of the organs and structures involved in reproduction and the formation and excretion of urine. This system performs important functions related to the elimination of the body's waste products and maintenance of homeostatic environment as well as functions related to reproduction.[1] The kidneys are also involved in regulating production of red blood cells, metabolizing hormones, and maintaining the acid–base balance of the blood.[2] Furthermore, part of normal kidney function requires unrestricted flow of urine out of the body. Figure 7–1 shows the female and male urinary systems. Table 7–1 shows the common signs and symptoms of urological dysfunction. Table 7–2 summarizes the conditions discussed in this chapter.

High-Yield Terms to Learn	
Pyelonephritis	Infection affecting the kidneys.
Hematuria	Blood in the urine.
Nocturia	Increased or unusual need to urinate at night time.
Cystitis	Infection of the bladder.
Adjuvant therapy	Treatment that is given in addition to the main treatment. In cancer, these are interventions done after surgery (usually chemotherapy and/or radiation) in attempt to remove all malignancy and/or prevent reoccurrence.
Benign prostatic hyperplasia (BPH)	Enlargement of the prostate gland in men.
Prostate-specific antigen (PSA) test	Blood test that detects PSA in the blood. PSA levels increase when the prostate is enlarged.
Transurethral resection of the prostate (TURP)	Surgical procedure where an instrument is inserted in the urethra and most of the prostate is removed (outer part is left).
Radical prostatectomy	Removal of the entire prostate gland and some surrounding tissues, including the seminal vesicles.
Androgen	Male hormone; increased levels of androgen may stimulate the growth of prostate cancer cells.
Urinary incontinence (UI)	An individual's inability to control the bladder, resulting in involuntary urine leakage.
Stress urinary incontinence (SUI)	Bladder leakage associated with exertion or physical activity.
Overactive bladder or urge incontinence	Results from the sudden contraction of the detrusor muscle causing a sudden and intense need to urinate that cannot be suppressed.
Dyspareunia	Pain during sexual intercourse.
Flatus	Gas or air in the gastrointestinal tract that is expelled through the anus.
Costovertebral angle	The angle formed on either side of the vertebral column between the last rib and the lumbar vertebrae. Tenderness in this region is indicative of renal disease.

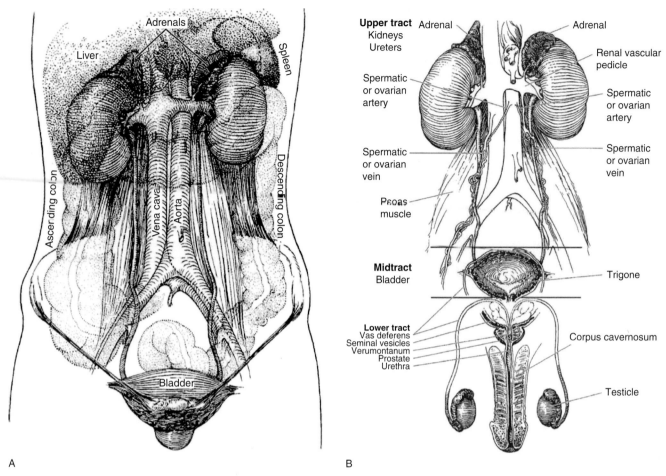

FIGURE 7–1 Female (**A**) and male (**B**) urinary system. (From McAninch JW, Lue TF. *Smith & Tanagho's General Urology*, 18th ed. New York, NY: McGraw-Hill, 2013. Figures 1–1 and 1–2.)

EXAMINATION

The physical therapist's examination includes taking the individual's history, conducting a standardized system review, and performing selected tests and measures to identify potential and existing movement-related disorders. During the history-gathering phase, the physical therapist may seek and receive information on genitourinary symptoms and complaints that may warrant referral for additional medical evaluation. The physical therapist may decide to use one, more than one, or portions of several specific tests and measures as part of the examination, based on the purpose of the visit, the complexity of the condition, and the directions taken in the clinical decision-making process.

Signs and symptoms of genitourinary disorders may include but are not limited to:

- Urgency and increased frequency of urination
- Dysuria

TABLE 7–1 Common signs and symptoms of urological dysfunction.

Sign or Symptom	Description	Common Cause
Dysuria	Pain and burning on urination	UTI
Frequency	An abnormally high amount of times that the patient needs to urinate	UTI, BPH, urological obstruction, IC
Hesitancy	Interrupted flow of a urinary system	BPH
Urgency	A feeling that urination will occur imminently	UTI, BPH, IC

UTI, urinary tract infection; BPH, benign prostatic hyperplasia; IC, interstitial cystitis.

From Capriotti T, Frizzell JP. Pathophysiology. *Introductory Concepts and Clinical Perspectives*. Philadelphia, PA: FA Davis; 2016, Table 23–1.

TABLE 7–2 Selected genitourinary conditions.

- Kidney failure
- Urinary tract infection
- Interstitial cystitis
- Bladder cancer
- Benign prostatic hyperplasia
- Prostate cancer
- Urinary incontinence

- Pyuria
- Hematuria
- Foul-smelling urine
- Positive urine culture
- Low-grade systemic fever
- Suprapubic tenderness
- Dyspareunia
- Stress incontinence
- Changes in voiding
- Nocturia
- Pain (referred to the back flank)
- Dehydration

Tests and measures that may be relevant to genitourinary disorders include but are not limited to:

- Palpation (bladder and kidney palpation that causes pain may indicate inflammation)
- Percussion (fist percussion over the costovertebral angle will elicit pain if infection is present)
- Auscultation (eg, listening for bruits [murmurs] in the blood flow to the kidneys from the abdominal aorta and renal arteries)

■ FOUNDATIONS FOR EVALUATION, DIFFERENTIAL DIAGNOSIS, PROGNOSIS AND INTERVENTIONS OF SELECTED GENITOURINARY PATHOLOGIES

Kidney Failure

Clinical Significance

Chronic kidney disease denotes the gradual decline in kidney function over time. In advanced stages of the condition, the body will be unable to eliminate dangerous levels of waste products, causing toxicity. End-stage renal disease (ESRD) will necessitate dialysis[3] and a kidney transplant.

Diagnostic Tests and Measures
Laboratory tests[4]

- Complete blood counts to identify blood urea and nitrogen (BUN), bicarbonate and serum albumin levels, lipid profile (also screens for cardiovascular disease), glomerular filtration rate
- Urinalysis
- Kidney biopsy

Imaging[5]

- Renal ultrasound

Clinical Findings, Secondary Effects, Complications[4,6]

1. Lethargy
2. Edema of the extremities
3. Weakness, excessive fatigue
4. Congestive heart failure
5. Increasing levels or urea in the blood, causing encephalopathy
6. Muscle cramping

Interventions/Treatment
Medical[7]

- Hemodialysis
- Kidney transplant
- Conservative management to treat the symptoms without dialysis or transplant

Pharmacological[8]—The aim of pharmacological management is to treat associated conditions due to failure of kidney function. These could include medications for hypertension, loss of bone and mineral contents in the body, hyperglycemia, and dyslipidemia, among others.

Physical Therapy—There is some evidence that exercise during hemodialysis sessions may help optimize function in people with ESRD undergoing dialysis. Exercise interventions include strengthening and aerobic exercises.[9]

Differential Diagnosis[10]

- Acute kidney injury
- Antiglomerular basement membrane disease
- Chronic glomerulonephritis
- Diabetic nephropathy
- Multiple myeloma
- Nephrolithiasis
- Nephrosclerosis

Urinary Tract Infection

Clinical Significance

Urinary tract infection (UTI) is the most common disorder affecting the urogenital system. The pathology refers to infectious conditions affecting any part of the urinary system—kidneys, ureters, bladder, and urethra.[11] UTI can be caused by offending bacteria, abnormal immune response reactions, drugs, radiation, or any other toxic substances.[1] Upper UTIs include infections involving the kidneys (pyelonephritis) or ureters, while lower UTIs include infections in the bladder (cystitis) or urethra (urethritis).[1] Depending on the urogenital structures affected, patients with UTIs may complain of flank pain, ipsilateral shoulder pain, low back pain, or pelvic/lower abdominal pain, and it is important for the physical therapist to determine the source of pain for patients with these complaints. UTI is most common in women. It has been noted that over 40% of women aged 20 to 40 years have had a lower UTI. This is because the rectum is closer to the urethra in females. *Escherichia coli* from the rectum can easily invade the female urogenital system, causing the condition. This condition is rare in males; therefore the healthcare practitioner needs to further investigate the urological system if a male patient has been diagnosed with lower UTI.[2]

Diagnostic Tests and Measures

Laboratory tests

- Complete blood count to identify infections
- Urine sample to check for blood in the urine (hematuria) or presence of infection
- To decrease the presence of contaminants that may affect the results, the urine must be collected "clean-catch" midstream[2]

Table 7–3 summarizes abnormal laboratory findings that may be identified on urinalysis.

Imaging[12,13]

- Computed tomography (CT) of the abdomen and/or urography with or without contrast, or magnetic resonance imaging (MRI)
- Intravenous pyelogram (IVP) can also be used to more closely assess the entire urogenital system and assess for kidney stones (it is important to check for allergies to the dye that will be used in the procedure)[2]
- Renal and bladder ultrasound

Clinical Findings, Secondary Effects, Complications[1,11,14]

1. Nocturia (increased or unusual need to urinate at night time)
2. Hematuria
3. Burning sensation when urinating
4. Fever, shaking, and chills
5. Nausea and vomiting
6. Pelvic/lower abdominal pain
7. Frequent, painful urination
8. Cloudy, bloody, dark and/or foul-smelling urine

Interventions/Treatment

Medical[15]—Mainly antibiotic treatment (see below), with antibiotic choice depending on the severity of the condition. The patient is instructed to hydrate frequently to assist in moving the flow of urine.

Pharmacological—Antibiotic therapy.

Physical therapy[1]—It is important for the physical therapist to identify possible systemic reasons for complaints of pain. Upper UTI may result in complaints of flank and ipsilateral shoulder pain, while lower UTI may result in pelvic or lower abdominal pain. These may mimic complaints of musculoskeletal pain.

Differential Diagnosis[16,17]

- Overactive bladder
- Vaginitis
- Urethral cancer
- Nephrolithiasis
- Urinary obstruction

Interstitial Cystitis

Clinical Significance

Interstitial cystitis is also known as painful bladder syndrome. This condition is characterized by a feeling of fullness in the bladder, causing urgency and frequency of urination.[18] The condition is often diagnosed primarily on the presence of symptoms.

TABLE 7–3 Abnormal laboratory findings on urinalysis.

Urinalysis Finding	Description	Common Cause
Bacteriuria	Bacteria in the urine that can be visualized on microscopy	UTI or asymptomatic bacteriuria (ASB)
Bilirubinuria	Bilirubin in the urine	Liver disorders Excessive hemolysis
Crystalluria	Crystals or pieces of a kidney stone in the urine; commonly calcium or uric acid	Nephrolithiasis or urolithiasis
Glucosuria	Glucose in the urine	Uncontrolled diabetes mellitus (DM)
Hematuria	Blood in the urine	UTI Nephrolithiasis or urolithiasis Urological malignancy
Ketonuria	Ketones in the urine	Fasting Starvation Uncontrolled DM
Leukocyte esterase	WBCs in the urine	UTI or ASB
Nitrites	Bacteria in the urine	UTI or ASB
Proteinuria (microalbuminuria)	A condition in which urine contains an abnormal amount of protein Normally urine should contain no more than 200 mg of protein per liter	Glomerular injury Kidney dysfunction caused by diabetes Kidney dysfunction caused by high blood pressure Inflammation of the kidney
Pyuria	WBCs (neutrophils) in the urine	UTI and ASB
Urinary casts	Cylindrical mucoprotein structures produced by the nephron tubules that appear in the urine Various casts found in urine sediment include hyaline, waxy, granular, fatty, crystal, RBC, WBC, bacterial, and epithelial	Nephrotic syndrome Dehydration Vigorous exercise Diuretics Tubular necrosis Autoimmune disorders Pyelonephritis Other kidney diseases

UTI, urinary tract infection; ASB, asymptomatic; DM, diabetes mellitus.

From Capriotti T, Frizzell JP. Pathophysiology. *Introductory Concepts and Clinical Perspectives.* Philadelphia, PA: FA Davis; 2016, Table 23–2.

Diagnostic Tests and Measures
Laboratory tests[2]

- Urinalysis
- Urine culture
- In females, hysteroscopy and laparoscopy may be needed to rule out endometriosis; in males, prostate disease may need to be ruled out[2]
- Cystoscopy can confirm any structural pathology on the walls of the bladder
- Potassium sensitivity test may show more urgency in urination with potassium than water[19]

Clinical Findings, Secondary Effects, Complications[2,19]

1. Pelvic pain
2. Perineal pain
3. Dysuria
4. Fullness of the bladder

Interventions/Treatment

Medical—The treatment is based on the postulated cause of the condition, so there is no universally accepted intervention. Bladder training and pelvic floor rehabilitation are common interventions. Dietary modifications may be implemented if certain foods have been shown to exacerbate the condition.

Pharmacological

- Anticholinergic drugs such as oxybutynin and tolterodine may be prescribed to manage urinary frequency.[19]
- Nonsteroidal anti-inflammatory drugs may be used to relieve pain.
- Pentosane polysulfate sodium (Elmiron), an FDA-approved drug for treating interstitial cystitis, may be used. It is postulated that this drug restores the inner surface of the bladder, thereby protecting the bladder wall from irritants that may trigger the signs and symptoms of the condition.

Physical therapy—Physical therapy may be helpful in alleviating symptoms in patients with interstitial cystitis, especially if there is an identified pelvic floor dysfunction. Specific interventions include manual therapy and soft tissue interventions, and also the use of physical and electrotherapeutic agents as appropriate.[20]

Bladder Cancer

Clinical Significance[21]

Bladder cancer is the most common of all urinary tract cancers. It affects older adults and men and is highly treatable when diagnosed early. This type of cancer affects males three times more than females, and Caucasians more than African Americans.[2] Cigarette smoking is a major risk factor in the development of bladder cancer. Environmental exposure in general accounts for about 80% of all bladder cancers.[2] Signs and symptoms of bladder cancer are similar to those of UTI, and that is the main reason for delayed diagnosis of bladder cancer, particularly for women.[2]

Diagnostic Tests and Measures
Laboratory tests[22]

- Cystoscopy is the diagnostic test of choice for assessing unexplained hematuria[2]
- Urinalysis
- Urine cytology
- Urine culture
- Urine tumor marker tests
- Biopsy (transurethral resection of bladder tumor [TURBT])

Imaging[22]

- Cystoscopy
- IVP or intravenous urogram (IVU) contrast radiographs of the urinary system
- CT urogram; CT-guided biopsy
- MRI urogram
- Ultrasound
- Chest x-rays and bone scans to determine metastasis to the lungs or bones

Clinical Findings, Secondary Effects, Complications[21,23]

1. The main symptom of bladder cancer is painless and intermittent hematuria
2. Pelvic pain
3. Frequent and painful urination
4. Urge to urinate even if the bladder is not full
5. Difficulty in urination
6. Low back pain

Interventions/Treatment

Medical[24]—Surgical management (removal of the cancerous growth). Partial cystectomy can be done when the growth is not very large, to remove part of the bladder wall and lymph nodes. Radical cystectomy (removal of the entire bladder and associated lymph nodes) may be necessary if the malignancy is large or in multiple sites in the bladder. In women, the reproductive structures (ovaries, fallopian tubes, uterus, cervix, and part of the vagina) are removed, while in males, the prostate and seminal vesicles are excised.

Pharmacological—In bladder cancer, chemotherapy can be administered in two ways. Intravesical chemotherapy is performed in very early stages of bladder cancer by administering the chemotherapy drugs directly into the bladder. In systemic chemotherapy, the drugs are administered intravenously or intramuscularly. In systemic administration, the effects go beyond the bladder to the other organ systems. Systemic chemotherapy is indicated in more advanced stages of bladder cancer, to shrink a large tumor prior to surgery or to kill other cancer cells that remain after other interventions (also termed adjuvant therapy).

Physical therapy—It is important for the physical therapist to provide interventions aimed at optimizing function in patients undergoing medical treatment for cancer. Common residual impairments following cancer surgery, radiation, or chemotherapy include limitations in range of motion and muscular weakness.

Differential Diagnosis[25,26]

- Benign prostatic hyperplasia (BPH)
- Bladder calculi
- Renal pelvic calculi
- Pyelonephritis
- Renal cancer

Benign Prostatic Hyperplasia

Clinical Significance[27]

BPH refers to enlargement of the prostate gland in men. An enlarged prostate can obstruct urinary flow and may cause pathologies in the kidney, bladder, or urinary tract. The pathological process involved in the hyperplasia of the prostate is not fully understood; however, it is postulated that the condition is due to the imbalance between cell proliferation and cell death. The increased size of the prostate can compress the urethra and obstruct the flow of urine. This causes the urine to be retained in the bladder, resulting in overdistention, increased frequency of urination, and increased frequency of emptying the bladder, especially at night (nocturia).[28] With significant distention of the bladder, even a slight increase in intra-abdominal pressure can cause overflow incontinence.[28]

Diagnostic Tests and Measures
Laboratory tests

- Urinalysis to identify infections
- Prostate-specific antigen (PSA) blood test—PSA levels increase when the prostate is enlarged
- Prostate biopsy to examine prostate tissue for the presence of cancer

Imaging[29]

- Transrectal ultrasound (TRUS) to assess and measure the prostate

Clinical Findings, Secondary Effects, Complications

1. Problems with urination: difficulty in initiation, weak stream, dribbling, increased frequency and nocturia, inability to fully empty the bladder
2. UTI
3. Hematuria

Complications arise due to obstruction of the urinary system caused by the enlarged prostate. These include urinary retention, UTIs, bladder stones, and bladder and kidney damage.

Interventions/Treatment[29,30]

Medical—The most common treatment is medication (see below). Surgical interventions can be done if the pharmacological interventions are unsuccessful. Transurethral resection of the prostate (TURP) is the surgical removal of the prostate.

Pharmacological—Pharmacological interventions include alpha blockers to relax prostate and bladder muscles to facilitate urination, 5-alpha reductase inhibitors to decrease the size of the prostate, or a combination of the two; tadalafil (Cialis) can also relax muscles of the bladder and prostate and helps in decreasing BPH symptoms.

Physical therapy—Physical therapists must be aware of the signs and symptoms of BPH and should refer patients with undiagnosed BPH for further medical evaluation if the person presents with signs and symptoms of BPH.

Differential Diagnosis[31]

- Prostate cancer
- Bladder cancer
- Prostatitis
- UTI in males

Prostate Cancer

Clinical Significance[32]

Prostate cancer is one of the most prevalent cancers in men. Patients are usually asymptomatic in the early stages of the disease and will start complaining of symptoms in the lower urinary tract, low back, hip, or lower extremity pain. Risk factors include increasing age, African American men and Caribbean men of African heritage, family history of prostate cancer, and several inherited gene mutations. Some factors that have been noted to possibly be associated with prostate cancer include high fat and red meat diet, obesity, smoking, exposure to certain chemicals, prostatitis, sexually transmitted infections, and previous vasectomy. A digital rectal exam (DRE) may identify potential bumps or hard areas in the prostate that may be cancerous.

Diagnostic Tests and Measures
Laboratory tests[33]

- PSA test (see preceding discussion)
- Prostate biopsy—a core needle biopsy, in which a hollow needle is introduced into the prostate and several samples of a small core of prostate tissue are extracted
- Lymph node biopsy

Imaging

- TRUS
- Bone scan to determine if the cancer has metastasized to the bone
- CT scan of the prostate
- MRI scan of the prostate

Clinical Findings, Secondary Effects, Complications[34,35]

1. Problems with urination: slow or weak stream, difficulty starting or stopping urination, nocturia, burning sensation when urinating
2. Hematuria
3. Blood in semen

4. Erectile dysfunction
5. Hip, back, or chest pain
6. Loss of appetite, weight loss
7. Nausea and vomiting

Interventions/Treatment

Medical[36]—Surgical removal of the prostate gland is a common intervention for prostate cancer that has not metastasized. Radical prostatectomy involves removal of the entire prostate gland and some surrounding tissues, including the seminal vesicles.

Radiation therapy can be done to kill cancer cells. This can be the first treatment for cancer or as part of adjuvant therapy.

Pharmacological[37]—Hormone therapy is performed to reduce the level of male hormones (androgens), as they stimulate growth of prostate cancer cells. The therapy is called androgen deprivation therapy (ADT) or androgen suppression therapy. Hormone therapy alone has not been found to completely cure prostate cancer.

Chemotherapy treatment is performed when the cancer has metastasized and hormone therapy is not achieving the desired results. Chemotherapy is thought to slow the progression of cancer but is unlikely to cure the condition. In addition, it is important to consider the deleterious side effects of chemotherapy.

Vaccine treatment is done in prostate cancer to provide a boost to the immune system to fight the prostate cancer cells.

Physical therapy—It is important for physical therapists to provide interventions aimed at optimizing function in patients undergoing medical treatment for cancer. Common residual impairments following cancer surgery, radiation, or chemotherapy include limitations in range of motion and muscular weakness.

Differential Diagnosis[38]

- BPH
- Bacterial prostatitis

Urinary Incontinence

Clinical Significance[1]

Urinary incontinence (UI) refers to an individual's inability to control the bladder, resulting in involuntary urine leakage.[39] UI is a major problem, especially in older institutionalized adults. UI ranges from leaking urine when coughing and sneezing to inability to get to the bathroom in time to urinate. Table 7–4 summarizes the types of incontinence.

Diagnostic Tests and Measures

Laboratory tests[40]

- Urinalysis—can identify signs of infection, blood, or other abnormalities in the urine
- Post-void residual measurement—is the amount of urine left in the bladder after an individual attempts to completely urinate

TABLE 7–4 Types of incontinence.

Type of Incontinence	Description
Stress incontinence	Involuntary leakage of urine as abdominal pressure rises, which typically occurs during coughing and sneezing. The leakage occurs because of either poor pelvic support or weakness in the urethral sphincter.
Urge incontinence, also called overactive bladder (OAB)	Detrusor muscle overactivity is the cause of the urine leakage. The cause is unclear, but IC is thought to be the etiology in some patients. The patient complains of feelings of urgency and frequency of urination many times a day.
Overflow incontinence	Chronic overdistention and urinary retention in the bladder results in overflow incontinence. BPH, which obstructs the urine outflow, is the most frequent cause in men. Failure of the detrusor muscle caused by damage of the pelvic spinal nerves can also cause this type of incontinence.
Neurogenic bladder	This disorder is the result of an interruption of the sensory nerve fibers between the bladder and the spinal cord or the afferent nerve tracts to the brain. Chronic overdistention of the bladder occurs.
Functional incontinence	Inability to hold urine caused by CNS problems such as stroke, psychiatric disorders, prolonged immobility, dementia, or delirium.
Mixed incontinence	Combination of stress incontinence and OAB.

From Capriotti T, Frizzell JP. Pathophysiology. *Introductory Concepts and Clinical Perspectives.* Philadelphia, PA: FA Davis; 2016, Table 23–3.

Clinical Findings, Secondary Effects, Complications

The primary types of UI include the following:

1. Stress urinary incontinence (SUI) is bladder leakage associated with exertion or physical activity.[41] This is due to a weak or damaged bladder or urethra.
2. Overactive bladder, or urge incontinence, results from the sudden contraction of the detrusor muscle causing a sudden and intense need to urinate that cannot be suppressed.[42]
3. Overflow incontinence results when the person is unable to completely empty the bladder, which in turn overflows and leaks out. The person does not have the sensation that the bladder is full or empty. Bacteria can grow in the stagnant urine left in the bladder, causing repeated UTIs.[1,43] This condition affects more men than women.[43]
4. Functional incontinence refers to physical (lack of mobility, arthritis) or mental (dementia) impairments that cause the involuntary leakage of urine.

Interventions/Treatment

Medical—Behavioral techniques such as bladder training and fluid and diet management can help with bladder control. Pelvic floor exercises may help regain control of muscles involved in urination. Electrical stimulation can also be helpful.

Pharmacological[40]—Medications commonly used to treat urinary incontinence include anticholinergics, alpha blockers, or topical estrogen.

Physical therapy—Physical therapy pelvic floor treatment may be able to help individuals with urinary incontinence to improve bladder control by specific exercises and other interventions. Exercises that target the pelvic floor musculature (primarily levator ani and urethral sphincter) are known as Kegel exercises. These exercises involve alternate relaxation and contraction of the urethral sphincter to start and stop urination while contracting the levator ani to prevent escape of flatus.

Differential Diagnosis[44]

- UTI
- Prostatitis
- Spinal cord condition
- Urinary obstruction

■ SUMMARY

Screening of the genitourinary system is key to identification of further need for medical referral. Understanding signs, symptoms, and pathologies related to genitourinary dysfunction will assist the physical therapist in identification of genitourinary structures that can cause pain that is referred to the abdomen and back.

REFERENCES

1. Goodman C, Heick J, Lazaro R. *Differential Diagnosis for Physical Therapists.* 6th ed. St. Louis, MO: Elsevier; 2017.
2. Capriotti T, Frizzell JP. *Pathophysiology. Introductory Concepts and Clinical Perspectives.* Philadelphia, PA: FA Davis; 2016.
3. Mayo Clinic. Chronic kidney disease. Available at: https://www.mayoclinic.org/diseases-conditions/chronic-kidney-disease/symptoms-causes/syc-20354521. Accessed March 8, 2018.
4. Medscape. Chronic kidney disease workup. Available at: https://emedicine.medscape.com/article/238798-workup. Accessed March 7, 2018.
5. End stage renal disease. Johns Hopkins Medicine. Available at: https://www.hopkinsmedicine.org/healthlibrary/conditions/kidney_and_urinary_system_disorders/end_stage_renal_disease_esrd_85,P01474. Accessed March 7, 2018.
6. Mayo Clinic. Chronic kidney disease. Available at: https://www.mayoclinic.org/diseases-conditions/chronic-kidney-disease/symptoms-causes/syc-20354521. Accessed March 8, 2018.
7. Choosing a treatment for kidney failure. Available at: https://www.niddk.nih.gov/health-information/kidney-disease/kidney-failure/choosing-treatment. Accessed March 7, 2018.
8. Schmid H, Schiffl H, Lederer SR. Pharmacotherapy of end-stage renal disease. *Expert Opin Pharmacother.* 2010 Mar; 11(4):597-613. doi: 10.1517/14656560903544494.
9. Goodman C, Fuller K. *Pathology: Implications for the Physical Therapist.* St. Louis, MO: Elsevier; 2015.
10. Medscape. Chronic kidney disease differential diagnoses. Available at: https://emedicine.medscape.com/article/238798-differential. Accessed March 7, 2018.
11. Mayo Clinic. Urinary tract infection. Available at: https://www.mayoclinic.org/diseases-conditions/urinary-tract-infection/symptoms-causes/syc-20353447. Accessed March 6, 2018.
12. Browne RF, Zwirewich C, Torreggiani WC. Imaging of urinary tract infection in the adult. *Eur Radiol.* 2004 Mar; 14(Suppl 3):E168-183.
13. Urinary tract infection. Available at: https://radiopaedia.org/articles/urinary-tract-infection. Accessed March 6, 2018.
14. WebMD. Your guide to urinary tract infections (UTIs). Available at: https://www.webmd.com/women/guide/your-guide-urinary-tract-infections#1. Accessed March 6, 2018.
15. Mayo Clinic. Urinary tract infection (UTI). Available at: https://www.mayoclinic.org/diseases-conditions/urinary-tract-infection/diagnosis-treatment/drc-20353453. Accessed June 20, 2018.
16. Epocrates. Urinary tract infections in women. Available at: https://online.epocrates.com/diseases/7735/Urinary-tract-infections-in-women/Differential-Diagnosis. Accessed March 6, 2018.
17. Medscape. Pediatric urinary tract infection differential diagnoses. Available at: https://emedicine.medscape.com/article/969643-differential. Accessed March 6, 2018.
18. Mayo Clinic. Interstitial cystitis. Available at: https://www.mayoclinic.org/diseases-conditions/interstitial-cystitis/symptoms-causes/syc-20354357. Accessed March 8, 2018.
19. Mayo Clinic. Interstitial cystitis. Available at: https://www.mayoclinic.org/diseases-conditions/interstitial-cystitis/diagnosis-treatment/drc-20354362. Accessed March 6, 2018.
20. Interstitial Cystitis Association. Physical therapy. Available at: https://www.ichelp.org/diagnosis-treatment/treatments/physicaltherapy/. Accessed March 6, 2018.
21. Mayo Clinic. Bladder cancer. Available at: https://www.mayoclinic.org/diseases-conditions/bladder-cancer/symptoms-causes/syc-20356104. Accessed March 6, 2018.
22. American Cancer Society. Tests for bladder cancer. Available at: https://www.cancer.org/cancer/bladder-cancer/detection-diagnosis-staging/how-diagnosed.html. Accessed March 6, 2018.
23. American Cancer Society. Signs and symptoms of bladder cancer. Available at: https://www.cancer.org/cancer/bladder-cancer/detection-diagnosis-staging/signs-and-symptoms.html. Accessed March 6, 2018.
24. American Cancer Society. Bladder cancer surgery. Available at: https://www.cancer.org/cancer/bladder-cancer/treating/surgery.html. Accessed March 6, 2018.
25. Bladder cancer differential diagnosis. Available at: https://www.wikidoc.org/index.php/Bladder_cancer_differential_diagnosis. Accessed March 6, 2018.
26. Oncology encyclopedia. Available at: http://oncolex.org/Bladder-cancer/Background/DifferentialDiagnoses. Accessed March 6, 2018.
27. Mayo Clinic. Benign prostatic hyperplasia (BPH). Available at: https://www.mayoclinic.org/diseases-conditions/benign-prostatic-hyperplasia/symptoms-causes/syc-20370087. Accessed March 6, 2018.
28. Porth C. *Essentials of Pathophysiology.* Philadelphia, PA: Wolters Kluwel; 2015.

29. Mayo Clinic. Benign prostatic hyperplasia (BPH). Diagnosis. Available at: https://www.mayoclinic.org/diseases-conditions/benign-prostatic-hyperplasia/diagnosis-treatment/drc-20370093. Accessed March 6, 2018.

30. Urology Care Foundation. What happens after treatment? Available at: https://www.urologyhealth.org/urologic-conditions/benign-prostatic-hyperplasia-(bph)/after-treatment. Accessed March 6, 2018.

31. Medscape. Benign prostatic hyperplasia (BPH) differential diagnoses. Available at: https://emedicine.staging.medscape.com/article/437359-differential. Accessed March 6, 2018.

32. American Cancer Society. What is prostate cancer? Available at: https://www.cancer.org/cancer/prostate-cancer/about/what-is-prostate-cancer.html. Accessed March 6, 2018.

33. American Cancer Society. Tests for prostate cancer. https://www.cancer.org/cancer/prostate-cancer/detection-diagnosis-staging/how-diagnosed.html. Accessed March 6, 2018.

34. American Cancer Society. Signs and symptoms of prostate cancer. Available at: https://www.cancer.org/cancer/prostate-cancer/detection-diagnosis-staging/signs-symptoms.html. Accessed March 6, 2018.

35. WebMD. Understanding prostate cancer – symptoms. Available at: https://www.webmd.com/prostate-cancer/guide/understanding-prostate-cancer-symptoms. Accessed March 6, 2018.

36. American Cancer Society. Surgery for prostate cancer. Available at: https://www.cancer.org/cancer/prostate-cancer/treating/surgery.html. Accessed March 6, 2018.

37. American Cancer Society. Chemotherapy for prostate cancer. Available at: https://www.cancer.org/cancer/prostate-cancer/treating/chemotherapy.html. Accessed March 6, 2018.

38. Medscape. Prostate cancer differential diagnoses. Available at: https://emedicine.medscape.com/article/1967731-differential. Accessed March 6, 2018.

39. Mayo Clinic. Urinary incontinence. Overview. Available at: https://www.mayoclinic.org/diseases-conditions/urinary-incontinence/symptoms-causes/syc-20352808. Accessed March 6, 2018.

40. Mayo Clinic. Urinary incontinence. Diagnosis. Available at: https://www.mayoclinic.org/diseases-conditions/urinary-incontinence/diagnosis-treatment/drc-20352814. Accessed March 6, 2018.

41. Medline Plus. Stress urinary incontinence. Available at: https://medlineplus.gov/ency/article/000891.htm. Accessed March 8, 2018.

42. Medicine.net. Overactive bladder. Available at: https://www.medicinenet.com/overactive_bladder/article.htm. Accessed March 6, 2018.

43. WebMD. Overflow incontinence. Available at: https://www.webmd.com/urinary-incontinence-oab/overflow-incontinence#1. Accessed March 6, 2018.

44. Medscape. Urinary incontinence differential diagnosis. Available at: https://emedicine.staging.medscape.com/article/452289-differential. Accessed on March 6, 2018.

QUESTIONS

1. Which of the following is FALSE regarding lower urinary tract infection?
   A. The most common offending organism is *E. coli*.
   B. Females are more likely to have lower UTI than males.
   C. Lower UTI in males typically resolves spontaneously.
   D. Urinalysis can be used to detect the presence of infection.

2. A physical therapist would like to determine possible non-musculoskeletal origins of ipsilateral shoulder pain. The therapist suspects the possibility of infection in the urogenital system. Nonmusculoskeletal flank pain is most associated with infection of which urogenital structure?
   A. Kidney
   B. Bladder
   C. Urethra
   D. Testes/ovaries

3. A physical therapist would like to determine possible non-musculoskeletal origins of ipsilateral shoulder pain. The therapist suspects the possibility of infection in the urogenital system. Nonmusculoskeletal low back or lower abdominal pain is most associated with infection of which urogenital structure?
   A. Kidney
   B. Ureter
   C. Bladder
   D. Testes/ovaries

4. A 75-year-old patient comes to physical therapy for balance and mobility exercises. He states that he has an enlarged prostate that causes difficulty in urination, made worse by his inability to ambulate to the bathroom quickly. An enlarged prostate is known by what other medical condition?
   A. Nephrolithiasis
   B. Pyelonephritis
   C. Prostatitis
   D. Benign prostatic hyperplasia

5. Which of the following blood tests can confirm the presence of an enlarged prostate?
   A. Thyroid-stimulating hormone (TSH)
   B. Prostate-specific antigen (PSA)
   C. Bladder tumor–associated antigen (BTA)
   D. Microalbumin urine test (MUT)

6. A physical therapist receives a referral to treat a patient who was recently admitted to an acute care hospital due to multiple incidents of falls in the past 3 days. Upon review of the medical chart, the patient was noted to have an infection affecting the kidneys. The medical term to indicate this condition is
   A. Glomerulonephritis
   B. Pyelonephritis
   C. Urethritis
   D. Cystitis

7. A patient was referred to physical therapy for mobility and ambulation training following complete removal of the prostate gland due to prostate cancer. Which surgical procedure was performed on the patient?
    A. Transurethral resection of the prostate (TURP)
    B. Transurethral needle ablation (TUNA)
    C. Radical prostatectomy
    D. Transurethral vaporization of the prostate

8. A patient with urinary incontinence was referred to physical therapy for treatment. On examination, the patient is unable to completely empty the bladder, which in turn overflows and leaks out. What type of urinary incontinence does the patient have?
    A. Stress urinary incontinence
    B. Overactive bladder
    C. Overflow incontinence
    D. Functional incontinence

9. Which of the following types of stress incontinence is more common in men than women?
    A. Stress urinary incontinence
    B. Overactive bladder
    C. Overflow incontinence
    D. Functional incontinence

10. A physical therapist is treating a patient with urinary incontinence (UI). Which type of UI results in incomplete emptying of the bladder, resulting in risk of urinary infection due to bacterial growth in the stagnant urine?
    A. Stress urinary incontinence
    B. Overactive bladder
    C. Overflow incontinence
    D. Functional incontinence

ANSWERS

1. The answer is **C**. While lower UTI is rare in males, a closer examination of the urogenital system is warranted on those who may have the disease, as it may be caused by a variety of pathologies.

2. The answer is **A**. Flank pain that is nonmusculoskeletal and possibly urogenital in origin is likely caused by an infection of the upper urinary tract (kidney or ureter).[1]

3. The answer is **C**. Low back or lower abdominal pain that is nonmusculoskeletal and possibly urogenital in origin is likely caused by an infection in the lower urinary tract (bladder or urethra).

4. The answer is **D**. Benign prostatic hyperplasia refers to a medical condition denoting an enlarged prostate.

5. The answer is **B**. Increased levels of prostate-specific antigen (PSA) can be indicative of an enlarged prostate.

6. The answer is **B**. Pyelonephritis pertains to the infection affecting the kidneys.

7. The answer is **C**. Radical prostatectomy refers to the complete removal of the prostate gland.

8. The answer is **C**. Overflow incontinence refers to inability to completely empty the bladder, which in turn overflows and leaks out. The person does not have the sensation that the bladder is full or empty.

9. The answer is **C**. Overflow incontinence occurs more in men than women.

10. The answer is **C**. In overflow incontinence, some urine is left in the bladder which can be breeding grounds for bacteria that may cause urinary tract infections.

CHECKLIST

When you complete this chapter, you should be able to:

❑ Identify the structures comprising the genitourinary system.

❑ Identify specific clinical findings of selected pathologies affecting the genitourinary system.

❑ Identify pertinent diagnostic tests and measures to confirm the presence of selected genitourinary pathologies.

❑ Discuss pertinent medical imaging modalities to confirm the presence of selected genitourinary pathologies.

❑ Identify appropriate pharmacological management of selected genitourinary conditions.

❑ List most common malignancies affecting the genitourinary system.

❑ Discuss the role of physical therapy in the medical management of selected genitourinary pathologies.

Non-Systems

Chris Childers and Ellen Lowe

■ SECTION A: EQUIPMENT, DEVICES AND TECHNOLOGY

The physical therapist has an extensive barrage of equipment devices and technology available. Definitions are as follows:

Adaptive devices: A variety of implements or equipment used to aid patients/clients in performing movements, tasks, or activities. Adaptive devices include:

- Environmental controls
- Hospital beds
- Raised toilet seats
- Seating systems

Assistive devices: A variety of implements or equipment used to aid patients/clients in performing movements, tasks, or activities. Assistive devices include:

- Canes
- Crutches
- Long-handled reachers
- Percussors and vibrators
- Power devices
- Static and dynamic splints
- Walkers
- Wheelchairs

The role of the physical therapist with respect to assistive devices is to choose the one that is most appropriate, and then teach the patient to use the device correctly. Table 8A–1 provides information on assistive devices for gait, including appropriate measurement of the device, and gait pattern most frequently used with the device. Tables 8A–2 and 8A–3 provide stair protocols and frequently used gait patterns.

Orthosis: An orthosis, or brace as it was historically called, is an external appliance that is worn by an individual to assist

their movement or to purposefully transfer load or weight-bearing forces.[1] See Table 8A–4 for more details. Orthotic devices include:

- Braces
- Casts
- Shoe inserts
- Splints

Prosthesis: A prosthesis replaces a missing portion of a limb. Primary LE prostheses include partial foot, transtibial and transfemoral. Physical therapists need to have a good understanding of the different types of socket, and the socks, sheaths, and liners used by the client.[1] The physical therapist also needs to understand gait abnormalities and probable causes, see Table 8A–5.

Protective devices:

- Cushions
- Helmets
- Protective taping

Personal protective equipment: see Section C.

Supportive devices:

- Compression garments
- Corsets
- Elastic wraps
- Mechanical ventilators
- Neck collars
- Serial casts
- Slings
- Supplemental oxygen
- Supportive taping

TECHNOLOGY

The rapid advances in technology benefit both physical therapists and their clients. Technology ranges from exoskeletons that allow paraplegic clients to walk, monitoring devices that prevent individuals with Alzheimer's from wandering out of their home, anatomy tables that replace cadavers, and equipment for biofeedback in the clinic ranging from pelvic floor contraction to balance and gait analysis. It is the responsibility of the physical therapist to learn about equipment and technology that is relevant to their clientele, and provide appropriate referral or guidance to individuals seeking more information about specific types of technology.

TABLE 8A–1 Gait devices.

Device	Unilateral/ Bilateral	Gait Patterns	Measurement	Typical Patient
Axillary crutches	Bilateral	Four point Two point Three point Modified three point	2 inches below axilla when correctly on the floor (2–4 inches lateral and 4–6 inches anterior to toes) and wrist crease at handle	Recent fracture Recent surgery Usually younger (under 65) Using three point or three-point modified when WB restrictions
	Unilateral	Modified four point Modified two point	As above	As above, progressing to a unilateral device with no WB restrictions
Forearm or Loftstrand crutches	Bilateral	Four point Two point Not recommended for three point or modified three point	Cuff distal to olecranon wrist crease at handle	Longer-term users such as chronic neurological patients but generally under 65
	Unilateral	Modified four point Modified two point	As above	As above requiring less support
Walkers Standard, front-wheeled, four-wheeled	Bilateral	Three point or modified three point gait just requiring support of bilateral device with no WB restrictions; is unnamed when using a walker	Wrist crease at handle	Generally over 65, may have WB restrictions or just instability
Single-point cane	Unilateral	Modified two point Modified four point	Wrist crease at handle	Adds some balance stability; least stable of all AD, used in opposite hand to affected leg if there is one leg affected Also used as a progression from a bilateral device when no WB restrictions apply
Wide- and short-based quad canes	Unilateral	Modified two point Modified four point	Wrist crease at handle	As above, but the wider base adds greater stability when there are balance deficits Often used with higher-functioning patients post CVA
Hemi walker	Unilateral	Modified four point Modified two point	Wrist crease at handle	Often used with patient post CVA for initial gait training Also used with patients post arm or shoulder injury or surgery who need increased stability using only one UE

WB, weight bearing; AD, assistive device; CVA, cerebrovascular accident; UE, upper extremity.

TABLE 8A–2 Stair protocol.

Stairs	First	Second	Third	Acronym
Ascending	Unaffected leg	Affected leg	Crutches or AD	GAS (good affected sticks)
Descending	Crutches or AD	Affected leg	Unaffected leg	SAG (sticks affected good)

TABLE 8A-3 Gait patterns.

Name of Gait Pattern	Bilateral or Unilateral Device	Description of Pattern	Comments
Four point	Bilateral	1 crutch 2 opposite foot 3 other crutch 4 other foot	Can be done with any bilateral device but with walkers it is not called a four-point gait unless using a reciprocal walker
Four-point modified	Unilateral	1 crutch 2 opposite foot 3 other foot	Any unilateral device can be used and is in the opposite hand to the affected LE
Two point	Bilateral	1 crutch and opposite foot together 2 other crutch and other foot together	Can be done with any bilateral device but not called two point if using a walker except for reciprocal walkers
Two-point modified	Unilateral	1 crutch and opposite foot together 2 other foot	Any unilateral device can be used and is in the opposite hand to the affected LE
Three point	Bilateral	1 crutches or walker 2 affected NWB leg swings through 3 hop forward on other leg	Only used when there is NWB on one side and must have bilateral device—crutches or walker
Three-point modified	Bilateral	1 crutches or walker 2 foot with weight restriction 3 other foot	Used with all other weight–bearing restrictions (other than NWB) and must have bilateral device—crutches or walker

NWB, non-weight bearing.

TABLE 8A-4 Orthosis.[1]

Type of Orthosis	Method of Control	Purpose
Ankle-foot orthosis	Limits plantar or dorsiflexion or assists motion	Control for foot drop, prevents toe drag
Knee-ankle-foot orthosis	Controls ankle and knee and often foot	Provides stability to the knee during gait
Hip-knee-ankle foot orthosis	Adds a pelvic band and hip joint	Adds hip control for greater stability
Trunk orthosis Corsets	Soft, non-rigid support	Primarily for abdominal compression
Rigid trunk orthosis	Rigid horizontal and vertical components	Limits movement of the trunk, often post-surgery of the spine
Cervical orthosis, soft or rigid	Fabric, foam, or a rigid plastic	Restriction of movement

TABLE 8A-5 Examples of gait deviations during prosthetic use.[1]

Gait Abnormality	Possible Prosthetic Causes	Other Possible Causes
Excessive knee flexion in early stance	Lack of plantarflexion Socket too anterior Socket too flexed	Flexion contracture Weak quadriceps muscles
Insufficient knee flexion in early stance	Excessive plantarflexion Socket too posterior Socket not flexed enough	Weak quadriceps Extensor spasticity
Early knee flexion in late stance	Dorsiflexion stop too soft Socket too anterior Socket too flexed	Flexion contracture
Delayed knee flexion in late stance	Dorsiflexion stop too stiff Socket too posterior Socket not flexed enough	Extensor spasticity

REFERENCE

1. O'Sullivan SB, Schmitz TJ, Fulk GD. *Physical Rehabilitation*. 6th ed. Philadelphia, PA: Davis Plus; 2013.

QUESTIONS

1. A patient is transitioning from using a front-wheeled walker to a single-point cane. Which of the following gait patterns is the therapist most likely to teach the patient?
   A. Two point
   B. Modified two point
   C. Three point
   D. Modified three point

2. A 24-year-old has just had ACL surgery, and is 50% partial weight bearing. Which of the following assistive devices and gait pattern would be most appropriate for this client?
   A. Front-wheeled walker and three-point gait
   B. Front-wheeled walker and modified three-point gait
   C. Axillary crutches and three-point gait
   D. Axillary crutches and modified three-point gait

3. A 75-year-old patient is non-weightbearing following an open reduction internal fixation on the right hip. Which of the following devices and gait pattern are most appropriate for this patient?
   A. Front-wheeled walker and four-point gait
   B. Front-wheeled walker and three-point gait
   C. Crutches and four-point gait
   D. Crutches and two-point gait

ANSWERS

1. The answer is **A**. This is the only gait pattern listed that uses a unilateral assistive device; all others require bilateral support.

2. The answer is **D**. The client is young and does not need the added support of a front-wheeled walker, and 50% weightbearing requires a modified three-point gait pattern.

3. The answer is **B**. The client is elderly so a more stable device would be appropriate, but more importantly a non-weightbearing gait pattern is always a three-point pattern.

■ SECTION B: THERAPEUTIC MODALITIES

INTRODUCTION TO THERAPEUTIC MODALITIES

In 2014, the American Physical Therapy Association (APTA) began recommending the use of the term "biophysical agents" to refer to physical agents and modalities. In addition, the APTA Choosing Wisely campaign addressed the use of biophysical agents. Their first recommendation states: "Don't employ passive physical agents except when necessary to facilitate participation in an active treatment program."[1] They further state that "The use of passive physical agents is not harmful to patients except when they communicate to patients that the passive, instead of active, treatment is appropriate." This highlights the need to give careful consideration to the clinical indications for application of biophysical agents. Clinical applications of biophysical agents include alteration of pain, improvement of skeletal muscle activity, and

High-Yield Terms to Learn

Acoustic streaming	The atmospheric pressure at sea level, equal to 1 ATA (760 mmHg).
Accommodation	The increased threshold of excitable tissue when a slowly rising stimulus is used. The quicker the rise time, the less the nerve can accommodate to the impulse.
Alternating current (AC)	The uninterrupted bidirectional flow of ions or electrons that must change direction at least one time per second.
Amplitude	The magnitude of current. Amplitude controls are often labeled intensity.
Asymmetrical waveform	Condition when the amplitude and duration characteristics between the two phases of the biphasic waveform differ in any manner.
Attenuation	A measure of the decrease in ultrasound energy by absorption, reflection, or refraction.
Beam nonuniformity ratio (BNR)	The ratio between spatial peak intensity and spatial average intensity of an ultrasound beam.
Burst	A series of pulses or brief periods of alternating current delivered consecutively and separated from the next series.

High-Yield Terms to Learn (*continued*)

Cavitation	Pulsation of gas bubbles in biological tissues in response to the passage of ultrasound.
Direct current	The continuous, unidirectional flow of charged particles for at least 1 second.
Duty cycle	The percentage of on time to the total time of electrical current multiplied by 100%.
Endorphins	Endogenous opioid-like peptides that reduce the perception of pain by binding to opioid receptors. (Also referred to as opiopeptins.)
Nerve conduction	The transmission of an electrical impulse along a nerve fiber.
Pizoelectric effect	The property of being able to generate electricity in response to a mechanical force, or being able to change shape in response to an electrical current (as in an ultrasound transducer).
Ramp-down time	The time it takes for the current to decrease from its maximum amplitude during the on time, back down to zero.
Ramp-up time	The time it takes for the current amplitude to increase from zero, at the end of the off time, to its maximum amplitude during the on time.

promotion of tissue healing. The physical therapist has a number of adjunctive interventions at his or her disposal. The use of these are determined by the goals of the intervention. In addition to articles cited, information comes from three text books frequently used in physical therapy programs.[2,3,4]

Various categories of physical agents are outlined in Table 8B–1.

TABLE 8B–1   Categories of physical agents.

Thermal	Thermotherapy
	Superficial agents
	Hot packs
	Paraffin
	Fluidotherapy
	Warm whirlpool
	Deep heating agents
	Ultrasound
	Diathermy
	Cryotherapy
	Ice pack
	Ice massage
	Cold whirlpool
Electromagnetic	Electrotherapy
	TENS
	NMES
	IFC
	HVPC
	Microcurrent
	Iontophoresis
	Diathermy (*although electromagnetic, diathermy does provide deep heat*)
	Ultraviolet
	Infrared
Mechanical	Traction
	Compression

TENS, transcutaneous electrical nerve stimulation; NMES, neuromuscular electrical stimulation; IFC, interferential current; HVPC, high-volt pulsed current.

THERMAL AGENTS

There are four major types of thermal modalities. These involve the transfer of thermal energy. See Table 8B–2.

Cryotherapy: The use of cold to induce therapeutic and physiological responses that result from decreased tissue temperature.

Thermotherapy: The application of therapeutic heat involving the transfer of thermal energy. Thermal effects can occur at a superficial or deep level.

TABLE 8B–2   Methods of heat transfer.

Method	Description	Examples
Conduction	Heat is transferred by direct contact of the modality to tissue	Hot packs/heating pads Paraffin Cold packs/ice bag Ice massage Warm or cold water immersion (if there is no agitation)
Convection	Moving fluid particles contact the skin, causing heating or cooling	Fluidotherapy Warm or cool whirlpool with agitation
Evaporation	Rapid evaporation of a liquid spray causes the skin temperature to drop, resulting in decreased pain sensation	Vapocoolant sprays
Radiation	Transfer of heat from a warmer source to a cooler source through a conducting medium such as air	Infrared lamp

TABLE 8B–3 Indications for cryotherapy and thermotherapy.

Cryotherapy	Thermotherapy
• Limitation of edema formation	• Pain reduction (analgesia)
• Pain reduction	• Increased joint range of motion
• Facilitation of skeletal muscle relaxation	• Decreased muscle spasm
• Limitation of secondary hypoxic tissue injury	

TABLE 8B–5 Effects of cryotherapy and thermotherapy.

Cryotherapy	Thermotherapy
• Vasoconstriction	• Vasodilation
• Decreased local tissue metabolism	• Increased metabolic rate
• Decreased inflammation	• Increased local nerve conduction
• Elevated pain threshold/ analgesia	• Increased collagen extensibility
• Decreased muscle spasm	• Increased collagen elasticity
• Reduced muscle efficiency	• Decreased joint stiffness
	• Increased muscle flexibility

Indications for cryotherapy and thermotherapy are listed in Table 8B–3. Contraindications for cryotherapy and thermotherapy are listed in Table 8B–4. Effects of cryotherapy and thermotherapy are listed in Table 8B–5.

The principle physiological effects of cold application are due to vasoconstriction, reduced metabolic function, and reduced motor and sensory nerve conduction velocities. The following list describes the major physiological effects of cold application:

• A rapid decrease in skin temperature where subcutaneous temperature falls less rapidly and displays a smaller temperature change. The ideal tissue temperature to achieve the optimal physiologic effects of cryotherapy is 15°C to 25°C.[5]

• A decrease in muscle and intra-articular temperature.

• Localized vasoconstriction of all smooth muscle by the central nervous system to conserve heat. Maximum vasoconstriction occurs at tissue temperatures of 15°C (59°F). Localized vasoconstriction is responsible for the decrease in the tendency toward formation and accumulation of edema, probably as a result of a decrease in local hydrostatic pressure. There is also a decrease in the amount of nutrients and phagocytes delivered to the area, thus reducing phagocytic activity.[2]

Localized analgesia:[6–12] The stages of analgesia achieved by cryotherapy are as follows:

• Stage 1: Cold sensation, which usually occurs within 3 minutes
• Stage 2: Burning or aching sensation, which usually occurs between 2 and 7 minutes

TABLE 8B–4 Contraindications for cryotherapy and thermotherapy.

Cryotherapy	Thermotherapy
• Cold hypersensitivity	• Potential hemorrhage
• Cold urticaria	• Thrombophlebitis
• Cold intolerance	• Vascular insufficiency
• Cryoglobulinemia	• Decreased thermal sensation
• Paroxysmal cold hemoglobinuria	• Impaired mentation
• Raynaud's disease or phenomenon	• Areas of infection or inflammation
• Over-regenerating peripheral nerves	• Areas of malignancy
• Area of circulatory compromise	• Recent application of liniments
• Peripheral vascular disease	

• Stage 3. Local numbness or analgesia, which usually occurs between 5 and 12 minutes
• Stage 4: Deep tissue vasodilation without increase in metabolism, which usually occurs between 12 and 15 minutes

The timing of these stages depends on the depth of penetration and varying thickness of adipose tissue. The patient should be advised regarding these various stages, especially in light of the fact that the burning/aching stage occurs before the therapeutic phases. Therapeutic effects of cold application include the following:

• Decreased cell permeability and decreased cellular metabolism, which results in a decreased demand for oxygen, which in turn limits further injury, particularly in the case of acute tissue damage.

• Decreased muscle spasm, which is produced through a raise in the threshold of activation of the muscle spindle.

• Decrease in the excitability of free nerve endings and peripheral nerve fibers, resulting in an increase in the pain threshold.[13,14]

Heat greatly influences the hemodynamic, neuromuscular, and metabolic processes of the body. Physiological effects of local heat include the following:[15–19]

• Skin temperature rises rapidly and exhibits the greatest temperature change. Subcutaneous tissue temperature rises less rapidly and exhibits a smaller change. Muscle and joint show less temperature change, if any, depending on size and structure. The increase in heat is dissipated through selective vasodilation and shunting of blood via reflexes in the microcirculation and regional blood flow.[20]

• Increase in local nerve conduction.

• Decreased muscle spasm, thereby facilitating stretching. The muscle relaxation likely results from a decrease in firing rates of the efferent fibers in the muscle spindle.

• Increased capillary permeability, cell metabolism, and cellular activity, which can increase the delivery of oxygen and chemical nutrients to the area while decreasing venous stagnation.[17,21]

• Increased analgesia through hyperstimulation of the cutaneous nerve receptors.

• An increase in tissue extensibility. In order to be therapeutic, the amount of thermal energy transferred to the tissue must be sufficient to stimulate without causing damage to the tissue. In an environment of connective tissue healing, the immature collagen bonds can be degraded by heat. This has obvious implications for the application of stretching techniques. Optimum results are obtained if the heat is applied during the stretch and

TABLE 8B-6 Clinical applications of whirlpool treatment according to temperature ranges.

Temperature	Degrees	Use
Very hot	104°F (40–43.4°C)	Short exposure of 7–10 minutes to increase superficial temperature
Hot	99–104°F (37–40°C)	Increase superficial temperature
Warm	96–99°F (35.5–37°C)	Increase superficial temperature where a prolonged exposure is wanted, such as to decrease spasticity of a muscle in conjunction with passive exercise
Neutral	92–96°F (33.5–35.5°C)	Patients who have an unstable core body temperature
Tepid	80–92°F (27–33.5°C)	May be used in conjunction with less vigorous exercise
Cool	67–80°F (19–27°C)	May be used in conjunction with vigorous exercise
Cold	57–67°F (13–19°C)	Used for longer exposure of 10–15 minutes to decrease superficial temperature
Very cold	32–55°F (0–13°C)	Used for short exposure of 1–5 minutes to decrease superficial temperature

the stretch is maintained until cooling occurs after the removal of the heat.[20]

Temperature ranges for application of whirlpool treatments are listed in Table 8B–6.

Hydrotherapy and fluidotherapy offer a number of advantages over other thermal modalities. They allow the patient to mobilize the affected part during the treatment. Most of the benefits associated with these modalities are related to the physical properties of fluids.

- Buoyancy: Water provides buoyance equal to the weight of the water displaced causing decreased weight bearing or gravitational effect on the body part(s) submerged.
- Hydrostatic pressure: Water exerts a circumferential pressure on the submerged body part(s) which can decrease edema and promote venous return.
- Resistance: Water provides resistance to movement of submerged body part(s) due to the cohesion of the water molecules and the force needed to separate them.

ELECTROTHERAPEUTIC MODALITIES

Electrical stimulation has a wide variety of applications in the physical therapy setting. Clinical applications of electrical stimulation are most commonly used to activate skeletal muscle for improving muscle performance or strengthening, to decrease pain, to improve blood flow, to decrease edema, or to facilitate

TABLE 8B-7 Electrotherapeutic modalities.

Indications	Precautions	Contraindications
Pain control Muscle contraction to • Increase strength • Improve ROM • Improve functional activity Tissue healing Improvement of blood flow Enhancement of transdermal drug delivery Decrease edema	Cardiac disease Patients with impaired mentation or in areas with impaired sensation Malignant tumors Areas of skin irritation or open wounds	Demand cardiac pacemaker or unstable arrhythmias Placement of electrodes over carotid sinus Areas where venous or arterial thrombosis or thrombophlebitis is present Pregnancy—over or around the abdomen or low back

tissue healing. Clinicians have a wide range of electrotherapeutic modalities at their disposal for treatment. Indications, precautions, and contraindications for electrotherapeutic modalities are listed in Table 8B–7.

Two common modes of electrotherapeutic modalities are transcutaneous electrical nerve stimulation (TENS), which is used for pain control (Table 8B–8), and neuromuscular electrical stimulation (NMES) (Table 8B–9), commonly used to improve strength, function, and range of motion (ROM).

High-Volt Pulsed Current

High-volt pulsed current (HVPC), also referred to as high-voltage galvanic therapy or high-voltage pulsed galvanic stimulation (HVPGS) utilizes a twin peak, monophasic, pulsed current. There is usually one large dispersive electrode along with one, two, or four active electrodes, with the active electrode being much smaller than the dispersive electrode.

Russian Current or Medium-Frequency Alternating Current

Russian current is a medium-frequency polyphasic waveform. The intensity is produced in a burst mode that has a 50% duty cycle, with a pulse width range of 50–200 microseconds, and an interburst interval of 10 milliseconds.[22] Medium-frequency currents can reduce resistance to current flow, making this type of current more comfortable than some others, especially if the current is delivered in bursts or if an interburst interval is used. Russian current is believed to augment muscle strengthening via polarizing both sensory and motor nerve fibers, resulting in tetanic contractions that are painless and stronger than those made voluntarily by the patient.

Interferential Current

Interferential current (IFC) works by combining two high-frequency alternating waveforms that are biphasic but that vary in relation to one another in amplitude, frequency, or both. Where these two distinct currents meet in the tissue, an electrical

TABLE 8B-8 Transcutaneous electrical nerve stimulation (TENS).

Mode of TENS	Conventional	Acupuncture-Like	Burst Train	Brief Intense
Frequency	80–110 Hz	<10 Hz (1–4 Hz)	100 Hz delivered at 2 Hz	100–150 Hz
Pulse duration	50–100 µs	150–200 µs	150–200 µs	150–200 µs
Amplitude	**Sensory level**	**Motor level**	**Motor level**	**Noxious level**
Mechanism of analgesia	Larger diameter peripheral nerve fibers neuromodulate pain via spinal neurochemical gating mechanism	Stimulates small diameter, high threshold peripheral afferents (A-delta) in order to activate extrasegmental descending pain inhibitory pathways	Simulates small diameter, high threshold cutaneous afferents (A-delta) to block transmission of nociceptive information in peripheral nerves and to activate extrasegmental analgesic mechanisms	
Advantages	Comfortable Fast-acting Can be used for acute or chronic since there is no motor response Can be worn continuously if needed	Amount of carryover can be up to 4 hours Minimal adaptation	Sometimes perceived as more comfortable than acupuncture-like TENS	Can be used during short minor, painful procedures Used when other TENS modes have not been successful Fast onset of analgesia
Disadvantages	Purely chemical response, so carryover is short Adaptation to stimulus is common	Motor response required, so may not be appropriate for acute conditions May limit functional activity Limited to 1 hour to reduce the potential of soreness from contractions Onset of analgesia delayed 20–30 minutes to allow for beta-endorphine release	Motor response required, so may not be appropriate for acute conditions May limit functional activity Limited to 1 hour to reduce the potential of soreness from contractions Onset of analgesia delayed 20–30 minutes to allow for beta-endorphine release	Uncomfortable Not used as first option Pain return is quite rapid

TABLE 8B-9 Neuromuscular electrical stimulation (NMES).

	To Strengthen Weakened Muscle	To Improve ROM (1 Muscle)	To Improve ROM (2 Muscles)	Functional Electrical Stimulation (FES)
Frequency	20–100 pps	50 pps	30–50 pps	30–4 pps
Pulse duration	200–600 µs	200–600 µs	200–600 µs	200–350 µs
Amplitude	To obtain strong muscle contraction (maximum tolerated or current necessary to achieve >50% MVC	Strong enough to move the body part through full available range of motion	Strong enough to move the body part through full available range of motion	To achieve –3/5 contraction
Ramp-up time	1–5 sec	3 sec	3 sec	0–1 sec
Ramp-down time	1–2 sec	0–1 sec	0–1 sec	0–1 sec
Duty cycle	1:3–1:5 with on-time up to 10 sec and off-time up to 50 sec	15 sec on/45 sec off	10 sec on (each channel)/10 sec off (each channel)	N/A stimulation is timed with demand of functional activity
Treatment time and duration	At least 10 contractions or up to 1 hour/day 3–5 times/week 4–8 weeks	30–60 minutes at least every other day	30–60 minutes at least every other day	Determined by muscle fatigue

MVC, Maximum Voluntary Contraction.

interference pattern is created based on the summation or the subtraction of the respective amplitudes or frequencies. Parameters for use of IFC can be found in Table 8B–10.

Iontophoresis

Transdermal iontophoresis is the delivery of ionic therapeutic agents through the skin by the application of a low-level electric current. Iontophoresis has proved to be valuable in the intervention of musculoskeletal disorders. Iontophoresis causes an increased penetration of drugs and other compounds into tissues by the use of an applied current through the tissue. The proposed mechanisms by which iontophoresis increases drug penetration are outlined in Table 8B–11.

Acoustic Radiation: Ultrasound

Ultrasound (US) is primarily used for its ability to deliver heat to deep musculoskeletal tissues such as tendon, muscle, and joint structures. The application of ultrasound requires a homogenous medium for effective sound wave transmission and to act as a lubricant. US produces a high-frequency alternating current. The waves are delivered through the transducer, which has a metal face-plate with a piezoelectric crystal cemented between two electrodes. This crystal can vibrate very rapidly, converting electrical energy to acoustical (sound) energy (via the reverse piezoelectric effect) with little dispersion of energy. The energy leaves the transducer in a straight line (collimated beam). As the energy travels further from the transducer, the waves begin to diverge.

The depth of penetration of the US depends on the absorption and scattering of the beam. Scar tissue, tendon, and cartilage demonstrate the highest absorption. Tissues that demonstrate poor absorption include bone, blood, adipose, and muscle.

Indications, precautions, and contraindications for US can be found in Table 8B–12. Depth of penetration is outlined in Table 8B–13 and recommended intensities are outlined in Table 8B–14.

Phonophoresis is a specific type of US application in which pharmacological agents are driven transdermally into the subcutaneous tissues. Both the thermal and mechanical properties of US have been cited as possible mechanisms for the pharmacological agents.

The efficacy or phonophoresis has not been conclusively established. The proposed indications include pain modulation and the decrease of inflammation in subacute and chronic musculoskeletal conditions. The method of application for phonophoresis is similar to the direct technique method of ultrasound except that a medicinal agent is use in the coupling medium to transmit the ultrasound beam. The typical treatment lasts 5 to 10 minutes and uses an intensity of 1 to 3 W/cm^2. Using lower intensity and a longer treatment time is thought to be more effective for introducing medication into the skin.

SPINAL TRACTION

Traction is a mechanical force applied to the body in a way that separates the joint surfaces and elongates surrounding soft tissue. Indications, contraindications, and precautions are listed in Table 8B–15. Recommended dosages are listed in Table 8B–16.

TABLE 8B–10 Interferential current.

	Frequency	Pulse Width
Muscle contraction	20–50 pps	100–300 μs
Pain management	50–120 pps	50–150 μs

TABLE 8B–11 Mechanisms of iontophoresis drug delivery.

The electrical potential gradient includes changes at the cellular level[23]
Pore formation occurs in the stratum corneum[24]
Hair follicles, sweat glands, and sweat ducts act as diffusion shunts for ion transport[25]

TABLE 8B–12 Ultrasound indications, precautions, and contraindications.

Indications	Precautions	Contraindications
Pain modulation	Acute inflammation	Healing fractures
Increased connective tissue extensibility	Breast implants in area of treatment	Impaired circulation
Reduction of soft tissue and joint restriction	Open epiphysis	Impaired cognitive function
Reduction of muscle spasm	Healing fractures	Impaired sensation
Remodeling of scar tissue		Thrombophlebitis
		Plastic components
		Area of malignancy
		Tuberculosis infection
		Hemorrhagic conditions
		Brain, ears, eyes, heart, cervical ganglia, carotid sinuses, reproductive organs, spinal cord, over cardiac pacemaker, over pregnant uterus

TABLE 8B–13 Ultrasound frequency.

Frequency	Depth of Penetration
1 MHz	Effective up to a depth of 5–8 cm
3 MHz	More superficial Effective to a depth of approximately 1–2 cm

The depth of penetration of the ultrasound beam is dependent upon the frequency.

TABLE 8B–14 Recommended intensity.

Intensity w/cm²	Purpose
0.1–1.0	Wound healing
0.5–1.0	Pain and spasm relief
0.5–1.5	Hematoma resorption
1.0–1.5	Increased plasticity of scar and connective tissue

The amount of tissue heating is dependent on the intensity of the ultrasound.

TABLE 8B–15 Spinal traction.

Indications	Precautions	Contraindications
Fluid exchange and nutrient transport within the disc	Structural diseases or conditions affecting the spine	Acute cervical trauma
Increase of intervertebral foramina dimensions	Medial disc protrusion	Whiplash
Reduction of disc herniation extension	Claustrophobia	Use of steroids or other medications that tend to compromise bone integrity
Relaxation of paraspinal muscle spasm	Inability to tolerate the desired position	Osteoporosis or osteopenia
Nerve root impingement	Disorientation	Rheumatologic disorders affecting connective tissues
Joint hypomobility	Chronic obstructive pulmonary disease (harnesses can be restrictive)	Rheumatoid arthritis
		Joint hypermobility/instability
		Pregnancy (lumbar)
		Prior stabilization or decompression
		Spinal implants
		Nonmechanical pain
		Peripheralization of symptoms with traction
		Uncontrolled hypertension

TABLE 8B–16 Traction dosage.

	Intensity	Duty Cycle	Duration
Cervical	10–25 lb	1:1 for mobility and facet problems	10–20 minutes (generally lower duration for static)
Lumbar	Up to ½ patient body weight	3:1 or static for disc problems	

TABLE 8B–17 Indications, precautions, and contraindications for intermittent pneumatic compression.

Indications	Precautions	Contraindications
• Edema reduction • Prevention of DVT • Venous stasis ulcers • Residual limb shaping after amputation • Control of hypertrophic scarring • Lymphedema	• Impaired sensation • Impaired mentation • Uncontrolled hypertension • Cancer • Stroke or significant peripheral nerves	• Heart failure • Pulmonary edema • Recent or acute DVT, thrombophlebitis, or pulmonary embolism • Obstructed lymphatic or venous return • Severe peripheral arterial disease • Ulcers resulting from venous insufficiency • Acute local skin infection • Significant hypoproteinemia • Acute trauma or fracture • Arterial revascularization

INTERMITTENT PNEUMATIC COMPRESSION

Intermittent pneumatic compression (IPC) is a mechanical force that increases external pressure on a body part. Indications, precautions, and contraindications can be found in Table 8B–17.

There is little agreement regarding IPC pressure or treatment times. In some machines the treatment cycles are preset, while others allow the therapist to determine the duty cycle. General guidelines accompany most machines.

STUDY PEARL

Temperature Conversions:
- Fahrenheit = (temperature in Celsius × 9/5) + 32 or (temperature in Celsius × 1.8) + 32
- Celsius = (temperature in Fahrenheit – 32) × 5/9 or (temperature in Fahrenheit – 32) × 0.55

STUDY PEARL

The effect of skin temperature on cutaneous blood flow involves the following:
- Normal cutaneous flow is 200 to 250 mL/min.
- At 15°C, maximal vasoconstriction is reached, with blood flow measured at 20 to 50 mL/min.
- Below 15°C, vasoconstriction is interrupted by rhythmic bursts of vasodilation occurring 3 to 5 times per hour and lasting 5 to 10 minutes. These bursts are more frequent and longer in individuals acclimated to the cold, making them less prone to frostbite injury.
- At 10°C, neurapraxia occurs, resulting in loss of cutaneous sensation.
- Below 0°C, negligible cutaneous blood flow allows the skin to freeze.
- Without circulation, skin temperature drops at a rate exceeding 0.5°C per minute.
- Smaller blood vessels (ie, microvasculature) freeze before large blood vessels.
- The venous system freezes before the arterial system because of lower flow rates.

STUDY PEARL

The use of ice by itself[6] or in conjunction with compression has been demonstrated to be effective in minimizing the amount of edema.[7] However, even though the immediate application of cold will help to control edema if applied immediately following injury, the gravity-dependent positions should be avoided with acute and subacute injuries because of the likelihood of additional swelling.

STUDY PEARL

Depth of penetration depends on the amount of cold, the length of the treatment time, the intensity and duration of the cold application, and the circulatory response of the body segment exposed.[5]

STUDY PEARL

The application of cold packs and ice bags over superficial peripheral nerves (ie, the deep peroneal [fibular] nerve and the fibular head) can result in temporary or permanent injury of these nerves.

STUDY PEARL

Prior to the application of cold, the area to be treated should be assessed for protective sensation to avoid skin damage.

STUDY PEARL

The choice of thermal modality depends on the goal of the treatment and the tissue to be treated. For example, if the primary treatment goal is a tissue temperature increase with a corresponding increase in blood flow to the deeper tissues, the clinician should choose a modality such as diathermy or ultrasound, which produces energy that can penetrate the cutaneous tissues and be directly absorbed by the deeper tissues.

STUDY PEARL

A decrease in diastolic blood pressure can occur during and following a heat application to a large body area.[5] Care should be taken when transferring any patient following such treatments.

STUDY PEARL

Prior to application of heat, the area to be treated should be assessed for protective sensation to avoid burning the patient.

STUDY PEARL

The skin normally looks pink or red following an application of heat. A dark red or mottled appearance indicates that too much heat has been applied and the treatment should cease.

STUDY PEARL

Wet heat produces a greater rise in local tissue temperature compared to dry heat at any given temperature.[26] However, at higher temperatures, wet heat is not tolerated as well as dry heat.

STUDY PEARL

Allowing a patient to lie on a hot pack or cold pack can weaken the seams and allow the substance inside to leak out.

STUDY PEARL

Patients lying on a hot pack should be assessed for tolerance more frequently than those patients who have the hot pack on top of them. The plastic on the plinth reflects the heat and does not allow it to dissipate as quickly, providing a higher dosage.

STUDY PEARL

Paraffin treatments provide six times the amount of heat available in water because the mineral oil in the paraffin lowers the melting point of the paraffin.[5] This provides the paraffin with a lower specific heat than water, allowing for a slower exchange of heat to the skin.

STUDY PEARL

The risk of burn with paraffin is substantial, and the clinician should weigh heavily the considerations between paraffin bath and warm whirlpool bath.

STUDY PEARL

When dipping into the paraffin, the first layer of wax should be the highest on the body segment and each successive layer lower than the previous one. This is to prevent subsequent layers from getting between the first layer and the skin and burning the patient.

STUDY PEARL

The phase duration contributes to the comfort of the stimulation, the amount of chemical change that occurs in the nerves, and nerve discrimination. A duration of 50 to 100 ms typically is used for sensory stimulation, and 220 to 300 ms is typically used for motor stimulation.[15]

STUDY PEARL

- Very short pulse durations with low intensities can depolarize sensory nerves.
- Longer pulse durations are required to stimulate motor nerves.
- Very long pulse durations with high intensities are needed to elicit a response from a denervated muscle.

STUDY PEARL

The effects of ultrasound are predominantly empirical and are based on reported biophysical effects within tissue,[27,28] and on anecdotal experience in clinical practice.[28–30]

STUDY PEARL

The greater ratio difference in the beam nonuniformity ratio (BNR), the more likely the transducer will have hot spots (areas of high intensity), which will increase the likelihood of patients experiencing a burning sensation.

STUDY PEARL

The entire ultrasound head does not emit ultrasound waves. This should factor in to the therapist's determination of an appropriate area for treatment. The area that does emit the sound waves is referred to as the effective radiating area (ERA).[31]

REFERENCES

1. Center for Integrity in Practice. Choosing wisely: the right care at the right time. Retrieved from http://integrity.apta.org/ChoosingWisely/. Accessed July 20, 2018.

2. Bellew JW, Michlovitz SL, Nolan TP. *Michlovitz's Modalities for Therapeutic Intervention.* Philadelphia, PA: FA Davis; 2016.

3. Cameron MH. *Physical Agents in Rehabilitation, From Research to Practice.* 4th ed. St. Louis, MO. Elsevier; 2012.

4. Bell GW, Prentice WE. Infrared modalities. In: Prentice WE, ed. *Therapeutic Modalities for Allied Health Professionals.* New York, NY: McGraw-Hill; 1998:201-262.

5. Zenlke JE, Andersen JC, Guion WK, et al. Intramuscular temperature responses in the human leg to two forms of cryotherapy: ice massage and ice bag. *J Orthop Sports Phys Ther.* 1998;27:301-307.

6. McMaster WC, Liddle S, Waugh TR. Laboratory evaluation of various cold therapy modalities. *AM J Sports Med.* 1978;6:291-294.

7. Knight KL. *Cryotherapy: Theory, Technique, and Physiology.* Chattanooga, TN: Chattanooga Publishing Company; 1985.

8. Daniel DM, Stone ML, Arendt DL. The effect of cold therapy on pain, swelling, and range of motion after anterior cruciate ligament reconstructive surgery. *Arthroscopy.* 1994;10:530-533.

9. Konrath GA, Lock T, Goitz HR, et al. The use of cold therapy after anterior cruciate ligament reconstruction. A prospective, randomized study and literature review. *Am J Sports Med.* 1996;24:620-633.

10. Michlovitz SL. The use of heat and cold in the management of rheumatic diseases. In: Michlovitz SL, ed. *Thermal Agents in Rehabilitation.* Philadelphia, PA: FA Davis; 1990:158-174.

11. Speer KP, Warren RF, Horowitz L. The efficacy of cryotherapy in the postoperative shoulder. *J Shoulder Elbow Surg.* 1996:5:62-68.

12. Knight KL. *Cryotherapy in Sports Injury Management.* Champaign, IL: Human Kinetics; 1995.

13. Knutsson E. Topical cryotherapy in spasticity. *Scand J Rehabil Med.* 1970;2:159-163.

14. Waylonis GW. The physiological effects of ice massage. *Arch Phys Med Rehabil.* 1967;48:42-47.

15. Knight KL, Aquino J, Johannes SM, et al. A re-examination of Lewis' cold induced vasodilation in the finger and ankle. *Athl Training.* 1890;15:248-250.

16. Clark D, Stelmach G. Muscle fatigue and recovery curve parameters at various temperatures. *Res Q.* 1966;468-479.

17. Baker R, Bell G. The effect of therapeutic modalities on blood flow in the human calf. *J Orthop Sports Phys Ther.* 1991;13:23.

18. Zankel H. Effect of physical agents on motor conduction velocity of the ulnar nerve. *Arch Phys Med Rehabil.* 1994;47:197-199.

19. Abramson DI, Bell B, Tuck S. Changes in blood flow, oxygen uptake and tissue temperatures produced by therapeutic physical agents: effect of indirect or reflex vasodilation. *AM J Phys Med.* 1961;40:5-13.

20. Frizzell LA, Dunn F. Biophysics of ultrasound. In Lehman JF, ed. *Therapeutic Heat and Cold.* 3rd ed. Baltimore, MD: Williams & Wilkins; 1982:353-385.

21. Barcroft H, Edholm OS. The effect of temperature on blood flow and deep temperature in the human forearm. *J Physiol.* 1943;102:5-20.

22. Gotlin RS, Hershkowtz S, Juris PM, et al. Electrical Stimulation effect on extensor lag and length of hospital stay after total knee arthroplasty. *Arch Phys Med Rehabil.* 1994;75:957.

23. Chein YW, Siddiqui O, Shi M, et al. Direct current iontophoretic transdermal delivery of peptide and protein drugs. *J Pharm Sci.* 1989;78:376-384.

24. Grimmes S. Pathways of ionic flow through human skin in vivo. *Acta Dermatol Venereol.* 1984;64:93-98.

25. Lee RD, White HS, Scott ER. Visualization if iontophoretic transport paths in cultured and animal skin models. *J Pharm Sci.* 1996;85:1186-1190.

26. Abramson DI, Tudk S, Lee SE, et al. Comparison of wet and dry heat in rising temperature of tissues. *Arch Phys Med Rehabil.* 1967;48:654.

27. Dyson M, Pond JB, Joseph J, et al. The stimulation of tissue regeneration by means of ultrasound. *Clin Sci.* 1968;35:273-285.

28. Dyson M, Suckling J. Stimulation of tissue repair by ultrasound: a survey of the mechanisms involved. *Physiotherapy.* 1978;64:105-108.

29. Aldes JH, Klaras TL. The use of ultrasonic radiation in the treatment of subdeltoid bursitis with and without calcaneous deposits. *West J Surg.* 1954;62:369-376.

30. Flax HJ. Ultrasound treatment for peritendinitis calcarea of the shoulder. *Am J Phys Med Rehabil.* 1964;42:117-124.

31. Dyson M. Mechanisms involved in therapeutic ultrasound. *Physiotherapy.* 1897;73:116-120.

QUESTIONS

1. A patient has just had a cast removed 6 weeks post Colles fracture. Which of the following modalities would be the BEST modality to increase ROM in the wrist and fingers?
   A. Fluidotherapy
   B. Heating pad
   C. Hot pack
   D. Paraffin

2. Which of the following locations are the optimal electrode placement for motor stimulation?
   A. One electrode on the functional motor point and the other over a more distal site on the extremity
   B. Electrodes as far away from each other as possible
   C. Distal to the muscle fibers
   D. One electrode on the functional motor point and the other on the muscle belly

3. A patient with severe rheumatoid arthritis is having an acute exacerbation resulting in neck pain with accompanying muscle guarding and spasm. Which of the following modalities and settings would be the BEST modality for pain control?
   A. Intermittent cervical traction at 12 lb with 1:1 duty cycle for 20 minutes
   B. Ultrasound at 1.5 w.cm^2, 1 MHz, 100% duty cycle for 7 minutes
   C. Moist hot pack to cervical spine for 20 minutes
   D. TENS to bilateral cervical spine pulse duration 60 ms, frequency 130 pps with amplitude modulation set to patient comfort with sensory stimulation for 30 minutes

4. A patient diagnosed with lateral epicondylitis has completed a therapeutic exercise program. The physical therapist instructs this patient on how to apply ice massage to the affected area. Which of the following is MOST appropriate?
   A. Continue with ice massage until a mild burning sensation is experienced
   B. Treatment time of 5 to 10 minutes
   C. Continue treatment until a response of numbness/tingling is experienced in the ring and little fingers
   D. Treatment time of 10 to 15 minutes

5. Ultrasound applied at 1.0 MHz is most effective at heating which of the following tissue types?
   A. Blood
   B. Fat
   C. Muscle
   D. Tendon

6. Although not clinically proven, it is generally recommended that when applying intermittent pneumatic compression, inflation pressure should not exceed:
   A. Diastolic blood pressure plus 10 mmHg
   B. Diastolic blood pressure minus 10 mmHg
   C. Systolic blood pressure plus 10 mmHg
   D. Systolic blood pressure minus 10 mmHg

ANSWERS

1. The answer is **A**. (*Michlovitz*, p. 79)[2]
   Although all modalities would provide heating for increase in tissue extensibility, fluidotherapy along with paraffin would allow increased exposure of irregular surfaces of fingers to heat over hot packs or heating pad. Fluidotherapy is the only modality that allows the patient to exercise during the treatment for optimal increase in ROM.

2. The answer is **D**. (*Michlovitz*, p. 296)[2]
   A. When placing electrodes for motor stimulation, a common mistake occurs when one electrode is placed over a motor point and the other is placed over a distal site on the extremity. The problem with this can be that the distal electrode is often placed away from the region of the motor nerve where the optimal response is obtained, rendering the stimulus less effective. Also, the distal electrode is often placed in a region where there is significantly less or no polarized muscle.
   B. Increasing the distance between electrodes increases the depth of penetration. If the muscle or muscle group is very superficial, as in the instance of wrist flexors, placing the electrodes too far apart can activate wrist extensors as well.
   C. During stimulation of muscle, if the patient's sensation goes straight from sensory to noxious, it is probably because one of the electrodes is not over an area of muscle tissue.
   D. Motor points are the locations where the greatest motor response is found for a given amount of stimulus. The other electrode should be placed over the muscle group rather than tendon area.

3. The answer is **D**.
   A. Cervical traction is contraindicated in patients with severe rheumatoid arthritis due to possible ligament instability (*Michlovitz*, p. 277).[2]
   B. Ultrasound at these parameters would produce tissue heating, which is contraindicated in acute inflammation (*Michlovitz*, p. 82).[2]
   C. Hot packs would produce tissue heating, which is contraindicated in acute inflammation (*Michlovitz*, p. 82).[2]
   D. These symptoms are likely to respond to pain modulation via TENS (Cameron, p. 263).[3]

4. The answer is **B**.
   A. A mild burning sensation is a normal sensation during an ice massage and should pass quickly. A prolonged phase may result if the area covered is too large or if a hypersensitive response is imminent (*Michlovitz*, p. 47).[2]
   B. A treatment time of 5 to 10 minutes is generally sufficient for a 10 cm × 15 cm area (*Michlovitz*, p. 47).[2]
   C. Cold application over an area of a superficial peripheral nerve can lead to neuropraxia or axonotmesis. Numbness/tingling in the ring and little finger could indicate damage to the ulnar nerve (*Michlovitz*, p. 43).[2]
   D. A treatment time of 5 to 10 minutes is generally sufficient for a 10 cm × 15 cm area (*Michlovitz*, p. 47).[2]

5. The answer is **B**. More dense connective tissues absorb ultrasound better than less dense tissues such as muscle or fat. Therefore, ultrasound is more effective at heating denser tissues (*Michlovitz*, p. 91).[10]
   A. Attenuation of ultrasound in blood is approximately 3%.
   B. Attenuation of ultrasound in fat is approximately 13%.
   C. Attenuation of ultrasound in muscle is approximately 24%.
   D. Attenuation of ultrasound tendon is approximately 59%, so of the choices, tendon tissue absorbs the highest percentage of heat.

6. The answer is **B**. Although studies suggest that pressure may not need to be that high, it is recommended that pressure not exceed patient diastolic blood pressure minus 10 mmHg, as pressure higher than that will restrict venous return (*Michlovitz*, p. 244).[2]

It is expected that a student who has completed or nearly completed a Doctor of Physical Therapy (DPT) curriculum would know the mechanics of application of the various physical agents available. *When you complete this section, you should be able to:*

❑ Determine the appropriate physical agents for patient application based on patient indications.

❑ Identify precautions and contraindications to application of physical agents.

❑ Select appropriate parameters for application of physical agents for a given patient.

■ SECTION C: PROTECTION AND PROFESSIONAL ROLES

PATIENT SAFETY

Within the medical profession there will always be a potential for emergency situations. Within an inpatient facility setting, it is the responsibility of the physical therapist to have a full understanding and awareness of the various "codes" that may be announced that directly influence patient safety. On hearing the code alarms, the physical therapist should follow facility protocols to ensure patient and staff safety. These "codes" can include patient abduction, on-site threat, environmental threat, and individual patient emergencies. Appropriate and correct action is required in all cases by the PT.

FALLS AND FALL RISK

All patients should be evaluated for fall risk at every visit, particularly those over the age of 65. The patient should not only be asked if they have experienced a fall since the previous visit, but the definition of a fall should also be clearly explained.

According to the World Health Organization, "A fall is defined as an event which results in a person coming to rest inadvertently on the ground or floor or other lower level." It does not have to result in injury, and many older adults will deny falling if they were not injured. It is therefore important to ensure that they understand what constitutes a fall and then determine if they have fallen.

Table 8C–1 shows protocols for a situation of a patient falling during therapy. During any family contact, no indication of guilt should be made, facts should be reported, and the family should be referred to appropriate management for follow-up as needed. Everything from the fall to the follow-ups should be carefully and accurately documented immediately to ensure accurate and full recollection of the incident. If incident was witnessed, be sure to get a statement from any witness.

RESTRAINTS

The Centers for Medicare and Medicaid Services (CMS) has very strict guidelines for the use of restraints in the skilled nursing arena. Each state has different interpretations of restraints, and local and state policies must be adhered to. The use of restraints is at times critical for patient safety; however, every effort has to have been made and documented to try less restrictive measures. Any inappropriate use of restraints, either chemical or physical, by a facility, caregiver, or family member, should be considered an act of abuse and be reported to the appropriate authorities using the correct policy per the facility, agency, or management guidelines. In many states, failure of a physical therapist to report possible abuse is a criminal offense.

ENVIRONMENTAL FACTORS

The environment can be both beneficial and detrimental to the health of a patient. A positive, well-lit, sunny, uncluttered setting can be positive and promote well-being. In contrast, a cluttered, dirty location can be hazardous for using assistive devices, can be unconducive to wound healing, and can increase the risk for falls and medical complications. It is the responsibility of all PTs to ensure that their working environment is clean, equipment is sanitized after each patient, and equipment is safe, in good working order, and is regularly checked for damage.

In the home setting, the physical therapist should conduct a thorough examination of the home and make recommendations for the removal of hazards such as throw rugs, electricity cords, clutter, etc., but keeping in mind that in the home health setting, the physical therapist is a guest of the patient, so any recommendations should be made tactfully and carefully, and it is the choice of the patient whether or not to comply. Clear documentation of recommendations should be made to ensure that patient safety was considered.

EMERGENCY PREPAREDNESS

It is the responsibility of every physical therapist to maintain current CPR certification and training, as well as basic first aid

TABLE 8C–1 Emergency response.

Location	Policies	Obvious Injury	No Obvious Injury	Follow-Up	Who to Contact
Outpatient clinic	Follow clinic policy and procedures	Call 911 for medical support	Get patient up, take vital signs; if normal, continue with caution and patient consent	Continue to monitor patient and only allow them to leave the clinic if you are sure they are stable and safe	Primary care physician Management of the facility
Home health setting	Follow agency policies and contact agency immediately	Call 911 for medical support	Get patient up, take vital signs; if normal, continue with caution	Continue to monitor patient throughout the session and do not leave the home until you are sure the patient is safe and stable and not alone	Home health agency Primary care physician Family as appropriate with patient consent
Inpatient setting	Follow facility protocols	Call nursing, emergency response team, and/or MD to the location	Call nursing and/or MD to the location Get patient up and continue per MD recommendations	Complete all facility paperwork and ensure that all appropriate follow-up calls will be made, or make them as needed	Ensure nursing have agreed to contact family and physician, otherwise PT may be required to do so. Document all calls made.

knowledge. In all settings the therapist should be aware of facility, agency, or management policies and protocols regarding disaster response and the role of the physical therapist in the situation. Within the home health setting, the physical therapist should be aware of the disaster levels of the patients and follow up after a natural disaster in the appropriate time frame. In the event that a facility has to be evacuated, the physical therapist should assist as needed, providing appropriate assistive device (AD) for ambulatory patients and coordinating with other members of the interdisciplinary team (IDT) to provide oxygen and other medical support as appropriate.

CARDIAC EVENTS

All patients should be constantly monitored for their response to activity when participating in physical therapy. Exercise protocols including maximum heart rates and response to activity should be adhered to. Patients on medications or pacemakers to control heart rate should be carefully monitored with perceived rate of exertion scales to ensure they are not overdoing physical activity.

Any unexpected event, such as obvious bleeding, severe dyspnea, changes in pallor, or profuse sweating, should be acted upon in the same way as a fall—see Table 8C–1. Facility protocols should be followed and inpatient facilities should involve nursing and MD, while outpatient and home health follow policies and determine whether to call 911 for additional medical support for the patient. In all cases, clear and accurate documentation of the event and the actions taken must be made immediately to ensure timely and accurate recall of the situation.

BODY MECHANICS AND INJURY PROTECTION

The physical therapist is responsible not only for the prevention of injury to self, but to their patients and other staff within the facility. The physical therapist will often be called on to demonstrate and train members of other departments with regard to correct lifting and transfer techniques. Strong emphasis should be made at all times that using appropriate equipment, such as Hoyer lifts, techniques such as two-person versus one-person, and lifting styles such as power lift or deep squat will prevent injuries, and even if these techniques take extra time or personnel, they should always be adhered to.

Lifting techniques such as the deep squat, power lift, straight leg lift, golfers lift, and stoop lift should all be taught to other personnel and modeled at all times by the members of the physical therapy department. Transferring patients should always include appropriate use of gait belt or equipment such as Hoyer lifts. One-person or two or more person transfers should be correctly used depending on the functional level of the patient. All staff within a facility should have received appropriate training with reverse demonstration in the use of mechanical lifting devices. It is often the role of the physical therapy department to provide this training. Facility policies and procedures must be adhered to. (See Figure 8C–1, algorithm for transfers.)

INFECTION CONTROL

Infection control is a critical component of the healthcare industry. The physical therapy department is a key area for infection risk, and equipment should routinely be sanitized after each patient use. Parallel bars should be wiped down after each patient, and Hoyer lift slings should be utilized according to facility policy—usually single-person use.

Hand Hygiene

Hand hygiene is critical and should be performed at a minimum between each patient contact, after eating, after touching soiled materials, after removing gloves, or after sneezing or blowing one's nose. Hand hygiene can be achieved through application and rubbing of hand sanitizer or through accurate hand washing.

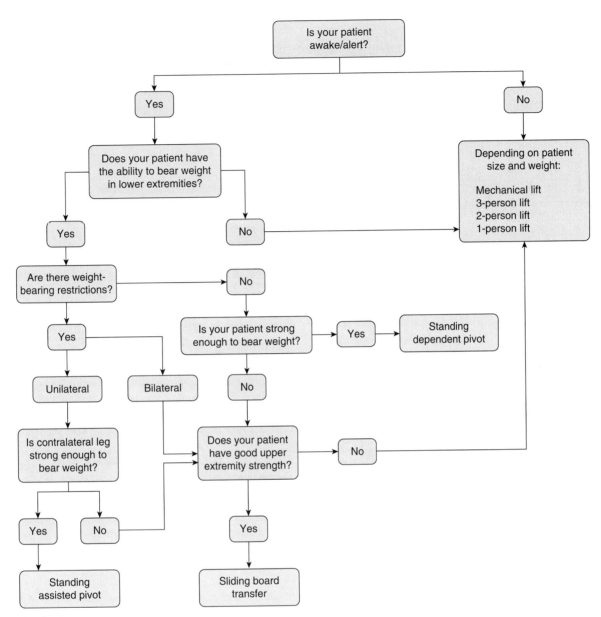

FIGURE 8C–1 Algorithm for transfers.

Hand washing should include at least 15 to 30 seconds of soap manipulation before rinsing.

According to a World Health Organization report, healthcare-associated infections are a major public health problem because they can increase morbidity and mortality and add a burden to the facility staff and patients. Most common infections include surgical incisions, GI infections, and respiratory and urinary tract infections. The very young, the very old, and those who are immune compromised are at the greatest risk for infections.

Precautions for Infection Control

Universal precautions (standard precautions) are designed to minimize the spread of infection through careful hand hygiene, correct disposal of needles or sharps, use of protective clothing including gloves and gown if physical contact with the patient is anticipated, and careful disposal of soiled linens and waste from the patient.

Transmission-based precautions are more specific precautions designed for each of the different modes of infection transmission, contact, droplet, airborne, common vehicle, and vector borne. Table 8C–2 provides the minimal recommendations, but equipment such as gloves can be added according to personal preference. It is also essential that all facility policies and procedures are followed.

ABUSE AND NEGLECT

Mandatory reporting procedures are in place at local, state, and federal levels to protect all of society but particularly the most vulnerable population, the young and the elderly. Correct reporting

TABLE 8C-2 Infection control.

Mode of Infection	Example of Disease	Protective Equipment	Transportation Limitations
Contact	Skin, GI, or wound infection	Gown if in direct contact Gloves	Minimize transport out of the room
Droplet	Meningitis, influenza, pneumonia	Mask if within 3 ft of the patient Gown and gloves not required	Minimize transport, mask on patient if leaving the room
Airborne	Measles, varicella, tuberculosis	Mask at all times Gown and gloves not required	Minimize transport, mask on patient if leaving the room
Common vehicle	Transmission by food, water, medication such as cholera	Will depend on the infection At a minimum, standard precautions	Minimize transport
Vector	Transmission by mosquito, fly, rats, such as malaria	Will depend on the infection At a minimum, standard precautions	

of abuse, following facility protocols and meeting local, state, and federal guidelines is critical. All abuse must be reported even if there is some level of doubt—that is for the authorities to determine. All facilities have abuse reporting policies which must be followed to meet the required standards.

Types of elder abuse include physical, financial, emotional/psychological, neglect, and sexual. These can occur within a facility setting, in the home, and in the community. They can involve facility staff, family members, or strangers. Often clients will talk to the physical therapist during their treatment sessions, and careful note and follow-up must be made if there is a suspicion of abuse or neglect. In the home health setting, careful observation of the interactions between the patient and caregivers can sometimes reveal potential abuse. Withholding medication, not allowing visitors or phone calls, failure to provide adequate nutrition, or failure to provide support for activities of daily living can all be considered signs of abuse, and should be reported to the agency or facility management per policy.

Child abuse categories are similar to elder abuse and include physical, emotional, and sexual as well as neglect. These too can occur in any setting, and typically occur in combination rather than in isolation, and if observed or suspected should be immediately reported per policy.

PATIENT CLIENT RIGHTS

Americans with Disabilities Act

The Americans with Disabilities Act (ADA) prohibits discrimination against those with disabilities with regard to employment, transportation, public accommodation, communication, and government activities. The Office of Disability Employment Policy (ODEP) provides information and technical assistance on the requirements of the ADA but does not enforce any part of the law. All physical therapy clinics and all medical facilities must meet ADA standards, and the ODEP can assist with ensuring that these standards are met.

Individuals with Disabilities Education Act

The Individuals with Disabilities Education Act (IDEA) of 2004 and resulting law ensures that children with disabilities receive the appropriate education provided by state and public agencies. This includes early intervention, special education, and related services. Currently over 6.5 million infants, toddlers, children, and youths with disability qualify under this act for special services.

Health Insurance Portability and Accountability Act

The Health Insurance Portability and Accountability Act (HIPAA) of 1996 ensures the protection of health information. The act sets standards for the use and disclosure of a person's health information, and failure to comply with the HIPAA rules is a federal offense. Privacy of health information includes discussing a patient with other people not authorized by the patient, including family members, leaving computers open and unmanned showing private health information, and talking about patients in an open area that can be overheard. In addition, the electronic transmission of medical information including fax, scans, emails, and texts is prohibited on open lines unless the information is encrypted. Any sharing of patient information should only be done with full awareness of the recipient and the mode of transmission. All healthcare professionals are required to be trained by their employers on all aspects of the HIPAA and its implementation. If a violation of the HIPAA is suspected it should immediately be reported to management per facility, agency, or corporate policy.

HUMAN RESOURCE LEGAL ISSUES

Occupational Safety and Health Administration

The Occupational Safety and Health Administration (OSHA) requires that under the laws of the US Department of Labor, all employers are responsible for provision of a safe and healthful workplace. To achieve this, employers must establish and enforce standards and provide training, education, and outreach assistance to their employees. The areas of consideration vary, depending on the type of work environment. There are strict laws for governing safety in agriculture, maritime work, construction, and the medical profession. As a physical therapist, it is critical to ensure that therapy working environments meet OSHA standards, and also to help other professionals be aware of health and safety issues in their lines of work.

Sexual Harassment

According to the US Equal Employment Opportunity Commission, it is unlawful for anyone, either applicant or employee, to be harassed in the workplace. This includes sexual harassment, which can be unwelcome sexual advances, request for sexual favors, or verbal or physical harassment of a sexual nature. Victim and harasser can be male or female, and can be the same sex. When frequent or severe enough to cause a hostile environment, or if it results in an adverse employment decision such as termination or demotion, it is illegal. Any suspicion of sexual harassment, whether personal or observed between others, should be reported per facility or management protocols.

DOCUMENTATION STANDARDS

The physical therapist is responsible for accurate and timely documentation of all occurrences, including screening, evaluation, treatments, and incident reporting. Each arena such as home health, inpatient, outpatient has its own unique aspects of documentation, and many corporations have additional documentation requirements for their employees.

The traditional SOAP note is still in use in many locations. In this style of documentation, the physical therapist uses the acronym for Subjective information (what the patient said about their current state, how they feel, how things are going), Objective (documentation of tests, measures, and interventions), Assessment (the patient's response to treatment, including post-treatment measurements), and Plan (the thought process for the next patient–therapist interaction).

Electronic medical records are found in many healthcare settings. These records often allow the physical therapist to readily access laboratory results, imaging, and consultations. It is illegal to access the medical record of personal family members and other individuals within the health setting unless the therapist is assigned to their care.

Electronic medical records often have check boxes, with optional narrative sections. The physical therapist should always use the narrative sections to ensure adequate detail is provided in the documentation. Litigation can take years, and a physical therapist facing an inquiry needs to be able to utilize their record from the event to accurately document what occurred. Falsification of medical records is illegal.

ROLES AND RESPONSIBILITIES OF OTHER HEALTHCARE PROFESSIONALS AND SUPPORT STAFF

The delegation of work to appropriate support staff is highly regulated at the state level. All practicing physical therapists should be familiar with their state regulations with respect to physical therapist assistants, technicians, and aides. Some states do not allow the use of aides, while other states allow them but with varying levels of supervisory regulation.

The interdisciplinary team is an important component of any patient care, particularly in the inpatient setting. Physical therapists should learn the roles of the different professionals and communicate appropriately. These include but are not limited to:

- Occupational therapy
- Speech and language therapy
- Nursing
- Social workers
- Dietician
- Orthotist and prosthetist
- Physician, surgeon, primary care physician, nurse practitioner

Documentation of all patient-related discussions with any of the above interdisciplinary team members must be completed, particularly when they relate to treatment intervention, such as changes in weightbearing status, use of orthotics, and changes in social settings that will affect discharge planning.

BIBLIOGRAPHY

IDEA, building the legacy. Retrieved from: http://idea.ed.gov/.

United States Department of Labor. Americans with Disabilities Act. Retrieved from https://www.dol.gov/general/topic/disability/ada. Accessed August 12, 2018.

US Department of health and human services. Health information privacy. Summary of the HIPPA privacy rule. Retrieved from: https://www.hhs.gov/hipaa/for-professionals/privacy/laws-regulations/. Accessed August 12, 2018.

US Department of Labor. Occupational safety and health administration. Retrieved from: https://www.osha.gov/law-regs.html. Accessed August 12, 2018.

US Equal employment opportunity commission. Sexual harassment. Retrieved from: https://www.eeoc.gov/laws/types/sexual_harassment.cfm. Accessed August 12, 2018.

World Health Organization Falls. Retrieved from: http://www.who.int/en/news-room/fact-sheets/detail/falls. Accessed August 12, 2018.

World Health Organization. Core components for infection prevention and control programs. Retrieved from: http://apps.who.int/iris/bitstream/10665/69982/1/WHO_HSE_EPR_2009.1_eng.pdf 2008. Accessed August 12, 2018.

QUESTIONS

1. A physical therapist arrives at a patient's home and finds the patient on the floor with an obvious injury to their right lower extremity. The caregiver is present but obviously distressed. Which of the following actions is most appropriate for the therapist to perform?
   A. Get the patient off the floor and take vital signs
   B. Call 911 and the home health agency for medical support
   C. Call the home health agency and report the incident
   D. Call 911 and leave the patient with the caregiver to wait for the paramedics

2. A physical therapist is working in a skilled nursing facility and has been informed that the patient has measles. Which of the following precautions are the minimum requirements for the therapist while working with this patient?
   A. Personal mask at all times
   B. Mask if within 3 feet of the patient
   C. Gown, gloves, and mask at all times
   D. Gown if in direct contact with patient

3. A physical therapist is working in the home of a patient with a long history of cardiac disease. The patient has recently had a pacemaker fitted and has been cleared for therapy to improve functional activity. Which of the following monitoring protocols is the most appropriate for the therapist to use with this patient?

   A. Take pulse and respiratory rate regularly throughout the session
   B. Continue working with patient to 80% heart rate max
   C. Do not exercise this patient as it is a contraindication
   D. Exercise the patient using the rate of perceived exertion (RPE) scale to monitor exertion

ANSWERS

1. The answer is **B**. If a patient has an obvious injury, medical support is critical and the home health therapist should call 911 but must also call the home health agency to report and complete paperwork as required. The patient and caregiver should not be left until after the paramedics have arrived.

2. The answer is **A**. Measles is an airborne infection, so a mask must be worn at all times when working with the patient. Gown and gloves are not required but can be used if the therapist or the facility require.

3. The answer is **D**. The pacemaker is designed to keep the patient's heart rate at a specific level regardless of exercise intensity, so monitoring pulse and aiming at 80% heart rate max is inappropriate. The use of the RPE scale is the safest way to exercise a patient with a fitted pacemaker.

■ SECTION D: RESEARCH AND EVIDENCE-BASED PRACTICE

INTRODUCTION

The ultimate purpose of a profession is to develop a knowledge base that will maximize the effectiveness of a practice. As our autonomy increases, so does the requirement for evidence that we are providing needed and quality care. In order for physical therapists to provide evidence-based care, evidence to support our choices must be available. In addition, therapists must possess the basic knowledge to interpret and analyze the available evidence.

RESEARCH TYPES

Research involves a controlled, systematic approach to obtain an answer to a question.[1] A number of research types are recognized:

- Experimental research: Involves the manipulation of a variable and then measuring the effects of this manipulation.[1] A variable is a measurement of phenomena that can assume more than one value or more than one category (see later).[1]
- Nonexperimental research: Does not manipulate the environment but may describe the relationship between different variables, obtain information about opinions or policies, or describe current practice.[1]

High-Yield Terms to Learn

Alternative hypothesis	Hypothesis stating the expected relationship between independent and dependent variables.
Clinical prediction rule	A statistical tool that quantifies the relative contribution of examination and history findings to determine a diagnosis, prognosis, or likely response to an intervention.
Concurrent validity	A type of measurement validity that describes the degree to which the outcomes of one test correlate with outcomes on a criterion test when both tests are given at relatively the same time.
Confidence interval	The range of values within which a population parameter is estimated to fall, with a specific level of confidence.

High-Yield Terms to Learn (*continued*)

Confounding	The contaminating effect of extraneous variables on interpretation of the relationship between independent and dependent variable.
Construct validity	A type of measurement validity; the degree to which a theoretical construct is measured by an instrument.
Content validity	The degree to which the items in an instrument adequately reflect the content domain being measured.
Evidence-based practice	The application of clinical decision-making for patient management based on research evidence, clinical expertise, patient values and preferences, and clinical circumstances.
Exploratory research	Research that has as its purpose the exploration of data to determine relationships among variables.
External validity	The degree to which results of a study can be generalized to persons or settings outside the experimental situation.
Extraneous variable	A variable that confounds the relationship between the independent and dependent variables.
Face validity	The assumption of validity of a measuring instrument based on its appearance as a reasonable measure of a given variable.
Gold standard	A measurement that defines the true value of a variable.
Independent variable	The variable that is presumed to cause, explain, or influence a dependent variable; a variable that is controlled by the researcher.
Internal validity	The degree to which the relationship between the independent and dependent variables is free from effects of extraneous factors.
Mean	A measure of central tendency, computed by summing the values of several observations and dividing by the number of observations.
Measurement error	The difference between an observed value for a measurement and the theoretical true score.
Median	A measure of central tendency representing the 50th percentile in a ranked distribution of scores.
Negative predictive value	In diagnostic testing, the proportion of subjects who are correctly identified as not having the condition of interest.
Null hypothesis	A statement of no difference or no relationship between variables.
Population	The entire set of individuals or units to which data will be generalized.
Positive predictive value	Estimate of the likelihood that a person who tests positive actually has the disease.
Power	The ability of a statistical test to find a significant difference that really does exist.
Random assignment	Assignment of subjects to groups using probability methods, where every subject has an equal chance of being assigned to each group.
Randomized controlled trial	An experimental study in which a clinical treatment is compared with a control condition, where subjects are randomly assigned to groups.
Reliability	The degree of consistency with which an instrument or rater measures a variable.
Research hypothesis	A statement of the researcher's expectations about the relationship between variables under the study.
Sensitivity	A measure of validity of a screening procedure based on the probability that someone with the disease will test positive.
Specificity	A measure of validity of a screening procedure based on the probability that someone who does not have the disease will test negative.
Standard deviation	A descriptive statistic reflecting the variability or dispersion of scores.
Systematic review	Review of a clearly formulated question that uses systematic and explicit methods to identify, select, and critically appraise relevant research.
Validity	The degree to which an instrument measures what it is intended to measure.
Variable	A characteristic that can be manipulated or observed and that can take on different values.

- Basic research: Generally thought of as laboratory-based research in which the researcher has control over nearly all aspects of the environment and subjects.[1]
- Clinical or applied research: Refers to research that seeks to solve practical problems by finding solutions to everyday problems, cure illness, and develop innovative technologies.

STATISTICS

Statistics is a branch of applied mathematics concerned with finding patterns in data and inferring connections between events.[2] A number of statistical terms and definitions are outlined in Table 8D–1.

> **STUDY PEARL**
>
> Much of the initial groundwork in statistics concerns making an accurate guess, or hypothesis.

TABLE 8D–1 Statistical terms and definitions.

Term	Definition
Abstract	A summary of the paper, usually between 100 and 500 words, that describes the most important aspects of the study, including: The problem investigated The subjects and instruments involved The design and procedures The major findings/conclusions
Conclusion	The conclusion responds to the original research question and hypothesis to describe what the study showed. It should bring coherence to the study.
Empirical methods	Research methods and data-gathering techniques supported by measurable evidence, not opinion or speculation.
Parameter	Numerical measurements describing some characteristic of the population.
Peer review	A process by which research studies are examined by an independent panel of researchers for review. The purpose of such a process is to open the study to examination, criticism, review, and replication by peer investigators and ultimately incorporate the new knowledge into the field.
Population	The population of a study refers to the group of people represented in a study. For example, if a researcher took a nationally representative sample of 1500 fourth-grade students, the sample is the 1500 fourth-grade students, but the population of the study would be fourth graders, in general.

Population and Samples

A population consists of all subjects (human or otherwise) that are being studied.

- Prevalence: The proportion of a population who has a particular disorder or condition at a specific point in time.
- Incidence: A rate of development of new cases of a disorder in a particular at-risk population over a given period of time.
- Parameter: A characteristic or measure obtained by using all the data values from a specific population.
- Sample: A group of subjects selected from a population.
- Statistic: A characteristic or measure obtained by using all the data values from a sample.

Variables

To gain knowledge about seemingly haphazard events, statisticians collect information called *variables*, which describe the event. Data are the values (measurements or observations) that the variables can assume.

> **STUDY PEARL**
>
> A valid informed consent for research purposes must include all of the following elements:
> - An understandable explanation of the purpose and procedures to be used
> - All reasonable and foreseeable risks
> - All potential benefits of participation

> **STUDY PEARL**
>
> The two traits of a variable that should always be achieved are:
> - Each variable should be *exhaustive*; it should include all possible answerable responses.
> - Each variable should be *mutually exclusive*; no respondent should be able to have two attributes simultaneously.

Variables can be classified as qualitative or quantitative.

- Qualitative: A variable that can be placed into a distinct category according to some characteristic or attribute, for example, gender.
- Quantitative: A variable that is numeric and can be ordered or ranked, for example, age, height, and weight. Quantitative variables can be further classified into two groups: discrete and continuous.[2]
  - Discrete: A variable that can assume only certain values that are countable, for example, the number of children in a family.
  - Continuous: A variable that can assume an infinite number of possible values in an interval between any two specific values, for example, temperature.

In addition to being classified as qualitative and quantitative, variables can be classified by how they are categorized, counted, or measured. This type of classification uses measurement scales. The four classic scales (or levels) of measurement are:[2]

- Nominal (classificatory; categorical): Classifies data into mutually exclusive, exhaustive categories in which no order or ranking can be imposed. Examples include arbitrary labels: zip codes, religion, and marital status.
- Ordinal (ranking): Classifies data into categories that can be ranked, although precise differences between the ranks do not exist, for example, letter grades (A, B, C, etc.) and body types (small, medium, large).
- Interval: Ranks data where precise differences between units of measure do exist, although there is no meaningful zero. Examples include temperature (degrees Centigrade, degrees Fahrenheit), IQ, and calendar dates.
- Ratio: Possesses all the characteristics of interval measurement, and a true zero exists. Examples include age and salary.

Types of Experiments

There are three basic types of statistical experiments: controlled, experimental, and field:

- Controlled: A controlled experiment generally compares the results obtained from an experimental sample against a control sample that is practically identical to the experimental sample except for the one aspect whose effect is being tested (the independent variable).
- Natural: An observational study in which the assignment of treatments to subjects has been haphazard. The assignment of treatments to subjects has not been made by the researchers or by randomization.
- Field: So named in order to highlight the contrast with laboratory experiments.

STUDY PEARL

Dependency refers to the "role" of the variable in the experiment or study.

Independent variable: A variable that is manipulated by the researcher; independent variables are controlled or fixed in order to observe their effect on dependent variables. For example, a treatment or program or cause.

Dependent variable: The variable that is measured by the researcher. For example, if a study examines the effects of iontophoresis on pain levels, the iontophoresis is the independent variable and the measurement of pain levels is the dependent variable.

Other types of variables include:

Random variable: One whose value is determined by chance.

Controlled variable: A variable that the researcher wants to remain constant.

Covariate: A phenomenon that affects the dependent variable and is not of interest to the researcher but that the researcher is unable to control.[1]

RESEARCH DESIGN

There are a number of primary types of research designs (Table 8D–2).

Control

Ideally, the researcher should attempt to remove the influence of any variable other than the independent variable in order to evaluate its effect on the dependent variable. An experimental design has the purpose of minimizing or controlling the effects on extraneous variables so that the relationship between the independent variable(s) and the dependent variable(s) can be ascertained.

Control Group

The control group is used as a standard for comparison with experimental groups in terms of age, abilities, race, etc. For example, a particular study may divide participants into two groups: an *experimental group* and a *control group*. The experimental group is given the experimental treatment under study, while the control group may be given either the standard treatment for the illness or a placebo. At the end of the study, the results of the two groups are compared.

Experimental Group

Study participants in the experimental group receive the drug, device, treatment, or intervention under study. In some studies, all participants are in the experimental group. In "controlled studies," participants will be assigned either to an experimental group or to a control group.

TABLE 8D-2 Research designs.

Controlled trials	These require the experimental procedure to be compared with a placebo or another previously accepted procedure. Controlled studies are more likely than uncontrolled studies to determine whether differences are due to the experimental treatment or to some extraneous factor.
Uncontrolled trials	These involve the investigators describing their experience with an experimental procedure; however, the experimental procedure is not formerly compared with a placebo or another previously accepted procedure.
Single-blind study	A study in which the investigator does not know if the subject is in the treatment group or the control group.
Double-blind study	A study in which neither the investigator nor the subject knows if the subject is in the treatment group or the control group.

From Dutton M. *McGraw-Hill's NPTE (National Physical Therapy Examination).* 2nd ed. New York, NY: McGraw-Hill; 2012:Table 3–2.

Placebo Effect

The placebo effect is the measurable, observable, or felt improvement in health not attributable to treatment. Experimental research uses placebos (usually sugar or starch pills) to test the effect of a medication. An inactive substance that looks like medicine but contains no medicine and has no treatment value (placebo) is administered to the patient. While participants in the control group are given the placebo, the other members of the study are given the actual medication.

Random Assignment

Random assignment is assignment by chance, like flipping a coin or pulling numbers out of a hat. This method is sometimes used to determine who is in the experimental group and who is in the control group. For example, in a study with random assignment to one of two groups, participants have a 50% chance of being assigned to either group.

> **STUDY PEARL**
>
> Bias or systematic error refers to the tendency to consistently underestimate or overestimate a true value.

DATA COLLECTION AND SAMPLING TECHNIQUES

Researchers use samples to produce a representative sample of the target population. To avoid any biasing of the collected information, samples must be collected in a systematic fashion.

Four basic methods of sampling are employed:

- Random sampling: All items have some chance of selection that can be calculated, thereby minimizing sampling bias.
- Systematic sampling: Sometimes referred to as *interval sampling*; means that there is a gap, or interval, between each selection (every 20th person).
- Stratified sampling: Sometimes called *proportional* or *quota* random sampling; involves dividing the population into homogeneous subgroups called strata and then taking a simple random sample from each subgroup. Stratified sampling assures that the overall population will be represented in addition to key subgroups of the population. For example, choosing only female patients.
- Cluster sampling: Involves dividing the population into groups, or clusters (such as geographic boundaries), and then randomly selecting sample clusters and using all members of the selected clusters as subjects of the samples. For example, it may not be possible to list all of the patients of a chain of physical therapy clinics. However, it would be possible to randomly select a subset of clinics (stage 1 of cluster sampling) and then interview a random sample of patients who visit those clinics (stage 2 of cluster sampling).

GRAPHICAL REPRESENTATION OF ORGANIZED DATA

The most convenient method of organizing data is to construct a frequency distribution.[3] Two types of frequency distributions are:[3]

- Categorical frequency distribution: Used for data that can be placed in specific categories, such as nominal- or ordinal-level data, for example, political affiliation.
- Grouped frequency distribution: Used when the range of data is large.

Data can be presented by constructing statistical charts and graphs. The choice of which chart or graph to use is determined by the type and breadth of the data, the audience it is directed to, and the questions being asked (Table 8D–3). The three most commonly used graphs in research include the histogram, frequency polygon, and cumulative frequency graph (ogive) (Figure 8D–1). In addition to these, the Pareto chart, the times series graph, and the pie graph are also used (see Figure 8D–1). In those cases where the researchers are interested in determining if a relationship between two variables (independent and dependent) exists, a scatterplot, or scatter diagram, can be used (see Figure 8D–1).

Sensitivity and Specificity

Sensitivity represents the proportion of a population with the target disorder, who has a positive result with the diagnostic test. A test that can correctly identify every person who has the target disorder has a sensitivity of 1.0. SnNout is an acronym for when Sensitivity of a symptom or sign is high, a Negative response rules out the target disorder. Thus, a "high" sensitive test helps rule out a disorder.

Specificity represents the proportion of the study population without the target disorder, in whom the test result is negative (Table 8D–4).[4] A test that can correctly identify every person who does not have the target disorder has a specificity of 1.0. SpPin is an acronym for when Specificity is extremely high, a Positive test result rules in the target disorder. Thus, a "high" specific test helps rule in a disorder or condition.

A test with a very high sensitivity but low specificity, and vice versa, is of little value, and the acceptable levels are generally set at between 50% (unacceptable test) and 100% (perfect test), with an arbitrary cutoff of about 80%.[4]

Validity

Validity is defined as the degree to which a test measures what it purports to be measuring, and how well it correctly classifies individuals with or without a particular disease.[5-7] Validity is directly related to the notion of sensitivity and specificity. There are several types of validity, including construct validity, face validity, content validity, external validity, concurrent validity, and criterion-referenced validity:

TABLE 8D-3 Statistical graphs.

Type of Display	Advantages	Disadvantages
Pictograph A pictograph uses an icon to represent a quantity of data values in order to decrease the size of the graph. A key must be used to explain the icon.	Easy to read Visually appealing Handles large data sets easily using keyed icons	Hard to quantify partial icons Icons must be of consistent size Best for only 2–6 categories Very simplistic
Line plot A line plot can be used as an initial record of discrete data values. The range determines a number line which is then plotted with X's for each data value.	Quick analysis of data Shows range, minimum and maximum, gaps and clusters, and outliers easily Exact values retained	Not as visually appealing as pictograph Best for under 50 data values Needs small range of data
Pie chart A pie chart displays data as a percentage of the whole. Each pie section should have a label and percentage. A total data number should be included.	Visually appealing Shows percent of total for each category	No exact numerical data Hard to compare two data sets The "Other" category can be a problem Total unknown unless specified Best for 3–7 categories Used only with discrete data
Map chart A map chart displays data by shading sections of a map, and must include a key. A total data number should be included.	Good visual appeal Overall trends show well	Needs limited categories No exact numerical values Color key can skew visual interpretation
Histogram A histogram displays continuous data in ordered columns. Categories are of a continuous measure such as time, inches, temperature, etc.	Visually strong Can compare to normal curve The vertical axis is usually a frequency count of items falling into each category	Cannot read exact values because data are grouped into categories More difficult to compare two data sets Used only with continuous data
Bar graph A bar graph displays discrete data in separate columns. A double bar graph can be used to compare two data sets. Categories are considered unordered and can be rearranged alphabetically, by size, etc.	Visually strong Can easily compare two or three data sets	Graph categories can be reordered to emphasize certain effects Used only with discrete data
Line graph A line graph plots continuous data as points and then joins them with a line. Multiple data sets can be graphed together, but a key must be used.	Can compare multiple continuous data sets easily Interim data can be inferred from graph line	Used only with continuous data
Frequency polygon A frequency polygon can be made from a line graph by shading in the area beneath the graph. It can be made from a histogram by joining midpoints of each column.	Visually appealing	Anchors at both ends may imply zero as data points Used only with continuous data
Scatterplot A scatterplot displays the relationship between two factors of the experiment. A trend line is used to determine positive, negative, or no correlation.	Shows a trend in the data relationship Retains exact data values and sample size Shows minimum/maximum and outliers	Hard to visualize results in large data sets Flat trend line gives inconclusive results Data on both axes should be continuous
Stem and leaf plot Stem and leaf plots record data values in rows, and can easily be made into a histogram. Large data sets can be accommodated by splitting stems.	Concise representation of data Shows range, minimum and maximum, gaps and clusters, and outliers easily Can handle extremely large data sets	Not visually appealing Does not easily indicate measures of centrality for large data sets
Box plot A box plot is a concise graph showing the five-point summary. Multiple box plots can be drawn side by side to compare more than one data set.	Shows five-point summary and outliers Easily compares two or more data sets Handles extremely large data sets easily	Not as visually appealing as other graphs Exact values not retained

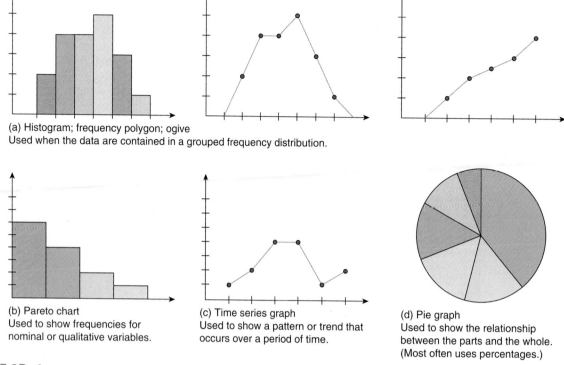

(a) Histogram; frequency polygon; ogive
Used when the data are contained in a grouped frequency distribution.

(b) Pareto chart
Used to show frequencies for
nominal or qualitative variables.

(c) Time series graph
Used to show a pattern or trend that
occurs over a period of time.

(d) Pie graph
Used to show the relationship
between the parts and the whole.
(Most often uses percentages.)

FIGURE 8D–1 Summary of graphs and uses of each. (Reproduced with permission from Bluman A. *Elementary Statistics: A Step by Step Approach*. 6th ed. New York, NY: McGraw-Hill; 2007:73.)

- Construct validity: The ability of a test to represent the underlying construct (the theory developed to organize and explain some aspects of existing knowledge and observations). Construct validity refers to overall validity.
- Face validity: The degree to which the questions or procedures incorporated within a test make sense to the users. The assessment of face validity is generally informal and nonquantitative, and is the lowest standard of assessing validity. It is based on the notion that the finding is valid "on the face of it." For example, if a weighing scale indicates that a normal-sized person weighs 2000 lb, that scale does not have face validity.
- Content validity: The assessment by experts that the content of the measure is consistent with what is to be measured. Content validity is concerned with sample-population representativeness, that is, the knowledge and skills covered by the test items should be representative of the larger domain of knowledge and skills. In many instances it is difficult, if not impossible, to administer a test covering all aspects of knowledge or skills. Therefore, only several tasks are sampled from the population of knowledge or skills. In these circumstances, the proportion of the score attributed to a particular component should be proportional to the importance of that component to total performance. In content validity, evidence is obtained by looking for agreement in judgments by judges. In short, one person can determine face validity, but a panel should confirm content validity.
- External validity: The degree to which study results can be generalized to different subjects, settings, and times.[8,9]
- Internal validity: The degree to which the reported outcomes of the research study are a consequence of the relationship between the independent and dependent variables and not the result of extraneous factors.
- Criterion-referenced validity: Determined by comparing the results of a test to those of a test that is accepted as a gold standard (a test which is accepted as being close to 100% valid).[4] There are three types of criterion-referenced validity: concurrent, predictive, and discriminant.
  - Concurrent: The degree to which the measurement being validated agrees with an established measurement standard administered at approximately the same time. Concurrent validity is a form of criterion validity.
  - Predictive: The extent to which test scores are associated with future behavior or performance.
  - Discriminant: The ability of a test to distinguish between two different constructs as is evidenced by a low correlation between the results of the test and those of tests of a different construct.

Diagnostic tests are used for the purpose of discovery, confirmation, and exclusion.[10] Tests for discovery and exclusion must have high sensitivity for detection, whereas confirmation tests require high specificity.[11] The sensitivity and specificity of any physical test to discriminate relevant dysfunction must be appreciated to make meaningful decisions.[12]

Prediction Value

The prediction value of a positive test indicates that those members of the study population who have a positive test outcome will have the condition under investigation (Table 8D–4).[4] The diagnostic power of the negative test outcome relates to those of

TABLE 8D-4   Concepts and definitions of sensitivity, specificity, and predictive values.

Concept	Definition
Sensitivity	Proportion of patients with a disease who test positive.
Specificity	Proportion of patients without the disease who test negative.
Positive predictive value (PPV)	Proportion of patients who actually have the disease who test positive. If the target disease is uncommon, there are many more false positive results and the PPV goes down.
Negative predictive value	Proportion of patients who do not actually have the disease and who test negative.

TABLE 8D-5   Kappa (κ) benchmark values.

Value (%)	Description
<40	Poor to fair agreement
40–60	Moderate agreement
60–80	Substantial agreement
>80	Excellent agreement
100	Perfect agreement

the study population with a negative test outcome who do not suffer from the condition under investigation.[4]

Likelihood Ratio

The likelihood ratio is the index measurement that is considered to combine the best characteristics of sensitivity, specificity, positive predictive value, and negative predictive value. Likelihood ratios are expressed as odds and are calculated from the values used to calculate sensitivity and specificity. The likelihood ratio indicates how much a given diagnostic test result will lower or raise the pretest probability of the target disorder.[4,13]

Reliability

Reliability is defined as the extent to which repeated measurements of a relatively stable phenomenon are close to each other.[14] Test-retest reliability is the consistency of repeated measurements that are separated in time when there is no change in what is being measured. Any difference between the two sets of scores represents measurement error, which can arise from a number of factors including intrarater variability, interrater reliability, or a lack of consistency of results. Reliability may be measured as repeatability between measurements performed by the same examiner (intrarater reliability), or between measurements by different examiners (interrater reliability). Instrument reliability deals with the tool used to obtain a measurement.

Reliability is quantitatively expressed by way of an index of agreement, with the simplest index being the percentage agreement value. The percentage agreement value is defined as the ratio of the number of agreements to the total number of ratings made.[15] However, because this value does not correct for chance agreement, it can provide a misleadingly high estimate of reliability.[6,15–17]

The results of an examination are of limited value if they are not consistently repeatable.[5,6] The kappa (κ) statistic is a chance-corrected index of agreement that overcomes the problem of chance agreement when used with nominal and ordinal data (Table 8D-5).[18] However, with higher-scale data such as ordinal

and parametric, it tends to underestimate reliability, in which case a weight kappa (ranked) or intraclass correlation coefficient (ICC—see later) (parametric) should be used.[19] Theoretically, κ can be negative if agreement is worse than chance. Practically, in clinical reliability studies, κ usually varies between 0.00 and 1.00.[19] The κ statistic does not differentiate among disagreements; it assumes that all disagreements are of equal significance.[19]

A number of calculations, including the Pearson product moment correlation coefficient and the ICC, can be used to assess reliability.

Threats to Validity and Reliability

The most common threats to validity and reliability are:

- Ambiguity—when correlation is taken for causation
- Errors of measurement—random errors or systematic errors
- History—when some critical event occurs between pretest and posttest
- Instrumentation—when the researcher changes the measuring device
- Maturation—when people change or mature over the research period
- Mortality—when people die or drop out of the research
- Regression to the mean—a tendency toward middle scores
- The John Henry effect—when groups compete to score well
- Sampling bias—the tendency of a sample to exclude some members of the sampling population and overrepresent others
- Setting—something about the setting or context contaminates the study
- The Hawthorne effect—a tendency of research subjects to act atypically as a result of their awareness of being studied

DESCRIPTIVE STATISTICS

Descriptive statistics describe what is, or what the data show. Descriptive statistics include the collection, organization, summarization, and presentation of data to reduce lots of data into a simpler summary.[2] For example, the grade point average (GPA) of a student describes the general performance of the student across a potentially wide range of course experiences.

Univariate analysis explores each variable in a data set separately, focusing on the following:

The Central Tendency

When populations are small, it is not necessary to use samples since the entire population can be used to gather information. Measures found by using all the data values in the population are called parameters. Measures of central tendency are measures of the location of the middle (or the center) of a distribution where data tend to cluster. Multiple metrics are used to describe this clustering, for example, mean, median, and mode:

- Mean: The arithmetic *mean* is what is commonly called the average. When the word "mean" is used without a modifier, it can be assumed that it refers to the arithmetic mean. The mean of a sample is typically denoted as $\bar{x}$. The mean is the sum of all the scores divided by the number of scores.
- Median: The median is the middle of a distribution. Half the scores are above the median and half are below. The median is less sensitive to extreme scores than the mean, and this makes it a better measure than the mean for highly skewed distributions (see later).
- Mode: The mode is the most frequently occurring score in a distribution. The advantage of the mode as a measure of central tendency is that its meaning is obvious. Further, it is the only measure of central tendency that can be used with nominal data.

Determination of Spread

Although measures of central tendency locate only the center of a distribution, other measures, such as a determination of the spread of a group of scores, are often needed to describe data. To examine the spread or variability of a data set, a number of measures are commonly used:[20]

- Range: The range is simply the highest value minus the lowest value.
- Variance: The average of the squares of the distance that each value is from the mean.
- Standard deviation (σ): The standard deviation (SD) shows the relation that the set of scores has to the mean of the sample—it is a determination of the spread of a group of scores or the average deviation of values around the mean. The SD is based on the distance of sample values from the mean and provides information about how tightly all the various examples are clustered around the mean in a set of data. When the examples are pretty tightly bunched together and the bell-shaped curve is steep, the SD is small. When the examples are spread apart and the bell curve is relatively flat, the SD is relatively large. Mathematically, the SD equals the square root of the mean of the square deviation, or the square root of the variance. The range can be used to approximate the SD by dividing the range value by 4.

Frequency Distribution

A frequency distribution is a tabulation of the values that one or more variables take in a sample. These values can be graphed, and frequency distributions can assume many shapes. Following are the most important shapes that are positively skewed, symmetric, and negatively skewed (Figure 8D–2) (see "Measures of Position," below):[20]

- Positively skewed: The majority of the data values fall to the left of the mean and cluster at the lower end of the distribution.
- Symmetric: The data values are evenly distributed on both sides of the mean.

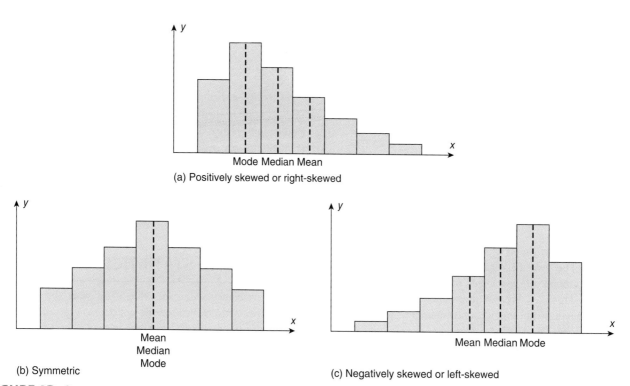

FIGURE 8D–2 Types of distributions. (Reproduced with permission from Bluman A. *Elementary Statistics: A Step by Step Approach*. 6th ed. New York, NY: McGraw-Hill; 2007:115.)

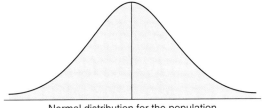

Normal distribution for the population

FIGURE 8D-3 Histogram showing a normal distribution. (Reproduced with permission from Bluman A. *Elementary Statistics: A Step by Step Approach.* 6th ed. New York, NY: McGraw-Hill; 2007:283.)

- Negatively skewed: The majority of the data values fall to the right of the mean and cluster at the upper end of the distribution.

STUDY PEARL

Normal distributions are a family of distributions that have a symmetrical and general shape, with values that are more concentrated in the middle than in the tails (Figure 8D-3). The standard normal distribution is a normal distribution with a mean of 0 and a standard deviation of 1.

Measures of Position

In addition to measures of central tendency and measures of variation, there are measures of position, which are used to locate the relative position of a data value in the data set.[20] One of the most common measures of position is the percentile. Percentiles divide the data set into 100 equal groups. The *N*th percentile is defined as the value such that *N* percent of the value lies below it. For example, a score in the 95th percentile represents the top 5% of scores.

- The lower quartile is defined as the 25th percentile—75% of the measures are above the lower quartile.
- The middle quartile is defined as the 50th percentile—the median of all the measures.
- The upper quartile is defined as the 75th percentile—25% of the measures are above the upper quartile.

STUDY PEARL

Variances and standard deviations are used to determine the spread of data. If the variance or standard deviation is large, the data are more dispersed. The measures of variance and standard deviation are also used to determine the consistency of a variable and the number of data values that fall within a specified interval in a distribution.

No variable fits a normal distribution perfectly, since a normal distribution is a theoretical distribution.[21] The mean, median, and mode of a

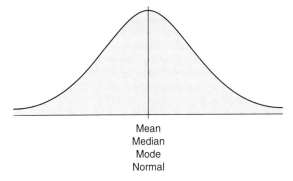

Mean
Median
Mode
Normal

FIGURE 8D-4 Normal distribution in relation to the mean, median, and mode. (Reproduced with permission from Bluman A. *Elementary Statistics: A Step by Step Approach.* 6th ed. New York, NY: McGraw-Hill; 2007:283.)

normal distribution have the same value due to the symmetry of the bell-shaped distribution (Figure 8D-4). The curve has no boundaries, and only a small fraction of the values fall outside of three SDs (a measure of how spread out a distribution is) above or below the mean:

- One SD away from the mean in either direction on the horizontal axis accounts for approximately 68% of the people in the group (Figure 8D-5).
- Two SDs away from the mean account for approximately 95% of the people (Figure 8D-5).
- Three SDs account for about 99% of the people (Figure 8D-5).
- The *z* value is actually the number of SDs that a particular *x* value is away from the mean.

STUDY PEARL

- Parametric statistical procedures, such as the ANOVA and *t*-test (see later), are performed on data that have a normal distribution, such as the distribution observed in a population.[1]
- Nonparametric procedures are performed on data that do not have a normal distribution, that is, a skewed distribution, as often is observed in a sample.[1]

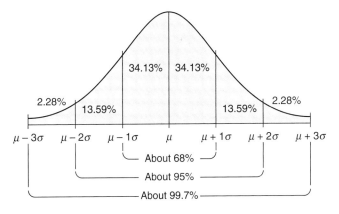

FIGURE 8D-5 Areas under a normal distribution curve. (Reproduced with permission from Bluman A. *Elementary Statistics: A Step by Step Approach.* 6th ed. New York, NY: McGraw-Hill; 2007:286.)

Skewness is a measure of the degree of asymmetry of a distribution. If the left tail (the tail at the small end of the distribution) is more pronounced than the right tail (the tail at the large end of the distribution), the function is said to have negative skewness (Figure 8D–6). If the reverse is true, it has positive skewness (Figure 8D–7). If the two halves of the curve are symmetrical (mirror images), the data distribution has zero skewness (Figure 8D–4).

In a distribution displaying perfect symmetry, the mean, the median, and the mode are all at the same point, and skewness is zero.

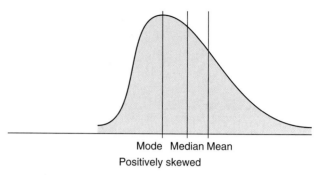

FIGURE 8D–7 Positively skewed distribution. (Reproduced with permission from Bluman A. *Elementary Statistics: A Step by Step Approach.* 6th ed. New York, NY: McGraw-Hill; 2007:283.)

Confidence Intervals

The sample mean will be, for the most part, somewhat different from the population mean due to sampling error.[22] An interval estimate of the parameter is an interval, or a range of values, used to estimate the parameter. This estimate may or may not contain the value of the parameter being estimated.[22] In interval estimates, the parameter is specified as being between two values.

The selection of a confidence level for an interval determines the probability that the confidence interval (CI) produced will contain the true parameter value. Common choices for the CI are 0.90, 0.95, and 0.99. These levels correspond to percentages of the area of the normal density curve. For example, a 95% CI covers 95% of the normal curve—the probability of observing a value outside of this area is less than 0.05.[4,13]

A confidence interval (CI) is a statistical range with a specified probability that a given parameter lies within the range. The confidence level of an interval estimate of a parameter is the probability that the interval estimate will contain a parameter, assuming that a large number of samples are selected and that the estimation process on the same parameter is repeated.[22]

Confidence Intervals for the Mean

When the SD is known and the variable is normally distributed, or when the SD is unknown and the sample size is ≥30, the standard normal distribution is used to find CIs for the mean.[22] However, in many situations, the population SD is not known and the sample size is less than 30. In such situations, the SD from the sample can be used in place of the population SD for CIs. A somewhat different distribution, called the t distribution (Figure 8D–8), must be used when the sample size is less than 30, and the variable is normally or approximately normally distributed (Table 8D–6).

Confidence Intervals for Variances and Standard Deviations

To calculate these CIs, the chi-square distribution is used. The chi-square variable is similar to the t variable in that its distribution is a family of curves based on the number of degrees of freedom.[22] Several of the distributions are shown in Figure 8D–9.

Inferential Statistics

Inferential statistics are used to try to reach conclusions that extend beyond the immediate data alone. Inferential statistics include making inferences from samples to populations, estimations and hypothesis testing, determining relationships, and

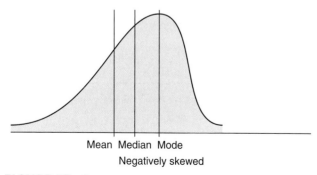

FIGURE 8D–6 Negatively skewed distribution. (Reproduced with permission from Bluman A. *Elementary Statistics: A Step by Step Approach.* 6th ed. New York, NY: McGraw-Hill; 2007:283.)

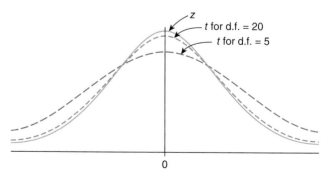

FIGURE 8D–8 The t family of curves. (Reproduced with permission from Bluman A. *Elementary Statistics: A Step by Step Approach.* 6th ed. New York, NY: McGraw-Hill; 2007:358.)

TABLE 8D-6 Similarities and differences between the *t* distribution and the standard normal distribution.

Similarities	Differences
Bell-shaped curve.	The variance is greater than one.
Symmetric about the mean: the mean, median, and mode are equal to 0 and are located at the center of the distribution.	The key distribution is actually a family of curves based on the concept of degrees of freedom, which is related to sample size.[a]
The curve never touches the *x*-axis.	As the sample size increases, the *t* distribution approaches the standard normal distribution.

[a]The degrees of freedom are the number of values that are free to vary after a sample statistic has been computed, and they tell a researcher which specific code to use when a distribution consists of a family of curves. For example, if the mean of 5 values is 10, then 4 of the 5 values are free to vary. But once 4 values are selected, the fifth value must be a specific number to get a sum of 50, since 50 ÷ 5 = 10. Hence the degrees of freedom are 5 − 1 = 4, and this value tells the researcher which *t* curve to use.

Reproduced with permission from Bluman AG. Confidence intervals and sample size. In: Bluman AG, ed. *Elementary Statistics: A Step by Step Approach.* 4th ed. New York, NY: McGraw-Hill; 2008:343-385.

making predictions.[2] Inferential statistics are based on probability theory.[2] Probability deals with events that occur by chance. Probability can be defined as the chance of an event occurring. The classical theory of probability states that the chance of a particular outcome occurring is determined by the ratio of the number of favorable outcomes (or successes) to the total number of outcomes. An event consists of a set of outcomes of a probability experiment. Probabilities can be expressed as fractions, decimals, or percentages.

- Probability sampling: Any method of sampling that utilizes some form of random selection, and uses a process or procedure that assures that the different units in the population have equal probabilities of being chosen.
- Nonprobability sampling: Does not require random selection of the parameters of the population to be identified. This type

of sampling is often utilized in physical therapy due to the increased difficulty of meeting the more rigid requirements of probability sampling.

Most of the major inferential statistics come from a general family of statistical models including the *t*-test, analysis of variance (ANOVA), and analysis of covariance (ANCOVA).

t-Test

The *t*-test is the most commonly used method to evaluate the differences in means between two groups when the SD is unknown, the sample size is less than 30, and the distribution of the variable is approximately normal. The groups can be independent (eg, blood pressure of patients who were given a drug vs a control group who received a placebo) or dependent (eg, blood pressure of patients "before" vs "after" they received a drug).

Analysis of Variance

ANOVA is a useful tool that helps the user to identify sources of variability from one or more potential sources, sometimes referred to as "treatments" or "factors." ANOVA is used rather than performing multiple *t*-tests because it protects against an inflation of α that would otherwise result from multiple *t*-tests.

STUDY PEARL

The *t*-test and ANOVA determine whether the difference(s) between the means of two (*t*-test) or more samples (ANOVA) could be due to random sampling error alone.

- A *t*-test is used with one independent variable with two levels (ie, there are two groups, such as control vs experimental).
- ANOVA is used when there is one independent variable with three or more levels (conditions), or there are two or more independent variables.

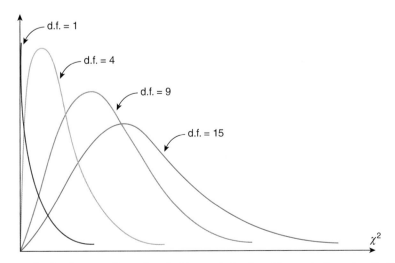

FIGURE 8D-9 The chi-square family of curves. (Reproduced with permission from Bluman A. *Elementary Statistics: A Step by Step Approach.* 6th ed. New York, NY: McGraw-Hill; 2007:374.)

By varying the factors in a predetermined pattern and analyzing the output, one can use statistical techniques to make an accurate assessment as to the cause of variation in a process. There are two common types of ANOVA, discussed below.

One-Way Analysis of Variance

The one-way ANOVA method of analysis requires multiple experiments or readings to be taken from a source that can take on two or more different inputs or settings. One-way ANOVA performs a comparison of the means of a number of replications of experiments performed where a single input factor is varied at different settings or levels. The object of this comparison is to determine the proportion of the variability of the data that is due to the different treatment levels or factors as opposed to variability due to random error. Basically, rejection of the null hypothesis indicates that variation in the outcome is due to variation between the treatment levels and not to random error. If the null hypothesis is rejected, there is a difference in the outcome of the different treatment levels at a significance α and it remains to be determined between which treatment levels the actual differences lie.

Two-Way Analysis of Variance

The two-way ANOVA method is an extension to the one-way ANOVA, in which comparisons can be made between two or more populations means with two or more independent variables (hence the name two-way), called factors.

Analysis of Covariance

ANCOVA is a test used to compare two or more treatment groups or conditions while also controlling for the effects of intervening variables (covariates), for example, two groups of subjects are compared on the basis of diet parameters using two different types of exercises; the subjects in one group are male and the subjects in the second group are female; gender then becomes the covariate that must be controlled during statistical analysis.

Intraclass Correlation Coefficient

The intraclass correlation coefficient (ICC) is a reliability coefficient calculated with variance estimates obtained through an ANOVA (Table 8D–7).[9] The ICC has been advocated as a statistic for assessing agreement or consistency between two methods of

measurement in conjunction with a significance test of the difference between means obtained by the two methods. The advantage of the ICC over correlation coefficients is that it does not require the same number of raters per subject, and it can be used for two or more raters or ratings.[9]

STUDY PEARL

- Spearman's rank correlation coefficient, or Spearman's rho (ρ), provides information as to the magnitude and direction of the association between two variables that are on an interval or ratio scale.
- The Pearson product-moment correlation coefficient (PPMCC, sometimes referred to as the Pearson correlation coefficient) measures the strength and direction of a *linear* relationship between the X and Y variables.[19] The PPMCC, which is denoted by the Greek letter "rho" (ρ), ranges from –1 to 1. A value of 1 implies a perfect relationship between X and Y:[19]
  - 0.00–0.25: Little or no relationship
  - 0.25–0.50: Fair relationship
  - 0.50–0.75: Moderate to good relationship
  - >0.75: Good to excellent relationship

STUDY PEARL

A statistical hypothesis is a conjecture about a population parameter. This conjecture may or may not be true.[23]

Hypothesis Testing

Statistical hypothesis testing is a decision-making process used for evaluating claims about a population.[23] Every hypothesis testing situation begins with a statement of a hypothesis.

There are two types of statistical hypothesis of each situation: the null hypothesis (H_0), and the alternative hypothesis (H_A).

1. Null hypothesis (H_0): A statistical hypothesis that states that there is no difference between a parameter and a specific value, or that there is no difference between two parameters.[23]
2. Alternative hypothesis (H_A): A statistical hypothesis that states the existence of a difference between a parameter and a specific value, or states that there is a difference between two parameters.[23]

Although the above definitions of null and alternative hypothesis use the word parameter, these definitions can be extended to include other terms such as distributions and randomness.[23]

In statistical hypothesis testing (Table 8D–8), the null hypothesis (H_0) is initially believed to be true, and the researcher sees if the data provide enough evidence to abandon the belief in H_0 in favor of the alternative hypothesis H_A. For example, in a jury trial there is a presumption of innocence (eg, the population means

TABLE 8D–7 Intraclass correlation coefficient benchmark values.

Value	Description
<0.75	Poor to moderate agreement
>0.75	Good agreement
>90	Reasonable agreement for clinical measurements

Data from Portney L, Watkins MP. *Foundations of Clinical Research: Applications to Practice.* Norwalk, CT: Appleton & Lange; 1993.

TABLE 8D-8 Guidelines for hypothesis testing.

1. Make a claim—a hypothesis that is assumed to be/is correct—the research hypothesis. For example, the research hypothesis could be "I wonder whether sleep deprivation would have an effect on mental performance."

2. State the null hypothesis and the alternative hypothesis. The null hypothesis (denoted H_0) is a statement about the value of a population parameter that MUST contain equality (=, $\leq$, $\geq$). For example, in the sleep deprivation study, the null hypothesis could be that sleep deprivation will have no effect on mental performance. The alternative hypothesis (denoted H_1) is the opposite statement—the one that must be true if the null hypothesis is false. The alternative hypothesis is a statement of what a statistical hypothesis test is set up to establish. In this example, the alternative hypothesis would be that sleep deprivation would have a positive or negative effect on mental performance. The goal is to ascertain a correct inference about the population that is being sampled with the experimental technique.

3. Decide on the appropriate test statistic. A test statistic is a quantity calculated from the sample of data and is determined by the assumed probability model and the hypotheses under question. Its value is used to decide whether or not the null hypothesis should be rejected in the hypothesis test.

4. Find the critical value for the test statistic and determine the critical region (see text).

5. Perform the calculations and state the conclusion.

of a control group and the experimental group are not different from each other). The null hypothesis is assumed to be true (the defendant is innocent) at the outset of inferential statistical analysis. The null hypothesis is only rejected in favor of the alternative hypothesis (eg, the two means differ) when the data provide the basis for "reasonable doubt about innocence," that is, based on the experimental data, it is more likely that the control and experimental groups are different from each other (Figure 8D–10).

Type I Errors

In a hypothesis test, a type I error occurs when the null hypothesis is rejected when it is in fact true; that is, H_0 is wrongly rejected.

	H_0 true	H_0 false
Reject H_0	**Error** Type I	Correct decision
Do not reject H_0	Correct decision	**Error** Type II

FIGURE 8D-10 Possible outcomes of a hypothesis test. (Reproduced with permission from Bluman A. *Elementary Statistics: A Step by Step Approach*. 6th ed. New York: McGraw-Hill; 2007:392.)

For example, in a clinical trial of a new drug, the null hypothesis might be that the new drug is no better, on average, than the current drug; that is H_0: There is no difference between the two drugs on average. A type I error would occur if we concluded that the two drugs produced different effects when in fact there was no difference between them (Figure 8D–11). A type I error is often considered to be more serious, and therefore more important to avoid, than a type II error (see next). The hypothesis test procedure is therefore adjusted so that there is a guaranteed "low" probability of rejecting the null hypothesis wrongly; this probability is never 0.

Type II Errors

In a hypothesis test, a type II error occurs when the null hypothesis H_0, is not rejected when it is in fact false. For example, in a clinical trial of a new drug, the null hypothesis might be that the new drug is no better, on average, than the current drug; that is H_0: There is no difference between the two drugs on average. A type II error would occur if it was concluded that the two drugs produced the same effect, that is, there is no difference between the two drugs on average, when in fact they produced different effects (Figure 8D–11). A type II error is frequently due to sample sizes being too small.

STUDY PEARL

Nothing can be proved absolutely. Likewise, the decision to reject or not reject the null hypothesis does not prove anything—the only way to prove something statistically is to use the entire population.[23] The question as to how large the difference is necessary to reject the null hypothesis is answered somewhat using the level of significance.

STUDY PEARL

- The critical or rejection region is the range of values of the test value that indicates there is a significant difference and that the null hypothesis should be rejected (Figure 8D-12); that is, the sample space for the test statistic is partitioned into two regions—one region (the critical region) will lead the researcher to reject the null hypothesis H_0, and the other will not. So, if the observed value of the test statistic is a member of the critical region, the researcher concludes "reject H_0"; if it is not a member of the critical region then the researcher concludes "do not reject H_0."

- The noncritical or nonrejection region is the range of values of the test value that indicates the difference was probably due to chance and that the null hypothesis should not be rejected.

	H_0 true (innocent)	H_0 false (not innocent)
Reject H_0 (convict)	Type I error 1.	Correct decision 2.
Do not reject H_0 (acquit)	Correct decision 3.	Type II error 4.

H_0: The defendant is innocent.
H_1: The defendant is not innocent.
The results of a trial can be shown as follows:

FIGURE 8D–11 Hypothesis testing and a jury trial. (Reproduced with permission from Bluman A. *Elementary Statistics: A Step by Step Approach*. 6th ed. New York, NY: McGraw-Hill; 2007:393.)

Significance Level

The level of significance (denoted α) is the maximum probability of wrongly rejecting the null hypothesis H_0, when it is in fact true (committing a type I error). In simple terms, α is the preset risk one is willing to take in committing a type I error with an inferential statistical test. It is the bar over which the data need to jump in order to reject the null hypothesis and be considered statistically significant. By convention, statisticians use three arbitrary significance levels (α): 0.10, 0.05, and 0.01 levels (although it can be any level, depending on the seriousness of the type I error).[23] That is, if the null hypothesis is rejected, the probability of a type I error will be 10%, 5%, or 1%, depending on which level of significance is used. For example, if the acceptable risk of committing a type I error is 5%, α is set to 0.05 (indicates that the expected difference due to chance is only 5 times out of every 100). While decreasing the α value reduces the risk of a type I error, decreasing it too much increases the chances of obtaining a type II error.

After a significance level is chosen, a critical value is selected from a table for the appropriate test. The critical value determines the critical and noncritical regions.

The critical value for any hypothesis test depends on the significance level at which the test is carried out, whether the test is one-tailed or two-tailed, and on the degrees of freedom (see next).

The critical value can be on the right side of the mean or on the left side of the mean for one tail test—its location depends on the inequality sign of the alternative hypothesis. To obtain the critical value, the researcher must choose an alpha level (Figure 8D–13).

STUDY PEARL

A *one-tailed* (one-sided) test indicates that the null hypothesis should be rejected when the test value is in the critical region on one side of the mean; the region of rejection is entirely within one tail of the probability distribution. A one-tailed test is either a right-tailed test or a left-tailed test, depending on the direction of the inequality of the alternative hypothesis.

A *two-tailed* (two-sided) test indicates that the null hypothesis can be rejected when there is a significant difference in either direction, above or below the mean; the region of rejection is located in either of the two critical regions (Figure 8D-14). An extreme test statistic in either tail of the distribution (positive or negative) will lead to the rejection of the null hypothesis of no difference.

The choice between a one-sided and a two-sided test is determined by the purpose of the investigation or prior reasons for using a one-sided test. In most scientific investigations, a conservative approach is used where the problem is formulated with a two-sided alternative hypothesis, allowing the data to determine precisely how the null hypothesis might be false.

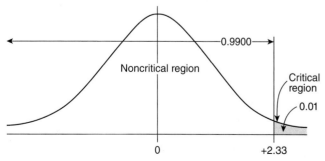

FIGURE 8D–12 Critical and noncritical regions for $\alpha = 0.01$ (right-tailed test). (Reproduced with permission from Bluman A. *Elementary Statistics: A Step by Step Approach*. 6th ed. New York, NY: McGraw-Hill; 2007:395.)

Probability (*p*) Value

The probability value (*p*-value) is used in statistics to describe the probability of something happening. A study will generally give a value of p for any conclusions drawn. The *p*-value is the probability of getting a sample statistic (such as the mean) or in a more extreme sample statistic in the direction of the alternative hypothesis when the null hypothesis is true—the risk of committing a type I error if the null hypothesis is rejected.

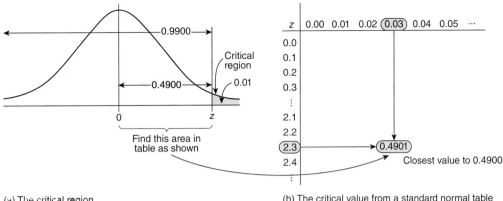

FIGURE 8D–13 Finding the critical value for α = 0.01 (right-tailed test). (Reproduced with permission from Bluman A. *Elementary Statistics: A Step by Step Approach*. 6th ed. New York, NY: McGraw-Hill; 2007:395.)

Small *p*-values suggest a very unusual observation under H_0 indicating that the null hypothesis is unlikely to be true. The smaller the *p*-value, the more convincing is the rejection of the null hypothesis. H_0 is rejected when the *p*-value is less than α.

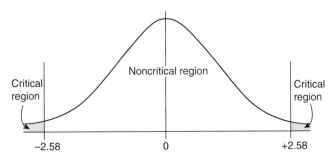

FIGURE 8D–14 Critical and noncritical regions for α = 0.01 (two-tailed test). (Reproduced with permission from Bluman A. *Elementary Statistics: A Step by Step Approach*. 6th ed. New York, NY: McGraw-Hill; 2007:395.)

The Power of a Hypothesis Test

The power of a statistical hypothesis test measures the test's ability to reject the null hypothesis when it is actually false—that is, to make a correct inference.

- The power of a hypothesis test is the probability of not committing a type II error. It is calculated by subtracting the probability of a type II error from 1.
- The maximum power a test can have is 1, whereas the minimum is 0.
- Ideally a test should have a high power, close to 1.

z-Test

The *z*-test is a statistical test of the mean of a population. It can be used when the sample size is ≥30, or when the population is normally distributed and the SD is known. For example, a *z*-test could be used if exam scores from a class of students are compared to a different class who took the same exam (when the population mean and SD are known). Z Statistic about using the standard normal table can be found at http://www.thepinsta.com/z-statistic-about-using-the-standard-normal-table_aQJ6tYlCANs2M5qdH2hotJtz0aE5iYExA3 40xbm%7CJxXJDFUKQYxYqVJVDH8PgV*i7r6GfeArPIOlW3w 9%7ChKeCg/a2YX6UD132AFbzLExvEYUF4UHmG44pF4m*LH KPdc8vVmsd8MIK32w5hlwafiQQQtbsC6Ylgm8dSBxmyzA2ei3A/.

CHOOSING THE CORRECT STATISTICAL CALCULATION

The choice of how to analyze data depends on the question being asked:[1]

- If the design is to learn about the association between two variables (eg, what is the relationship between arm girth and elbow flexor strength), a correlation coefficient should be calculated.
- If the question deals with prediction (eg, if the patient has knee range of motion of 10°–50° on the second postoperative day, how many days will the patient likely remain in the hospital?), a regression analysis is appropriate.
- If the question is whether a treatment has an effect or shows a difference (eg, does spinal traction reduce the signs and symptoms of a cervical root compression?), a chi-square, ANOVA, or *t*-test is appropriate.

- For a correlation study to determine the degree of association, a Spearman rho is used for ordinal data, whereas a Pearson correlation coefficient is calculated for interval data.
- If the question is whether two groups differ on the dependent variable, and the data are normally distributed with equal variances, a t-test is appropriate.

STUDY PEARL

Sackett and colleagues[24] define best evidence as:

- Clinically relevant research, often from the basic sciences, but especially from patient-centered clinical research
- The accuracy and precision of diagnostic tests
- The power of prognostic markers
- The efficacy and safety of therapeutic, rehabilitative, and preventive regimens

USE OF EVIDENCE-BASED PRACTICE

Evidence-based practice (EBP), the integration of three key elements—best research evidence, clinical expertise, and patient values—is having an increasing impact on the profession of physical therapy.

When integrating evidence into clinical decision making, an understanding of how to appraise the quality of the evidence offered by clinical studies is important. Judging the strength of the evidence becomes an important part of the decision-making process.

SCIENTIFIC RIGOR BY TYPE OF RESEARCH DESIGN

Unfortunately, many of the experimental studies that deal with physical therapy topics are not well-designed trials. Awareness of the distinction between efficacy and effectiveness is important for therapists attempting to translate evidence to practice.

STUDY PEARL

Clinical prediction rules (CPR) are tools designed to assist clinicians in decision making when caring for patients. However, although there is a growing trend to produce a number of CPRs in the field of physical therapy, few CPRs presently exist.

- **Efficacy:** Refers to outcomes of interventions provided in a controlled setting under experimental conditions. When attempting to apply the results of an efficacy study, a therapist must consider whether subject characteristics and the manner in which intervention was provided generalize to patients on their caseloads and how to adapt the intervention to constraints within their practice settings.[25]
- **Effectiveness:** Refers to outcomes of interventions provided within the scope of clinical practice.

Sackett[26] proposed a five-level system that relates the experimental design to levels of evidence and grades of recommendation (Table 8D–9). A grade A recommendation (the randomized controlled trial) (Table 8D–10) indicates that outcomes are supported by at least one level I study. A grade B recommendation indicates outcomes are supported by at least one level II study. A grade C recommendation indicates that outcomes are supported by level III, IV, or V studies.

STUDY PEARL

Randomized controlled trials and systematic reviews provide the strongest, most relevant evidence to inform practice (Table 8D–11).

Evidence-based practice is a four-step process:

1. A clinical problem is identified and an answerable research question is formulated.
2. A systematic literature review is conducted and evidence is collected.
3. The research evidence is summarized and critically analyzed.
4. The research evidence is synthesized and applied to clinical practice.

TABLE 8D-9 A hierarchy of evidence grading.

	Level of Evidence Grading = A	Level of Evidence Grading = B	Level of Evidence Grading = C	Level of Evidence Grading = D	Level of Evidence Grading = E
Type of Study	Randomized controlled trial	Cohort study	• Nonrandomized trial with concurrent or historical controls • Case study • Study of sensitivity and specificity of a diagnostic test • Population-based descriptive study	• Cross-sectional study • Case series • Case report	• Expert consensus • Clinical experience

Data from Sackett DL. Rules of evidence and clinical recommendations on the use of antithrombotic agents. *Chest.* 1986;89:2S-3S.

TABLE 8D-10 The randomized controlled trial.

An experimental design in which subjects are randomly assigned to an experimental or control group permitting the strongest inferences about cause and effect. Typically volunteers agree to be randomly allocated to groups receiving one of the following:

- Treatment and no treatment
- Standard treatment and standard treatment plus a new treatment
- Two alternate treatments

The common feature is that the experimental group receives the treatment of interest, and the control group does not. At the end of the trial, outcomes of subjects in each group are determined—the difference in outcomes between groups provides an estimate of the size of the treatment effect.

- Less exposed to bias
- Ensures comparability of groups
- Provide evidence of efficacy

Data from Maher CG, Herbert RD, Moseley AM, et al. Critical appraisal of randomized trials, systematic reviews of randomized trials and clinical practice guidelines. In: Boyling JD, Jull GA, eds. *Grieve's Modern Manual Therapy: The Vertebral Column.* Philadelphia, PA: Churchill Livingstone; 2004:603-614; Petticrew M. Systematic reviews from astronomy to zoology: myths and misconceptions. *BMJ.* 2001;322: 98-101; Palisano RJ, Campbell SK, Harris SR. Evidence-based decision-making in pediatric physical therapy. In: Campbell SK, Vander Linden DW, Palisano RJ, eds. *Physical Therapy for Children.* St. Louis: W.B. Saunders; 2006:3-32.

TABLE 8D-11 Systematic reviews.

Systematic review	Review of the literature conducted in a way that is designed to minimize bias—"a study of studies."
	Recently published reviews can be used to assess the effects of health interventions, the accuracy of diagnostic tests, or the prognosis for a particular condition.
	Usually involve criteria to determine which studies will be considered, the search strategy used to locate the studies, the methods for assessing the quality of the studies, and the process used to synthesize the findings of individual studies.
	Particularly useful for busy clinicians who may be unable to access all the relevant trials in an area and may otherwise need to rely upon their own incomplete surveys of relevant trials.
	NB: A systematic review is only as good as the quality of each study.
Meta-analysis	A mathematical synthesis of the results of two or more research reports. A meta-analysis can be performed on studies that used reliable and valid measures and report some type of inferential statistic (eg, *t*-test, ANOVA).

Data from Maher CG, Herbert RD, Moseley AM, et al. Critical appraisal of randomized trials, systematic reviews of randomized trials and clinical practice guidelines. In: Boyling JD, Jull GA, eds. *Grieve's Modern Manual Therapy: The Vertebral Column.* Philadelphia, PA: Churchill Livingstone; 2004:603-614; Petticrew M. Systematic reviews from astronomy to zoology: myths and misconceptions. *BMJ.* 2001;322: 98-101; Palisano RJ, Campbell SK, Harris SR. Evidence-based decision-making in pediatric physical therapy. In: Campbell SK, Vander Linden DW, Palisano RJ, eds. *Physical Therapy for Children.* St. Louis: W.B. Saunders; 2006:3-32.

TABLE 8D-12 Clinical practice guidelines.

Recommendations for management of a particular clinical condition

Intended to provide current standards for quality practice in order to improve effectiveness and efficiency of health care

Involve compilation of evidence concerning needs and expectations of recipients of care, the accuracy of diagnostic tests, effects of therapy, and prognosis

Usually necessitates the results from one or sometimes several systematic reviews

May be presented as clinical decision algorithms

Can provide a useful framework upon which clinicians can build clinical practice

Data from Maher CG, Herbert RD, Moseley AM, et al. Critical appraisal of randomized trials, systematic reviews of randomized trials and clinical practice guidelines. In: Boyling JD, Jull GA, eds. *Grieve's Modern Manual Therapy: The Vertebral Column.* Philadelphia, PA: Churchill Livingstone; 2004:603-614.

Practice guidelines are systematically developed statements to assist patient and practitioner decisions about the management of a health condition (Table 8D–12).[25] In general, practice guidelines include recommendations for the following:[25]

- Who should receive the intervention?
- Expected outcomes.
- Documentation including selection of reliable and valid tests and measures.
- Utilization of services (frequency and duration, number of visits).
- Procedural interventions.
- Coordination of care.
- Discharge planning.

In 1998, an international group of researchers and policymakers formed the Appraisal of Guidelines for Research and Evaluation (AGREE) collaboration in order to improve the quality and effectiveness of clinical practice guidelines.[25]

STUDY PEARL

The critically appraised topic (CAT) provides a format for therapists to summarize the research evidence from a literature search conducted as part of clinical practice.[27] A CAT is a one- to two-page summary of research related to a focused clinical question that includes implications for practice.[25]

INSTRUMENTATION GOLD STANDARD

The instrumentation gold standard can be defined as an instrument with established validity that can be used as a standard for assessing or comparing other instruments.

REFERENCES

1. Underwood FB. Clinical research and data analysis. In: Placzek JD, Boyce DA, eds. *Orthopaedic Physical Therapy Secrets*. Philadelphia, PA: Hanley & Belfus; 2001:130-139.

2. Bluman AG. The nature of probability and statistics. In: Bluman AG, ed. *Elementary Statistics: A Step by Step Approach*. 4th ed. New York, NY: McGraw-Hill; 2008:1-32.

3. Bluman AG. Organizing data. In: Bluman AG, ed. *Elementary Statistics: A Step by Step Approach*. 4th ed. New York, NY: McGraw-Hill; 2008:33-100.

4. Van der Wurff P, Meyne W, Hagmeijer RHM. Clinical tests of the sacroiliac joint, a systematic methodological review. Part 2: validity. *Man Ther*. 2000;5:89-96.

5. Feinstein AR. *Clinimetrics*. Westford, MA: Murray Printing Company; 1987.

6. Marx RG, Bombardier C, Wright JG. What we know about the reliability and validity of physical examination tests used to examine the upper extremity. *J Hand Surg*. 1999;24A:185-193.

7. Roach KE, Brown MD, Albin RD, et al. The sensitivity and specificity of pain response to activity and position in categorizing patients with low back pain. *Phys Ther*. 1997; 77:730-738.

8. Domholdt E. *Physical Therapy Research: Principles and Applications*. Philadelphia, PA: WB Saunders. 1993.

9. Huijbregts PA. Spinal motion palpation: a review of reliability studies. *J Man Manip Ther*. 2002;10:24-39.

10. Feinstein AR. Clinical biostatistics XXXI. On the sensitivity, specificity, and discrimination of diagnostic tests. *Clin Pharmacol Ther*. 1975;17:104-116.

11. Anderson MA, Foreman TL. Return to competition: functional rehabilitation. In: Zachazewski JE, Magee DJ, Quillen WS, eds. *Athletic Injuries and Rehabilitation*. Philadelphia, PA: WB Saunders; 1996:229-261.

12. Jull GA. Physiotherapy management of neck pain of mechanical origin. In: Giles LGF, Singer KP, eds. *Clinical Anatomy and Management of Cervical Spine Pain. The Clinical Anatomy of Back Pain*. London, UK: Butterworth-Heinemann. 1998:168-191.

13. Jaeschke R, Guyatt G, Sackett DL. Users guides to the medical literature. III. How to use an article about a diagnostic test. B. What are the results and will they help me in caring for my patients? *JAMA*. 1994;27:703-707.

14. Wright JG, Feinstein AR. Improving the reliability of orthopaedic measurements. *J Bone Joint Surg*. 1992;74B:287-291.

15. Haas M. Statistical methodology for reliability studies. *J Manip Physiol Ther*. 1991;14:119-132.

16. Cooperman JM, Riddle DL, Rothstein JM. Reliability and validity of judgments of the integrity of the anterior cruciate ligament of the knee using the Lachman's test. *Phys Ther*. 1990;70:225-233.

17. Shields RK, Enloe LJ, Evans RE, et al. Reliability, validity, and responsiveness of functional tests in patients with total joint replacement. *Phys Ther*. 1995;75:169.

18. Laslett M, Williams M. The reliability of selected pain provocation tests for sacroiliac joint pathology. *Spine*. 1994;19:1243-1249.

19. Portney L, Watkins MP. *Foundations of Clinical Research: Applications to Practice*. Norwalk, CT: Appleton & Lange; 1993.

20. Bluman AG. Measures of central tendency. In: Bluman AG, ed. *Elementary Statistics: A Step by Step Approach*. 4th ed. New York, NY: McGraw-Hill; 2008:101-176.

21. Bluman AG. The normal distribution. In: Bluman AG, ed. *Elementary Statistics: A Step by Step Approach*. 4th ed. New York, NY: McGraw-Hill; 2008:281-341.

22. Bluman AG. Confidence intervals and sample size. In: Bluman AG, ed. *Elementary Statistics: A Step by Step Approach*. 4th ed. New York, NY: McGraw-Hill; 2008:343-385.

23. Bluman AG. Hypothesis testing. In: Bluman AG, ed. *Elementary Statistics: A Step by Step Approach*. 4th ed. New York, NY: McGraw-Hill; 2008:387-455.

24. Sackett DL, Strauss SF, Richardson WS, et al. *Evidence Based Medicine: How to Practice and Teach EBM*. 2nd ed. Edinburgh, Scotland: Churchill Livingstone; 2000.

25. Palisano RJ, Campbell SK, Harris SR. Evidence-based decision-making in pediatric physical therapy. In: Campbell SK, Vander Linden DW, Palisano RJ, eds. *Physical Therapy for Children*. St. Louis: Saunders; 2006:3-32.

26. Sackett DL. Rules of evidence and clinical recommendations on the use of antithrombotic agents. *Chest*. 1986;89: 2S-3S.

27. Fetters L, Figueiredo EM, Keane-Miller D, et al. Critically appraised topics. *Pediatr Phys Ther*. 2004;16:19-21.

QUESTIONS

1. The strongest support for use of a selected treatment technique would be provided by which of the following types of study?
   A. Individual randomized controlled trial
   B. Individual cohorts study
   C. Individual case-control study
   D. Case series

2. A study examines the effect of ultrasound intensities on the pain level of patients with plantar fasciitis. In this study "pain level" is which of the following types of variable?
   A. Attribute variable
   B. Dependent variable
   C. Dichotomous variable
   D. Independent variable

3. When a therapist refers to the relationship between goniometric measurement results and the measurements of radiographic images whose validity is known, this is best described as which of the following types of validity?
   A. Content validity
   B. Construct validity
   C. Concurrent validity
   D. Predictive validity

4. A therapist is performing ROM of knee flexion following knee arthroplasty. The therapist wants to know the most common threshold for meaningful change to determine if treatment is beneficial to this patient. Which of the following definitions best describes this threshold?
   A. Standard error of measurement
   B. Minimal clinical important difference
   C. Minimal detectable difference
   D. Standard deviation

5. If the Fall Risk Assessment and Screening is negative for patient falls in 99% of individuals without a history of falling, then the measurement of balance in this test is considered to be which of the following definitions?
   A. Sensitive
   B. Specific
   C. Reliable
   D. Valid

ANSWERS

1. The answer is **A**. (Chart in Portney and Watkins, p 362; Levels of Evidence.)[19]
A hierarchy has been developed by the Oxford Centre for Evidence-Based Medicine to categorize studies by levels of evidence (https://www.cebm.net/2016/05/ocebm-levels-of-evidence/).
   A. The highest level of evidence is the randomized controlled trial. These are considered Level 1 studies.
   B. Individual cohort studies are classified as Level 2 studies.
   C. Individual case-control studies are classified as Level 3.
   D. Case series are classified as Level 4.

2. The answer is **B**. (Portney and Watkins, pp 129-130).[19]
   A. The dependent variable is the response (pain level) that is assumed to be caused by another (independent) variable.
   B. The independent variable is presumed to cause, explain, or influence a dependent variable. It is a variable that is manipulated or controlled by the researcher.
   C. A dichotomous variable is used when qualitative variable such as gender can take on only two values.
   D. An attribute variable is an independent variable with levels that cannot be manipulated or assigned by the researcher but that represent subject characteristics such as age.

3. The answer is **C**. (Portney and Watkins, p 102).[19]
   A. Content validity refers to the degree to which the items in an instrument adequately reflect the content domain being measured.
   B. Construct validity indicates the degree to which a theoretical construct is measured by the instrument.
   C. Concurrent validity is demonstrated when a test score correlates well with a measure that has previously been validated.
   D. Predictive validity is a form of measurement in which an instrument is used to predict some future performance.

4. The answer is **B**. (Portney and Watkins, p 647).[19]
   A. Standard error of measurement estimates the standard error in a set of repeated scores.
   B. The minimal clinical important difference is the smallest change in an outcome measure that is perceived as beneficial by the patient and that would lead to a change in the patient's medical management, assuming an absence of excessive side effects and costs.
   C. Minimal detectable difference is the smallest amount of change that can be considered above the threshold of error expected in the measurement.
   D. Standard deviation reflects the variability or dispersion of scores around the mean.

5. The answer is **B**. (Portney and Watkins, p 620).[19]
The validity of a diagnostic test, such as the "Fall Risk Assessment and Screening," is evaluated by its accuracy in assessing the presence or absence of a target condition such as falls. A test is considered specific when the test is negative in persons who do not have the condition. A highly specific test will rarely be positive when a person does not have the condition.
   A. Sensitivity is the probability of obtaining a positive test among individuals who have the disease.
   B. Specificity is the probability of obtaining a negative test among individuals without the condition. Since 99% of individuals who had no history of falls tested negative, this test is highly specific.
   C. Reliability refers to the extent to which a test or measurement is consistent on repeated trials. In this situation, there is no indication that the Fall Risk Assessment and Screening is administered multiple times.
   D. Validity refers to the degree to which a test or measurement accurately reflects the specific concept the clinician is attempting to measure. In this example, the data do not provide useful information for assessing the extent to which the Fall Risk Assessment and Screening is a valid way to identify individuals who are at risk for falling.

CHECKLIST

When you complete this section, you should be able to:

❑ Evaluate the quality of a research study based on scientific rigor by type of research design, level of evidence, and methods.

❑ Identify application and significance of various statistical analyses.

❑ Describe data collection and sampling techniques.

❑ Identify the characteristics of various graphic representations.

❑ Apply descriptive statistics and measures appropriately.

■ SECTION E: TEACHING AND LEARNING

INTRODUCTION

Education can be defined as any act or experience that has a formative effect on the mind, character, or physical ability of an individual.

Learning refers to the ways people acquire, process, store, and apply new information. Learning is most effective when an individual is ready to learn; that is, when one wants to know something.

MOTIVATION

Motivation plays a critical role in the learning process, and success motivates more than failure (Table 8E–1). Basic principles of motivation exist that are applicable to learning in any situation.

The environment can be used to focus the patient's attention on what needs to be learned. For example, interesting visual aids, such as booklets, posters, or practice equipment, motivate learners by capturing their attention and curiosity.

Incentives, including privileges and receiving praise from the educator, motivate learning. Both affiliation and approval are strong motivators.

Internal motivation is longer lasting and more self-directive than is external motivation, which must be repeatedly reinforced by praise or concrete rewards.

MASLOW'S HIERARCHY OF NEEDS

Maslow's hierarchy of needs is based on the concept that there is a hierarchy of biogenic and psychogenic needs that humans must progress through. Maslow hypothesizes that the higher needs in this hierarchy only come into focus once all the needs that are lower down in the pyramid are mainly or entirely satisfied. Maslow's hierarchy is often depicted as a pyramid consisting of five levels (Figure 8E–1). The lower levels (physiological and safety needs) are referred to as *deficiency needs*, while the top three levels (love/belonging, status, and self-actualization needs) are referred to as a *being needs*. According to Maslow, in order for an individual to progress up the hierarchy to the being needs, the deficiency needs must be met. Growth forces (eg, personal growth, integration, and fulfillment) create upward movement in the hierarchy, whereas regressive forces (eg, sickness, discomfort, lack of security) push predominant needs further down the hierarchy.

DOMAINS OF LEARNING

Bloom identified three domains of educational activities.[1]

- **Cognitive:** Mental skills (knowledge)
  - Involves knowledge and the development of intellectual skills.
  - Includes the recall or recognition of specific facts, procedural patterns, and concepts that serve in the development of intellectual abilities and skills.
  - There are six major categories (degrees of difficulties) starting from the simplest behavior to the most complex, with the

High-Yield Terms to Learn

Active learning	The process of having students engage in some activity that forces them to reflect upon ideas and how they are using those ideas. Requiring students to regularly assess their own degree of understanding and skill at handling concepts or problems in a particular discipline. The attainment of knowledge by participating or contributing. The process of keeping students mentally, and often physically, active in their learning through activities that involve them in gathering information, thinking and problem solving.
Affective domain	Actions or behaviors are controlled by feelings, attitudes or values.
Cognitive domain	Actions or behaviors are controlled by knowledge or understanding.
Decision making	Reason that results in action.
Learning style	The preferred way in which a person absorbs, processes, comprehends, and retains knowledge.
Passive learning	A method of learning or instruction where students receive information from the instructor and internalize it, and where the learner receives no feedback from the instructor.
Problem solving	Making, implementing, and evaluating decisions relating to some aspect of physical therapy.
Psychomotor domain	Manual or physical skills.
Reflection	The internal process of examining an experience that raises an issue of concern.
Sensory motor learning	Improvement, through practice, in the performance of sensory-guided motor behavior.[1]
Teaching style	The general principles, pedagogy, and management strategies used for classroom instruction.

TABLE 8E–1 Learning theories.

Theory	Principle Elements	Strategies	Prominent Theorists	Clinical Application
Algo-heuristic	Identifying the mental processes (conscious and subconscious) that underlie expert learning, thinking, and performance in any area. All cognitive activities can be analyzed into operations of an algorithmic, semi-algorithmic, heuristic, or semi-heuristic nature. Teaching students how to discover processes is more valuable than providing them with already formulated processes.	Once discovered, the operations and their systems can serve as the basis for instructional strategies and methods.	L. Landa	Performing a task or solving a problem always requires a certain system of elementary knowledge units and operations.
Androgyny	Adults need to know why they need to learn something, and need to learn experientially as they approach learning as problem solving. Adults learn best when the topic is of immediate value.	There is a need to explain why specific things are being taught (eg. certain commands, functions, operations, etc). Learning activities should be in the context of common tasks to be performed instead of memorization. Instruction should take into account the wide range of different backgrounds of learners; learning materials and activities should allow for different levels/types of previous experience with computers. Since adults are self-directed, instruction should allow learners to discover things for themselves, providing guidance and help when mistakes are made.	M. Knowles	Can be applied to any form of adult learning. Has been used extensively in the design of organizational training programs.
Adult learning	Integrates other theoretical frameworks for adult learning such as andragogy (Knowles), experiential learning (Rogers), and lifespan psychology. Consists of two classes of variables: personal characteristics (aging, life phases, and developmental stages) and situational characteristics (part-time vs full-time learning, and voluntary vs compulsory learning).	The three personal characteristics must be taken into consideration. Aging results in the deterioration of certain sensory-motor abilities (eg. eyesight, hearing, reaction time) while intelligence abilities (eg. decision-making skills, reasoning, and vocabulary) tend to improve.	K.P. Cross	Adult learning programs should adapt to the aging limitations of the participants, while capitalizing on the experience of participants. Adults should be challenged to move to increasingly advanced stages of personal development.

(Continued)

TABLE 8E-1 Learning theories. (Continued)

Theory	Principle Elements	Strategies	Prominent Theorists	Clinical Application
Behaviorist (stimulus-response theory)-operant conditioning	Learning is a function of a change in overt behavior. Changes in behavior are the result of an individual's response to events (stimuli) and their consequences that occur in the environment. The response of one behavior becomes the stimulus for the next response. Learning occurs when an individual engages in specific behaviors in order to receive certain consequences (learned association). Behavior can be controlled or shaped by operant conditioning. Desired or correct behaviors are identified so that frequent and scheduled reinforcements (positive reinforcement) can be given to reinforce the desired behaviors. Negative behaviors are ignored (negative reinforcement) so that these behaviors become weakened to the point where they disappear (extinction).	Positive reinforcement is used through the use of rewards that are meaningful to the individual. Timing of reinforcement. Continuous reinforcement: A behavior is reinforced every time it occurs. Partial reinforcement: A behavior is reinforced intermittently. Fixed interval: The period of time between the occurrences of each instance of reinforcement is fixed or set. Variable interval: The period of time between the occurrences of each instance of reinforcement varies around a constant average.	B.F. Skinner, G. Watson	Limited clinical use: behavior modification techniques may be used when working with adults with impaired or limited cognitive abilities or young children. Repetition is a necessary prerequisite for learning.
Classical conditioning	First model of learning to be studied in psychology. Demonstrates the environment's control over behavior. Type of associative learning—relates the capacity of animals/humans to learn new stimuli and connect them to natural reflexes, allowing non-natural cues to elicit a natural reflex. The conditioned stimulus, or conditional stimulus, is an initially neutral stimulus that elicits a response—known as a conditioned response—that is learned by the organism. Conditioned stimuli are associated psychologically with conditions such as anticipation, satisfaction (both immediate and prolonged), and fear. The relationship between the conditioned stimulus and conditioned response is known as the conditioned (or conditional) reflex. The process by which an individual learns to associate an unconditional stimulus with a conditional stimulus but receives no benefit from doing so.	Therapies associated with classical conditioning are aversion therapy, flooding, systematic desensitization, and implosion therapy. Much of what we like or dislike is a result of classical conditioning.	I. Pavlov, J.B. Watson	These techniques have been criticized for being unethical since they have the potential to cause trauma. Perhaps the strongest application of classical conditioning involves emotion. Common experience and careful research both confirm that human emotion conditions vary rapidly and easily, particularly when the emotion is intensely felt or negative in direction, it will condition quickly.
Cognitive dissonance	There is a tendency for individuals to seek consistency among their cognitions (ie, beliefs, opinions). When there is an inconsistency between attitudes or behaviors (dissonance), something must change to eliminate the dissonance. In the case of a discrepancy between attitudes and behavior, it is most likely that the attitude will change to accommodate the behavior.	There are three ways to eliminate dissonance: Reduce the importance of the dissonant beliefs. Add more consonant beliefs that outweigh the dissonant beliefs. Change the dissonant beliefs so that they are no longer inconsistent.	L. Festinger	Dissonance theory is especially relevant to decision making and problem solving.

Theory	Description	Application	Author(s)	Notes
Cognitive flexibility	Focuses on the nature of learning in complex and ill-structured domains. Emphasis is placed upon the presentation of information from multiple perspectives and use of many case studies that present diverse examples. Effective learning is context-dependent. Stresses the importance of constructed knowledge; learners must be given an opportunity to develop their own representations of information in order to properly learn.	Learning activities must provide multiple representations of content. Instructional materials should avoid oversimplifying the content domain and support context-dependent knowledge. Instruction should be case-based and emphasize knowledge construction, not transmission of information. Knowledge sources should be highly interconnected rather than compartmentalized.	R. Spiro, P. Feltovitch, R. Coulson	Limited: Cognitive flexibility theory is especially formulated to support the use of interactive technology.
Cognitive load	Learning happens best under conditions that are aligned with human cognitive architecture. The contents of long-term memory are sophisticated structures (schema) that permit us to perceive, think, and solve problems, rather than a group of rote-learned facts. Schemas are acquired over a lifetime of learning, and may have other schemas contained within themselves. The difference between an expert and a novice is that a novice hasn't acquired the schemas of an expert.	Change problem-solving methods to use goal-free problems or worked examples. Eliminate the working memory load associated with having to mentally integrate several sources of information by physically integrating those sources of information. Eliminate the working memory load associated with unnecessarily processing repetitive information by reducing redundancy. Increase working memory capacity by using auditory as well as visual information under conditions where both sources of information are essential (ie, nonredundant) to understanding.	J. Sweller	Cognitive load theory has many implications in the design of learning materials, such as handouts and home exercise programs
Constructivist theory	Learning is an active process in which learners construct new ideas or concepts based upon their current/past knowledge. Cognitive structure (ie, schema, mental models) provides meaning and organization to experiences and allows the individual to "go beyond the information given."	Instruction must be concerned with the experiences and contexts that make the student willing and able to learn (readiness). Instruction must be structured so that it can be easily grasped by the student (spiral organization). Instruction should be designed to facilitate extrapolation and or fill in the gaps (going beyond the information given).	J. Bruner	Much of this theory is linked to child development
Experiential learning	Two types of learning: Cognitive (meaningless)—academic knowledge such as learning vocabulary or multiplication tables. Experiential (significant)—applied knowledge such as personal change and growth.	Significant learning takes place when the subject matter is relevant to the personal interests of the student. Learning that is threatening to the self (eg, new attitudes or perspectives) is more easily assimilated when external threats are at a minimum. Learning proceeds faster when the threat to the self is low. Self-initiated learning is the most lasting and pervasive.	C. Rogers	Applies primarily to adult learners and adult learning.

(Continued)

TABLE 8E–1 Learning theories. (Continued)

Theory	Principle Elements	Strategies	Prominent Theorists	Clinical Application
Genetic epistemology	Cognitive structures (ie, development stages) are patterns of physical or mental action that underlie specific acts of intelligence and correspond to stages of child development. There are four primary cognitive structures: Sensorimotor stage (0–2 years)—intelligence takes the form of motor actions. Preoperation period (3–7 years)—intelligence is intuitive in nature. Concrete operational stage (8–11 years)—cognition is logical but depends upon concrete referents. Formal operations (12–15 years)—thinking involves abstractions.	Children will provide different explanations of reality at different stages of cognitive development. Cognitive development is facilitated by providing activities or situations that engage learners and require adaptation (ie, assimilation and accommodation). Learning materials and activities should involve the appropriate level of motor or mental operations for a child of given age; avoid asking students to perform tasks that are beyond their current cognitive capabilities. Use teaching methods that actively involve students and present challenges.	J. Piaget	The theory has been applied extensively to teaching practice and curriculum design in elementary education.
Modes of learning	Three modes of learning: Accretion: The addition of new knowledge to existing memory, the most common form of learning Structuring: Involves the formation of new conceptual structures or schema. Tuning: The adjustment of knowledge to a specific task usually through practice, the slowest form of learning and accounts for expert performance.	Instruction must be designed to accommodate different modes of learning. Practice activities affect the refinement of skills but not necessarily the initial acquisition of knowledge.	D. Rumelhart, D. Norman	Multiple applications to physical therapy—general model for human learning.
Humanist	Emphasis placed on personal freedom, dignity of the individual, and the learner's needs and feelings during the learning process. The learner experiences unconditional positive regard, acceptance, and understanding. Promotes active rather than passive learning.	Teacher must function as a facilitator and resource finder. Learning must address relevant problems and issues.	A.H. Maslow	Used in clinical situations that emphasize self-discovery, self-appropriated learning, and experimental learning.
Social learning	The social learning theory emphasizes the importance of observing and modeling the behaviors, attitudes, and emotional reactions of others. Social learning theory explains human behavior in terms of continuous reciprocal interaction between cognitive, behavioral, and environmental influences.	The highest level of observational learning is achieved by first organizing and rehearsing the modeled behavior symbolically and then enacting it overtly. Coding modeled behavior into words, labels, or images results in better retention than simply observing. Individuals are more likely to adopt a modeled behavior if it results in outcomes they value, or if the model is similar to the observer and has admired status and the behavior has functional value.	A. Bandura	Applied extensively to the understanding of aggression and psychological disorders, particularly in the context of behavior modification.

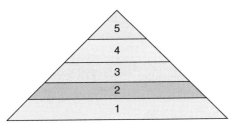

5. Actualization
4. Status (esteem)
3. Love/belonging
2. Safety
1. Physiological (biological needs)

FIGURE 8E-1 Maslow's hierarchy of needs.

first one having to be mastered before the next one can take place (Table 8E–2)

- **Affective:** Growth in feelings or emotional areas (attitude) (Table 8E–3)
  - Includes the manner in which matters are dealt with from an emotional aspect
  - Includes feelings, values, appreciation, enthusiasms, motivations, and attitudes
- **Psychomotor:** Manual or physical aspects (skills)
  - Includes physical movement, coordination, and use of the motor-skill areas
  - Development of these skills requires practice and is measured in terms of speed, precision, distance, procedures, or techniques in execution

The seven major categories of activities in the psychomotor domain are listed from the simplest to the most complex (Table 8E–4).

Decision Making

Most theories accept the idea that decision making consists of a number of steps or stages, such as recognition, formulation, the generation of alternatives, an information search, then selection, and finally action. Furthermore, it is well-recognized that routine cognitive processes such as memory, reasoning, and concept formation play a primary role in decision making. In addition, decision-making behavior is affected (usually adversely) by anxiety and stress.

Problem Solving

Problem-solving skills appear to be related to many other aspects of cognition such as schema (the ability to remember similar problems), pattern recognition (recognizing familiar problem elements), and creativity (developing new solutions). The issue of transfer is highly relevant to problem solving.

Sensory Motor Learning

Motor skills can be classified as continuous (eg, tracking), discrete (eg, skills that have a definite beginning and end), or procedural (eg, typing). Behavioral psychology emphasizes the use of practice variables in sensory-motor skills such as massed (concentrating

TABLE 8E-2 Cognitive domain.

Category	Examples and Key Words
Knowledge: Recall data or information.	Able to recite a poem; quote prices from memory. Key Words: defines, identifies, labels, lists, matches, names, outlines, recalls, recognizes, reproduces, selects
Comprehension: Understand the meaning, translation, interpolation, and interpretation of instructions and problems.	Able to rewrite a policy and procedures manual; can explain the steps for performing a complex task. Key Words: comprehends, distinguishes, estimates, explains, interprets, paraphrases, predicts, summarizes
Application: Use a concept in a new situation or unprompted use of an abstraction. Apply what was learned in the classroom to novel situations in the workplace.	Can use a manual to set up a video recorder, can apply the laws of statistics to evaluate a research study. Key Words: applies, computes, constructs, demonstrates, manipulates, modifies, operates, prepares, produces, relates, shows, solves
Analysis: Separate material or concepts into component parts so that its organizational structure may be understood. Distinguish between facts and inferences.	Can fix a piece of exercise equipment by using logical deduction; can gather information and select the required tasks for staff training. Key Words: analyzes, breaks down, compares, contrasts, differentiates, distinguishes, identifies, illustrates, infers, outlines, separates
Synthesis: Build a structure or pattern from diverse elements. Put parts together to form a whole, with emphasis on creating a new meaning or structure.	Can design or revise a process to perform a specific task, is able to integrate training from several sources to solve a problem. Key Words: categorizes, combines, compiles, composes, creates, devises, designs, generates, modifies, rearranges, reconstructs, reorganizes, summarizes
Evaluation: Make judgments about the value of ideas or materials.	Can select the most effective solution; hire the most qualified candidate; explain and justify a new budget. Key Words: appraises, compares, concludes, contrasts, critiques, discriminates, interprets, justifies, summarizes

TABLE 8E-3 Affective domain: the five major categories from the simplest behavior to the most complex.

Category	Example and Keywords
Receiving phenomena: Awareness, willingness to hear, selected attention.	Able to listen to others with respect; listen for and remember the name of newly introduced people. Key words: chooses, describes, follows, identifies, locates, names, points to, selects
Responding to phenomena: Active participation on the part of the learner. Attends and reacts to a particular phenomenon. Learning outcomes may emphasize compliance in responding, willingness to respond, or satisfaction in responding (motivation).	Is an active participant in staff discussions and is able to deliver an in-service presentation. Asks many questions about new ideas, concepts in order to fully understand them. Key words: answers, assists, complies, conforms, discusses, labels, performs, practices, reads, recites, reports, tells, writes
Valuing: The worth or value a person attaches to a particular object, phenomenon, or behavior. This can range from simple acceptance to the more complex state of commitment.	Is sensitive toward individuals and various cultural differences. Informs management on matters that one feels strongly about Key words: completes, demonstrates, differentiates, initiates, invites, joins, justifies, proposes, reports, selects, shares
Organization: Organizes values into priorities by contrasting different values, resolving conflicts between them, and creating a unique value system. The emphasis is on comparing, relating, and synthesizing values.	Able to recognize the need for balance between freedom and responsible behavior. Accepts professional ethical standards. Prioritizes time effectively to meet the needs of the organization, family, and self. Key words: adheres, alters, arranges, combines, compares, completes, defends, generalizes, identifies, integrates, modifies, organizes, relates, synthesizes
Internalizing values (characterization): Has a value system that controls their behavior. The behavior is pervasive, consistent, predictable, and most importantly, characteristic of the learner. Instructional objectives are concerned with the individual's general patterns of adjustment (personal, social, emotional).	Demonstrates self-reliance and can work independently, but also cooperates in group activities as a team player. Uses an objective approach in problem solving. Values people for what they are, not how they look. Key words: discriminates, displays, influences, listens, modifies, performs, proposes, qualifies, questions, revises, solves, verifies

TABLE 8E-4 Psychomotor domain.

Category	Examples and Key Words
Perception: The ability to use sensory cues to guide motor activity.	Able to detect nonverbal communication cues; can estimate where a moving ball will land and can move to the correct location to catch the ball. Key Words: chooses, detects, differentiates, distinguishes, identifies, isolates, relates, selects
Set: Readiness to act—includes mental, physical, and emotional sets.	Knows and acts upon a sequence of steps in a construction process. Is able to recognize own abilities and limitations. Key Words: initiates, displays, explains, proceeds, reacts, states, volunteers
Guided response: The early stages in learning a complex skill that includes imitation and trial and error.	Can perform an exercise as demonstrated; follows instructions well. Key Words: copies, traces, follows, reproduce
Mechanism: This is the intermediate stage in learning a complex skill.	Can use a personal computer effectively; able to perform simple DIY projects at home; can drive a car. Key Words: assembles, calibrates, constructs, dismantles, fixes, manipulates, measures, mends, organizes
Complex overt response: The skillful performance of motor acts that involve complex movement patterns in a quick, accurate, and highly coordinated manner and with a minimum expenditure of energy.	Can parallel park a car into a tight spot. Displays skill and competence while playing sports. Key Words: the same as for Mechanism, except that the performance is quicker, better, more accurate, etc.
Adaptation: Skills are well developed and the individual can modify movement patterns to fit special requirements.	Responds effectively to unexpected experiences; able to modify instructions to meet the needs of the learners. Key Words: adapts, alters, changes, rearranges, reorganizes, revises, varies
Origination: Can create new movement patterns to fit a particular situation or specific problem.	Able to independently develop a new and comprehensive training program or exercise protocol. Key Words: arranges, builds, combines, composes, constructs, creates, designs, initiates

the teaching or practice in a short period of time) versus spaced (distributing the teaching or practice over a longer period of time) practice, part versus whole task learning, and feedback/reinforcement schedules. Long-term retention of motor skills depends upon regular practice. Learning and retention of sensory-motor skills is improved by both the quantity and quality of feedback (knowledge of results) during training. Two ways in which learning/teaching of motor skills can be facilitated include:

- Slowing down the rate at which the information is presented
- Reducing the amount of information that needs to be processed

STUDY PEARL

Some form of guided learning seems most appropriate when high proficiency in a new skill is involved. On the other hand, if the task is to be recalled and transferred to a new situation, then some type of problem-solving strategy may be better.

There is evidence that mental rehearsal, especially involving imagery, facilitates performance. This may be because it allows additional memory processing related to physical tasks (eg, the formation of schema) or because it maintains arousal or motivation for an activity.

STUDY PEARL

Many forms of sensory-motor behavior are learned by imitation, especially complex movements such as dance, signing, crafts, or manual-therapy techniques.

LEARNING STYLES

There are several different theories regarding learning styles. However, it is not feasible to incorporate every learning theory into every session. One approach classifies learning styles as follows:[2]

- Accommodators. These learners look for the significance of the learning experience. These learners enjoy being active participants in their learning, and will ask many questions such as "What if?" and "Why not?"
- Divergers. These learners are motivated to discover the relevance of a given situation, and prefer to have information presented to them in a detailed, systematic, and reasoned manner.
- Assimilators. These learners are motivated to answer the question, "What is there to know?" They like accurate, organized delivery of information and they tend to respect the knowledge of the expert. These learners are perhaps less "instructor intensive" than some other learning styles. They will carefully follow

prescribed exercises, provided a resource person is clearly available and able to answer questions.
- Convergers. These learners are motivated to discover the relevancy or "how" of a situation. The instructions given to this type of learner should be interactive, not passive.

Another series of learning styles that are used frequently were devised by Taylor,[3] who proposed that there are three common learning styles:

- Visual. As the name suggests, the visual learner assimilates information by observation, using visual cues and information such as pictures, anatomical models, and physical demonstrations.
- Auditory. Auditory learners prefer to learn by having things explained to them verbally.
- Tactile. Tactile learners, who learn through touch and interaction, are the most difficult of the three groups to teach. Close supervision is required with this group until they have demonstrated to the clinician that they can perform the exercises correctly and independently. Proprioceptive neuromuscular facilitation (PNF) techniques, with the emphasis on physical and tactile cues, often work well with this group.

Analytical Learner

The analytical/objective learner processes information in a step-by-step order, perceives information in an objective manner, and is able to use facts and easily understand the relationships between them. This type of learner perceives information in an abstract, conceptual manner; information does not need to be related to personal experience. As this type of learner may have difficulty comprehending the big picture, a step-by-step learning process with some form of structure is recommended.

Intuitive/Global Learner

The intuitive/global learner processes information all at once, and not in an ordered sequence. Global learners are spontaneous and intuitive, and tend to learn in layers, absorbing material almost randomly without seeing connections, and then suddenly "getting it." The learning of this type reflects personal life experiences and is thus subjective. As this type of learner tries to relate the subject matter to things they already know, information needs to be presented in an interesting manner using attractive materials.

Reasoning: Inductive versus Deductive Reasoning

Inductive and deductive reasoning are two methods of logic used to arrive at a conclusion based on information assumed to be true. Both are used in research to establish hypotheses.

- Deductive reasoning: Involves a hierarchy of statements or truths and the arrival at a specific conclusion based on generalizations.
- Inductive reasoning: Essentially the opposite of deductive reasoning. It involves trying to create general principles by starting with many specific instances.
- Initiative: Active versus passive learning.

- Active/aggressive learner: Exhibits initiative, actively seeks information; may reach conclusions quickly before all information is gathered.
- Passive learner: Often exhibits little initiative; responds best to direct learning.

TEACHING STYLES

Bicknell-Holmes and Hoffman[4] describe a variety of teaching methods that correlate with most learning styles. These techniques involve active, or discovery, learning—the patient is able to actively participate in the learning process, which is in direct contrast with a teaching method such as lecturing, where the patient is a passive observer. Discovery learning has certain attributes:

- Emphasizes learning over content
- Uses failure as an opportunity to learn
- More is learned by doing than by watching
- Involves patients in higher levels of cognitive processing

Some of the methods of discovery learning include:

- Case-based learning: A fairly common active learning strategy in which the patient is able to participate in the decision-making or problem-solving process.
- Incidental learning: Learning is linked to game-like scenarios.
- Learning by exploring: A collection of questions and answers on a particular topic are organized into a system and patients can explore the various topics at their own pace.
- Learning by reflection: A type of active learning that involves higher level cognitive skills—patients are expected to model certain skills or concepts they have acquired through their instructor or through another system of learning.
- Simulation-based learning: The clinician creates an artificial environment in which patients can practice skills or apply concepts that they have learned, without the pressure of a real-world situation.
- Real-life examples: Using real-life problems and examples in a variety of scenarios (buying a house/car; using a bus schedule, etc).
- Relevant instruction: Instruction should be practical and the examples and exercises should be important and meaningful to the patients, because patients often need to know why they need to learn a particular skill or concept, or how it will be useful to them in their everyday lives.
- Humor: To help keep the patients engaged and interested and to make their sessions more enjoyable.

Improving Compliance with Learning and Participation

A number of factors have been outlined to improve compliance, including:

- Involving the patient in the intervention planning and goal setting
- Realistic goal setting for both short- and long-term goals
- Promoting high expectations regarding final outcome
- Promoting perceived benefits

- Projecting a positive attitude
- Providing clear instructions and demonstrations with appropriate feedback
- Keeping the exercises pain-free or with a low level of pain
- Encouraging patient problem solving

Community and Staff Education

The strengths and weaknesses of various teaching methods when presenting community education programs or when educating staff are outlined in Table 8E–5.

Using Visual Aids

A number of guidelines when using visual aids are outlined in Table 8E–6.

REFLECTION

Boyd and Fales[6] defined reflection as the process of examining an experience that raises an issue of concern. It is an internal process we use to help refine our understanding of an experience which may lead to changes in our perspectives. Literature suggests that expert clinicians routinely use the reflective process. In their study of expert clinicians, Jensen et al.[7] noted that the use of the reflective process was a key factor that set expert clinicians apart from their peers. Reflection is integral to clinical decision making.

Element	Definition
Reflection-in-action	Analyzing the effectiveness of one's own cues and handling as well as patient performance and behaviors; decisions are made and interventions may be modified
Reflection-on-action	Thinking about clinician-patient interaction and performance once the treatment session is over
Reflection-for-action	Thinking about one's own prior experiences that lead to ways of thinking about clinical decision-making and professional practice that is broader than one-on-one practice

CULTURAL INFLUENCES

It is important that clinicians are sensitive to cultural issues in their interactions with patients. Cultural influences shape the framework within which people view the world, define and organize reality, and function in their everyday life.

Individuals often group themselves on the basis of cultural similarities, and as a result, form cultural groups. Cultural groups share behavioral patterns, symbols, values, beliefs, and other characteristics that distinguish them from other groups.

At the group level, cultural differences are generally variations of differing emphasis or value placed on particular practices.

TABLE 8E–5 Teaching methods.

Teaching Method	Strengths	Weaknesses	Preparation
Lecture	Presents factual material in a direct, logical manner Contains experience which inspires Useful for large groups	Experts are not always good teachers Audience is passive Learning is difficult to gauge Communication is one-way	Needs clear introduction and summary Needs time and content limit to be effective Should include examples, anecdotes
Lecture with discussion	Involves audience, at least after the lecture Audience can question, clarify, and challenge	Time may limit discussion period Quality is limited to quality of questions and discussion	Requires that questions be prepared prior to discussion
Panel of experts	Allows experts to present different opinions Can provoke better discussion than a one-person discussion Frequent change of speakers keeps attention from lagging	Experts may not be good speakers Personalities may overshadow content Subject may not be in logical order	Facilitator coordinates focus of panel; introduces and summarizes Briefs panel
Brainstorming	Listening exercise that allows creative thinking for new ideas Encourages full participation because all ideas equally recorded Draws on group's knowledge and experience Spirit of congeniality is created One idea can spark off other ideas	Can be unfocused Needs to be limited to 5–7 minutes People may have difficulty getting away from known reality If not facilitated well, criticism and evaluation may occur	Facilitator selects issue Must have some ideas if group needs to be stimulated
Videotapes/slides	Entertaining way of teaching content (colorful) and raising issues Keeps group's attention Looks professional Stimulates discussion Demonstrates three-dimensional movement	Can raise too many issues to have a focused discussion Discussion may not have full participation Only as effective as following discussion Can be expensive	Need to set up equipment Effective only if facilitator prepares questions to discuss after the show
Discussion	Pools ideas and experiences from group Effective after a presentation, film, or experience that needs to be analyzed Allows everyone to participate in an active process	Not practical with more than 20 people Few people can dominate Others may not participate Is time consuming Can get off the track	Requires careful planning by facilitator to guide discussion Requires question outline
Small group discussion	Allows participation of everyone People often more comfortable in small groups Can reach group consensus	Needs careful thought as to purpose of group Groups may get sidetracked	Need to prepare specific tasks or questions for group to answer
Role-playing	Introduces problem situation dramatically Provides opportunity for people to assume roles of others and thus appreciate another point of view Allows for exploration of solutions Provides opportunity to practice skills	People may be too self-conscious Not appropriate for large groups People may feel threatened	Trainer has to define problem situation and roles clearly Trainer must give very clear instructions
Case studies	Develops analytic and problem-solving skills Allows for exploration of solutions for complex issues Allows patient to apply new knowledge and skills	People may not see relevance to own situation Insufficient information can lead to inappropriate results	Case must be clearly defined Case study must be prepared
Guest speaker	Personalizes topic Breaks down audience's stereotypes	May not be a good speaker	Contact speakers and coordinate Introduce speaker appropriately

TABLE 8E–6 Guidelines for the use of visual aids.

Overheads	Flip Charts	Slides
Use the most professional lettering available. Use transparencies of one color only and secure transparencies to cardboard frames (if available). Number each transparency. Prior to the session, check overheads for readability of type size by audience at far end of room. Printing should be no smaller than 1/4″ high. Information should be placed on the top two-thirds of the transparency. Be familiar with the operation of the projector and make sure projector works. Have extra bulbs available. While presenting, be certain neither you nor the projector blocks anyone's view. Use a pencil rather than a finger to note a detail on the transparency. If you have a list of points, black out all but the first point, then move the cover sheet one point at a time.	Choose a chart size that is appropriate for the design, your height, and the size of the audience. Draw the art to fit the vertical shape of the chart. Make the lettering dark enough and large enough to be read by everyone in the audience. During preparation, leave several blank pages between each written page to allow for corrections and additions. For the final presentation, remove all but one blank page at the beginning so that you can turn to that blank page when there is no relevant visual. Securely attach the chart to the easel and adjust the easel height for the presentation. When writing on the flip chart, don't speak to the chart.	Slides should be used instead of flip charts if the group is large. Design the visuals for continuous viewing and as notes. Maintain continuity—have all slides horizontal or vertical, not mixed. Allow sufficient production time. Place no more than 15 words per slide. Use black or blue background with bright colors. Check the position and order of the slide in the carousel or tray. Use a conventional pointer. Keep as many lights on as possible.

REFERENCES

1. Bloom BS. *Taxonomy of Educational Objectives, Handbook I: The Cognitive Domain*. New York, NY: David McKay Publications; 1956.

2. Litzinger ME, Osif B. Accommodating diverse learning styles: designing instruction for electronic information sources. In: Shirato L, ed. *What is Good Instruction Now? Library Instruction for the 90s*. Ann Arbor, MI: Pierian Press; 1993.

3. Taylor JA. A practical tool for improved communications. *Supervision*. 1999;59:18-19.

4. Bicknell-Holmes T, Hoffman PS. Elicit, engage, experience, explore: discovery learning in library instruction. *Reference Services Review*. Emerald, Simmons College Library. 2000: 313-322.

5. Plack M, Driscoll M. *Teaching and Learning in Physical Therapy: From Classroom to Clinic*. Thorofare, NJ: Slack Incorporated. 2017.

6. Boyd E, Fales A. Reflective learning: key to learning from experience. *J Hum Psychol*. 1893:23:99-117.

7. Jensen GM, Gywer J, Hack LM, Shepard KF. *Expertise in Physical Therapy*. Boston, MA: Butterworth-Heinemann; 1999.

QUESTIONS

1. Which of the following steps would be considered the first step in developing a mutually agreeable plan of care that optimizes patient adherence?
   A. Assess readiness
   B. Develop a plan of care
   C. Provide intervention and education
   D. Develop shared meaning through dialogue

2. While treating a patient, the physical therapist realizes that he/she needs to adjust his/her handling technique to enhance patient response. In which type of reflection would this be considered?
   A. Premise reflection
   B. Reflection-in-action
   C. Reflection-on-action
   D. Reflection-for-action

3. A patient who is in the Developing Competency Stage on the Novice to Expert Continuum will require which of the following levels of guidance?
   A. Details and close supervision
   B. Guidance through practice and feedback
   C. Methods to integrate activity into their everyday life.
   D. Challenge to adapt activity to novel and complex situations

ANSWERS

1. The answer is **C**. Plack and Driscoll (p 221)[5] provide a table listing the steps for developing a care plan that promotes patient adherence. The steps to this plan are:

   - Step 1 Develop a shared meaning through dialogue
   - Step 2 Develop a plan of care
   - Step 3 Assess readiness
   - Step 4 Provide intervention and education
   - Step 5 Check for understanding
   - Step 6 Check for adherence and optimize motivation
   - Step 7 Reinforce adherence

2. The answer is **B**. (Plack and Driscoll, pp 37-41).[5]
  A. Premise reflection occurs when the individual recognizes and begins to explore or critique his or her own assumptions, values, beliefs, and biases.
  B. Reflection-in-action involves analyzing the effectiveness of one's own cues, handling skills and patient performance and behaviors; decisions are made and interventions may be modified.
  C. Reflection-on-action is thinking about clinician-patient interaction and performance once the treatment session is over. Plan of care can be modified based on the assessment made.
  D. Reflection-for-action is thinking about prior experiences that have similarities to the current patient you are about to treat and devising a treatment based on those experiences.

3. The answer is **B**. (Plack and Driscoll, p 138).[5]
  A. Details and close supervision are required for teaching patients in the novice stage.
  B. Guidance through practice and feedback are characteristics required by patients in the developing competency stage.
  C. and **D.** Methods to integrate activity into everyday life and challenge to adapt activity to novel and complex situations are strategies employed for patients in the expert stage of the continuum.

CHECKLIST

When you complete this section, you should be able to:

❑ Compare and contrast various learning theories.

❑ Apply Maslow's Hierarchy of Needs to patient performance.

❑ Use Bloom's Taxonomy to construct patient goals appropriate for their level of performance.

❑ Apply the concept of learning styles to improve patient education.

❑ Design appropriate visual aids for a given audience.

❑ Apply reflective elements to clinical practice.

9

Special Topics: Geriatrics

Chris Childers and Jim Mathews

■ CLINICAL APPLICATION OF FOUNDATIONAL SCIENCES

In 2011, the Federation of State Boards of Physical Therapy (FSBPT) issued a conservative estimate that older adults (ages 65–85) accounted for 40% of all physical therapy services and contributed to both the large growth in the profession[1,2] and the projected future shortages of physical therapists (Figure 9–1). In addition, the **old-old** were, and continue to be, the fastest growing **component age group** in the United States.[3]

Caring for this aging tsunami[3] requires the entry-level physical therapist to: (1) differentiate normal expected changes from unexpected changes, (2) care-plan and create interventions across the patient-client life spectrum while collaborating with families and interprofessional teams, (3) provide caregiver, family, and patient-client support and training, and (4) advocate for both health promotion and safety.[4] Chronic conditions such as heart disease,

High-Yield Terms to Learn

Ageism	Age discrimination; occurs when bias is the primary motivation behind acts against a person or group.
Agnosia	Failure to recognize or identify objects despite intact sensory function.
Apraxia	Impaired ability of previously learned motor activities yet intact motor function.
Component age groups	Chronological age is defined as age in years, and is therefore easily determined. For convenience and simplicity, the following terms are used for the component age groups: • Middle-age: 45 to 64 years • Young-old: 65 to 74 years • Old: 75 to 84 years • Old-old: 85 to 99 years • Oldest-old: 100+ years
Concreteness	Recognizing concrete concepts but not abstract concepts or words.
Dementia-related memory loss	Initially short-term with progression to include long-term memory.
Durable power of attorney for health care	"Durable power" allows a patient to name a "patient advocate" to act on behalf of the patient and carry out his or her wishes.
Geriatrics	The branch of medicine that focuses on health promotion and the prevention and treatment of disease and disability in later life.
Gerontology	The study of the aging process and the science related to the care of the elderly.
Life expectancy	Life expectancy, the number of years an individual can expect to live, is based on average life spans. Men generally have lower life expectancy rates than women at every age.
Life span	Maximum life span: the greatest age attainable by any member of a species. Average life span: the average age reached by members of a population. This figure has shown changes over time, largely due to medical advances. The average life span was 47 years in 1900 and 75 years in 1990. As of the year 2017, in the United States the life expectancy for females was 81 years. For males the comparable figure was 77.

High-Yield Terms to Learn (*continued*)

Living will	A living will allows a patient to state his or her wishes in writing but does not name a patient advocate.
Morbidity	Morbidity (from Latin *morbidus*: sick, unhealthy) refers to the number of people who have a disease (prevalence) as compared to the total number of people in a population at a particular point in time. The term morbidity can also refer to: • The state of being diseased • The degree or severity of a disease • The incidence of a disease (the number of new cases in a particular population during a particular time interval)
Mortality	Mortality refers to the number of deaths (from a disease or in general) per 1000 people and is typically reported on an annual basis. Reductions in mortality have resulted in impressive increases in life expectancy that have contributed to the growth of the older population, especially at the oldest ages.
Visuospatial impairment	Diminished ability to identify stimuli and their locations.

stroke, diabetes, and arthritis are projected to continue to grow (Figure 9–2) in aging adults, requiring the competent skilled services of the physical therapist to reduce **morbidity** and **mortality**.

EXAMINATION

During the initial assessment, the physical therapist must differentiate the effects of aging, inactivity, and disease from the underlying impairments and functional limitations that result in movement dysfunctions. The following sections look at expected and unexpected changes that occur with aging to better understand how to differentiate between them, and ultimately to provide individualized care.

Muscular Changes

Expected

• Reduction in type II muscle number and size.[5]
   • Accounts for age-related differences in muscle mass (33% loss by age 70).

• Caused by many factors (immune/hormone/vascular/neurological changes with aging).
• Exercise training can increase muscle size via hypertrophy of remaining type II fibers.
• Exercise not likely to stimulate increased number of type II fibers.
• Differs from disuse atrophy, which affects both fiber types.[6]
• No difference in gender as to the onset age and magnitude of muscle function loss.[7]
• Decreased peak anaerobic muscle power.
• Decreased muscular strength.
• Decreased speed of movement.
• Decreased flexibility
   • Shoulder and hip flexibility decline significantly after age 70.[8]
   • Losses in flexibility should not impact daily function or lead to disability.
   • Levels of physical activity do not seem to prevent normal aging changes.[8]

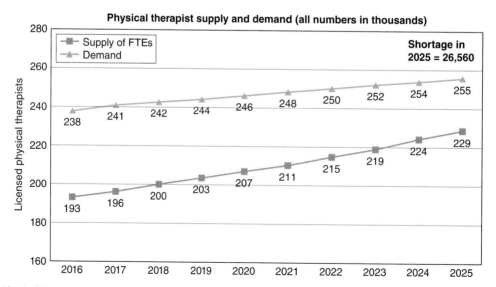

FIGURE 9–1 Physical therapist supply and demand. 2016 Projections using attrition rate of 3.5%. FTE, full-time employees. (Used with permission from http://www.apta.org/WorkforceData/ModelDescriptionFigures/.)

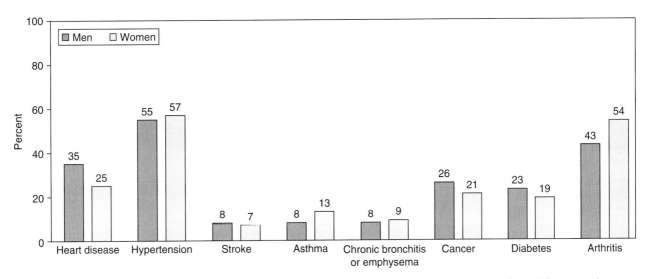

FIGURE 9–2 Chronic health conditions. (From Centers for Disease Control and Prevention. National Center for Health Statistics.)

- Fatigue at cellular level
  - Less peripheral blood circulation = decreased oxygen to muscles.[9]
  - Thicker collagen causes less muscle elasticity.[10]
  - Reduced ATPase and proteins.[11]
  - Mitochondria decreased and/or dysfunctional = decline in oxidative capacity.[12]

Unexpected
- Sarcopenia
  - Greater reduction in type II number and size.
  - Loss of muscle function; ie, strength and power.[13]
  - Occurs in 33% of community-dwelling older adults.[13]
  - Responds well to resistance exercise training for ≥3 months.[13]
  - Major contributor to debility, disease, and death.[13]
- Muscular contractures
  - Loss of range of motion of a joint that impacts function or leads to disability.[14]
  - This type of loss is related to shortened muscle or tendon versus joint deformity.
  - Prevalent in immobile patients.[14]
- Disuse atrophy
  - Loss of type I and type II fibers from inactivity or being bed-bound.

KEY CONCEPT

Early mobility is imperative, as are both aerobic and resistance exercises, to counteract both the expected and unexpected changes that can occur with aging. Yoga, tai chi, water aerobics, swimming, and traditional resistance programs are beneficial.

Collagenous and Cardiopulmonary Changes

Expected
- Loss of water from the cellular matrix.[15]
  - Shrinkage of articular cartilage (eg, intervertebral discs).
  - Decreased shock absorption (caution with plyometric exercises).
  - Reduction in joint range of motion.
- Increased number of collagen crosslinks.[16]
  - "Stiffer" tissues, greater passive tension within tissues.
  - More effort required to move.
  - Loss of end range of motion.
  - Greater heart muscular effort for less cardiac output (see cardiovascular below).
- Loss of elastic fibers.[16]
  - Sagging skin.
  - Sagging organs, constipation, prolapse.
  - Less pliability in ligaments and tendons.
- Cardiovascular
  - Decreased maximal aerobic capacity.
  - Decreased heart rate (HR), decreased peak HR.
  - Decreased maximal cardiac output, stroke volume, and maximal O_2 consumption.
  - Decreased maximal skeletal muscle blood flow.
  - Decreased capillary density.
  - Increased HR and blood pressure (BP) responses to exercise.
  - Increased thickening of left ventricle and heart valves.
- Pulmonary
  - Decreased vital capacity.
  - Decreased elasticity of lungs.
  - Decreased vital capacity and tidal volumes.
  - Increased stiffness of chest wall.
  - Increased respiratory rate.

Unexpected

- Arterial ruptures: plaque buildup can cause less pliable arteries to rupture.[17]
- Hernias: inguinal and abdominal hernias may contribute to urinary tract infection (UTI); limit lifting.[18]
- Gastroesophageal reflux disease (GERD).
- Heart attack (myocardial infarction [MI]).
- Congstive heart failure (CHF).
- Chronic obstructive pulmonary disease (COPD).
- Hypertension (HTN).
- Venous insufficiency.
- Intermittent claudication.
- Organ transplants.
- Respiratory failure (RF).
- Emphysema/bronchitis.
- Asthma.
- Pneumonia.
- Arrhythmias/pacemakers/bypasses/stents/ablations/valve replacements.

KEY CONCEPT

Conditions such as pneumonia, COPD, and CHF have high **mortality** rates, while caring for **morbidities** of survivors is done at a high financial cost to the individual and society. Physical therapists play a key role in prevention and optimal management of such diseases.

Endocrine, Metabolic, Integumentary, and Exocrine Changes

Expected

- Proportion of body composition from fat increases, versus muscle, which decreases.
  - Increase from 15% fat of 20 year old to nearly 30% for 70 year old.
  - May obtain nearly 50% in 80-year-old females.
  - Majority of fat increase is peritoneal fat.
  - Increased risk for diabetes, cancer, metabolic syndromes, and heart disease.
  - Increased epicardia fat.
- Decreased metabolism.
  - Decreased total body water.
  - Decreased appetite.
  - Decreased protein synthesis rate.
- Reduced epithelial cell turnover rate.
  - Bruise more easily.
  - Thinner skin with skin tears.
  - Dry mouth, eyes, throat, and skin.

Unexpected

- Malnutrition.
- Diabetes/hyper- and hypoglycemia.

- Dehydration.
- Vitamin D deficiency.
- Nonhealing wounds.
- Amputations.
- Obesity.

Skeletal and Articular Changes

Expected

- Osteopenia: Loss of bone volume and lower bone mineral density (BMD).
- Females lose about 30% of bone mass by age of 70; males lose about 15% by age of 70.
- Decreased tensile strength of bone.
- Reduced thickness and resilience of articular cartilage—decreased joint space.
- Degeneration of joints is not uncommon with aging (90%), most with abnormal images.
- Altered arthrokinematics and force transmissions.
- Reduced height.
- Joint flexibility reduced by 25% to 30% over the age of 70.

Unexpected

- Fractures.
- Kyphosis.
- Osteoporosis (affects more than 30% of women over the age of 65).
- Spinal stenosis with paresis and loss of lordosis.
- Osteoarthritis.
- Abnormal postures.
- Loss of functional range of motion.
- Low back pain.
- Joint replacements.

KEY CONCEPT

Osteoporosis, osteoarthritis, and hip fractures can severely impact function.

Neurological Changes

Expected

- Loss of neurons, neuronal myelin, and axons (Table 9–1).
- Reduced motor reaction time/reduced strength (ventral horn and BA 4,6 neurons).
- Reduced autonomic responses (sympathetic and parasympathetic)
- Reduced somatic sensations (dorsal horn neurons and BA 3,1,2).
- Reduced primary sensations (tastes, sight, smell, hearing—reduced cranial nerves).
- Reduced coordination (shrinking of cerebellum, reduced vestibular nerve).

TABLE 9–1 Expected neural changes.

Neuronal Change w/Aging	Declines
Grey matter—declining number of neurons	**Cognitive:** Memory, attention, perception, learning, problem solving, planning, awareness, thought, language, consciousness, body scheme **Sensory:** All sensations **Motor:** Coordination, motor plan, skill acquisition, and movement timing
White matter—declining myelin on remaining neurons	Slow reaction time (motor); slower sensation sense (sensory)

Adapted from Nichols-Larsen DS et al. *Neurologic Rehabilitation: Neuroscience and Neuroplasticity in Physical Therapy Practice.* New York, NY: McGraw Hill Professional; 2015:Table 17–1.

- Reduced reaction time and memory (shrinking brain).
- Reduced perception of temperature, abnormal pain sensitization (anterolateral system [ALS] and brain).
- Reduced neuroplasticity.
- Dopamine level depletion.
- Decrease in nerve conduction velocity by about 0.4% a year after age 70.
- Decreasing reflexes 70 to 80 years old: ankle jerk is absent (70%).
- Increased postural sway (less in women than in men with linear increase with age).
- Changes in sleep patterns.

Unexpected

- Multiple sclerosis (MS).
- Stroke (cerebrovascular accident [CVA]); for each successive decade after age 55, the stroke rate more than double in both men and women.[19]

TABLE 9–2 Alzheimer's disease - Progression.

Stage of Alzheimer's Disease	Deficits
Early stage	Problems in retaining new information, forgetfulness, social withdrawal, may stop participating in activities and hobbies they formerly loved. Moody, time-disoriented, and exhibiting poor judgment.
Intermediate stage	Behavioral and personality changes, **apraxia, agnosia, concreteness of thought, memory loss, visual-spatial deficits**, pronounced and psychotic symptoms. Exhibits changes in gait with confusion of day/night. Late in this stage there may be excessive wandering and weight loss problems—patient may forget how and when to eat. Care is required at this stage.
Late stage	Loss of many functional abilities; ie, motor function no longer preserved. Declines in walking, continence, and basic mobility. High risk for contractures, decubitus ulcers, anorexia, and injuries.

TABLE 9–3 Differentiating dementia, delirium, and depression.

Factor	Dementia	Delirium	Depression
Onset	Insidious (unknown)	Acute	Acute
Conscious state	Impaired	Highly variable	Unusual
Mood	Stable	Highly variable	Depressed with daily variations
Duration	Long term and progressive	Short term (days; eg, post-operative state)	Short—weeks
Features	↓ Short > long-term memory loss	Short attention span	Short-term memory loss
Sleep/wake	Get day/night mixed up	Highly variable	Sleep too long, or not sleeping (insomnia)

Adapted from Nichols-Larsen DS et al. *Neurologic Rehabilitation: Neuroscience and Neuroplasticity in Physical Therapy Practice.* New York, NY: McGraw Hill Professional; 2015:Table 17–4.

- Insomnia.
- Hydrocephalus.
- Hematomas.
- Tremors.
- Seizures.
- Parkinson's disease (PD).
- Alzheimer's disease (AD) (Table 9–2).
- Dementia/delirium/depression (Table 9–3).

KEY CONCEPT

Expected neurological changes with aging requires that the physical therapist assess for changes in cognition, and sensory and motor function as well as develop individualized plans of care in a respectful, clear manner. Unexpected changes may require longer durations of care, care-giver training, behavioral management, and adaptive and maintenance-type care.

Immune/Lymphatic Changes

Expected

- More easily develop an inflammatory response.
- Bacteria can escape from lymphatic vessels.

Unexpected

- Cancer (a type of hyperplastic pathology).
- Diabetes.
- Chronic infection/inflammation.[20]

Seventy percent of all cancer-related deaths occur in people over 65, making identification and collaboration with a healthcare team imperative for early treatment.[21]

Renal/Urogenital Changes

Expected
- Declining renal function with age-related to loss of nephron.
- Reduced filtration rate of kidneys.
- Loss of thirst.
- Menopause in women 45 to 65 years old with loss of estrogen.
- Menopause often comes with hot flashes, anxiety, and depression.
- Men gradually lose testosterone; however, not sperm production.
- Weakening of pelvic floor muscles.

Unexpected
- End-stage renal disease (ESRD).
- Hemodialysis.
- Peritoneal dialysis.
- Catheters (indwelling, Foley).
- Urinary incontinence, any form, more prevalent stress incontinence in women.
- Urinary retention and prostate cancer (males).

KEY CONCEPT

Dehydration and incontinence are not expected, but their prevalence in both males and females remains high. Having the ability to address these issues with geriatric clients and having access to water and restrooms are all essential in the delivery of geriatric physical therapy care.

■ FOUNDATIONS OF EVALUATION, DIFFERENTIAL DIAGNOSIS, PROGNOSIS, AND INTERVENTIONS

BEHAVIORAL MANAGEMENT TECHNIQUES—INDICATED WITH COGNITIVE DECLINES OR PSYCHIATRIC DECLINES

- Stay calm and exemplify calm behavior.
- Reassure and acknowledge their feelings.
- Listen to what they are saying and maintain eye contact.
- Simplify your instructions and if possible the environment.

- Try distraction.
- Explain what you are about to do; allow for processing time.
- Reorient without arguing or demanding that they understand.
- Slow down; with severe dementia allow up to 1 minute for response.
- Avoid change in caregivers and the environment in which they live.
- Encourage familiarity with consistent caregivers.
- Use touch to connect with the person but do not use it to restrain or control them.
- Educate and support family.

KNOW THE ABSOLUTE CONTRAINDICATIONS TO EXERCISES

- Severe coronary artery disease with unstable angina pectoris.
- Acute MI (<2 days after infarction).
- Severe valvular heart disease.
- Rapid or prolonged atrial or ventricular arrhythmias/tachycardias.
- Uncontrolled HTN.
- Profound orthostatic hypotension.
- Acute thrombophlebitis.
- Acute pulmonary embolism (<2 days after event).
- Avoid ageism, for example, elderly should not be exercised or achieve goals.

FALL MANAGEMENT AND PREVENTION

- Common causes of falls[22]
  - Accidents and environmental hazards
  - Gait disturbance, balance disorders or weakness, pain related to arthritis
  - Vertigo (central and/or peripheral causes)
  - Medications and substance abuse
  - Cognitive impairments
  - Postural (orthostatic) hypotension
  - Visual disorder
  - Loss of range of motion and/or strength in ankles
  - Central nervous system disorder
  - Syncope
  - Epilepsy
- Assess root cause of falls (Figure 9–3)
- Design interventions that address the causes (Table 9–4)
- Care-plan across the **life-spectrum** and differentiate expected effects of aging to unexpected[23]

KEY CONCEPT

Falls are the leading cause of fatalities in seniors, and remain the leading cause for injuries at great costs to the patient and society. Gait changes are often an early manifestation of pathology.

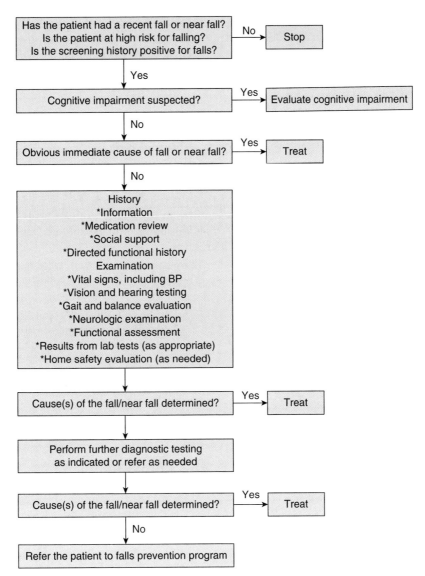

FIGURE 9–3 An algorithm for the evaluation of falls. (From Dutton M. *McGraw-Hill's NPTE (National Physical Therapy Examination)*. 2nd ed. New York, NY: McGraw-Hill; 2012:Figure 14–1.)

TABLE 9–4 Fall risk interventions.

Risk Factors	Interventions
Postural (orthostatic) hypotension SBP drops >20 mmHg OR DBP <90 mmHg in standing	Ankle pumps/elevate head of bed Recommend decrease in dosage of hypertension meds, or medications to increase blood pressure Pressure stockings
On four or more medications	Have MD review if all are still needed
Environmental hazards	Home safety assessment; make adaptations as needed, remove obstacles like throw rugs, improve lighting, etc.
Gait impairments	Gait training, assistive devices, and therapeutic exercises
Balance and/or transfer losses	Balance exercises, therapeutic activities, environmental alterations, and neuromuscular re-education
Impairments in range of motion or strength	Therapeutic exercises

SBP, systolic blood pressure; DBP, diastolic blood pressure.

Data from Tinetti ME, Baker DI, McAvay G, et al. A multifactorial intervention to reduce the risk of falling among elderly people living in the community. *N Engl J Med*. 1994;331 (13):821-827.

Due to the systemic, cellular, and biomechanical changes that occur with normal aging it is not surprising that most older adults having **at least one chronic condition**. Optimal aging should be considered in the care of aging adults to prevent loss of function and becoming frail.

COLLABORATE INTERPROFESSIONALLY

- Referral and consultations based on needs from the biopsychosocial model.[24]
- Nutritional assessment of a patient's nutritional status with dietician or nutritionist.
- Communication with social worker for elderly food programs (eg, Meals on Wheels).
- Recommendations for occupational therapy assess meal preparation and activities of daily living.
- Aspiration, coughing with eating, and fever ideal for swallow assessment by Speech Language Pathologist (SLP).
- Advanced directives generally need involvement of teams when:
  - Terminal illness is expected in a relatively short time.
  - Permanent disability in an intolerable situation is expected.

Provide Caregiver/Family Support and Training

- Consult **durable power of attorney for health care.**
- Consult with someone familiar with **Living Will** to ensure that the care of a physical therapist is indicated in the Living Will.
- Seek to modify restraints (environmental and chemical).
- Involve the family as needed.
- Provide follow-up and track performance.
- Educate caregivers, friends, and family on HEP.

Evidenced-based exercise programs such as the Otago Exercise Program require considerable training and tracking to be done effectively, which may require investment and authorization for multiple family visits.[23]

Advocate for Health Promotion and Safety

- Advocacy is important due to pervasive **ageism**.
- Culturally, **ageism** can come in subtle forms, such as slurs and lack of inclusion.

- Need to advocate and educate on exercise safety.
- Appropriate and safe use of assistive devices.
- Home/living environment.
- Chronic conditions are higher in lower income populations: inner city and rural.
- Life expectancy and lifespan are significantly lower for African Americans.
- Environment, education, nutrition, and access to healthcare services are barriers.
- Help prevent social isolation.
- Provide empowerment.
- Involve patient in decision-making.
- Be the patient's advocate for needed services.
- Provide opportunities for socialization and encouragement.

Across an individual's lifespan, changes that occur may require differing adaptations, increased caregiver support, professional consultations, modifications, and new adaptive equipment like wheelchairs. Advocating for such things takes time to do but is invaluable to the patient to reach their maximum quality of life and safety.

REFERENCES

1. Bradley KM, Caramagno J, Waters S, Koch A; Federation of State Boards of Physical Therapy. Analysis of practice for the physical therapy profession: entry-level physical therapists. Available at https://www.fsbpt.org/Portals/0/documents/free-resources/PA2011_PTFinalReport 20111109.pdf. Published November 9, 2011.
2. World Confederation for Physical Therapy. Resources and information: older people. Available at: http://www.wcpt.org/node/47941. Accessed March 1, 2018.
3. Avers D. Infusing an optimal aging paradigm into an entry-level geriatrics course. *J Phys Ther Educ*. 2014;28(2):22.
4. Wong R, Avers D, Barr J, Ciolek C, Klima D, Thompson M. Essential competencies in the care of older adults at the completion of the entry-level physical therapist professional program of study. Available at https://geriatricspt.org/pdfs/AGPT-PT-Essential-Competencies.pdf. Accessed March 1, 2018.
5. Nilwik R, Snijders T, Leenders M, et al. The decline in skeletal muscle mass with aging is mainly attributed to a reduction in type II muscle fiber size. *Exp Gerontol*. 2013;48(5):492-498.
6. Demontis F, Piccirillo R, Goldberg AL, Perrimon N. Mechanisms of skeletal muscle aging: insights from Drosophila and mammalian models. *Dis Model Mech*. 2013;6(6):1339-1352.
7. Daly RM, Rosengren BE, Alwis G, Ahlborg HG, Sernbo I, Karlsson MK. Gender specific age-related changes in bone density, muscle strength and functional performance in the elderly: a-10 year prospective population-based study. *BMC Geriatr*. 2013;13(1):71.

8. Stathokostas L, McDonald MW, Little R, Paterson DH. Flexibility of older adults aged 55-86 years and the influence of physical activity. *J Aging Res.* 2013;2013:743843.

9. Heinonen I, Koga S, Kalliokoski KK, Musch TI, Poole DC. Heterogeneity of muscle blood flow and metabolism: influence of exercise, aging and disease states. *Exerc Sport Sci Rev.* 2015;43(3):117.

10. Wilson SL, Guilbert M, Sulé-Suso J, et al. 2014. A microscopic and macroscopic study of aging collagen on its molecular structure, mechanical properties, and cellular response. *FASEB J.* 2014;28(1):14-25.

11. de Lores Arnaiz GR, Ordieres MGL. Brain Na+, K+-ATPase activity in aging and disease. *Int J Biomed Sci.* 2014;10(2):85.

12. Kalyani RR, Corriere M, Ferrucci L. Age-related and disease-related muscle loss: the effect of diabetes, obesity, and other diseases. *Lancet Diabetes Endocrinol.* 2014;2(10):819-829.

13. Cruz-Jentoft AJ, Landi F, Schneider SM, et al. Prevalence of and interventions for sarcopenia in ageing adults: a systematic review. Report of the International Sarcopenia Initiative (EWGSOP and IWGS). *Age Ageing.* 2014;43(6):748-759.

14. Offenbächer M, Sauer S, Rieb J, et al. Contractures with special reference in elderly: definition and risk factors – a systematic review with practical implications. *Disabil Rehabil.* 2014;36(7):529-538.

15. Guccione AA, Avers D, Wong R. *Geriatric Physical Therapy.* eBook. Elsevier Health Sciences; 2011.

16. Guilbert M, Roig B, Terryn C, et al. Highlighting the impact of aging on type I collagen: label-free investigation using confocal reflectance microscopy and diffuse reflectance spectroscopy in 3D matrix model. *Oncotarget.* 2016;7(8):8546.

17. Plenz GA, Deng MC, Robenek H, Völker W. Vascular collagens: spotlight on the role of type VIII collagen in atherogenesis. *Atherosclerosis.* 2003;166(1):1-11.

18. Mandal PP, Komut O, Mondal A, Banerjee M, Nizami NE, Tamang R. Study of the relationship between presence of bilateral inguinal hernia and intensity of lower urinary tract symptoms in a tertiary care centre of Eastern India. *J Contemp Med Surg Radiol.* 2017;2(3):89-93.

19. Michael KM, Shaughnessy M. Stroke prevention and management in older adults. *J Cardiovasc Nurs.* 2006;21(5):S21-S26.

20. Campisi J. Aging, cellular senescence, and cancer. *Annu Rev Physiol.* 2013;75:685-705.

21. Berger NA, Savvides P, Koroukian SM, et al. Cancer in the elderly. *Trans Am Clin Climatol Assoc.* 2006;117:147-55.

22. National Council on Aging. Falls prevention facts. Available at: https://www.ncoa.org/news/resources-for-reporters/get-the-facts/falls-prevention-facts/. Accessed on March 4, 2018.

23. Shubert TE, Smith ML, Ory MG, et al. Translation of the Otago Exercise Program for adoption and implementation in the United States. *Front Public Health.* 2015;3:152.

24. American Physical Therapy Association (APTA). Guide to Physical Therapist Practice 3.0. ISBN: 978-1-931369-85-5. doi: 10.2522/ptguide3.0_978-1-931369-85-5.

QUESTIONS

1. Which of the following muscular changes is considered a normal reaction to aging?
   A. Reduced type II muscle number and size
   B. Reduced type I muscle number and size
   C. Increased type II muscle number and size
   D. Increased type I muscle number and size

2. Which of the following locations are most likely to decrease in flexibility as a normal response to aging?
   A. Shoulder and elbow
   B. Shoulder and hip
   C. Hip and ankle
   D. Knee and elbow

3. Which of the following conditions is most likely to cause fatigue at cellular level in the aging adult?
   A. Increased peripheral blood circulation
   B. Decreased collagen levels
   C. Increased ATPase and proteins
   D. Decreased or dysfunctional mitochondria

4. Sagging skin and organs potentially leading to prolapse are a result of which of the following collagenous changes?
   A. Loss of water from the cellular matrix
   B. Increased collagen crosslinks
   C. Loss of elastic fibers
   D. Decreased collagen crosslinks

5. Which of the following changes is most likely to occur in the aging adult?
   A. Increased epicardial fat
   B. Increased total body water
   C. Increased appetite
   D. Increased protein synthesis

6. A physical therapist is working with a patient with known Alzheimer's disease. The patient has obvious visual-spatial deficits and some gait abnormalities. Which stage of the disease is most likely being demonstrated by this patient?
   A. Early stage
   B. Intermediate stage
   C. Late stage
   D. Unable to stage

7. Which of the following deficits will be most noticed with a loss of white matter in the brain as a result of normal aging?
   A. Changes in problem solving
   B. Increased sensory awareness
   C. Variations in skill acquisition
   D. Slower reaction times

8. Which of the following group of symptoms will be seen in a patient experiencing delirium?
   A. Impaired consciousness, excessive sleep, depressed mood
   B. Highly variable consciousness, short attention span, variable sleep patterns
   C. Impaired consciousness, highly variable mood, insomnia
   D. Highly variable consciousness, insomnia, short attention span

9. A patient complains of experiencing incontinent episodes because she is unable to get to the bathroom quickly enough and her arthritis limits her ability to quickly adjust her clothing. Which type of incontinence is this patient most likely experiencing?
   A. Stress
   B. Urge
   C. Functional
   D. Mixed

10. Which of the following interventions would be the most appropriate for a client with age-related osteoporosis of the thoracic spine?
   A. Trunk flexion exercises
   B. Trunk extension exercises
   C. High-intensity interval training
   D. No intervention is appropriate

ANSWERS

1. The answer is **A**. Normal aging expects a reduction in type II muscle number and size. Size can be increased with training with a hypertrophy reaction, but numbers are unlikely to improve with exercise or activity.

2. The answer is **B**. These areas generally lose significant flexibility with aging but do not normally reduce functional levels.

3. The answer is **D**. There is decreased, not increased peripheral blood circulation, there is increased collagen, which makes the muscle less elastic, and there is decreased ATPase and protein.

4. The answer is **C**. Loss of elastic fibers causes sagging skin and organs and decreased pliability in tendons and ligaments. Crosslinks increase with aging and cause stiffer tissue and water decreases causing decreased shock absorption and range of motion.

5. The answer is **A**. All other issues listed are typically decreased in the older adult population.

6. The answer is **B**. Visual spatial deficits and gait abnormalities decline in the intermediate stage. During the late stages of Alzheimer's there is significant loss of motor function and the patient is unlikely to be ambulatory.

7. The answer is **D**. The key to loss of white matter is the loss of myelin, which therefore slows down the neural pathways. There are changes in problem solving and skill acquisition related to loss of grey matter, and sensory changes will be slowed, not increased.

8. The answer is **B**. This list includes all aspects of delirium where the client presents with highly variable levels of consciousness, short attention span, and variable sleep patterns. Impaired consciousness is associated with dementia; too much sleep or insomnia are associated with depression as well as depressed mood.

9. The answer is **C**. The patient is lacking in gait speed and fine motor ability to reach the bathroom and adjust clothing. Therefore, she is most likely suffering from functional incontinence. Stress incontinence occurs with increased intra-abdominal pressure such as coughing or sneezing. Urge is the experience of the sudden need to urinate with increased frequency. Mixed is a combination of urge and stress.

10. The answer is **B**. Clients with thoracic osteoporosis should have interventions that focus on extension. Flexion exercise and high intensity will increase the risk for fracture. However, clients with osteoporosis will benefit from appropriate interventions.

CHECKLIST

When you complete this chapter, you should be able to:

❑ Outline expected changes with aging and role of ageism.

❑ Compare expected physiological changes to unexpected changes with aging.

❑ Compare strategies/interventions for fall prevention and reduction.

❑ Outline ways to advocate for the geriatric patient.

❑ Differentiate chronic diseases that are common (although not expected) with aging.

CHAPTER 9 Summary Table

Major Concept	Description
Ageism	Seniors will often encounter ageism daily from their families, their friends, society, themselves, and the healthcare system. The physical therapist needs to encourage these individuals through the use of exercise, a focus on quality of life, and the benefits of increased mobility.
Assessment	Assessing for expected and unexpected changes is pivotal in developing an individualized and effective plan of care.
Early mobility	Early mobility is needed for geriatric patients in order to avoid continued muscle loss, pneumonia, wounds, osteoclastic activity, and cardiopulmonary decline.
Chronic diseases	Many persons over the age of 65 develop one or more chronic diseases, which can lead to many needs on the biopsychosocial model. This in turn requires the physical therapist to consider outside consultations and interprofessional care delivery.
Falls and prevention	In geriatric care, falls are major source to injury, debility, and even mortality. Using good assessment skills to find the cause of falls and designing interventions that are focused on improving these causes can have great benefit to the client.
Successful aging	Cognitive, physical, and sensory declines are part of normal aging; however, normal aging allows one to live a good quality of life even into the ninth decade of life, challenging the notions and biases on aging. Unexpected changes need to be addressed early to prevent loss of quality of life and independence.

Special Topics: Pediatrics

Annie Burke-Doe

■ CLINICAL APPLICATION OF FOUNDATIONAL SCIENCES

Pediatric physical therapy is a specialty practice that addresses the needs of the child and family. Care is provided through support, guidance, and interventions that are family-centered, culturally appropriate, age appropriate (0–21 years), and that improve quality of life and function. Pediatric treatment settings can vary among the acute neonatal intensive care unit, the acute hospital, an outpatient setting, school, and home, to address a few. Pediatric therapists treat infants and children with disabilities, typical developing children, and adolescents and young adults with and without disabilities. Some unique aspects of pediatric physical therapy include the understanding of child development as it relates to behavior management, developmental models, family

interactions, social trends, reimbursement issues, and the requirements of working in diverse areas. Table 10–1 describes typical development. Physical therapy models of delivery can include the therapist working independently (unidisciplinary), the therapist evaluating the patient and then meeting with other professionals to discuss the case (multidisciplinary), joint examination with other professionals (transdisciplinary), and working with equal participation in serving the child and family (collaborative).

EXAMINATION

The physical therapist examination includes taking the individual's history, which will include the family as appropriate, conducting a standardized systems review, and performing selected tests

High-Yield Terms to Learn	
Intraventricular hemorrhage (IVH)	Also known as **intraventricular** bleeding, is a bleeding into the brain's ventricular system, where the cerebrospinal fluid is produced and circulates through toward the subarachnoid space. It can result from physical trauma or from **hemorrhaging** in stroke.
Periventricular leukomalacia (PVL)	A type of brain injury that affects infants. The condition involves the death of small areas of brain tissue around fluid-filled areas called ventricles. The damage creates "holes" in the brain.
Norm-referenced tests (NRT)	A type of **test**, assessment, or evaluation that yields an estimate of the position of the **tested** individual in a predefined population, with respect to the trait being measured.
Standardized tests	Any form of test that (1) requires all test takers to answer the same questions, or a selection of questions from common bank of questions, in the same way, and that (2) is scored in a "standard" or consistent manner, which makes it possible to compare the relative performance of individual students or groups of students. While different types of tests and assessments may be "standardized" in this way, the term is primarily associated with large-scale tests administered to large populations of students, such as a multiple-choice test given to all the eighth-grade public-school students in a particular state, for example.
APGAR score	An objective score of the condition of a baby after birth. This score is determined by scoring the heart rate, respiratory effort, muscle tone, skin color, and response to a catheter in the nostril.
Retinopathy of prematurity (ROP)	A potentially blinding disease caused by abnormal development of retinal blood vessels in premature infants. The retina is the inner layer of the eye that receives light and turns it into visual messages that are sent to the brain.
Hyperbilirubinemia	A condition in which there is too much bilirubin in the blood. When red blood cells break down, a substance called bilirubin is formed. Babies are not easily able to get rid of the bilirubin and it can build up in the blood and other tissues and fluids of the baby's body.

High-Yield Terms to Learn (*continued*)

Sensory processing disorder (SPD)	A condition that exists when multisensory integration is not adequately processed in order to provide appropriate responses to the demands of the environment. It is still debated as to whether SPD is an independent disorder or the observed symptoms of various other, more well-established, disorders.
Respiratory distress syndrome (RDS)	A breathing disorder that affects newborns. RDS rarely occurs in full-term infants. The disorder is more common in premature infants born about 6 weeks or more before their due dates.
Cyanosis	A bluish color of the skin and the mucous membranes due to insufficient oxygen in the blood. For example, the lips can develop cyanosis when exposed to extreme cold. Cyanosis can be present at birth, as in a "blue baby," an infant with a malformation of the heart that permits into the arterial system blood that is not fully oxygenated.
Baclofen	A muscle relaxer and an antispastic agent. Baclofen is used to treat muscle symptoms caused by multiple sclerosis, including spasm, pain, and stiffness. Baclofen is sometimes used to treat muscle spasms and other symptoms in people with injury or disease of the spinal cord.
Diazepam	First marketed as Valium, is a medication of the benzodiazepine family that typically produces a calming effect. It is commonly used to treat a range of conditions including anxiety, alcohol withdrawal syndrome, benzodiazepine withdrawal syndrome, muscle spasms, seizures, trouble sleeping, and restless legs syndrome.
Dantrolene	**Dantrolene** sodium is a postsynaptic muscle relaxant that lessens excitation-contraction coupling in muscle cells. It achieves this by inhibiting Ca^{2+} release from sarcoplasmic reticulum stores by antagonizing ryanodine receptors.
Tizanidine	A short-acting muscle relaxant, is used to treat spasticity. Learn about side effects, interactions and indications.
Botox	A highly purified preparation of botulinum toxin A, a toxin produced by the bacterium *Clostridium botulinum*. Botox is injected in very small amounts into specific muscles as a treatment for spasticity.
Antalgic	Counteracting or avoiding pain, as a posture or gait assumed to lessen pain.
Tonic seizures	During a tonic seizure, the individual's muscles initially stiffen, and they lose consciousness. The eyes roll back into the head as the muscles (including those in the chest, arms, and legs) contract and the back arches. As the chest muscles tighten, it becomes harder for the individual to breathe—the lips and face may take on a bluish hue, and the individual may begin to make gargling noises.
Clonic seizures	During a **clonic seizure**, the individual's muscles begin to spasm and jerk. The elbows, legs, and head will flex and then relax rapidly at first, but the frequency of the spasms will gradually subside until they cease altogether. As the jerking stops, it is common for the person to let out a deep sigh, after which normal breathing resumes.
Gowers' sign	A medical sign that indicates weakness of the proximal muscles, namely those of the lower limb. The sign describes a patient who must use their hands and arms to "walk" up their own body from a squatting position due to lack of hip and thigh muscle strength.

and measures to identify potential and existing movement-related disorders. During the history-gathering phase, the physical therapist may seek and receive information on other systems symptoms and complaints that may warrant referral for additional medical evaluation. The physical therapist may decide to use one, more than one, or portions of several specific tests and measures as part of the examination, based on the purpose of the visit, the complexity of the condition, and the directions taken in the clinical decision-making process.

Tests and measures for the pediatric population are vast and can include assessment in behavior, intelligence, gross and fine motor, and adaptability to various environments, and are often norm- or criterion-referenced.[1] Norm-referenced tests are standardized tests on groups of individual populations they are designed to test. This allows the clinician to determine the exact developmental age of the child compared to performance typically expected. Criterion-referenced tests measure the child's development on skills in terms of absolute mastery levels. These tests have reference points that may not be dependent on a reference group—the child is competing against himself or herself rather than a reference group.

Signs and symptoms of atypical development in the pediatric population may include but are not limited to:

- Impairment of body function and structures (physiology and anatomical structures)
- Changes in muscle tone (hypotonic, hypertonic)
- Presence of spasticity
- Impaired age-appropriate development (delay in gaining milestones)
- Quiet, unresponsive baby

TABLE 10–1 Developmental charts.

1–2 months

Activities to be observed:

- Holds head erect and lifts head.
- Turns from side to back.
- Regards faces and follows objects through visual field.
- Drops toys.
- Becomes alert in response to voice.

Activities related by parent:

- Recognizes parents.
- Engages in vocalizations.
- Smiles spontaneously.

3–5 months

Activities to be observed:

- Grasps cube—first ulnar then later thumb opposition.
- Reaches for and brings objects to mouth.
- Makes "raspberry" sound.
- Sits with support.

Activities related by parent:

- Laughs.
- Anticipates food on sight.
- Turns from back to side.

6–8 months

Activities to be observed:

- Sits alone for a short period.
- Reaches with one hand.
- First scoops up a pellet, then grasps it using thumb opposition.
- Imitates "bye-bye."
- Passes object from hand to hand in midline.
- Babbles.

Activities related by parent:

- Rolls from back to stomach.
- Is inhibited by the word *no*.

9–11 months

Activities to be observed:

- Stands alone.
- Imitates pat-a-cake and peek-a-boo.
- Uses thumb and index finger to pick up pellet.

Activities related by parent:

- Walks by supporting self on furniture.
- Follows one-step verbal commands; eg, "Come here," "Give it to me."

1 year

Activities to be observed:

- Walks independently.
- Says "mama" and "dada" with meaning.
- Can use a neat pincer grasp to pick up a pellet.
- Releases cube into cup after demonstration.
- Gives toys on request.
- Tries to build a tower of two cubes.

Activities related by parent:

- Points to desired objects.
- Says one or two other words.

18 months

Activities to be observed:

- Builds tower of three to four cubes.
- Throws ball.
- Seats self in chair.
- Dumps pellet from bottle.

Activities related by parent:

- Walks up and down stairs with help.
- Says 4–20 words.
- Understands a two-step command.
- Carries and hugs doll.
- Feeds self.

24 months

Activities to be observed:

- Speaks short phrases, two words or more.
- Kicks ball on request.
- Builds tower of six to seven cubes.
- Points to named objects or pictures.
- Jumps off floor with both feet.
- Stands on either foot alone.
- Uses pronouns.

Activities related by parent:

- Verbalizes toilet needs.
- Pulls on simple garment.
- Turns pages of book singly.
- Plays with domestic mimicry.

30 months

Activities to be observed:

- Walks backward.
- Begins to hop on one foot.
- Uses prepositions.
- Copies a crude circle.
- Points to objects described by use.
- Refers to self as *I*.
- Holds crayon in fist.

Activities related by parent:

- Helps put things away.
- Carries on a conversation.

3 years

Activities to be observed:

- Holds crayon with fingers.
- Builds tower of 9–10 cubes.
- Imitates three-cube bridge.
- Copies circle.
- Gives first and last name.

Activities related by parent:

- Rides tricycle using pedals.
- Dresses with supervision.

(Continued)

TABLE 10–1 Developmental charts. (*Continued*)

3–4 years

Activities to be observed:

- Climbs stairs with alternating feet.
- Begins to button and unbutton.
- "What do you like to do that's fun?" (Answers using plurals, personal pronouns, and verbs.)
- Responds to command to place toy *in*, *on*, or *under* table.
- Draws a circle when asked to draw a person.
- Knows own sex. ("Are you a boy or a girl?")
- Gives full name.
- Copies a circle already drawn. ("Can you make one like this?")

Activities related by parent:

- Feeds self at mealtime.
- Takes off shoes and jacket.

4–5 years

Activities to be observed:

- Runs and turns without losing balance.
- May stand on one leg for at least 10 seconds.
- Buttons clothes and laces shoes. (Does not tie.)
- Counts to four by rote. "Give me two sticks." (Able to do so from pile of four tongue depressors.)
- Draws a person. (Head, two appendages, and possibly two eyes. No torso yet.)
- Knows the days of the week. ("What day comes after Tuesday?")
- Gives appropriate answers to: "What must you do if you are sleepy? Hungry? Cold?"
- Copies + in imitation.

Activities related by parent:

- Self-care at toilet. (May need help with wiping.)
- Plays outside for at least 30 minutes.
- Dresses self except for tying.

5–6 years

Activities to be observed:

- Can catch ball.
- Skips smoothly.
- Copies a + already drawn.
- Tells age.
- Concept of 10 (eg, counts 10 tongue depressors), may recite to higher number by rote.
- Knows right and left hand.
- Draws recognizable person with at least eight details.
- Can describe favorite television program in some detail.

Activities related by parent:

- Does simple chores at home (eg, taking out garbage, drying silverware).
- Goes to school unattended or meets school bus.
- Good motor ability but little awareness of dangers.

6–7 years

Activities to be observed:

- Copies a Δ.
- Defines words by use. ("What is an orange?" "To eat.")
- Knows if morning or afternoon.
- Draws a person with 12 details.
- Reads several one-syllable printed words. (My, dog, see, boy.)

7–8 years

Activities to be observed:

- Counts by 2s and 5s.
- Ties shoes.
- Copies a ◊.
- Knows what day of the week it is. (Not date or year.)
- No evidence of sound substitution in speech (eg, *fr* for *thr*).
- Draws a man with 16 details.
- Reads paragraph #1 Durrell:

Reading:

- Muff is a little yellow kitten. She drinks milk. She sleeps on a chair. She does not like to get wet.

Corresponding arithmetic:

$$\begin{array}{cccc} 7 & 6 & 6 & 8 \\ +4 & +7 & -4 & -3 \end{array}$$

Adds and subtracts single-digit numbers.

8–9 years

Activities to be observed:

- Defines words better than by use. ("What is an orange?" "A fruit.")
- Can give an appropriate answer to the following:
- "What is the thing for you to do if …
  - —you've broken something that belongs to someone else?"
  - —a playmate hits you without meaning to do so?"
- Reads paragraph #2 Durrell:

Reading:

A little black dog ran away from home. He played with two big dogs. They ran away from him. It began to rain. He went under a tree. He wanted to go home, but he did not know the way. He saw a boy he knew. The boy took him home.

Corresponding arithmetic:

$$\begin{array}{cccc} & 67 & & \\ 67 & 16 & 14 & -84 \\ +4 & +27 & -8 & -36 \end{array}$$

Is learning borrowing and carrying processes in addition and subtraction.

9–10 years

Activities to be observed:

- Knows the month, day, and year.
- Names the months in order. (15 seconds, 1 error.)
- Makes a sentence with these three words in it (item 1 or 2 below; can use words orally in proper context):
  - 1. work … money … men
  - 2. boy … river … ball
- Reads paragraph #3 Durrell:

Reading:

- Six boys put up a tent by the side of a river. They took things to eat with them. When the sun went down, they went into the tent to sleep. In the night, a cow came and began to eat grass around the tent. The boys were afraid. They thought it was a bear.
- Should comprehend and answer the question: "What was the cow doing?"

Corresponding arithmetic:

$$\begin{array}{ccc} 5204 & 23 & 837 \\ -530 & \times 3 & \times 7 \end{array}$$

Learning simple multiplication.

(Continued)

TABLE 10-1 Developmental charts. (*Continued*)

10–12 years	12–15 years
Activities to be observed:	**Activities to be observed:**
• Should read and comprehend paragraph #5 Durrell:	• Reads paragraph #7 Durrell:
Reading:	***Reading:***
• In 1807, Robert Fulton took the first long trip in a steamboat. He went one hundred and fifty miles up the Hudson River. The boat went five miles an hour. This was faster than a steamboat had ever gone before. Crowds gathered on both banks of the river to see this new kind of boat. They were afraid that its noise and splashing would drive away all the fish.	• Golf originated in Holland as a game played on ice. The game in its present form first appeared in Scotland. It became unusually popular and kings found it so enjoyable that it was known as "the royal game." James IV, however, thought that people neglected their work to indulge in this fascinating sport so that it was forbidden in 1457. James relented when he found how attractive the game was, and it immediately regained its former popularity. Golf spread gradually to other countries, being introduced in America in 1890. It has grown in favor until there is hardly a town that does not boast of a private or public course.
• Answer: "What river was the trip made on?"	• Ask to write a sentence: "Golf originated in Holland as a game played on ice."
• Ask to write the sentence: "The fishermen did not like the boat."	• Answers questions:
Corresponding arithmetic:	• "Why was golf forbidden by James IV?"
420 9)72 31)62	• "Why did he change his mind?"
×89	***Corresponding arithmetic:***
Should do multiplication and simple division.	4762÷536 ❑ 7 1/6
	+❑ −3 1/6
	Reduce fractions to lowest forms.
	Does long division, adds and subtracts fractions.

Modified with permission from Leavitt SR, Gofman H, Harvin D, Hutchings JJ. Use of developmental charts in teaching well-child care. *J Pediatr.* 1963;62:278-9.

• Lack of language development
• Limitations in comprehension
• Limitations in social interactions

Tests, measures (Table 10–2), and screening that may be relevant to the pediatric population will be based on history and systems review and may include but are not limited to:

• Impairment level measures (joint motion, muscle function)
• Functional limitations (activity-based measures, often standardized measures)
• Disability (participation assessment)
• Reflexes (Table 10–3 describes primitive reflexes)
• Determination of developmental age (Table 10–1)
• Infant assessments
  • APGAR score—a measure of the physical condition of a newborn infant
  • Behavioral assessment—Brazelton Neonatal Behavioral Assessment Scale
  • General Movements Assessment
  • Movement Assessment of Infants (MAI)
  • Alberta Infant Motor Scale
• Comprehensive developmental assessments
  • Bayley Scales of Infant Development II
  • Peabody Development Motor Scales (PDMS-2)
  • Bruininks Oseretsky Test of Motor Proficiency (BOT-2)
• Assessments designed for children with disabilities
  • Gross Motor Function Measure (cerebral palsy)
  • Pediatric Evaluation of Disability Inventory (PEDI)

• School based
  • School Function Assessment
  • Hawaiian Early Learning Profile
• Sensory integration
  • Pediatric Clinical Test of Sensory Interaction for Balance
  • Sensory Integration and Praxis tests
• Pain scales
  • Faces Pain Scale
  • Neonatal Infant Pain Scale
  • Faces, Legs, Activity, Cry, Consolability Behavioral pain Scale (FLACC)
• Visual assessment
  • Developmental Test of Visual Motor Integration
  • Developmental Test of Visual Perception

■ FOUNDATIONS OF EVALUATION, DIFFERENTIAL DIAGNOSIS, PROGNOSIS, AND INTERVENTIONS

PREMATURITY

Clinical Significance

Prematurity is defined as neonates born at less than 37 weeks' gestation (40 is typical gestation). Most of the difficulties associated with prematurity (preterm) occur in infants with birth

TABLE 10-2 Test and measure in pediatrics.

Test and Measure	Relevance to Pediatric Physical Therapy
Aerobic capacity/ endurance	Children with respiratory conditions such as bronchopulmonary dysplasia or cystic fibrosis, or who have ventilation assist needs should be tested in this area. In addition, those children whose movement is severely restricted by neuromotor conditions or musculoskeletal conditions such as juvenile chronic arthritis (JCA), osteogenesis imperfecta, or arthrogryposis may warrant testing in this area.
Anthropometric characteristics	Cartilage models of the long bones appear by the 6th week of gestation and primary centers of ossification appear in almost all bones of the limbs by the 12th week, and in the vertebrae by the 7th or 8th week. Children with conditions that affect growth such as pituitary gland dysfunction or bone disease such as osteogenesis imperfecta will have bone growth impairments. Indirectly, cardiac or renal conditions can also retard growth. Growth can also fall below norms in children with cerebral palsy. Growth charts with plots of height, weight, and frontal-occipital circumference are maintained by physicians and nurses. Body composition, the ratio of fat mass to fat-free mass, impacts performance on tests of aerobic and muscular fitness. Obesity in American children is a growing concern and points to a community health role of the pediatric physical therapist to improve fitness in children. Baseline measurement may include girth and body fat tests.
Arousal, attention, and cognition	This aspect is commonly addressed by other disciplines using tests such as the Brazelton Neonatal Assessment of Behavior Scale (BNABS), the Assessment of Preterm Infant Behavior (APIB), and the Movement Assessment of Infants (MAI).
Assistive and adaptive devices	Children with all types of conditions and varying severity of involvement can have assistive device needs ranging from temporary crutches to sophisticated power-driven wheelchairs. Adaptive devices may be needed at certain times for children who experience pain associated with JCA, or for children with spinal cord injuries, traumatic brain injuries, or severe cerebral palsy. Some standardized tests include testing with and without equipment, such as found on the Gross Motor Function Measure (GMFM), the Pediatric Evaluation of Disability Inventory (PEDI), and the School Function Assessment (SFA).
Circulation	Testing in this area is important for children with cardiac conditions, lymphatic conditions, respiratory conditions including bronchopulmonary dysplasia, diabetes, and certain genetic syndromes involving the circulatory or lymphatic systems. In addition, children with obesity should have baseline measures of at least pulse rate and blood pressure completed.
Cranial and peripheral nerve integrity	The pediatric physical therapist does not routinely examine cranial nerve integrity in children, as this is often done by other disciplines with whom the physical therapist collaborates. Nonetheless, the pediatric physical therapist should be aware of the clinical signs and symptoms that may indicate cranial and peripheral nerve involvement. For example, absence or asymmetry of smiling, or other facial reactions may indicate facial nerve problems. Testing is also important for children who have severe neurological involvement following traumatic brain injury or near drowning, or in later stages of progressive disorders.
Environmental, home, and work (job/school/ play) barriers	Results of these tests are often used to suggest modifications to the environment. Specific examples in pediatric physical therapy are the PEDI and the SFA.
Ergonomics and body mechanics	For children, consideration includes classroom placement for listening, attending, or functioning, as well as the height of the seat in class and whether or not foot support is provided. This section may also include assessment of safety at school; dexterity in coordination for pointing to objects on the language board, or using hand controls on a power wheelchair; analyzing preferred postures for performance of tasks and activities; and how varied body or equipment placement improves performance or posture, or minimizes fatigue.
Gait, locomotion, and balance	Once walking has begun, clinicians will most often use observation to describe the gait pattern. The 30-Second Walk Test is an example of a quick appraisal of a child's functional performance with gait, specifically the distance the child can walk in 30 s.[c] Balance testing may be done using the original or Modified Functional Reach test, or the Pediatric Clinical Test for Sensory Interaction in Balance (PCTSIB). The Bruininks Oseretsky Test of Motor Proficiency has a subtest on balance. Similarly, the Gross Motor Scale of the Peabody Developmental Motor Scales (PDMS) has five categories, of which "balance" is one.
Integumentary integrity	The assessment of skin integrity in children is particularly important in cases of suspected abuse.
Joint integrity/ mobility	Joint integrity measurements of children are mostly subjective. Two tests of hip joint integrity in infants under age 6 months are used to detect hip dysplasia associated with subluxation or dislocation.
Motor function (motor control and motor learning)	Recently, the functional-ecological theories of motor control addressing function, practicality, culture, and environment seem to have attracted the greatest attention clinically. Testing of motor control may be subjective or objective, and typically focuses on a very specific aspect of motor performance. Motor learning cannot be measured directly; instead it is inferred from behavior.

(Continued)

TABLE 10-2 Test and measure in pediatrics. (*Continued*)

Test and Measure	Relevance to Pediatric Physical Therapy
Muscle performance (including strength, power, and endurance)	Muscle tone abnormalities are common in children with impaired neuromotor development and range from hypertonicity, spasticity, and rigidity to hypotonicity, hypotonia, and flaccidity. Muscle tone can be judged subjectively by observation of posture and movement as well as by hands-on examination of a muscle's response to stretch. The muscle tone section of the MAI can also be used. Methods of strength testing in children include manual muscle testing, or the appraisal of functional skills that require strength.
Neuromotor development and sensory integration	A number of standardized tests exist for the assessment of motor milestone development, most of which are based on knowledge of normal development. For example, the Alberta Infant Motor Scale (AIMS) provides motor milestone information and is extremely valuable for describing motor function in the child who is under 19 months old or who has not yet achieved walking.
Orthotic, protective, and supportive devices	Children with cerebral palsy and myelomeningocele commonly use orthotic devices. Children who incur burns may wear compression garments. Infants with congenital club foot deformity may undergo serial casting.
Pain	The pain-o-meter, in which children are asked to show on a scale their level of pain, has been employed with children with JCA. Visual analogue scales for pain have also been employed so children can judge their own pain levels. In pediatrics, managing pain and other sensations under one category—sensory integrity—is common for most reporting purposes.
Posture	Postural control shows a distinct, continuous developmental progression and is a critical component of skill acquisition. The development of postural control appears to follow a cephalocaudal sequence starting with the head. Delayed or abnormal development of postural control limits a child's ability to develop age-appropriate motor skills, including independent mobility and manipulation skills. Causes of poor postural control can include spasticity, insult to the motor or sensory component of the central and peripheral nervous system, Down syndrome, cerebral palsy, abnormalities of muscle structure and function, and decreased strength. *Note:* Resting posture in recumbent, sitting, and standing positions may result in contractures. Parents can be asked about the duration of time that the child spends in postures such as supine lying so that recommendations can be made.
Prosthetic requirements	Children with congenital amputations comprise the largest percentage of children with limb deficiencies. The examination should describe the child's level of accommodation to the prosthetic device and the time spent with or without the device.
Range of motion	Atypical neuromuscular activity during the years of musculoskeletal growth can result in modeling errors that can cause joint dysfunction and disability. Lower limb rotational deformities are also common in children with neuromuscular disorders. Range of motion may be tested passively, by moving the child's limb, or actively, by letting the child perform the movement. For example, children with JCA are often tested actively to concurrently judge the effective range of motion, whereas children with cerebral palsy (CP) are often tested passively or by both means to distinguish true available motion from poor control, spasticity, or weakness.
Reflex integrity	In pediatrics, reflexes may be classified as diagnostic or developmental. Diagnostic reflexes include reflexes that might be used in a neurologic examination at any age such as muscle stretch reflexes, clonus, Babinski, or variations of the Babinski reflex. Developmental reflexes tend to be more specific to neurologic examination of the developing infant and young child. This cluster of reflexes include attitudinal, righting, protection, and equilibrium reactions. Rather than specifically testing the primitive reflexes, many clinicians use visual appraisal of posture and movement to ascertain their persistence or influence.
Self-care and home management (including activities of daily living [ADL] and instrumental activities of daily living [IADL])	A tool such as the Transdisciplinary Play-Based Assessment[d,e] can be used. In addition, two standardized functional tests in pediatrics provide information pertinent to this area: the PEDI and the SFA. Another test, the Canadian Occupational Performance Measure,[f-i] is designed to help establish goals by identifying functional limitations in daily life and rating them in importance to reducing disability in daily roles.
Sensory integrity (including proprioception and kinesthesia)	In very young children, sensation cannot be tested in the same way it is tested in adults. Rather, the examiner must look at the child's facial expression or other body reactions to judge sensory integrity. For older children, more sophisticated tests of sensation and sensory perception are embedded in the Sensory Integration and Praxis Test (SIPT). This test, which requires special training and advanced clinical skills, evaluates sensory processing deficits related to learning and behavior problems, including visual, tactile, and kinesthetic perception as well as motor performance.

(*Continued*)

TABLE 10–2 Test and measure in pediatrics. (*Continued*)

Test and Measure	Relevance to Pediatric Physical Therapy
Ventilation and respiration (gas exchange)	The majority of clinical tests in this area produce objective data on pulmonary function such as obtained with a spirometer (measures air volume after maximal inspiration), and the oximeter (measures oxygen saturation in the blood). Infants with respiratory distress syndrome (RDS) or bronchopulmonary dysplasia (BPD), children with cystic fibrosis or asthma, children with cardiac conditions, and those who are ventilator dependent definitely should be examined in this area.

[a]Data from Knutson LM. Examination, evaluation, and documentation for the pediatric client. In: Damiano D, ed. *Topics in Physical Therapy: Pediatrics*. Alexandria, VA: American Physical Therapy Association; 2001:1-36.

[b]Data from Clayton-Krasinski D, Klepper S. Impaired neuromotor development. In: Cameron MH, Monroe LG, eds. *Physical Rehabilitation: Evidence-Based Examination, Evaluation, and Intervention*. St Louis, MO: Saunders/Elsevier; 2007:333-366.

[c]Data from Campbell SK, Kolobe TH, Osten ET, et al. Construct validity of the test of infant motor performance. *Phys Ther*. 1995;75:585-596.

[d]Data from Lotan M, Manor-Binyamini I, Elefant C, et al. The Israeli Rett Syndrome Center. Evaluation and transdisciplinary play-based assessment. *Sci World J*. 2006;6:1302-1313.

[e]Data from Linder TW. *Transdisciplinary Play-Based Assessment*. Baltimore, MD: Paul H Brookes; 1996.

[f]Data from Verkerk GJ, Wolf MJ, Louwers AM, et al. The reproducibility and validity of the Canadian Occupational Performance Measure in parents of children with disabilities. *Clin Rehabil*. 2006;20:980-988.

[g]Data from Eyssen IC, Beelen A, Dedding C, et al. The reproducibility of the Canadian Occupational Performance Measure. *Clin Rehabil*. 2005;19:888-894.

[h]Data from Carswell A, McColl MA, Baptiste S, et al. The Canadian Occupational Performance Measure: a research and clinical literature review. *Can J Occup Ther*. 2004;71:210-222.

[i]Data from Law M, Baptiste S, McColl M, et al. The Canadian occupational performance measure: an outcome measure for occupational therapy. *Can J Occup Ther*. 1990;57:82-87.

From Dutton M. *McGraw-Hill's NPTE (National Physical Therapy Examination)*. 2nd ed. New York, NY: McGraw-Hill; 2012:Table 16-18.

TABLE 10–3 Primitive reflexes.

Reflex	Description
Rooting	Response to light tactile stimulation near the mouth. Infant moves head in direction of the stimulus and opens the mouth. Usually disappears around 9 months of age.
Sucking	Response to nipple or finger in mouth. Can be assessed as to whether it is sustainable and consistent.
Moro	One hand supports the infant's head in midline, the other supports the back. The infant is raised to 45 degrees and the head is allowed to fall through 10 degrees. Mature response is abduction then adduction of the limbs. Usually disappears around 3–6 months of age.
Palmar/plantar grasp	Stimulus applied to palm of hand or soles of feet. The response is a grasping of the digits. Usually disappears around 2–3 months of age.
Tonic labyrinthine	Prone position facilitates flexion. Supine position facilitates extension.
Asymmetric tonic neck reflex (ATNR)	Related to position of head turn: • Extension of extremities on face side. • Flexion of extremities on skull side. Usually disappears around 2–7 months of age.
Babinski	The foot twists in and the toes fan out in response to a stroke of the sole of the foot. Usually disappears around 6–9 months of age.
Symmetric tonic neck reflex (STNR)	Infant positioned in quadruped. Arm and head do the same thing, legs do the opposite; eg, head is extended, arms extend, and legs flex.
Crossed extension	Pressure applied to sole of the foot produces flexion and extension of the opposite leg.
Proprioceptive placing	Pressure applied to dorsum of the foot or hand. Response is flexion, followed by extension of the extremity to bring the foot/hand on top of the stimulating surface. Usually disappears around 1 month of age.
Positive supporting	Pressure applied to sole of the foot produces extension of the extremity for weight bearing. Also known as primary standing.
Neonatal stepping	Walking motion produced as the infant is moved along a surface while being held under the arms. Also known as automatic walking.

Data from Capute AJ, Palmer FB, Shapiro BK, et al. Primitive reflex profile: a quantitation of primitive reflexes in infancy. *Dev Med Child Neurol*. 1984;26:375-383; Damasceno A, Delicio AM, Mazo DF, et al. Primitive reflexes and cognitive function. *Arq Neuropsiquiatr*. 2005;63:577-582; Schott JM, Rossor MN. The grasp and other primitive reflexes. *J Neurol Neurosurg Psychiatry*. 2003;74:558-560; Zafeiriou DI. Primitive reflexes and postural reactions in the neurodevelopmental examination. *Pediatr Neurol*. 2004;31:1-8.

TABLE 10-4　Determination of gestational age.

- Menstrual age: the age of a fetus or newborn, in weeks, from the first day of the mother's last normal menstrual period.
- Gestational age: also known as fetal age, is the time measured from the first day of the woman's last menstrual cycle to the current date—the time inside the uterus. A pregnancy of normal gestation is approximately 40 weeks, with a normal range of 38-42 weeks.
- Preterm: born before 37 weeks of gestational age.
- Post term: born after 42 weeks.
- Conceptional age: the age of a fetus or newborn in weeks since conception.
- Chronological age: the time elapsed from date of birth to present day.
- Corrected age: based on the age the child would be if the pregnancy had actually gone to term. The corrected age, generally used for the first 2 years of life, can be calculated as the chronological age minus the number of weeks/months premature.

From Dutton M. *McGraw-Hill's NPTE (National Physical Therapy Examination)*. 2nd ed. New York, NY: McGraw-Hill; 2012:Chapter 16.

weights of 1500 g (3 lb, 5 oz) or less, usually in those born at less than 32 weeks of gestational age. Causes of prematurity include but are not limited to poor prenatal care, multiple fetuses, placental abnormalities, preeclampsia, increased maternal age, comorbidity of mother, and unhealthy lifestyle.[2] Gestational age and birth weight should be assessed and interpreted (Table 10-4).

Diagnostic Tests and Measures

Laboratory tests—Laboratory tests are completed to improve the outcome. Tests include blood glucose to maintain proper glucose levels, complete blood count for red cell measurement (anemia, polycythemia, infection), Coombs test for blood type, electrolyte levels, and metabolic screening.

Imaging—Chest radiographs, cranial ultrasonography.

Clinical Findings, Secondary Effects, Complications

1. Intraventricular hemorrhage
2. Periventricular leukomalacia
3. Retinopathy of prematurity (ROP)
4. Hyperbilirubinemia
5. Global hypotonia, with the level of hypotonia related to the degree of prematurity
6. Posturing of the extremities in extension and abduction, with decreased flexor patterns and midline orientation
7. Absent, reduced, or inconsistent primitive reflexes
8. Minimal spontaneous movement
9. Dysfunction of sensory organization
10. Difficulty moving between states of deep sleep, light sleep, alertness
11. Thermoregulation problems
12. Respiratory distress syndrome (RDS) (lack of surfactant)
13. Fluid, electrolyte, and glucose management

Interventions/Treatment

Medical—Medical treatment will include stabilization in the delivery room with prompt respiratory and thermal management. The American Academy of Pediatrics has established guidelines. Skin care, fluid and electrolyte management, and feeding will be addressed. Medical treatment is based on needs assessment.

Pharmacological—Prematurity is not a specific illness. Medications will be prescribed for a purpose.

Physical therapy—The physical therapist can provide consultation, handling, and development for specific needs of the preterm infant. The therapist will observe the infant and monitor for tolerance to handling and behavioral states of alertness, drowsiness, and sleep. Muscle tone, symmetry, reflexes, feeding, and breathing are assessed, and once examination and evaluation are completed interventions will be determined based on the infant's individual needs. Interventions may include positioning, range of motion, active movement, back-to-sleep education, illness prevention, and equipment needs, use, and monitoring as appropriate.

Differential Diagnosis

- Extremely low birth weight infant
- Fetal growth restriction

Selected Overview of Other Common Conditions Related to the Neonate Pulmonary System

Cyanosis

Newborns with significant cyanosis should be evaluated by the appropriate medical staff expeditiously. The numerous reasons for cyanosis in neonates and infants include pulmonary, hematologic, toxic, and cardiac causes.[3] Diminished pulses in all extremities indicate poor cardiac output or peripheral vasoconstriction. Absent or diminished femoral pulses suggest the presence of ductal-dependent cardiac lesions (eg, coarctation of the aorta). Although hypertension is uncommon in newborns, it is rarely idiopathic.

Respiratory Distress Syndrome

Originally described in adults, acute respiratory distress syndrome (ARDS), which is also known as *hyaline membrane disease*, occurs in all ages. The clinical signs depend on the type, acuity, and severity of the initial insult, but include dyspnea/tachypnea, flaring of the nostrils, use of accessory muscles, and diffuse rales. The prognosis of infants with RDS varies with the severity of the original disease, but RDS is the leading cause of neonatal death and morbidity.[4]

Bronchopulmonary Dysplasia

Bronchopulmonary dysplasia (BPD) is a chronic lung disease of infancy, which begins with the destruction of the respiratory tract cilia followed by necrosis of the cells of the respiratory epithelium as distal as the bronchioles. The chronic lack of oxygenation often impairs neuromotor development.

Bronchiolitis

Bronchiolitis is an acute, infectious, inflammatory disease of the upper and lower respiratory tract resulting in obstruction of the small airways.[5-7] Although it may occur in all age groups, the larger airways of older children and adults better accommodate mucosal edema, and severe symptoms are usually only evident in young infants. Respiratory syncytial virus (RSV) is the most commonly isolated agent. The disease is highly contagious. Viral shedding in nasal secretions continues for 6 to as long as 21 days after the development of symptoms. Hand washing and the use of disposable gloves and gowns may reduce nosocomial spread. Eighteen to twenty percent of hospitalized infants with RSV bronchiolitis develop apnea. Diagnosis is based on the infant's age, seasonal occurrence, and physical findings. Physical examination often reveals otitis media, retractions, fine rales, and diffuse, fine wheezing. The severity of the disease is directly related to post-conceptual age. Infants less than 6 months of age are the most severely affected due to smaller, more easily obstructed airways and a decreased ability to clear secretions. First infections are usually most severe, with subsequent attacks generally milder.

Periventricular Leukomalacia

Periventricular leukomalacia (PVL), a bilateral white matter lesion, is the most common ischemic brain injury in premature infants.[8] PVL may result from hypotension, ischemia, and coagulation necrosis at the border or watershed zones of deep penetrating arteries of the middle cerebral artery. Decreased blood flow affects the white matter at the superolateral borders of the lateral ventricles. The site of injury affects the descending corticospinal tracts, visual radiations, and acoustic radiations. Initially, most premature infants are asymptomatic. If symptoms occur, they usually are subtle. Symptoms may include decreased tone in lower extremities, increased tone in neck extensors, apnea and bradycardia events, irritability, pseudobulbar palsy with poor feeding, and clinical seizures.

Periventricular Hemorrhage-Intraventricular Hemorrhage

Periventricular hemorrhage-intraventricular hemorrhage (PVH-IVH) remains a significant cause of both morbidity and mortality in infants who are born prematurely. PVH-IVH is thought to be caused by capillary bleeding. Two major factors that contribute to the development of PVH-IVH are (1) loss of cerebral autoregulation and (2) abrupt alterations in cerebral blood flow and pressure. Sequelae of PVH-IVH include lifelong neurological deficits, such as cerebral palsy (CP), mental retardation, and seizures. PVH-IVH is diagnosed primarily using brain imaging studies, usually cranial ultrasonography. As PVH-IVH can occur without clinical signs, serial examinations are necessary for the diagnosis.

Cardiovascular System

Patent Ductus Arteriosus

Patent ductus arteriosus (PDA) is the fifth or sixth most common congenital cardiac defect. It involves the persistence of a normal fetal structure between the left pulmonary artery and the descending aorta beyond 10 days of life. Signs and symptoms include, but are not limited to, tachypnea, tachycardia, diaphoresis, and cyanosis.

Tetralogy of Fallot

Tetralogy of Fallot (TOF) is a complex of anatomic abnormalities arising from the maldevelopment of the right ventricular infundibulum. Cyanosis develops within the first few years of life, or at birth, which may demand surgical repair. The rare patient may remain marginally and imperceptibly cyanotic, or acyanotic and asymptomatic, into adult life.

Musculoskeletal System

Congenital Muscular Torticollis

Congenital muscular torticollis (CMT) refers to presentation of the neck in a twisted or bent position due to a unilateral shortening of the sternocleidomastoid (SCM) muscle. The position adopted by the head and neck is one of side-bending of the neck to the same side as the contracture with rotation of the neck to the opposite side as the contracture. In addition, the infant may exhibit asymmetric neck extension and forward head posture (FHP) due to upper cervical extension. There is little agreement as to the etiology of CMT. Theories include direct injury to the SCM muscle (due to birth trauma or intrauterine mispositioning), abnormal vascular patterns, rupture of the muscle, infective myositis, fibrosis of the SCM, neurogenic injury, and hereditary factors.

Talipes Equinovarus (Clubfoot)

Clubfoot, or talipes equinovarus, is a congenital deformity consisting of hindfoot equinus, hindfoot varus, and forefoot varus. Can be classified as postural or positional (not true clubfeet) or fixed or rigid (are either flexible [ie, correctable without surgery] or resistant [ie, requires surgical release]). Treatment consists of manipulation (reducing the talonavicular joint by moving the navicular laterally and the head of the talus medially) and serial casting, which is most effective if started immediately after birth.

Developmental (Congenital) Dysplasia of the Hip

Developmental dysplasia of the hip involves an abnormal development of the acetabulum and the proximal femur, the labrum, capsule, and other soft tissues of the hip, which results in a failure of the femoral head to rest correctly in the acetabulum of the pelvis. Although the condition may occur at any time from conception to skeletal maturity, it occurs more frequently in early life. Two terms are used to describe this condition: the traditional term *congenital hip dysplasia (CHD)* and the current term *developmental dysplasia of the hip (DDH)*. The hip may be dislocated, dislocatable, or subluxated. The signs and symptoms that may be found in the newborn include asymmetric fat folds in the thigh or extra skin folds on the involved side. Positive Ortolani test/Barlow maneuver signs may be present. In the older child, the signs and symptoms usually include legs that are unequal in length and a positive Galeazzi sign. The treatment[9] of this condition depends on the child's age. From birth to 9 months, the Pavlik harness has traditionally been used. The harness restricts hip extension and adduction and allows the hip to be maintained in flexion and abduction, the "protective" position. The position of flexion and abduction enhances normal acetabular development, and the kicking motion allowed in this position stretches the contracted hip adductors and promotes spontaneous reduction of the dislocated hip. In infants older than 9 months of age who are beginning to walk independently, an abduction orthosis can be used as an alternative to the Pavlik harness.

Neurologic System

Hydrocephalus

Hydrocephalus is an abnormal accumulation of cerebrospinal fluid (CSF) within the ventricles inside the brain.[10-14] Intracranial pressure (ICP) rises if production of CSF exceeds absorption. This occurs if CSF is overproduced, resistance to CSF flow is increased, or venous sinus pressure is increased. Congenital hydrocephalus is thought to be caused by a complex interaction of environmental and perhaps genetic factors. Acquired hydrocephalus may result from intraventricular hemorrhage, meningitis, head trauma, tumors, and cysts. Symptoms in infants include poor feeding, irritability, reduced activity, and/or vomiting. The symptoms in children include a slowing of mental capacity, drowsiness, headaches, neck pain, visual disturbances, and gait disturbance.

Arthrogryposis

Arthrogryposis, or arthrogryposis multiplex congenita, encompasses nonprogressive neurological conditions that are characterized by multiple joint contractures and rigid joints found throughout the body at birth.[15-19] The pathogenesis of arthrogryposis has not been determined but is thought to be due to a combination of fetal abnormalities, maternal disorders (eg, infection, drugs, trauma, and other maternal illnesses), and genetic inheritance. Although joint contractures and associated clinical manifestations vary from case to case, there are several common characteristics: the involved extremities are fusiform or cylindrical in shape with thin layers of subcutaneous tissue and absent skin creases. The deformities are usually symmetric, and the severity increases distally, with the hands and feet typically being the most deformed. The patient may have joint dislocations, especially the hips, and occasionally at the knees.

Brachial Plexus Injury

Brachial plexus injury occurs most commonly in larger babies during delivery. Associated injuries include fractured clavicle, fractured humerus, subluxation of cervical spine, cervical cord injury, and facial palsy. Erb's palsy (C5-C6) is the most common and is associated with lack of shoulder motion. The involved extremity lies adducted, prone, and internally rotated. Moro, biceps, and radial reflexes are absent on the affected side. Grasp reflex is usually present. Five percent of patients have an accompanying (ipsilateral) phrenic nerve paresis. Klumpke paralysis (C7-C8, T1) is rare, resulting in weakness of the intrinsic muscles of the hand; grasp reflex is absent. If cervical sympathetic fibers of the first thoracic spinal nerve are involved, Horner syndrome is present.

Spina Bifida

Spina bifida includes a continuum of congenital anomalies of the spine due to insufficient closure of the neural tube and failure of the vertebral arches to fuse.[20-26] Spina bifida is classified into aperta (visible or open) and occulta (not visible or hidden). The three main types of spina bifida are listed in Table 10-5. Spina bifida aperta is often used interchangeably with myelomeningocele, which is an open spinal cord defect that usually protrudes dorsally. The neurological complications associated with spina bifida are outlined in Table 10-6. Interventions are based on clinical findings.

TABLE 10-5 The three main types of spina bifida.

Type	Description
Spina bifida occulta	"Occulta" means hidden; thus the defect is not visible.
	Rarely linked with complications or symptoms.
	Usually discovered accidentally during an x-ray or MRI for some other reason.
Meningocele (spina bifida aperta)	The membrane that surrounds the spinal cord may enlarge, creating a lump or "cyst." This is often invisible through the skin and causes no problems.
	If the spinal canal is cleft, or "bifid," the cyst may expand and come to the surface. In such cases, since the cyst does not enclose the spinal cord, the cord is not exposed.
	The cyst varies in size, but it can almost always be removed surgically if necessary, leaving no permanent disability.
Myelomeningocele (spina bifida aperta)	The most complex and severe form of spina bifida. A section of the spinal cord and the nerves that stem from the cord are exposed and visible on the outside of the body, or, if there is a cyst, it encloses part of the cord and the nerves.
	Usually involves neurological problems that can be very serious or even fatal.
	This condition accounts for 94% of cases of true spina bifida.
	The most severe form of spina bifida cystica is myelocele, or myeloschisis, in which the open neural plate is covered secondarily by epithelium and the neural plate has spread out onto the surface.

From Dutton M. *McGraw-Hill's NPTE (National Physical Therapy Examination)*. 2nd ed. New York, NY: McGraw-Hill; 2012:Table 16-24.

TABLE 10–6 Neurological complications associated with spina bifida.

Complication	Description
Syringomeningocele	The Greek word *syrinx*, meaning tube or plate, is combined with *meninx* (membrane) and *kele* (tumor); the term thus describes a hollow center with the spinal fluid connecting with the central canal of the cord enclosed by a membrane with very little cord substance.
Syringomyelocele	Protrusion of the membranes and spinal cord lead to increased fluid in the central canal, attenuating the cord tissue against a thin-walled sac.
Diastematomyelia	From the Greek root *diastema* (interval) and *myelon* (marrow). Is accompanied by a bony septum in some cases.
Myelodysplasia	From the Greek term *myelos*, meaning spinal cord, with *dys* for difficult and *plasi* for molding. This is a defective development of any part of the cord.
Arnold-Chiari deformity	Malformation of the cerebellum with elongation of the cerebellar tonsils. The cerebellum is drawn into the fourth ventricle. The condition also is characterized by smallness of the medulla and pons, and internal hydrocephalus. In fact, all patients with spina bifida cystica (failure to close caudally) have some form of Arnold-Chiari malformation (failure to close cranially). The Chiari II malformation is a complex congenital malformation of the brain, nearly always associated with myelomeningocele. This condition includes downward displacement of the medulla, fourth ventricle, and cerebellum into the cervical spinal canal, as well as elongation of the pons and fourth ventricle, probably due to a relatively small posterior fossa. Signs and symptoms include stridor, apnea, irritability, cerebellar ataxia, and hypertonia.
Craniorachischisis (total dysraphism)	A condition in which the brain and spinal cord are exposed. This often results in early spontaneous abortion, often associated with malformations of other organ systems.
Tethered cord	A longitudinal stretch of the spinal cord that occurs with growth resulting in progressive loss of sensory and motor function, long tract signs, and changes in posture and gait. Presence may be signaled by foot deformities previously braced easily, new onset of hip dislocation, or worsening of a spinal deformity, particularly scoliosis. Progressive neurologic defects in growing children may suggest a lack of extensibility of the spine or that it is tethered and low lying in the lumbar canal with the potential for progressive irreversible neurologic damage and requiring surgical release.
Hydrocephalus	Characterized by a tense, bulging fontanel and increased occipital frontal circumference. Signs and symptoms include decreased upper extremity coordination, disturbed balance, strabismus, and ocular problems. Medical intervention involves placement of a shunt between ventricle and heart/abdomen.
Neurogenic bowel and bladder	Incontinence.

Data from Ali L, Stocks GM. Spina bifida, tethered cord and regional anaesthesia. *Anaesthesia.* 2005;60:1149-1150; Dias L. Orthopaedic care in spina bifida: past, present, and future. *Dev Med Child Neurol.* 2004;46:579; Mitchell LE, Adzick NS, Melchionne J, et al. Spina bifida. *Lancet.* 2004;364:1885-1895; Shaer CM, Chescheir N, Erickson K, et al. Obstetrician-gynecologists' practice and knowledge regarding spina bifida. *Am J Perinatol.* 2006;23:355-362; Spina bifida. *Nurs Times.* 2005;101:31; Verhoef M, Barf HA, Post MW, et al. Functional independence among young adults with spina bifida, in relation to hydrocephalus and level of lesion. *Dev Med Child Neurol.* 2006;48:114-119; Woodhouse CR. Progress in the management of children born with spina bifida. *Eur Urol.* 2006;49:777-778.

Cerebral Palsy

CP is non-progressive damage to the cerebral cortex and other parts of the brain that occurs during prenatal, perinatal, or postnatal period. CP is diagnosed when a child does not reach motor milestones while also exhibiting abnormal muscle tone or movement pattern dysfunctions such as asymmetry. Despite advances in neonatal care, CP remains a significant clinical problem. In most cases of CP, the exact cause is unknown but is most likely multifactorial. CP can be classified in several ways, including a diagnosis based on the area of the body exhibiting motor impairment: monoplegia (one limb), diplegia (lower limbs), hemiplegia (upper and lower limbs on one side of the body), and quadriplegia (all limbs). Other classifications and manifestations are represented in Table 10–7.

Clinical Significance

Disturbances include:

1. Primary impairments of the muscular system include insufficient muscle force generation, spasticity, abnormal extensibility, and exaggerated or hyperactive reflexes.

2. Primary impairments of the neuromuscular system include poor selective control of muscle activity, reduced anticipatory regulation, and a decreased ability to learn distinctive movements.

Diagnostic Tests and Measures

Laboratory tests—Blood and urine tests to rule out metabolic disorders.

Imaging—X-ray, ultrasound, electroencephalography, CT, MRI.

Clinical Findings, Secondary Effects, Complications

Secondary impairments of the skeletal system include malalignment such as torsion or hip deformities.

Interventions/Treatment

Medical—Diagnosis will consist of observation, history, and a neurological exam.[27] Pharmacological, neurosurgical, and

TABLE 10-7 Cerebral palsy classifications and manifestations.

	Spastic	Athetoid	Ataxic	Hypotonic
Muscle stiffness	Excessively stiff and taut, especially during attempted movement	Low	Variable	Diminished resting muscle tone and decreased ability to generate voluntary muscle force
Posture	Abnormal postures and movements; mass patterns of flexion/extension	Poor functional stability, especially in proximal joint	Low postural tone with poor balance	Variable
Visual tracking	Some deficits	Poor visual tracking	Poor visual tracking, nystagmus	Variable
Muscle tone	Increase in antigravity muscles Imbalance of tone across joints that can cause contractures and deformities	Fluctuates, but generally decreased—floppy baby syndrome	Slightly decreased	Minimal to none
Initiating movement	Difficult	No problems	No problems	Difficult
Sustaining movement	Able to in some	Unable	No problems	Unable
Terminating movement	Unable	Variable	No problems	Uncontrolled
Muscle co-activation	Abnormal	Poorly timed	No problems	None
ROM limitations	Passive ROM, overall decreased	Hypermobile	In spine	Hypermobile

From Dutton M. *McGraw-Hill's NPTE (National Physical Therapy Examination)*. 2nd ed. New York, NY: McGraw-Hill; 2012:Table 16–32.

orthopedic surgeries may be recommended at some point. Orthotic interventions may be recommended.

Pharmacological

- Skeletal muscle relaxants (baclofen, diazepam, dantrolene, tizanidine)
- Antispasticity medications (baclofen, diazepam, dantrolene, tizanidine, Botox)

Physical therapy—In few conditions do physical therapists play such a central role[28] or have as much potential to influence the outcome of children's lives. Children with CP have variable but significant disruptions in the categories of recreation, community roles, personal care, education, mobility, housing, and nutrition, and are most associated with locomotion capabilities. The clinician must be able to identify the abilities as well as participation restrictions, activity limitations, and impairment of body structure and function of the patient. At all ages, examination of impairment involves qualitative, and when possible, quantitative assessment of single-system and multisystem impairments. Common physical therapy equipment is described in Table 10–8.

Differential Diagnosis

- Genetic disorders or syndromes
- Metabolic disorders

SELECTED OVERVIEW OF OTHER COMMON CONDITIONS RELATED TO THE CHILD

Cystic Fibrosis

Cystic fibrosis (CF), an autosomal recessive disorder involving multiple organ systems (lungs, liver, intestine, pancreas) and exocrine gland dysfunction, can result in chronic respiratory infections, pancreatic enzyme insufficiency, and associated complications in untreated patients. The root cause of CF is a malfunction of the epithelial cells' ability to conduct chloride that results in water transport abnormalities, resulting in viscous secretions occurring in the respiratory tract, pancreas, gastrointestinal tract, sweat glands, and other exocrine tissues. This increased viscosity makes the secretions difficult to clear. The clinical characteristics of CF are listed in Table 10–9. Sweat chloride analysis is critical to distinguish CF from other causes of severe pulmonary and pancreatic insufficiencies.[29] CF is a disorder that often requires management by a multidisciplinary team. The goals of the intervention are maintenance of adequate nutritional status, prevention of pulmonary and other complications, encouragement of physical activity, and provision of adequate psychosocial support.

In the neonate, because the lungs are morphologically normal at birth, the most frequently seen symptoms are meconium ileus, malabsorption of nutrients, and failure to thrive, all of which are

TABLE 10–8 Pediatric adaptive equipment.

Equipment	Type	Description
Standers	*Supine version:* User enters the device on their backs, then they are strapped in and brought upright. Used when more support is needed posteriorly.	Promotes weight-bearing and stretching, and, depending on the child's diagnosis, can help with the proper formation of the hip joint and building bone density. Promotes bone mineralization and respiratory, bowel, and bladder function. Helps teach mobility skills.
	Prone version: Loads from the chest, and patient is strapped from behind. Used for cases when greater head and trunk control is needed.	Allows child to gain important emotional and social support by enabling them to interact with the rest of the world from a "normal" position.
Sidelyers		Used in cases when the patient has a tonic labyrinthine reflex (TLR), which can elicit more extensor tone in supine, and more flexor tone in prone.
Adaptive seating		Seating can be customized to meet the specific support and posture needs of the individual. As a general rule, seating systems should be customized to maintain the head in neutral position, the trunk upright, and the hips, knees, and ankles in correct alignment. For children with cerebral palsy, seating systems can be designed with a sacral pad and knee-block to correct pelvic tilt, decrease pelvic rotation, and abduct/derotate the hip joint.
Orthoses	Various	Orthoses are frequently required to maintain functional joint positions, especially in nonambulatory or hemiplegic patients. Frequent reevaluation of orthotic devices is important, as children quickly outgrow them and can undergo skin breakdown from improper use. AFOs are commonly used. Submalleolar orthosis is used for forefoot and midfoot malalignment.

AFO, ankle-foot orthosis.

From Dutton M. *McGraw-Hill's NPTE (National Physical Therapy Examination)*. 2nd ed. New York, NY: McGraw-Hill; 2012:Table 16–21.

TABLE 10–9 Clinical manifestations of cystic fibrosis.

System	Signs and Symptoms
Gastrointestinal tract	Intestinal, pancreatic, and hepatobiliary Meconium ileus Recurrent abdominal pain and constipation Diabetes Patients may present with a history of jaundice or gastrointestinal tract bleeding Minimal weight gain—failure to thrive (FTT)
Integumentary	Salty perspiration ("Kiss your Baby week" for early detection) Clubbing of nail beds Central and peripheral cyanosis
Respiratory tract	Wheezing, rales, or rhonchi Chronic or recurrent cough, which can be dry and hacking at the beginning and can produce mucoid (early) and purulent (later) sputum Recurrent pneumonia, atypical asthma, pneumothorax, hemoptysis, are all complications and may be the initial manifestation Dyspnea on exertion, history of chest pain, recurrent sinusitis, nasal polyps, and hemoptysis may occur Pulmonary artery hypertension Cor pulmonale Bronchospasm
Urogenital tract	Males are frequently sterile because of the absence of the vas deferens Undescended testicles or hydrocele may exist

Data from Lucas SR, Platts-Mills TA. Physical activity and exercise in asthma: relevance to etiology and treatment. *J Allergy Clin Immunol*. 2005;115:928-934; Mintz M. Asthma update: part I. Diagnosis, monitoring, and prevention of disease progression. *Am Fam Physician*. 2004;70:893-898; Ram FS, Robinson SM, Black PN, et al. Physical training for asthma. *Cochrane Database Syst Rev*. 2005;CD001116; Welsh L, Kemp JG, Roberts RG. Effects of physical conditioning on children and adolescents with asthma. *Sports Med*. 2005;35:127-141.

associated with the gastrointestinal tract. However, within a few months some infants may develop signs of impaired respiratory function.[30]

Torsional Conditions

These include in-toeing or out-toeing, probably the most common reason for elective referral of a child to an orthopedist. Clinical examination of the child with in-toeing or out-toeing should include documentation of the foot progression angle (FPA) in standing or walking, hip rotation range of motion, thigh-foot axis, and alignment of the foot.[31]

FPA, also known as *the angle of gait*, is defined as the angle between the longitudinal axis of the foot and a straight line of progression of the body in walking.[32] While observing gait, the clinician assigns a value to the angle of both the right and left foot. In-toeing is expressed as a negative value (eg, –20 degrees), and out-toeing is expressed as a positive value (eg, +20 degrees). FPA is variable during infancy, but during childhood and adult life it shows little change, with a mean of +10 degrees and a normal range of –3 to +20 degrees.[32]

Hip rotation range of motion is measured most accurately in the prone position (or with the anxious young child being held facing the parent's chest), with the hip in a position of neutral flexion/extension. If the hip is in anteversion (anteverted), the patient will usually have more hip internal rotation than external rotation, assuming no soft tissue tightness. The sum of hip internal rotation and external rotation is usually 120 degrees up to age 2 years; over age to it is 95 to 110 degrees.[33]

Thigh-foot axis is a reflection of the version of the tibia, which is assessed using the thigh-foot angle (the angular difference between the longitudinal axes of the thigh and the foot, as measured in the prone position with the knee flexed). Tibial torsion can also be described as the angle formed by a straight-line axis through the knee and the axis through the medial and lateral malleoli. By convention, internal tibial torsion is expressed as a negative value, while external tibial torsion is expressed as a positive value. Scoles[34] described the following approximate thigh-foot normative angles:

- Birth: –15 degrees (normal range –30 to +20 degrees)
- Age 3: +5 degrees (normal range –10 to +20 degrees)
- Mid-childhood to skeletal maturity: +10 degrees (normal range –5 to +30 degrees)

Controversy exists regarding the appropriate treatment of internal tibial torsion because the natural history of the condition is a gradual improvement in most cases. In some cases a Friedman counter splint or a Denis Browne bar may be prescribed for night wear for approximately 6 months.

Slipped Capital Femoral Epiphysis

Slipped capital femoral epiphysis (SCFE) is a disorder of epiphyseal growth that represents a distinctive type of instability of the proximal femoral growth plate due to a Salter-Harris type 1 fracture through the proximal femoral physis.[31,35-40] The cause of SCFE is uncertain, although it has been established that stress around the hip causes a shear force to be applied at the growth plate, which causes the epiphysis to move posteriorly and medially. In addition, the position of the proximal physis normally changes from horizontal to oblique during preadolescence and adolescence, redirecting the hip forces. The patient usually has an antalgic limp and pain in the groin, often referred to the anteromedial aspect of the thigh and knee. The leg is usually held in external rotation, both when supine and when standing. There may be tenderness to palpation on the anterior and lateral aspect of the hip. Decreased hip motion is noted in flexion, abduction, and internal rotation. With attempts to flex the hip, the legs move into external rotation. Knowledge of SCFE and its manifestations will facilitate prompt referral by the clinician to an orthopedic surgeon. Diagnosis can be confirmed using both anteroposterior (AP) pelvis and lateral frog-leg radiographs of both hips. CT is a sensitive method of measuring the degree of tilt and detecting early disease, but it is rarely needed. MRI depicts the slippage earliest, and MRI can demonstrate early marrow edema and slippage.

Legg-Calvé Perthes Disease

Legg-Calvé-Perthes disease (LCPD) is an idiopathic osteonecrosis of the capital femoral epiphysis of the femoral head.[41-47] LCPD has an unconfirmed etiology, but may involve an interruption of the blood supply to the capital femoral epiphysis, bone infarction, and revascularization as new bone ossification starts. Changes to the epiphyseal growth plate can occur secondary to a subchondral fracture. When a subchondral fracture occurs, it is usually the result of normal physical activity, not direct trauma to the area. Patients frequently have a painful limp (pain in the groin, hip, or knee), a positive Trendelenburg sign (hip abduction weakness), and limited hip range of motion, especially in hip abduction and internal rotation.[31]

Osgood Schlatter Disease

Osgood-Schlatter (OS) disease is a benign, self-limiting traction apophysis at the knee, which is one of the most common causes of knee pain in the adolescent.[48] OS occurs during periods of rapid growth; the contraction forces of the quadriceps are transmitted through the patellar tendon onto a small portion of the tibial tuberosity that is only partially developed, which can result in a partial avulsion fracture through the ossification center. Eventually, secondary heterotopic bone formation occurs in the tendon near its insertion, producing a visible lump.

Down Syndrome (Trisomy 21)

The extra chromosome 21 that occurs in Down syndrome affects almost every organ system and results in a wide spectrum of phenotypic consequences. Impairments associated with this condition include hypotonia, decreased force generation of muscles, congenital heart defects, visual and hearing losses, and cognitive deficits (mental retardation).

Seizure Disorders

Seizures can be defined as neurologic manifestations of involuntary and excessive neuronal discharge.[49-51] The symptoms depend on the part of brain that is involved and may include an altered level of consciousness, tonic-clonic movements of some or all body parts, or visual, auditory, or olfactory disturbance. Differential diagnosis includes epilepsy, drugs (noncompliance with prescription, withdrawal syndrome, overdose, multiple drug abuse), hypoxia, brain tumor, infection (eg, meningitis), metabolic disturbances (eg, hypoglycemia, uremia, liver failure, electrolyte disturbance), and head injury. Most seizures in children involve loss of consciousness and tonic-clonic movements, but auditory, visual, or olfactory disturbance, behavioral change, or absences in attention may also occur. The various types of seizures are outlined in Table 10–10.

Duchenne Muscular Dystrophy

The muscular dystrophies (MD) associated with defects in dystrophin range greatly, from the very severe Duchenne muscular dystrophy (DMD) to the far milder Becker muscular dystrophy (BMD).[52-61] DMD, the best-known form of muscular dystrophy, is due to a mutation in a gene on the X chromosome that prevents the production of dystrophin, a normal protein in muscle. DMD

TABLE 10–10 Seizure disorders.

Type	Description
Generalized	Affects both hemispheres Characterized by change in level of consciousness Bilateral motor involvement
Simple partial	Affects only part of brain (focal, motor, or sensory) Formerly called focal seizures May progress to generalized seizures The history is important, because the anticonvulsants used for partial seizures differ from those used for generalized seizures
Complex partial	Partial seizure with affective or behavioral changes
Febrile	Associated with temperature >38°C Occurs in children <6 years old (prevalence is 2%–4% among children <5 years old) No signs or history of underlying seizure disorder Often familial Uncomplicated and benign if seizure is of short duration (<5 minutes) Involves tonic-clonic movements

Data from Camfield P, Camfield C. Advances in the diagnosis and management of pediatric seizure disorders in the twentieth century. *J Pediatr.* 2000;136:847-849; Nelson LP, Ureles SD, Holmes G. An update in pediatric seizure disorders. *Pediatr Dent.* 1991;13:128-135; Sanger MS, Perrin EC, Sandler HM. Development in children's causal theories of their seizure disorders. *J Dev Behav Pediatr.* 1993;14:88-93; Tharp BR. An overview of pediatric seizure disorders and epileptic syndromes. *Epilepsia.* 1987;28(suppl 1):S36-S45.

affects boys, and very rarely, girls. DMD typically manifests with weakness in the pelvis and upper limbs, resulting in frequent falling, an inability to keep up with peers while playing, and an unusual gait (waddling). Around the age of 8 years, most patients notice difficulty climbing stairs or rising from the ground. Because of this proximal lower back and extremity weakness, parents often note that the child pushes on his knees in order to stand (Gowers' sign). The posterior calf is usually enlarged as a result of fatty and connective tissue infiltration, or by compensatory hypertrophy of the calves secondary to weak tibialis anterior muscles. Respiratory muscle strength begins a slow but steady decline. The forced vital capacity gradually wanes, leading to symptoms of nocturnal hypoxemia such as lethargy and early morning headaches. As DMD progresses, a wheelchair may be required. Most patients with DMD die in their early twenties because of muscle-based breathing and cardiac problems.

Rheumatology: Juvenile Rheumatoid Arthritis

Juvenile rheumatoid arthritis (JRA) is a group of diseases that are associated with chronic joint inflammation. JRA is a persistent arthritis, lasting at least 6 weeks, in one or more joints of a child (younger than 16 years of age), when all other causes of arthritis have been excluded.[62,63] The exact etiology of JRA is unclear, but it is an autoimmune inflammatory disorder. General history and observation of JRA includes morning stiffness, gait deviations, and severe joint pain. JRA is thought to be triggered by a preceding illness.

Hematopoietic System: Hemophilia

Hemophilia is the most common inherited coagulation (blood clotting) disorder. It is inherited as a sex-linked autosomal recessive trait. Because the genes involved are located on the X-chromosome, males are affected because they have only one X-chromosome. Hemophilia, which is caused by an abnormality of plasma-clotting proteins necessary for blood coagulation,[64] is characterized by prolonged bleeding, although the blood flow is not any faster than what occurred in a normal person at the same injury. Two primary types exist, hemophilia A (classic hemophilia—factor VIII deficiency) and hemophilia B (Christmas disease—factor IX deficiency). The classification of the severity of hemophilia has been based on either clinical bleeding symptoms or on plasma procoagulant levels, which are the most widely used criteria. The trademark characteristic of hemophilia is hemorrhage into the joints, which is painful and leads to long-term inflammation and deterioration of the joint. This in turn results in permanent deformities, misalignment, loss of mobility, and extremities of unequal lengths.

■ SUMMARY

Pediatrics is a specialty in physical therapy. Most pediatric physical therapists get advanced training to understand the unique aspects of this population.

REFERENCES

1. Connolly BH. Tests and assessment. In: Connolly BH, Montgomery PC, eds. *Therapeutic Exercise in Developmental Disabilities*. Thorofare, NJ: SLACK; 2001:15-33.

2. Furdon SA. Medscape prematurity. Updated: Oct 13, 2017. In: Nimavat, DH, ed. https://emedicine.medscape.com/article/975909-overview#a5. Accessed May 15, 2018.

3. Grifka RG. Cyanotic congenital heart disease with increased pulmonary blood flow. *Pediatr Clin North Am*. 1999;46:405-425.

4. Kahn-D'Angel L, Unanue-Rose RA. The special care nursery. In: Campbell SK, Vander Linden DW, Palisano RJ, eds. *Physical Therapy for Children*. 3rd ed. St. Louis, MO: Saunders; 2006:1053-1097.

5. Clover RD. Clinical practice guideline for bronchiolitis: key recommendations. *Am Fam Physician*. 2007;75:171.

6. Perrotta C, Ortiz Z, Roque M. Chest physiotherapy for acute bronchiolitis in paediatric patients between 0 and 24 months old. *Cochrane Database Syst Rev*. 2007;CD004873.

7. Lieberthal, A. S et al. Diagnosis and management of bronchiolitis. *Pediatrics*. 2006;118:1774-1793.

8. Sugai K, Ito M, Tateishi I, et al. Neonatal periventricular leukomalacia due to severe, poorly controlled asthma in the mother. *Allergol Int*. 2006;55:207-212.

9. Leach J. Orthopedic conditions. In: Campbell SK, Vander Linden DW, Palisano RJ, eds. *Physical Therapy for Children*. 3rd ed. St. Louis, MO: Saunders; 2006:481-515.

10. Kinsman D. The child with hydrocephalus or myelomeningocele. II. Comprehensive physical therapy program. *Phys Ther*. 1966;46:611-615.

11. Fredrickson D. The child with hydrocephalus or melomeningocele. I. Initial and continuing physical therapy evaluation. *Phys Ther*. 1966;46:606-611.

12. Andersson S, Persson EK, Aring E, et al. Vision in children with hydrocephalus. *Dev Med Child Neurol*. 2006;48:836-841.

13. Bergsneider M, Egnor MR, Johnston M, et al. What we don't (but should) know about hydrocephalus. *J Neurosurg*. 2006;104:157-159.

14. Rizvi R, Anjum Q. Hydrocephalus in children. *J Pak Med Assoc*. 2005;55:502-507.

15. Mallia Milanes G, Napolitano R, Quaglia F, et al. Prenatal diagnosis of arthrogryposis. *Minerva Ginecol*. 2007;59:201-202.

16. Mennen U, van Heest A, Ezaki MB, et al. Arthrogryposis multiplex congenita. *J Hand Surg [Br]*. 2005;30:468-474.

17. Bernstein RM. Arthrogryposis and amyoplasia. *J Am Acad Orthop Surg*. 2002;10:417-424.

18. Hardwick JC, Irvine GA. Obstetric care in arthrogryposis multiplex congenita. *BJOG*. 2002;109:1303-1304.

19. O'Flaherty P. Arthrogryposis multiplex congenita. *Neonatal Netw*. 2001;20:13-20.

20. Shaer CM, Chescheir N, Erickson K, et al. Obstetrician-gynecologists' practice and knowledge regarding spina bifida. *Am J Perinatol*. 2006;23:355-362.

21. Woodhouse CR. Progress in the management of children born with spina bifida. *Eur Urol*. 2006;49:777-778. Epub Feb 6, 2006.

22. Verhoef M, Barf HA, Post MW, et al. Functional independence among young adults with spina bifida, in relation to hydrocephalus and level of lesion. *Dev Med Child Neurol*. 2006;48:114-119.

23. Ali L, Stocks GM. Spina bifida, tethered cord and regional anaesthesia. *Anaesthesia*. 2005;60:1149-1150.

24. Spina bifida. *Nurs Times*. 2005;101:31.

25. Mitchell LE, Adzick NS, Melchionne J, et al. Spina bifida. *Lancet*. 2004;364:1885-1895.

26. Dias L. Orthopaedic care in spina bifida: past, present, and future. *Dev Med Child Neurol*. 2004;46:579.

27. Goodman CC. Pathology of the nervous system. In: *Pathology for the Physical Therapist*. Chapter 35.

28. Olney SJ, Wright MJ. Cerebral palsy. In: Campbell SK, Vander Linden DW, Palisano RJ, eds. *Physical Therapy for Children*. St. Louis, MO: Saunders. 2006:625-664.

29. Shah U, Moatter T. Screening for cystic fibrosis: the importance of using the correct tools. *J Ayub Med Coll Abbottabad*. 2006;18:7-10.

30. Agnew JL, Ashwell JA, Renaud SL. Cystic fibrosis. In: Campbell SK, Vander Linden DW, Palisano RJ, eds. *Physical Therapy for Children*. 3rd ed. St. Louis, MO: Saunders. 2006:819-850.

31. Leach J. Orthopedic conditions. In: Campbell SK, Vander Linden DW, Palisano RJ, eds. *Physical Therapy for Children*. 3rd ed. St. Louis, MO: Saunders. 2006:481-515.

32. Staheli LT. Rotational problems of the lower extremity. *Orthop Clin North Am*. 1987;18:503-512.

33. Engel GM, Staheli LT. The natural history of torsion and other factors influencing gait in childhood. A study of the angle of gait, tibial torsion, knee angle, hip rotation, and development of the arch in normal children. *Clin Orthop Relat Res*. 1974;99:12-17.

34. Scoles PV. *Pediatric Orthopaedics in Clinical Practice*. 2nd ed. Chicago, IL: Year Book. 1988.

35. Kalogrianitis S, Tan CK, Kemp GJ, et al. Does unstable slipped capital femoral epiphysis require urgent stabilization? *J Pediatr Orthop B*. 2007;16:6-9.

36. Kamarulzaman MA, Abdul Halim AR, Ibrahim S. Slipped capital femoral epiphysis (SCFE): a 12-year review. *Med J Malaysia*. 2006;61(suppl A):71-78.

37. Flores M, Satish SG, Key T. Slipped capital femoral epiphysis in identical twins: is there an HLA predisposition? Report of a case and review of the literature. *Bull Hosp Jt Dis*. 2006;63:158-160.

38. Aronsson DD, Loder RT, Breur GJ, et al. Slipped capital femoral epiphysis: current concepts. *J Am Acad Orthop Surg*. 2006;14:666-679.

39. Umans H, Liebling MS, Moy L, et al. Slipped capital femoral epiphysis: a physeal lesion diagnosed by MRI, with radiographic and CT correlation. *Skeletal Radiol*. 1998;27:139-144.

40. Busch MT, Morrissy RT. Slipped capital femoral epiphysis. *Orthop Clin North Am*. 1987;18:637-647.

41. Herring JA, Kim HT, Browne R. Legg-Calve-Perthes disease. Part II: Prospective multicenter study of the effect of treatment on outcome. *J Bone Joint Surg Am*. 2004;86-A:2121-2134.

42. Herring JA, Kim HT, Browne R. Legg-Calve-Perthes disease. Part I: Classification of radiographs with use of the modified lateral pillar and Stulberg classifications. *J Bone Joint Surg Am*. 2004;86-A:2103-2120.

43. Moens P, Fabry G. Legg-Calve-Perthes disease: one century later. *Acta Orthop Belg.* 2003;69:97-103.

44. Thompson GH, Price CT, Roy D, et al. Legg-Calve-Perthes disease: current concepts. *Instr Course Lect.* 2002;51:367-384.

45. Gross GW, Articolo GA, Bowen JR. Legg-Calve-Perthes disease: imaging evaluation and management. *Semin Musculoskelet Radiol.* 1999;3:379-391.

46. Roy DR. Current concepts in Legg-Calve-Perthes disease. *Pediatr Ann.* 1999;28:748-752.

47. Townsend DJ. Legg-Calve-Perthes disease. *Orthopedics.* 1999;22:381.

48. Mital MA, Matza RA. Osgood-Schlatter's disease: the painful puzzler. *Physician Sports Med.* 1977;5:60.

49. Camfield P, Camfield C. Advances in the diagnosis and management of pediatric seizure disorders in the twentieth century. *J Pediatr.* 2000;136:847-849.

50. Tharp BR. An overview of pediatric seizure disorders and epileptic syndromes. *Epilepsia.* 1987;28(suppl 1):S36-S45.

51. Nelson LP, Ureles SD, Holmes G. An update in pediatric seizure disorders. *Pediatr Dent.* 1991;13:128-135.

52. Eagle M, Bourke J, Bullock R, et al. Managing Duchenne muscular dystrophy—the additive effect of spinal surgery and home nocturnal ventilation in improving survival. *Neuromuscul Disord.* 2007;17:470-475.

53. King WM, Ruttencutter R, Nagaraja HN, et al. Orthopedic outcomes of long-term daily corticosteroid treatment in Duchenne muscular dystrophy. *Neurology.* 2007;68:1607-1613.

54. Freund AA, Scola RH, Arndt RC, et al. Duchenne and Becker muscular dystrophy: a molecular and immunohistochemical approach. *Arq Neuropsiquiatr.* 2007;65:73-76.

55. Zhang S, Xie H, Zhou G, et al. Development of therapy for Duchenne muscular dystrophy. *Zhongguo Xiu Fu Chong Jian Wai Ke Za Zhi.* 2007;21:194-203.

56. Velasco MV, Colin AA, Zurakowski D, et al. Posterior spinal fusion for scoliosis in Duchenne muscular dystrophy diminishes the rate of respiratory decline. *Spine.* 2007;32:459-465.

57. Main M, Mercuri E, Haliloglu G, et al. Serial casting of the ankles in Duchenne muscular dystrophy: can it be an alternative to surgery? *Neuromuscul Disord.* 2007;17:227-230.

58. Karol LA. Scoliosis in patients with Duchenne muscular dystrophy. *J Bone Joint Surg Am.* 2007;89(suppl 1):155-162.

59. Grange RW, Call JA. Recommendations to define exercise prescription for Duchenne muscular dystrophy. *Exerc Sport Sci Rev.* 2007;35:12-17.

60. Deconinck N, Dan B. Pathophysiology of Duchenne muscular dystrophy: current hypotheses. *Pediatr Neurol.* 2007;36:1-7.

61. Wagner KR, Lechtzin N, Judge DP. Current treatment of adult Duchenne muscular dystrophy. *Biochim Biophys Acta.* 2007;1772:229-237.

62. Duffy CM, Arsenault L, Duffy KN, et al. The Juvenile Arthritis Quality of Life Questionnaire—development of a new responsive index for juvenile rheumatoid arthritis and juvenile spondyloarthritides. *J Rheumatol.* 1997;24:738-746.

63. Brewer EJ, Jr, Bass J, Baum J, et al. Current proposed revision of JRA criteria. JRA Criteria Subcommittee of the Diagnostic and Therapeutic Criteria Committee of the American Rheumatism Section of The Arthritis Foundation. *Arthritis Rheum.* 1977;20:195-199.

64. Goodman CC. The cardiovascular system. In: Goodman CC, Boissonnault WG, Fuller KS, eds. *Pathology: Implications for the Physical Therapist.* 2nd ed. Philadelphia, PA: Saunders. 2003:367-476.

QUESTIONS

1. A physical therapist initiates an examination of an infant. The infant is observed sitting alone without support, reaching with one hand and waving "bye-bye." The infant is demonstrating typical development for which of the following ages:
   A. 1 to 2 months
   B. 3 to 5 months
   C. 6 to 8 months
   D. 9 to 11 months

2. Your neighbor has discussed concern that their 4-month-old infant daughter has not been able to demonstrate the same gross motor activities as the same age cousin. You start by asking the neighbor if the infant can perform which of the milestones consistent with 4 months of age:
   A. Transitions sitting to crawling
   B. Stands with assistance
   C. Raises self to sit
   D. Pivots in prone position

3. Determination of pain is a key aspect of child examination. An appropriate pain assessment for a 13-month-old includes which of the following?
   A. Parents should determine pain levels
   B. Faces pain scale
   C. Visual analog scale
   D. Face, Legs, Activity, Cry, Consolability behavioral scale

4. The best measure to determine the quantity of movement in children with cerebral palsy or down syndrome is:
   A. Gross Motor Function Measure
   B. Denver Developmental Screening Test
   C. Peabody Developmental Motor Scales
   D. Test of Gross Motor Development

5. The physical therapist is observing a child limping while walking on a firm surface. The child demonstrates a shortened stance phase but has level hips. Physical examination reveals range of motion limitation a tenderness at the hip only. Which gait type has the therapist identified?
   A. Abductor lurch
   B. Antalgic
   C. Equines
   D. Circumduction

6. A 5-year-old child presents to the clinic with joint inflammation involving many joints. Physical examination findings include limitations in range of motion of the same joints, weakness, and significant pain. The parents report the child requires assistance with self-care and that handwriting has been difficult. Imaging reveals joint space narrowing. This description is most likely indicative of which of the following pediatric diseases affecting connective tissue?

A. Ehlers-Danlos syndrome
B. Juvenile idiopathic arthritis
C. Pediatric lupus erythematous
D. Hemophilia

7. During a school screening, a 10-year-old girl presents with a rib hump during the Adams Forward Bend test. Further testing with a sociometer was performed. Which of the following results should be referred to the physician?
A. 1- to 4-degree scoliometer trunk rotation angle
B. 5- to 9-degree scoliometer trunk rotation angle
C. 10-degree scoliometer trunk rotation angle
D. >15 degree scoliometer trunk rotation angle

8. A 3-year-old child with developmental hip dysplasia presents to the clinic with gross motor delay. During treatment, the unstable hip joint should avoid which end-of-range hip positions?
A. Extension
B. Flexion
C. External rotation
D. Abduction

9. Gowers' sign used by children with muscular dystrophy compensates for:
A. Distal weakness
B. Proximal weakness
C. Distal contractures
D. Proximal contractures

10. Congenital muscular torticollis is a nonprogressive unilateral contracture of the sternocleidomastoid muscle. Typical neonatal cervical range of motion is:
A. 25 degrees cervical rotation and 20 degrees of lateral flexion
B. 50 degrees cervical rotation and 35 degrees of lateral flexion
C. 90 degrees cervical rotation and 50 degrees of lateral flexion
D. 100 degrees or more cervical rotation and 65 degrees of lateral flexion

11. Brachial plexus injuries occur when nerve roots are damaged causing transient or permanent nerve damage. A teenager who spent the evening drinking fell from a height but was able to break the fall by holding on to a metal railing, stretching his neck and arm forcefully. He now presents with shoulder internal rotation and adduction, the wrist flexed and fingers extending. This position is characteristic of:
A. Total plexus palsy
B. Erb's palsy
C. Klumpke's palsy
D. Ulnar nerve palsy

12. "W" sitting is used by children to assist with stability when sitting on the floor. Risk that are associated with prolonged used of "W" sitting include which of the following?
A. Limited unilateral use of the upper extremities
B. Laxity of muscles at hips
C. No hand preference
D. Over-strengthening of core muscles

ANSWERS

1. The answer is **C**. Six to eight-month milestones include sitting alone, reaching with one hand, and waving goodbye.

2. The answer is **D**. Pivoting in prone is a customary developmental milestone between ages 4 to 5 months, other answers are consistent with older infants.

3. The answer is **D**. Faces, Legs, Activity, Cry, Consolability behavioral scale is used for a child who is preverbal and cannot participate in a self-reporting scale. All other options require the child to report their pain.

4. The answer is **A**. Gross Motor Function Measure was developed for use in children with cerebral palsy and Down syndrome. All other measures are norm-referenced test not specifically designed for cerebral palsy and Down syndrome.

5. The answer is **B**. Antalgic gait includes a shorted stance, tenderness, and reduced range on physical examination. Abductor lurch would present with a Trendelenburg sign, equinus would have heel cord contracture or limitations, and circumduction gait may be due to limb length discrepancy or weakness.

6. The answer is **B**. Juvenile idiopathic arthritis is believed to be an autoimmune dysfunction related to interleukin 1. Joint inflammation involving few or many joints with joint synovium proliferation causes overgrowth (pannus), which can erode the adjacent cartilage, causing joint narrowing and destruction. Significant pain is present. Ehlers-Danlos includes developmental delay, hyperextensibility of the skin and joints, scarring, hernias, easy bruising, and muscle hypotonia. The primary symptoms of pediatric lupus erythematous are inflammation, oral and nasal rash or ulcers, kidney dysfunction, headaches, cerebral vascular injury, and cognitive dysfunction. Pain, fatigue, and other discomfort may impact physical function. Hemophilia is a pathology associated with missing proteins required for blood clotting leading to chronic bleeding. Joint destruction leading to premature arthritis and chronic pain occurs. Muscle atrophy and range of motion limitations are noted.

7. The answer is **C**. Ten-degree or greater scoliometer trunk rotation angle should be referred to the physician.

8. The answer is **A**. Extreme or forceful extension should be avoided, as it may lead to dislocation. The most common intervention is the Pavlik harness, which maintains the hip in flexion, adduction, and slight external rotation.

9. The answer is **B**. Gowers' sign used by children with muscular dystrophy compensates for proximal muscle weakness.

10. The answer is **D**. Typical neonates should have 100 degrees or more cervical rotation and 65 degrees of cervical lateral flexion.

11. The answer is **B**. Erb's palsy presents with shoulder internal rotation and adduction, the wrist flexed and fingers extending. Klumpke's palsy has motor deficits that affect muscles of the hand and lateral sensation of the medial arm. Total plexus palsy affects all the muscles of the arm and hand. Ulnar nerve palsy would present with a loss of sensation in the hand, especially the ring and little fingers, as well as loss of coordination in the fingers.

12. The answer is **C.** In a "W" sitting position, a child has too much trunk control and stability. It is very easy to use either hand to accomplish tasks, limiting the development of hand preference. The wide sitting stance of the W position makes it easier to keep the body upright. Children sitting in a W position do not have to use their core muscles as much and will not develop them as they would in other sitting positions. The W position makes it difficult for children to rotate their upper bodies and reach across to either side with one or both arms, allowing them to use the upper extremity unilaterally with ease. If a child is prone to muscle tightness or hypertonia, sitting in a W position will increase tightness in hips, knees, and ankles.

CHECKLIST

When you complete this chapter, you should be able to:

❏ List developmental milestones with the appropriate age range of acquisition.

❏ Identify time course and presentation of primitive reflexes.

❏ Compare techniques to determine gestational age.

❏ Outline signs, symptoms, and clinical presentation of various pediatric pathologies.

❏ Compare developmental outcome measures and determine population for use.

❏ Identify common pediatric durable medical equipment and their use.

❏ Compare seizure disorders.

Index

Note: Page numbers followed by *f* and *t* indicate figures and tables, respectively. A *b* following a page number indicates a boxed feature.